D0161364

OXYGEN TRANSPORT TO
TISSUE XVIII

ADVANCES IN EXPERIMENTAL MEDICINE AND BIOLOGY

OXYGEN TRANSPORT TO TISSUE XVIII

Edited by

Edwin M. Nemoto
University of Pittsburgh
Pittsburgh, Pennsylvania

and

Joseph C. LaManna
Case Western Reserve University
Cleveland, Ohio

Consulting Editors

Christopher Cooper
David Delpy
Karlfried Groebe
Thomas K. Hunt
Peter Keipert
Avrahim Mayevsky
Roland N. Pittman
William L. Rumsey
Peter Vaupel
David F. Wilson

PLENUM PRESS • NEW YORK AND LONDON

Library of Congress Cataloging-in-Publication Data

Oxygen transport to tissue XVIII / edited by Edwin M. Nemoto and
   Joseph C. LaManna ; consulting editors, Christopher Cooper ... [et
   al.].
        p. cm. -- (Advances in experimental medicine and biology ; v.
   411)
   "Proceedings of the 23rd Annual Meeting of the International
Society on Oxygen Transport to Tissue, held August 23-27, 1995, in
Pittsburgh, Pennsylvania"--T.p. verso.
   Includes bibliographical references and index.
   ISBN 0-306-45516-1
   1. Tissue respiration--Congresses. 2. Ischemia--Congresses.
I. Nemoto, Edwin Mamoru, 1942-   . II. LaManna, Joseph C.
III. International Society on Oxygen Transport to Tissue. Meeting
(23rd : 1995 : Pittsburgh, Pa.) IV. Series.
   [DNLM: 1. Oxygen--metabolism--congresses. 2. Biological
Transport--physiology--congresses. 3. Oxygen Consumption-
-physiology--congresses.   W1 AD559 v.411 1997 / QV 312 09787 1997]
QP177.0975   1997
612.2'6--dc21
DNLM/DLC
for Library of Congress   97-4326
                                                              CIP

Proceedings of the 23rd annual meeting of the International Society on Oxygen Transport to Tissue, held August 23 – 27, 1995, in Pittsburgh, Pennsylvania

ISBN 0-306-45516-1

© 1997 Plenum Press, New York
A Division of Plenum Publishing Corporation
233 Spring Street, New York, N. Y. 10013

10 9 8 7 6 5 4 3 2 1

INTERNATIONAL SOCIETY ON OXYGEN TRANSPORT TO TISSUE

1995

SPONSORS

The ISOTT and the local organizing committee gratefully acknowledge the generous financial support of the following companies:

- ALLIANCE PHARMACEUTICAL CORP.
- BLOOD SUBSTITUTES OF BAXTER HEALTHCARE CORP.
- EPPENDORF
- JOHNSON & JOHNSON

- Baxter Healthcare Corp., Cardiovascular Group—Edwards Critical Care Division
- Haemonetics Corp.
- Medical Systems Corp.
- Somanetics
- UpJohn
- Hamamatsu Photonics K.K.

PREFACE

The 23rd annual meeting of the International Society on Oxygen Transport to Tissue took place from August 23–27, 1995, at the Station Square Sheraton along the shores of the Monongahela River where it meets with the Allegheny and Ohio Rivers to form the "Point" of the city of Pittsburgh. Pittsburgh was a convenient location for the meeting being between both the East and West coasts of the United States and between the Asian and European continents. It is easily accessible by air via its large international airport. In addition, Pittsburgh has just recently undergone a transition from the steel mills and industries of old to an age of computers and biotechnology as evidenced by the new Biotechnology Center of the University of Pittsburgh where a lunch and tour were provided for interested participants. On the tour, the participants got to see the mix of projects ranging from molecular biology to clinical projects studying membrane oxygenators, ventricular assist devices, oxygen carriers, and more, representing the forefront of research on oxygen delivery systems to tissue.

This small 300-member society of physicists, chemists, clinicians, engineers, biochemists, and biological scientists is responsible for some of the major developments in the delivery of oxygen to tissues such as: (1) Microelectrodes for oxygen, carbon dioxide, and various ions; (2) Fluorocarbons; (3) Methods of tissue oxygen mapping; (4) Blood substitutes; and (5) Noninvasive near infrared spectroscopy or cerebral oximetry, clearly attesting to the success of this peculiar blend of scientists, engineers, mathematicians, and clinicians. One hundred fifty registrants with 115 free presentations participated in this meeting to continue the tradition of open debate and scientific exchange in free presentations highlighted by special invited lectures aimed at bringing new areas of focus. Lectures on positron emission tomography and functional magnetic resonance imaging brought to this society for the first time, emphasized the application of these powerful imaging techniques in assessing regional brain oxygen metabolism and function. A lecture on angiogenesis emphasized the dynamic processes occurring within tissues in adapting to oxygen deficiency while a lecture on metabolic compartmentation reminded us of the heterogeneity and compartmentation of not only tissue oxygenation and perfusion, but also metabolism at the cellular level. Lectures on hemoglobinopathies and potential mechanisms of amelioration in addition to the development of oxygen carriers bring to the fore the potential for molecular biology in addressing problems in tissue oxygenation. Finally, lectures on the chemistry of nitric oxide and other oxygen radicals, and the role of free radicals in tissue oxygenation brought to fore, other roles of oxygen in regulating tissue oxygenation and its potentially detrimental effects.

To encourage the participation of young scientists and clinicians in the society, two awards are presented at each meeting. Dr. Clare E. Elwell of the Department of Medical

Physics was the winner of the Melvin H. Knisely Award for her contributions in near infrared (NIR) spectroscopy and consistent productivity in the field and to the society. Dr. Phillip E. James was awarded the Lubber's award for his paper entitled, "Intrarenal PO_2 Measured by EPR Oximetry and the Effects of Bacterial Endotoxin."

In the area of assessing tissue oxygenation, the free papers revealed the clinical application of NIR spectroscopy and cerebral oximetry, a brain-child of this society, in various clinical states, touching the surface of this potentially valuable monitoring technique in noninvasive monitoring. The early development of NIR for optical imaging was also presented. The use of NIR phosphors was also developed for tissue oxygen mapping attaining greater penetration into the tissue. Several papers from one group highlighted the application of electron paramagnetic resonance (EPR) oximetry to the measurement of tissue oxygenation using paramagentic materials introduced into the tissue. Highlighting one aspect of bioengineering in molecular biology from the industrial aspect, a group of papers focused on all aspects of protein kinase C separation and production on an industrial level from transgenic animals. As in the past, various aspects of tissue oxygen delivery and measurements of tissue oxygenation were presented as it relates to the brain, heart, and tumors in terms of oxygen delivery with oxygen carriers, tissue adaptation to hypoxia by angiogenesis, and the role of leukocytes and the immune response to tissue hypoxia and injury. Finally, the continued role of nitric oxide and oxygen free radicals to tissue injury and regulation of tissue oxygenation was also explored.

Following the meeting in Pittsburgh, some of the ISOTT members attended a satellite meeting on "Adaptation to Hypoxia" at Case Western Reserve University in nearby Cleveland, Ohio. A total of 70 attendees discussed hypoxic adaptation from the cellular level to macro adaptations in human populations living at high altitude for generations.

The editors wish to thank the local organizing committee for their painstaking work in reviewing and grading the abstracts presented and their enthusiastic support. We also thank the consulting editors for their work on the manuscripts and by doing so, have provided peer-review. We owe special thanks to Ms. Laraine Visser for her meticulous work in editing all of the manuscripts and the staff of Plenum Press who have been very cooperative and have done a great job. Finally, we would like to especially thank the staff of the Continuing Education Center of the University of Pittsburgh Medical Center, and in particular, Ms. Diane Applegate.

CONTENTS

Part 2. Myocardial Hypoxia-Ischemia

Part 3. Tissue Oxygen Distribution

Part 4. Tissue Oxygenation in Tumors

Part 5. Oxygen Supply–Demand

Part 6. Angiogenesis and Microcirculation

Part 7. Oxygen Carriers

Part 8. Anticoagulants and Tissue Oxygenation

Part 9. Near Infrared Spectroscopy

Part 10. Nitric Oxide and Free Radicals

Part 11. Measurement of Tissue Oxygen

CALCIUM-DEPENDENT O_2 SENSITIVITY OF CAT CAROTID BODY

D. G. Buerk,[1,2,3] S. Osanai,[1] D. K. Chugh,[1] A. Mokashi,[1] and S. Lahiri[1]

[1]Departments of Physiology
[2]Bioengineering
[3]Institute for Environmental Medicine
University of Pennsylvania School of Medicine
Philadelphia, Pennsylvania 19104–6086

INTRODUCTION

Mechanisms for the chemosensory response to hypoxia in the carotid body (CB) are not fully known. Two theories have been proposed (see Lahiri, 1994). The metabolic hypothesis states that available energy is reduced when O_2 is low, causing depolarization and Ca^{2+} release, and release of neurotransmitters. The membrane chromophore hypothesis is a possible mechanism involving O_2-sensitive ion channels. Through binding to the chromophore (presumably a protein in the cell membrane), a decrease in O_2 can decrease K^+ conductance, leading to depolarization and activation of Ca^{2+} channels. Although the proposed mechanisms are different, a common feature to both hypotheses is that neurotransmitter release is mediated by Ca^{2+}.

In the current study, O_2 consumption was quantified from measurements with O_2 microelectrodes in cat CBs perfused with physiological concentrations of Ca^{2+} (2.2 mM) or with Ca^{2+}-free solutions. The O_2 sensitivity (relationship between chemosensory discharge and tissue PO_2) was found to depend on the Ca^{2+} concentration in the perfusate. With Ca^{2+}-free perfusate, the neural discharge (ND) frequency response to hypoxia was reduced and the O_2 sensitivity curve was shifted to the left of control. However, the O_2 consumption rate was unaffected by the presence or absence of Ca^{2+} in the perfusate.

METHODS

The experimental apparatus and physiological preparation used for studies with isolated, perfused and superfused cat CBs are described in detail by Iturriaga *et al.* (1991). We used a flow interruption method to determine O_2 consumption from the tissue PO_2 disappearance rate measured by recessed gold cathode (Whalen-type) PO_2 microelectrodes

Oxygen Transport to Tissue XVIII, edited by Nemoto and LaManna
Plenum Press, New York, 1997

inserted into the CB, as described in a previous *in vitro* study (Buerk *et al.*, 1994). The flow interruption technique can also be used *in vivo* with an appropriate analysis that includes the effects of oxyhemoglobin (Buerk *et al.*, 1989).

The CB was perfused with normoxic, normocapnic solutions from a constant-pressure (80 Torr) gravity driven reservoir maintained at 37 °C. Effluent was removed by continuous suction. The control perfusate was a modified Tyrode's solution containing (in mM) 112 NaCl, 4.7 KCl, 2.2 $CaCl_2$, 1.1 $MgCl_2$, 22 sodium glutamate, 21 $NaHCO_3$, 5.0 N-2-hydroxyethyl piperazine-N-2-esthanesulfonic acid (HEPES), and 5.0 glucose. In the Ca^{2+}-free perfusate, 2.2 mM $CaCl_2$ was replaced with 3.3 mM $MgCl_2$. Control and Ca^{2+}-free solutions were equilibrated by bubbling with compressed gasses containing 5% CO_2 and 20% O_2. Perfusate pH was 7.39 - 7.40 at 37 °C.

The sinus nerve was desheathed, placed on a platinum electrode and lifted up into a layer of paraffin oil which floated above the preparation. Neural discharge (ND) was measured using a differential AC-amplifier with band-pass (10 Hz to 1 kHz) and notch (60 Hz) filters. The ND frequency was electronically discriminated, and an analog signal proportional to the number of impulses per sec was recorded. A digital record of the ND frequency was also continuously printed during the course of the experiment. Analog signals for the PO_2 microelectrode and ND were tape recorded for later playback through a computer controlled data acquisition system with 12 bit accuracy at sampling rates ranging from 2 to 20 Hz. After a series of control flow interruption measurements were made, the CB was then switched to Ca^{2+}-free perfusion for another series of flow interruption measurements. The sequence was repeated after returning to control perfusate.

RESULTS

A total of 235 flow interruption measurements from 16 cat CB experiments were digitized by computer. Data were analyzed for the tissue PO_2 and baseline ND before stopping flow, and for the rate of O_2 disappearance (dPO_2/dt) and peak ND after stopping flow. The tissue PO_2 was also determined at the time when 50% of the change in ND frequency was reached.

Representative examples of simultaneous ND (top panels, A, C) and tissue PO_2 (bottom panels, B, D) measurements with control and Ca^{2+}-free perfusates are shown in Figure 1. In the left panels (A, B), flow interruption measurements during perfusion with control solution are shown before switching to Ca^{2+}-free perfusate at t = 0. The first flow interruption measurements in Ca^{2+}-free perfusate were made approximately 2 min later. After switching to Ca^{2+}-free perfusate, the baseline ND (lower sets of dashed lines in A) decreased slightly, from 60 to 50 impulses/sec. The maximum ND (upper sets of dashed lines) was also slightly lower, from 460 to 450 impulses/sec. Midpoints for the ND responses are also marked (middle sets of dashed lines). The O_2 disappearance rates (dPO_2/dt, dashed lines in B) were -2.3 and -2.0 Torr/sec respectively. Symbols are shown for the tissue PO_2 when the ND increased to 50% of maximum, at 34 Torr (open circle) for control, and 18 Torr (open square) for Ca^{2+}-free perfusion.

The ND responses became slower and the maximum ND decreased for each successive flow interruption measurement. The last measurement in this series is shown in the right panels (C, D) of Figure 1. After about 45 min of perfusion with Ca^{2+}-free solution, ND responses were markedly attenuated, rising from the baseline around 45 to about 105 impulses/sec (dashed lines in C). The O_2 disappearance rate (dashed line in D) was -1.5

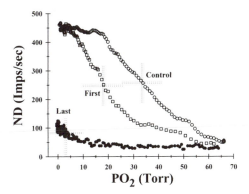

Figure 1. Neural discharge (ND, top panels) and tissue PO$_2$ (bottom) measured in cat carotid body during short periods of flow interruption with control and Ca^{2+}-free perfusate (switched at t = 0 in A, B). Dashed lines in A, C show baseline, midpoint and maximum ND. Dashed lines in B, D show O$_2$ disappearance rate (dPO$_2$/dt). Last flow interruption measurements (C, D) were made after 45 min of Ca^{2+}-free perfusion.

Torr/sec and the tissue PO$_2$ at 50% of the maximum ND response was around 3 Torr (solid circle, D).

The decrease in the ND responses and changes in the relationships with tissue PO$_2$ are shown in Figure 2 for the control (open circles), first (open squares) and last (solid circles) Ca^{2+}-free measurements in the preceding Figure. The 50% changes in ND at the tissue PO$_2$s where they occurred are marked by the intersecting dashed lines. Note that there was a leftward shift in the O$_2$ sensitivity after only 2 min of Ca^{2+}-free perfusion (first), with a marked leftward shift for the last data set.

Similar changes in O$_2$ sensitivity were seen in all 16 CB experiments, with the tissue PO$_2$ at 50% of the ND response ranging in the 20 to 50 Torr range for controls, eventually falling to around 5 Torr or lower after 30 to 45 min of Ca^{2+}-free perfusion. Overall results are summarized in Table 1. There were no significant differences in the average tissue PO$_2$

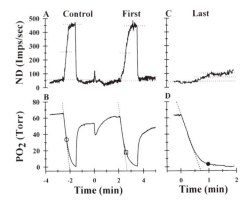

Figure 2. O$_2$ sensitivity curves showing the relationship between neural discharge and tissue PO$_2$ during the control and Ca^{2+}-free flow interruption measurements shown in Figure 1. Dashed lines show the midpoint (50%) ND response and tissue PO$_2$ where it occurred. Perfusion with Ca^{2+}-free solution caused a progressive reduction in the maximum ND and leftward shift in O$_2$ sensitivity for successive flow interruption measurements, with the 50% ND response occurring at lower tissue PO$_2$ values.

Table 1. Summary of flow interruption measurements with normal (2 mM Ca^{2+})
and Ca^{2+}-free perfusion (N = 16 CBs)

Calcium in perfusate	2 mM	0 mM	t-test
Number of measurements	122	113	
PO_2 (Torr) ± SE	59.3 ± 4.7	59.9 ± 5.6	N.S.
dPO_2/dt (Torr/sec) ± SE	-4.35 ± 0.54	-4.08 ± 0.52	N.S.
VO_2 (mL O_2/100 g/min) ± SE	0.736 ± 0.091	0.690 ± 0.088	N.S.

between control and or Ca^{2+}-free perfusates, or in average O_2 disappearance rates or calculated O_2 consumption rates.

DISCUSSION

We observed a progressive decline in the chemosensory response to hypoxia as extracellular Ca^{2+} was removed, without changes in O_2 consumption. A similar, slow decline in hypoxic responses to flow interruption with zero Ca^{2+} was also reported by Shirahata and Fitzgerald (1991). This progressive decline appears to be consistent with gradual depletion of Ca^{2+} from an intracellular pool. The release of Ca^{2+} from intracellular stores was proposed by Duchen and Biscoe (1992) based on their measurements of changes in $[Ca^{2+}]_i$ with hypoxia in isolated rabbit glomus cells after removing $[Ca^{2+}]_e$. The present study demonstrates that the slower response is not due to lower metabolism (implying that energy requirements are the same), and is the first to show that the removal of $[Ca^{2+}]_e$ caused a shift in O_2 sensitivity.

One possible explanation for the shift in O_2 sensitivity is an alteration in dopamine (DA) or other substances that may modulate hypoxic chemotransduction. It is well known that DA release is coupled to hypoxia (Gonzalez *et al.*, 1992) although its importance has been questioned (Sun and Reis, 1994). Combined Ca^{2+}-fluorescence and electrochemical studies with isolated rabbit glomus cells have shown that DA is released when cytosolic Ca^{2+} is elevated either by a hypoxic stimulus or by direct membrane depolarization (Urena *et al.*, 1994). In our laboratory, Buerk *et al.* (1995) have quantified DA release during flow interruption in the cat CB preparation using an electrochemical microsensor. Further experimental work is needed to investigate whether DA affects Ca^{2+}-dependent changes in O_2 sensitivity.

ACKNOWLEDGMENTS

This research was supported by NIH grants HL-43413–06 and HL-50180–02.

REFERENCES

Buerk, D.G., Nair, P.K. and W.J. Whalen. (1989). Two-cytochrome model for carotid body $P_{ti}O_2$ and chemosensitivity changes after hemorrhage. J. Appl. Physiol., 67:60–66.

Buerk, D.G., Itturiaga, R. and S. Lahiri. (1994). Testing the metabolic hypothesis of O_2 chemoreception in the cat carotid body *in vitro*. J. Appl. Physiol., 76:1317–1323.

Buerk, D.G., Lahiri, S., Chugh, D. and A. Mokashi. (1995). Electrochemical detection of rapid dopamine release kinetics during hypoxia in perfused/superfused cat carotid bodies. J. Appl. Physiol., 78:830–837.

Duchen, M.R. and T.J. Biscoe. (1992). Relative mitochondrial membrane potential and $[Ca^{2+}]_i$ in type I cells isolated from the rabbit carotid body. J. Physiol. London, 450:33–61.

Gonzalez, C., Almaraz, L., Obeso, A. and R. Rigual. (1992). Oxygen and acid chemoreception in the carotid body chemoreceptors. Trends in Neurolog. Sci., 15:146–153.

Iturriaga, R., Rumsey, W.L., Mokashi, A., Spergel, D., Wilson, D.F., and S. Lahiri. (1991). *In vitro* perfused-superfused cat carotid body for physiological and pharmacological studies. J. Appl. Physiol., 70:1393–1400.

Lahiri, S. (1994). Chromophores in O$_2$ chemoreception: The carotid body model. News in Physiol. Sci., 9:161–165.

Shirahata, M., and R.S. Fitzgerald. (1991). Dependence of hypoxic chemotransduction in cat carotid body on voltage-gated calcium channels. J. Appl. Physiol., 71:1062–1069.

Sun, M-K., and D.J. Reis. (1994). Dopamine or transmitter release from rat carotid body may not be essential to hypoxic chemoreception. Am. J. Physiol., 267:R1632-R1639.

Urena, J., Fernandez-Chacon, R., Benot, A.R., Alvarez de Toledo, G., and J. Lopez-Barneo. (1994). Hypoxia induces voltage-dependent Ca^{2+} entry and quantal dopamine secretion in carotid body glomus cells. Proc. Natl. Acad. Sci., USA, 91:10208–10211.

PERFUSION MRI ASSESSMENT OF CEREBRAL BLOOD FLOW AND CO$_2$ REACTIVITY AFTER CONTROLLED CORTICAL IMPACT IN RATS

Michael L. Forbes,[1] Kristy S. Hendrich,[6] Joanne K. Schiding,[1] Donald S. Williams,[6] Chien Ho,[6,7] Steven T. DeKosky,[1,2,4] Donald W. Marion,[1,2,5] and Patrick M. Kochanek[1,2,3]

[1]Safar Center for Resuscitation Research
[2]The University of Pittsburgh Brain Trauma Research Center
[3]Departments of Anesthesiology/Critical Care Medicine
[4]Psychiatry
[5]Neurosurgery
University of Pittsburgh
Pittsburgh, Pennsylvania 15260
[6]The Pittsburgh NMR Center for Biomedical Research
[7]Department of Biological Sciences
Carnegie Mellon University
Pittsburgh, Pennsylvania 15213

1. INTRODUCTION

Contemporary animal models of traumatic brain injury (TBI)[1,2,3] have provided insight into the mechanisms of brain injury by modeling features such as diffuse axonal injury and contusion. These models have also facilitated the study of the cellular and molecular mechanisms of secondary injury[3,4,5] and have contributed to the development of clinical trials[6].

However, our understanding of the cerebral circulation after TBI in these models remains limited. This is due to the lack of a technique that provides serial regional cerebral blood flow (rCBF) measurements in the rat. As a result, basic cerebrovascular issues such as the effect of the manipulation of P$_a$CO$_2$ after severe (TBI) remain incompletely understood.

The ideal technique for measuring CBF after TBI should be [1] **non-invasive**, allowing for serial measurements, [2] **quantitative**, and [3] **produce an accurate flow map**, due to the regional heterogeneity of posttraumatic CBF. Current techniques for measuring rCBF in rats such as laser doppler flowmetry, microspheres and autoradiography all fail to meet these criteria on at least one account.

Oxygen Transport to Tissue XVIII, edited by Nemoto and LaManna
Plenum Press, New York, 1997

We report for the first time the measurement of rCBF after TBI using the entirely non-invasive arterial spin-labeled perfusion MRI technique [7]. We hypothesize that [a] perfusion MRI can serially and non-invasively measure rCBF and [b] will serially measure the response of the cerebral vasculature to a reduction in P_aCO_2.

2. METHODS AND MATERIALS

2.1. Brain Trauma Model

Nine male Sprague-Dawley rats (300–350 gm; 5 sham, 4 TBI) underwent anesthesia and surgical preparation using 4% isofluorane induction in $N_2O:O_2$ (2:1), orotracheal intubation and mechanical ventilation. The isofluorane was reduced to 2% followed by sterile surgical placement of a femoral arterial catheter. Penicillin (Bicillin 100,000 U. IM Upjohn, Kalamazoo, MI) and gentamicin (10 mg/kg IM, Elkins-Sinn, Cherry Hill, NJ) were given to minimize iatrogenic infection risk.

We used the controlled cortical impact (CCI) model[1] of TBI as recently modified[2]. CCI uses a pneumatically driven piston device that reliably and reproducibly delivers a focal contusion to the exposed dura overlying the cortex. The depth, duration and velocity of the impact are preset.

The rat was placed in a stereotactic frame and the scalp was retracted, exposing the left parietal bone. A 1.0 x 0.5 cm craniotomy was made using a high speed dental drill under a binocular operating microscope. A burr hole was made 5.0 mm anterior and 2.0 mm lateral to the bregma in the ipsilateral skull and a temperature probe (0.009 inch diameter) was inserted stereotactically 2 mm deep into the cortex. A 30 minute equilibration period occurs after the brain temperature reaches $37 \pm 0.5°C$ and the brain is maintained at this temperature. The bone flap was left in place to allow equilibration and optimization of arterial blood gasses (ABGs) followed by isofluorane reduction to 1%. For both groups, target values for the ABGs were a P_aCO_2 between 35–45 torr and a P_aO_2 of > 100 torr. The bone flap and the temperature probe were removed and a CCI, 4 m/s, 2.5 mm depth was delivered onto the exposed dura overlying the left parietal cortex. The bone flap was replaced and sealed with dental cement and the scalp was resutured. In the sham group, all anesthesia and surgery was identical to the TBI group, without CCI. The femoral line and brain temperature probe were removed and the rat was allowed to recover over 1 h. After extubation, supplemental O_2 was delivered for 30 min. Once recovered, the rat was returned to its cage with full access to food and water.

2.2. Perfusion MRI Method

Perfusion MRI by arterial spin labeling[7] is a novel technique for the serial, non-invasive measurement of rCBF. It quantifies rCBF as a function of the reduction in magnetization of tissue due to inflowing labeled blood. Perfusion MRI was performed using the Bruker Biospec (Bruker Instruments, Billerica, MA) 4.7 Tesla magnet with a 40 cm bore and 15 cm gradient insert. The data acquisition plane was defined using multislice, coronal spin-echo images at the level of the left parietal cortex. After spin inversion at the carotid level, a labeled image was obtained. This was followed by a control image with no spin inversion. Using Equation 1, a quantitative map of CBF was generated for each rat.

$$\mathbf{CBF} = \lambda/T_{1obs} \bullet (M_C - M_L)/(2\alpha \bullet M_C) \qquad (1)$$

where:

$\lambda =$	Blood-brain partition coefficient for water
$T_{1obs} =$	Spin-Lattice Relaxation time for tissue water in the presence of flow
$M_C =$	Magnetization intensity of the control image
$M_L =$	Magnetization intensity of the labeled image
$\alpha =$	Degree of arterial spin labeling

T_{1obs} (1.6 sec)and α (0.8), were measured previously in a separate group of rats. A value of 0.9 mL/gm was assumed for λ[7].

2.3. Image Acquisition Protocol

Twenty-four hours after TBI, the rats were taken to the MRI Center where they were reanesthetized with 5% halothane and $N_2O:O_2$ (2:1) . The halothane was reduced to 1.5% for the placement of the femoral arterial line. The halothane was turned off when the rats are placed in the magnet. A continuous infusion of pancuronium (1:10 dilution of pancuronium:saline at 3.3 mL/h) was given for paralysis while the images were being acquired. Blood gases, rectal temperature and mean arterial blood pressure (MABP) were continuously monitored.

In this study the target range for normal ventilation (NV) was 30–40 torr, while the target for hyperventilation (HV) was 15–25 torr. After NV was established, rCBF was measured in duplicate by perfusion MRI (2000 ms recovery time, 30 ms echo time, 5 cm field of view, 2 mm slice thickness and a 128 x 64 matrix size). The tidal volume and ventilator rate were increased accordingly to obtain HVand rCBF was measured, again in duplicate.

2.4. Data Analysis

Regions of interest (ROI) were defined on the control (anatomic) images using image analysis software stimulate 3.6.1, kindly provided by John Strupp (Center for Magnetic Resonance Research, University of Minnesota Medical School, Minneapolis, Mn). ROIs were defined as the left and right parietal cortex (LCtx, RCtx, respectively) and included the contusion. Perfusion maps were generated as described above and mean CBF was calculated within each ROI. When motion artifacts were detected, the map was excluded from the study. This resulted in the exclusion of 6 of 36 maps. At least one map was retained for each condition in each rat. When both perfusion maps were motion-free, the average of 2 measurements was computed. Within group comparisons were made using the paired t-test while comparisons between groups were made using the unpaired t-test.

Table 1. Physiologic parameters during perfusion MRI data acquisition

Sham	NV	HV	TBI	NV	HV
pO_2	85.1 ± 5.2	$*116.3 \pm 6.2$	pO_2	80.8 ± 8.9	$*129.6 \pm 5.9$
pCO_2	38.0 ± 2.4	$*22.7 \pm 1.8$	pCO_2	38.6 ± 1.9	$*19.6 \pm 0.8$
MABP	140.0 ± 7.6	$*152.5 \pm 5.4$	MABP	146.3 ± 4.8	143.1 ± 4.8
$Temp_{core}$	35.1 ± 1.1	36.9 ± 0.1	$Temp_{core}$	36.6 ± 0.1	37.2 ± 0.3

(all values mean ± SEM) * $p < 0.05$ NV -vs- HV values

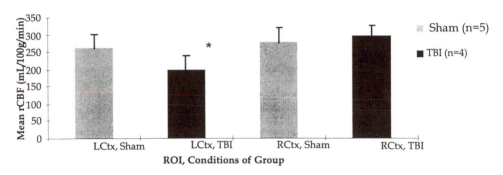

Figure 1. Mean rCBF values during NV in the LCtx and RCtx in sham and TBI groups.

3. RESULTS

3.1. Physiologic Parameters

Table 1 depicts mean physiologic parameters during perfusion imaging. There was no significant difference between TBI and sham for any physiologic parameter at any time. P_aCO_2 was reduced by HV, as expected *(p < 0.05 HV -vs- NV)* in both groups. While MABP in the sham group and P_aO_2 in both groups increased *(p < 0.05 HV -vs- NV)* it is unlikely that these differences are physiologically important.

3.2. Mean rCBF Measurements

Figure 1 shows the mean rCBF values during NV in the LCtx and RCtx in sham and TBI groups. At 24 h after CCI there was no significant difference in rCBF in the RCtx between sham and TBI groups. However, rCBF in the LCtx was reduced after TBI (LCtx -vs- RCtx *p <0.05).*

3.3. Assessment of rCBF as a Function of P_aCO_2

During HV, there was a reduction in rCBF in the LCtx and RCtx in both TBI and sham groups. (See Table 2).

An example of the CBF response of the cerebral circulation to reduction in P_aCO_2, as assessed in our model, is shown in Figure 2. These are representative perfusion maps in the same rat 24 h after TBI during NV and HV. Black depicts low flow while white de-

Table 2. Effect Of HV on rCBF, assessed by perfusion MRI

ROI	LCtx rCBF		RCtx rCBF	
P_aCO_2	*NV*	*HV*	*NV*	*HV*
Sham	262 ± 42	*143 ± 15	280 ± 41	*142 ± 10
TBI	200 ± 41	*104 ± 21	296 ± 33	*119 ± 19

p < 0.05 HV-vs- NV, data are Mean ± SEM

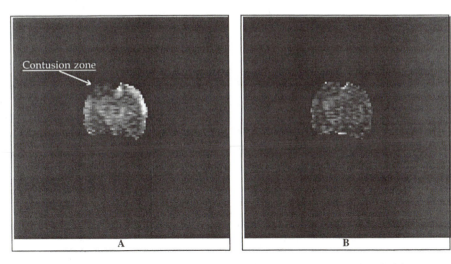

Figure 2. Perfusion maps from TBI study during normal (A) and reduced (B) $PaCO_2$.

picts high flow. Image A shows the area of focal contusion and accompanying low flow area in a slice through the contused area, the left medial parietal cortex. Image B shows CBF during HV. Note the global reduction of flow during HV. It appears that the contusion zone is not expanded during HV. These images, to our knowledge, are the first *in vivo* description of regional CO_2 responsivity in the rat after TBI.

4. CONCLUSIONS

We have demonstrated that perfusion MRI is feasible for the measurement of rCBF and the response of the cerebral vasculature to CO_2 reduction in the rat. At 24 h after CCI, CBF was reduced in the injured LCtx (Figs. 1,2) but not the RCtx relative to shams. This is consistent with findings obtained by autoradiography.

Hyperventilation produced a reproducible reduction in cortical flow. Perfusion MRI holds promise as the single technique currently available that allows serial non-invasive assessment of rCBF and produces maps of CBF in rodents. It was effective in the assessment of CO_2 responsivity in our model and may ultimately have utility in determining the efficacy of a number of therapeutic interventions.

6. ACKNOWLEDGMENTS

This project is supported by The Society of Critical Care Medicine Established Investigator Award, The Laerdal Foundation (P.K.), Children's Hospital of Pittsburgh (M.F.), NIH (P.K. & C.H.) Grant #s RR-10962, RR-03631 (C.H.) and the NINDS Grant # 2P50 NS30318–04A1 (P.K. & C.H.).

5. REFERENCES

1. Lighthall JW: Controlled Cortical Impact: A New Experimental Brain Injury Model. *J Neurotrauma* 5: 1–15, 1988
2. Kochanek PM, Marion DW, Zhang W, Schiding JS, White M, Palmer AM, Clark RSB, O'Malley ME, Styren SD, Ho C, DeKosky ST: Severe Controlled Cortical Impact in Rats: Assessment of Cerebral Edema, Blood Flow and Contusion Volume *J Neurotrauma* 12: 1015–26, 1996
3. Saunders ML, Miller JD, Stablein D, Allen G: The Effects of Graded Experimental Trauma On Cerebral Blood Flow And Responsiveness To CO_2 *J Neurosurg* 51:18–26, 1979
4. Kontos HA, Wei EP: Superoxide Production In Experimental Brain Injury. *J Neurosurg* 64(5): 803–7, 1986
5. Meis G, Ishimaru S, Xie , Seo K, Hossman KA: Ischemic Thresholds of Cerebral Protein Synthesis and Energy State Following Middle Cerebral Artery Occlusion in Rat. *J Cereb Blood Flow Me*tab 11:753–61, 1991
6. Muizelaar JP, Marmarou A, Young HF, Choi SC, Wolf A, Schneider RL, Kontos HA: Improving The Outcome Of Severe Head Injury With The Oxygen Radical Scavenger Polyethylene Glycol-Conjugated Superoxide Dismutase: A Phase II Trial. *J Neurosurg* 78(3):375–82, 1993
7. Williams DS, Detre JA, Leigh JS, Koretsky AP: Magnetic Resonance Imaging of Perfusion Using Spin Inversion of Arterial Water. *Proc Natl Acad Sci USA* 89:212–16, 1992

HISTOLOGICAL ASSESSMENT OF RODENT CNS TISSUES TO EPR OXIMETRY PROBE MATERIAL[*]

P. J. Hoopes,[1] K. J. Liu ,[3] G. Bacic ,[3] E. L. Rolett ,[2] J. F. Dunn, [3] and
H. M. Swartz [3]

Departments of Medicine
[1]Radiation Oncology
[2]Cardiology
[3]Radiology
Dartmouth Medical School
Hanover, New Hampshire

ABSTRACT

The effects of the paramagnetic oxygen sensing material, lithium phthalocyanine (LiPc) and fusinite were assessed in the brain of Mongolian gerbils and the spinal columns of rats respectively, to determine if there are histologically discernible changes in the tissue surrounding the probe material. This information is essential for the evaluation of the role of EPR oximetry in the measurement of pO_2 in the CNS; the technique has great potential value for such measurements because it reports on the pO_2 accurately and sensitively and, after the initial placement, measurements can be made repeatedly without invasive procedures or anesthesia. Histologic assessments demonstrated the inert nature of both the fusinite and LiPc EPR probes in rodent CNS tissue over relatively long (2 month) time periods. The fusinite suspensions and LiPc crystals (size range of approximately 100–200 μm) remained well localized to the point of injection and created mild acute tissue reaction on implantation (which appeared to resolve quickly) and virtually no tissue reaction at later times. The majority of the implanted fusinite and LiPc material was present extracellularly in the brain and spinal cord. MRI provided an accurate, noninvasive

* This work was supported in part by Grant GM51630 from DHHS/NIH/GM.

Oxygen Transport to Tissue XVIII, edited by Nemoto and LaManna
Plenum Press, New York, 1997

assessment of probe placement and was able to investigate pathologic effects (hemorrhage, edema, necrosis) associated with the probe placement and treatment effects.

1. INTRODUCTION

The brain and spinal cord have a high metabolic rate and depend primarily on aerobic metabolism. Therefore, these tissue are very sensitive to changes in oxygen status and pathologic changes that can occur if there are significant changes in the delivery and/or utilization of oxygen in local regions of brain or spinal cord. Complex and effective physiologic controls have evolved to enable the brain and spinal cord to maintain adequate levels of oxygen. Knowledge of the control mechanisms for maintaining local partial pressure of oxygen (pO_2) and conditions which lead to their failure to prevent pathologic changes is incomplete. This deficiency is due, in part, to the difficulty in making measurements of local pO_2 under various physiological and pathophysiological conditions. Such knowledge seems essential for devising optimal strategies for diagnosis and therapy for the many processes which can lead to hypoxic changes in the brain and spinal cord, especially for ischemia- reperfusion type injuries.

Methods of measuring oxygen have recently been reviewed by Chapman (1). The *in vivo* methods can be divided into those that are invasive, such as the use of microelectrodes, or noninvasive, such as nuclear magnetic resonance spectroscopy (MRS). The invasive methods appear to give better determinations of the actual pO_2, but because of their invasiveness may perturb the phenomena they are being used to measure and they cannot be repeated at frequent intervals. Other techniques such as cryospectrophotometry or the use of fluorescent dyes may give accurate results but require the acquisition of biopsies to obtain information on pO_2. The most common way to measure brain pO_2 has been to use oxygen sensitive electrodes, by insertion of small microelectrodes (2) or by surface multielectrode arrays (3). The former may cause mechanical injury to the tissue and repeated measurements at the same site are not possible. The latter method cannot make accurate measurements of local pO_2 deep in brain tissue. A noninvasive optical method has been developed recently, using the oxygen quenching of phosphorescence (4), but it requires intravenous injection of porphyrins and measurements are limited a depth of 1 mm from the surface. Near infrared spectroscopy also has been used, but it measures cerebral blood flow and saturation of hemoglobin, not the interstitial pO_2 (5).

Recently there has been significant progress in the use of electron paramagnetic resonance (EPR, or completely equivalently, electron spin resonance or ESR) spectroscopy for measurements of oxygen in vivo in conscious animals (6). This has resulted from the development of low frequency EPR instruments (1 GHz or lower) suitable for use with living subjects (7,8) and the development of new stable paramagnetic particles (fusinite, India ink, lithium phthalocyanine) with oxygen sensitive EPR spectra (9,10, 11). These particles combine several desirable properties as probes of the pO_2 including high sensitivity to the pO_2, resistance to chemical reactions, and a high degree of inertness in biological systems. The exact location of the paramagnetic particles in tissues can be determined by magnetic resonance imaging (MRI) (12). These developments have established EPR oximetry as a versatile tool for sensitive, noninvasive, and reproducible measurements of pO_2 in a variety of biological systems.

A critical factor in the use of electron paramagnetic resonance (EPR) oximetry is the accurate placement of the probe (oxygen sensitive paramagnetic material) and assessment of the tissue reaction to the probe material. The studies reported here, performed in rodent brain and spinal cord, were designed to assess: a) the acute and chronic tissue effects of EPR oximetry probe material placement and residence, and b) the accuracy and sensitivity of MRI as a noninvasive tool for determination of EPR probe placement and correlation of histologic and imaging tissue effects.

The gerbil brain and the rat spinal cord were chosen as models for these experiments because of the importance of making measurements of pO_2 in the CNS. The Mongolian gerbil is commonly used to study occlusive cerebral ischemia due to its unique neurologic vasculature allowing production of unilateral and bilateral ischemia. A relatively high percentage of Mongolian gerbils have an incomplete Circle of Willis, which allows for the production of unilateral cerebral ischemia (via unilateral carotid occlusion) and near complete loss of cerebral blood flow (in the frontal lobes) when both carotids are occluded (13–16). Irradiation of the rat spinal cord is a well studied model for radiation myelopathy and a model which has proven predictive value for radiation myelopathy in man.

2. METHODS

2.1. General Procedure

The historical assessments were carried out in the context of experiments to investigate acute ischemia in the brain and long-term effects of irradiation in the spinal cord. The probe, fusinite or lithium phthalocyanine, was implanted in the cerebral cortex through a small hole in the cranium or in the spinal cord through the dura (following laminectomy) using specific land marks for consistent implantation. The EPR spectra of the probes were measured to obtain cerebral and spinal cord parenchymal pO_2 values in both anesthetized and unanesthetized animals using a low frequency EPR spectrometer. Probe placement was confirmed by MRI imaging (using a 12 cm bore 7.0 T SMIS MRI/MRS unit) and by gross and histologic exam following removal and sectioning of the brain/spinal cord at sacrifice. Additionally, MRI was used to assess and compare ischemic and/or irradiation damage such as necrosis, demyelination, hemorrhage, and edema. Following treatment and EPR/MRI exams, the brains and spinal cords were histologically assessed using light microscopy and a variety of relevant histochemical stains.

2.2. Animal Models

Because some of the most interesting and important studies of pO_2 in the brain are related to ischemia we have chosen the Mongolian Gerbil for the studies in the brain, since its unique anatomical differences make it an ideal model for studying forebrain ischemia. Due to the absence of posterior communicating arteries in 50–70% of the animals, complete ischemia can be produced by occlusion of the common carotid arteries. Permanent bilateral ligation is fatal because there is no connection between the basilar artery and the carotid circulation (13, 14). In a smaller percentage (approx. 50%) of male Mongolian gerbils the occlusion of one common carotid artery produces unilateral forebrain ischemia. The gerbils normally tolerate this procedure well, however a significant percentage of the animals will exhibit minor neurologic deficits. The most reliable histopathologic changes, following the aforementioned vascular occlusive procedures is the loss of pyramidal cells in the CA1 region of the hippocampus following limited (5 minute, bilateral occlusion) ischemia. Following a longer, 30 minute, bilateral occlusion ultrastructural alterations in the CA1, CA3, and dentate gyrus of the hippocampus include: shifted nuclei, absent or altered

Golgi complexes, swelling of the molecular layer, enlargement of the perikaryon and peri-vascular processes of the astrocytes in the deeper layers of the cortex, and enlargement of the endoplasmic reticulum in the neurons have been demonstrated (15, 16).

2.3. MRI

Probe placement was confirmed by MRI (using a 12 cm bore 7.0 T SMIS MRI/MRS unit) and by gross and histologic exam following removal and sectioning of the brain/spinal cord at sacrifice. Additionally, the MRI was used to assess tissue damage and to compare changes such as ischemia, necrosis, demyelination, hemorrhage and edema with other assessment techniques such as histology. An MRI unit of this type is capable of assessing tissue images (slices) in the range of 100 μ or less. These images demonstrate resolution closely comparable to routine histologic sections. Additionally, the MRI is noninvasive and can show pathophysiologic changes not easily determined by histology. Mosely et al. (17) have demonstrated the potential for characterizing stroke (focal ischemia) with diffusion-weighted imaging at very detailed resolution (magnetic resonance microscopy). The shielded gradients necessary for magnetic resonance microscopy are also well suited for running diffusion sequences. Using a 7-Tesla system fields of 90 gauss/cm can be obtained with short echoes. Images acquired with a TR = 1000 msec, a TE of 40 msec and a diffusion-weighted coefficient of greater than 1000 sec/mm^2 are able to produce a 1 mm slice thickness with an in plane resolution of less than 80 micron. These types of studies now make following the precise pathophysiology and pathologic outcome of an ischemic episode possible in a noninvasive setting. To date, only few MRI studies of chronic progressive radiation myelopathy (CPRM) have been published (18,19). The characteristic findings at the early stage were: swelling of the spinal cord and a high-signal intensity area on T2-weighted images encompassing long segments of the cord often extending beyond the boundaries of the radiation field (20 / 26). All stages of radiation injury have in common an increase in free tissue water which helps produce the hypodensity on CT and increased T_1 and T_2 on MRI. This may be the result of endothelial cell damage, which causes increased capillary permeability and vasogenic edema or demyelination, which leads to the replacement of hydrophobic myelin by water (20). One of the most common findings in radiation myelopathy is a focal cord enhancement on T1-weighted images following administration of Gd-DTPA. Later atrophy of the cord was noted without abnormal signal intensity. In an only MRI study of CPRM in rabbits, high-intensity lesions were recognized on T_2W images prior to or with the onset of radiation myelopathy, but it is not known how early the MR lesion appears or how the lesion changes with time.

2.4. Histopathology

Following the ischemia or radiation treatments and EPR, MRI and/or blood flow exams, the animals are sacrificed with an overdose of barbiturate. The brains and spinal cords are removed, immersion fixed in 10% neutral buffered formalin, sectioned in the same plane as the MRI images and processed for slide preparation and staining. The sections are made at the site of the implant and serially throughout the treated and/or imaged area. Routine histologic stains include hematoxylin and eosin, cresyl violet (neurons) and luxol fast blue/PAS (normal and degenerating myelin). Histologic slides are examined morphologically using light microscopy with the general goal of being able to visualize the probe material in unperturbed (by the sectioning process) section of tissue that is cut thin enough to offer good morphologic resolution. There are two potential difficulties in

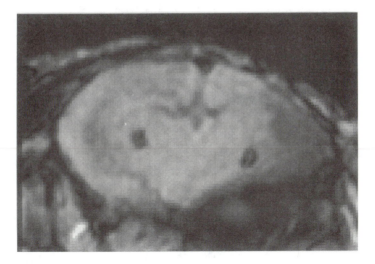

Figure 1. 7.0 T MRI of LiPc crystals implanted in both hemispheres of a Mongolian gerbil brain. The two crystals produced independent EPR - oxygen readings allowing simultaneous assessment of the ischemic and nonischemic hemispheres in the unilateral carotid occlusion ischemia experiments in these animals .

cutting histologic sections with probe material: 1) the possibility that the sections are not cut in the proper region of tissue which contains the probe material, and 2) the possibility that the microtome blade does not pass easily through the probe material and tears the tissue by dragging and displacing the material. In order to alleviate these the problems, it is important to: 1) trim the tissues in the proper orientation and thickness (generally 6–8 micron) with the probe material visible on the face of the tissue to be cut, 2) imbed the tissues in the appropriate position, so that the tissue face to cut has the probe material just beneath the surface.

3. RESULTS

3.1. Histology, EPR-pO$_2$ MRI, and Blood Flow Assessments of Gerbil Brain Ischemia

Histologic assessments demonstrated the inert nature of the fusinite probe in the gerbil brain and that the fusinite remained well localized to the point of injection over a 60 day time period. There is little or no inflammation or tissue effect associated with intermediate term implantation of the fusinite EPR probe (Figure 2). In other studies in our laboratory using both LiPc and fusinite probes in the rat brain, we have found that both fusinite and LiPc probe material remain primarily extracellular, however, a comparatively greater percentage of the fusinite is found intracellularly. This occurrence may be due to the relatively smaller particulate size of the fusinite (compared to the LiPc crystals). Cerebral damage resulting from unilateral occlusive ischemia requires approximately 7 days to fully develop in the gerbil model. The hippocampus is the region of the brain that is most sensitive to ischemia and the loss of CA-1 hippocampal neurons was the predominant histologic effect noted in the majority of the animals. Although almost all animals included in this study lost hippocampal neurons in the ischemic hemisphere, the extent of cerebral

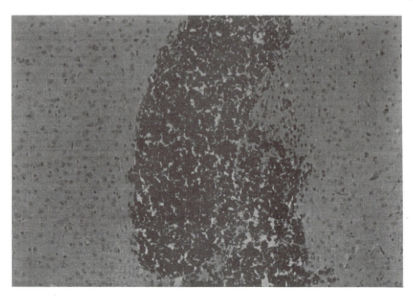

Figure 2. High magnification (60 x) photomicrograph demonstrating the fusinite material 60 days following implant in the cerebral cortex of a Mongolian gerbil. The fusinite is stereotactically implanted with a 27 gauge needle to depth of approximately 3 mm. There is extremely minimal tissue reaction surrounding the fusinite, therefore the distance from the fusinite to the normal brain parenchyma is minimal. Hematoxylin & Eosin stain.

damage (including focal demyelination, axon loss and focal necrosis) in this model appeared to be somewhat more variable than suggested in some early literature. This finding, along with anesthesia-induced pO_2 variations could help explain some of the variations in histologic damage we observed. EPR measurements showed that cerebral pO_2 decreased from ~ 35 mmHg in an unanesthetized animal, to ~ 25 mmHg in an anesthetized animal, and further to ~ 12 mmHg in the ischemic (carotid occlusion) cerebrum. The MRI also allowed us to document placement and position of the probe material. As shown in figure 1, we were able to place the LiPc probe material in both cerebral hemispheres of a subset of Mongolian gerbil brains. The two crystals produced independent EPR-oxygen readings, allowing simultaneous assessment of the ischemic and nonischemic hemispheres in the unilateral carotid occlusion ischemia experiments in these animals. Blood flow measurements (laser Doppler, ml/100 gm tissue/min), assessed by interstitial probe placement in the cerebral tissue, reflected normal and ischemic conditions. Cerebral blood flow in the affected hemisphere decreased by ~ 40% following unilateral carotid occlusion.

3.2. Histology, EPR-pO_2, MRI, and Blood Flow Assessments of Irradiated Rat Spinal Cord

In our spinal cord experiments, the LiPc crystals are placed directly into the rat spinal cord parenchyma (following a dorsal laminectomy) using a 26–28 gauge needle. We have been able to record valid pO_2 measurements in the rat spinal cord throughout a 30 day post implantation period and are continuing to look at longer implantation times. Our histologic studies (light microscopy) have shown that the effect of the laminectomy and the LiPc implantation procedure on spinal cord function has been negligible in irradiated and unirradiated animals and that there is virtually no long-term tissue reaction as as-

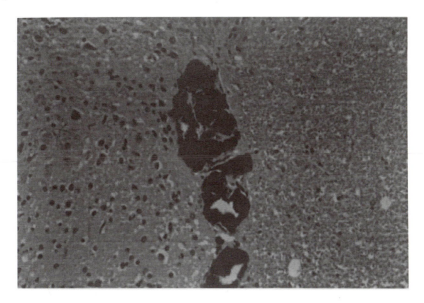

Figure 3. High magnification (60 x) photomicrograph demonstrating the a LiPc crystal implanted in the dorsal white matter of a rat spinal cord 14 days following the implant. The LiPc crystal is positioned at the junction of the gray (left) and white matter (right). There is no inflammatory or foreign body tissue reaction associated with the crystal. The crystal material is directly adjacent to the parenchymal tissue. Although we do not have histologic assessment of chronic LiPc implants in the rat spinal cord, long term implants in gerbil brain have produced almost no inflammatory or foreign body type reactions. Hematoxylin & Eosin stain.

sessed by light microscopy (Figure 3). As expected, we have observed occasional foci of demyelination and hemorrhage in the irradiated cords, however these areas have not been specifically associated with the probe material. In general, we have found that the majority of the LiPc material remains extracellular, however, occasional resident phagocytic cells contain small fragments of the probe material. Although we have not documented hemorrhage surrounding the probe material in our spinal cord studies, we have seen minimal focal hemorrhage surrounding the LiPc probe material in rat brains examined up to 96 hours following implantation. It seems likely that this type of reaction also occurs in the rat spinal cords and our ongoing studies are designed to examine this finding. EPR based pO_2 measurements in the rat spinal cord recorded values of ~ 30 mmHg when the animal is under gas anesthesia and 20 mm Hg when the animal is under barbiturate anesthesia. Spinal cord pO_2 values were found to be similar before irradiation and following irradiation (30 Gy) at 20 minutes and 7 days and only slightly decreased at 30 days post irradiation. Spinal cord blood flow (laser Doppler, ml/100 gm tissue/min) determinations, made by placing a surface probe directly on the spinal cord dura in the region of irradiated or nonirradiated cord tissue, were similar before and 20 minutes following irradiation. There was a slight decrease in blood flow 7 and 30 days post irradiation

4. CONCLUSIONS

1. Histologic assessments of rodent brain and spinal cord tissues following no treatment, vascular occlusion (gerbil brain) and radiation (rat spine) have dem-

onstrated the stability, inert nature (very little inflammation and/or tissue reaction) and pO_2 measuring ability of both the fusinite and LiPc EPR probe material over relatively long (1–2 month) time periods. In some cases we have noted minor hemorrhage associated with the probe implant. Although this hemorrhage appears to resolve quickly(~5 days or less) it could impair the accuracy of pO_2 readings immediately following implantation.

2. The majority of implanted fusinite and LiPc material is present extracellularly in the brain and spinal cord; however, some material is present intracellularly in resident phagocytic cells, which at the time of our histologic observations, are generally in close association with the probe material at the site of the implant. Although our fusinite and LiPc studies were not designed to be directly comparable with respect to animal model and time endpoint, fusinite (possibly due to a smaller size) appears to be more readily taken into cells (phagocytized).

3. Although CNS tissues are relatively homogeneous, variation in vascular anatomy could lead to erroneous oximetry data if oximetry probes are not properly placed. Therefore, the use of MRI as a noninvasive tool to assess probe placement is critical for accurate EPR oximetry studies. 7.0 T MRI is capable of providing a sensitive, accurate and noninvasive pathophysiologic assessment of tissue effects (e.g. ischemia, hemorrhage, demyelination, edema, necrosis), in the brain and spinal cord of rodents. The obvious advantage of this assessment technique is that it can be performed at will over long periods in the same animal and offers resolution which compares favorably with histology.

REFERENCES

1. Chapman J. Measurement of tumor hypoxia by invasive and non-invasive procedures: a review of recent clinical studies. *Radiother Oncol* 1991; 20 (Suppl 1): 13–19.
2. Nair, P.K., Buerk, D.G. and Halsey, J.H., Comparison of oxygen metabolism and tissue pO2 in cortex and hippocampus of gerbil brain, *Stroke,* 18 (1987) 616–662.
3. Grota, J. , Zimmer, K. and Schubert, R., Tissue oxygenation in normal and edematous brain cortex during arterial hypocapnia, *Adv. Exp. Med. Biol.,* 180 (1984)179–184.0.
4. Wilson, D.F., Gomi, S., Pastuszko, A. and Grindberg, J.H., Oxygenation of the cortex of the brain of cats during occlusion of the middle cerebral artery and reperfusion, *Adv. Exp. Med. Biol.,* 317 (1992) 689–694.
5. Elwell, C.E., Cope, M., Edwards, A.D., Wyatt, J.S., Reynolds, E.O.R. and Deply, D.T., Measurements of cerebral blood flow in adult humans using near infrared spectroscopy-methodology and possible errors, *Adv. Exp. Med. Biol.,* 317 (1992) 235–245.
6. Swartz, H.M. and Walczak, T., In vivo EPR: prospects for the 90's, *Phys. Med.,* 9 (1993) 41–48.
7. Colacicchi, S., Alecci, M., Gualtieri, G., Quaresima, V., Urisini, C.L., Ferrari, M. and Sotgiu, A., New experimental procedures for in vivo L-band and radio frequency EPR spectroscopy/imaging, *J. Chem. Soc. Perkin Trans.,* 2 (1993) 2077–2082.
8. Nilges MJ, Walczak T and Swartz HM, 1 GHz in vivo ESR spectrometer operating with surface pulse. *Phys Med* 1989; 5: 195–201.
9. Liu, K.J., Gast, P., Moussavi, M., Norby, S.W., Vahidi, N., Walczak, T., Wu, M. and Swartz, H.M., Lithium phthalocyanine: a probe for electron paramagnetic resonance oximetry in viable biological systems, *Proc. Natl. Acad. Sci. USA,* 90 (1993) 5438–5442.
10. Swartz, H.M., Liu, K.J., Goda, F. and Walczak, T., India ink: a potential clinically applicable EPR oximetry probe, *Magn. Reson. Med.,* 31 (1994) 229–232.
11. Vahidi, N., Clarkson, R.B., Liu, K.J., Norby, S.W., Wu, M. and Swartz, H.M., In vivo and in vitro EPR oximetry with fusinite: a new coal-derived, particulate EPR probe, *Magn. Reson. Med.,* 31 (1994) 139–146.
12. Bacic, G, Liu, KJ, O'Hara, JA, Harris, RD, Szybinski, K, Goda, F and Swartz, HM, Oxygen tension in a murine tumor: a combined EPR and MRI study, *Magn. Reson Med,* 30 (1993) 568–572.

13. Levine S and Sohn D, Cerebral ischemia in infant and adult gerbils, *Arch Path* 1969; 87: 315–317.

14. DeLeo JA, Floyd RA and Carney JM, Increased in vitro lipid peroxidation of gerbil cerebral cortex as compared with rat, *Neuroscience Letters* 1986; 67: 63–67.

15. Abel MS and McCandless DW, Metabolic profile of hippocampal regions after bilateral ischemia and recovery. *Neurochem Res* 1982; 7: 789–797.

16. Bubis JJ, Fujimoto T, Ito, U Mrsulja BJ, Spatz M and Klatzo I, Experimental cerebral ischemia in Mongolian gerbils, *Acta Neuropath* 1976; 36: 285–294.

17. Moseley ME, Cohen Y, Montorovich J et al. Early detection of regional cerebral ischemia in cats; comparison of diffusion and T2 weighted MRI and spectroscopy. *Magn Reson Imag* 1990; 14:330–345.

18. Glockner JF, Swartz HM. In vivo EPR oximetry using two novel probes: fusinite and lithium phthalocyanine. In: eds. Erdmann W, Bruley DF. *Oxygen transport in tissue.* New York: Plenum Publishing Corporation 1992; 229–245.

19. Wang PJ, Shen WC, Jan JS. MR imaging in radiation myelopathy. *AJNR* 1992; 13:1049–1055.

20. Zweig G, Russell EJ. Radiation myelopathy of the cervical spinal cord: MR findings. *AJNR* 1990; 11:1188–1190.

4

REGIONAL DIFFERENCES IN METABOLISM AND INTRACELLULAR pH IN RESPONSE TO MODERATE HYPOXIA

J. C. LaManna, M. A. Haxhiu, K. L. Kutina-Nelson, S. Pundik, B. Erokwu, and N. S. Cherniack

School of Medicine
Case Western Reserve University
Cleveland, Ohio 44106

1. INTRODUCTION

It is well known that hypoxia induces increased respiration through activation of peripheral chemoreceptor reflex pathways. But, in the absence of afferent inputs from peripheral chemoreceptors, systemic hypoxia causes depression of breathing activity. Evidence of hypoxic depression of respiration also can be observed in animals and in humans with intact peripheral chemoreceptors.The effects of central hypoxia on respiratory activity require more time to develop than the effects of hypoxic stimulation through peripheral chemoreceptors, suggesting the involvement of relatively slow metabolic processes. The mechanism by which hypoxia causes central depression of breathing is not known, but several possibilites can be suggested.

Decreased oxygen availability promotes the metabolic production of lactic acid by glycolysis within the cells, which reduces the excitability of CNS neurons.[1] Lactic acid may diffuse into the extracellular fluid, or cells may actively transport H^+ outward.

Intracellular pH plays an important role as a feed-back mechanism in controlling energy metabolism, cell volume regulation, spatial buffering, neurotransmitter synthesis and release, and neurotransmitter receptor function.[2] Hypoxic acidosis might act indirectly through inhibition of glutamate receptors.[3,4] In regions where pH remained moderately acid, NMDA receptor would remain inactive even if glutamate levels were raised. Monaghan and Cotman [5] have reported the distribution of NMDA receptors in the brain in respiratory related brainstem regions. Because the NMDA receptor pathway plays a significant role in cardiovascular and respiratory activity including respiratory timing,[6] pH-induced changes in the NMDA receptor function might partly mediate hypoxia-induced respiratory modulation. Thus, tissue patterns of acidosis are an important variable determining neuronal responses to hypoxia. Whether spatial differences exist in intracellular pH within

Oxygen Transport to Tissue XVIII, edited by Nemoto and LaManna
Plenum Press, New York, 1997

neuronal networks involved in regulation of breathing activity occurs during hypoxia-induced respiratory depression is not known.

Although cell ATP concentrations are buffered by phosphocreatine, if hypoxia is prolonged and severe, a decrease in cellular ATP will occur. ATP can either directly modulate the channel as a ligand or play a role in Na channel modulation by phosphorylation. Recently, it has been shown that excitability of neurons could be altered via sodium channel modulation as well as modulation of the hyperpolarizing ATP-sensitive K^+ channels,[7,8] the closure of which is ATP- dependent. In addition, the ATP-sensitive K^+ channel affinity for ATP is pH-dependent, decreasing with increasing acidosis.[9] Thus, higher concentrations of ATP would be required to keep the channel closed in acidic conditions.

Whether hypoxia-induced decreases in PCr and ATP are closely related in the brainstem neuronal network involved in breathing and cardiovascular control is not known. Furthermore the relationships among regional alterations in intracellular pH, PCr and ATP are not well established. Despite the importance of pHi and of energetic sources in brain function, regional changes in these variables in relation of respiratory depression induced by oxygen deprivation have not been studied. This could be partly due to the lack of quantitative methods for their simultaneous measurements. Techniques which can be used for determination of intracellular pH , like 31P-NMR,[10] microelectrodes,[11] and optical probes, i.e. absorption,[12] and fluorescent [13,14] dye, have differential advantages and disadvantages with respect to invasiveness, cost, ease of calibration, sensitivity, spatial and temporal resolution.[15]The development of the quantitative method for pHi determination using the absorption properties of the vital dye neutral red [15] has progressed to the point where the method has been used to reliably determine intracellular pH in intact rat brains,[2,16,17] and in brain slice preparations.[2,18]

To demonstrate the feasibility of the experimental paradigm, and as an initial test of the hypothesis that metabolic changes within the brain stem in response to hypoxia are coordinated processes that play an important role in the global behavior of respiratory and cardiovascular outputs, we determined the specific regional metabolic response patterns within two regions of the the medulla oblongata, rostral ventrolateral medulla (RVL) and nucleus tractus solitarius (NTS), to a decreased PaO_2 under eucapnic conditions.

2. METHODS

2.1. Animals and Surgical Preparation

Male Sprague-Dawley rats were anesthetized with urethane (1.3 g/kg, ip). The femoral artery was cannulated to measure arterial pressure and heart rate and to withdraw samples for blood gas analysis. The external jugular vein was cannulated for administration of fluid and drugs. Animals were tracheotomized and ventilated with 100 % O_2, to avoid superposition of secondary effects on the immediate respiratory changes induced by hypoxia. The volume and the pump rate were adjusted to the body weight and breathing frequency. The body temperature of the animals was maintained at 37–38°C. To expose the ventrolateral medulla, a ventral midline incision was made in the neck. The esophagus and the trachea were transected and the proximal portions of both were reflected cranially. After removing overlying muscles, a wide craniotomy was performed, the ventral aspect of the medulla exposed and covered with warm artificial cerebrospinal fluid, as earlier described.[19] The vagus nerves were isolated and cut, in order to eliminate input from lung mechanoreceptors and prevent eventual entrainment of respiratory output to the ventilator.

Respiratory output was obtained by recording the electromyographic activity of the diaphragm (D_{EMG}). Bipolar stainless steel twisted wires, with wire tips 1 mm apart, were implanted via an abdominal incision, which was later sutured closed, into the costal part of the diaphragm near the lateral position of central tendon. The electrical activity was amplified with an AC coupled amplifier having a band pass filter setting of 3 Hz-3 kHz (Grass Instruments, Model PH 511). Signal was full wave rectified and then processed by a moving averager with a 100 ms time constant. Diaphragm EMG activity was recorded simultaneously with blood pressure on a 6 channel Gould stripchart recorder. The rate of ventilator was adjusted to give arterial CO_2 ($Pa\,CO_2$) around 35–38 mmHg. At least 60 min was allowed for recovery from surgery. Arterial blood was taken, 0.1 ml for analyses of blood gases and pH, and then saline solution of neutral red (2%) was slowly injected intravenously 2 ml over 20 min. Before the end of infusion, the inspired gas was switched from oxygen to the hypoxic gas mixture (8% O_2 in N_2). When cessation of breathing activity occurred (see Figure 1) brain stem was frozen in situ. Control animals were ventilated with oxygen through all experimental procedures.

2.2. *In Situ* Fixation of Brainstem

In situ fixation was performed by funnel freezing of the brainstem with liquid nitrogen.[20] Just before freezing, a plastic funnel was placed over the medulla and a seal was made around the base with stopcock grease to prevent leakage of liquid nitrogen. Liquid nitrogen was then poured into the funnel and the funnel maintained at least one third full for 6 to 7 minutes after which the rat was immersed in liquid nitrogen. Frozen rats were stored at -80 °C until further processing.

2.3. Intracellular pH Determination

The brains of the frozen rats were removed in a glove box maintained at -30 °C , and 20 um coronal sections were performed through the entire brainstem in a cryomicrotome. During sectioning, photographic slides using Fujichrome 50 'Velvia' 35 mm color slide film in a Nikon F2 camera with a macro lens, close-up bellows and a ring flash, were made of the block face of the frozen experimental brain alongside a frozen, unstained rat brain or frozen homogenate which act as a spectrophotometric "blank". These slides were then examined under a microscope (Olympus Inc., Model SIT 68) and initially processed through an analog processor (Dage MTI Inc., Model DSP 100). Interference band-pass filters at 450 and 550 mm were alternately placed between the light

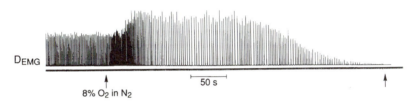

D_{EMG}

|← 50 s →|

↑
8% O_2 in N_2

Figure 1. Diaphragm electromyogram recorded during an hypoxic cycle as indicated by the arrows. The activity is observed to initially increase in frequency, then strength. A prolonged slowing follows until the strength drops to zero.

source of the microscope and the photographic slide to obtain images at the peak absorbance wavelengths for the acid and base forms of neutral red. Wratten gelatin filters (Kodak, #78A) were also placed between the light source and the photographic slides to equalize the transmission at 450 and 550 mm. Eight-bit images of the blank and experimental brains were captured using NIH Image (v 1.55) and processed using Alice v 2.3 (formerly Digital Image Processing Station, Hayden Image Processing Group, Boulder, CO) on a Macintosh IIci computer. This latter program provides for image math functions and maintains 16 bits during all calculations which avoids the problem of roundoff error when optical densities and standard calibration curve equations are applied to the image. Intracellular pH images are based on the standard reflectance curve for brain pastes: pH =[(Absorbance$_{550}$/Absorbance$_{450}$)-10.5]/-1.3. Intracellular pH values are reported as mean ± sem from investigator selected regions of interest, or as histogram distributions of individual pixels, each approximately .01 mm by .01 mm in size. Details of the methods and review of the physical, chemical, and biological characteristics of the dye have been documented.[2,12,15] Briefly, the dye administered intravenously is taken up rapidly into brain due to high lipid solubility. It is concentrated in all the cell types in the cytoplasmic organellar membranes where it is responsive to the cytoplasmic compartment. The cell membrane, nucleus and nuclear membrane, and myelin remain unstained. It is important to note that because it is a ratio method it is concentration independent, as long as a minimum amount of dye is present. The method is quantitative with respect to pH over the range of at least 6.0 to 8.0.

2.4. Metabolite Assays

Twenty micron sections of the frozen brains were collected and lyophilized for metabolite determinations. PCr and ATP were determined by microquantitative histochemistry on the freeze-dried sections as described previously.[21,22] Discrete samples, corresponding to regions of interest used for pHi analyses, were dissected in a low humidity room with the aid of a dissection microscope. The 0.1 to 1.0 μg tissue samples were weighed on a quartz fiber balance. The tissue samples were assayed for ATP and PCr, using the luciferin-luciferase method; Lactate was assayed using enzymatic cycling as previously described.[21,22]

3. RESULTS

In the rats, switching the inspired gas from oxygen to the hypoxic gas mixture (8% O_2 in N_2) was associated with an expected reduction of arterial PaO$_2$ (435 ± 14 vs 36 ± 2 mmHg; $p < 0.01$), slight change in PaCO$_2$ (37 ± 3 vs 35 ± 3; $p > 0.1$) , and significant fall in pH (7.37 ± .03 vs 7.23 ± .02; $p < 0.05$). As shown in Figure 1, exposure to isocapnic

Table 1. Brainstem regional pHi and metabolites (nm/mg dry wt.; mean ± sem)

		pHi	Lactate	PCr	ATP
RVL	Control	7.19 ± 0.12 (4)	17.8 ± 9.5 (7)	19.5 ± 3.7 (7)	6.6 ± 0.5 (7)
	Hypoxic	6.96 ± 0.04 (9)	53.6 ± 8.3 (8)	5.0 ± 1.0 (8)	4.1 ± 0.6 (8)
NTS	Control	7.21 ± 0.14 (4)	17.0 ± 6.8 (7)	16.1 ± 3.5 (7)	6.0 ± 0.5 (7)
	Hypoxic	6.95 ± 0.04 (9)	53.4 ± 7.3 (8)	5.0 ± 0.6 (8)	4.2 ± 0.5 (8)

hypoxia caused an initial increase in respiratory frequency, followed by an increase in amplitude, and then decrease in rate of breathing, reduction of peak activity and apnea. At the time of apnea, which occurred on average after about 8 to 15 minutes, the brain was frozen in situ and prepared according to the above described protocols.

3.1. Distribution of Intracellular pH during Deprivation Induced Respiratory Depression

Table 1 reports the intracellular pH in control rat brainstem and in hypoxic rat brainstem in the RVL and the compact portion of the nucleus ambiguus, and the NTS. Figure 2 illustrates the studied regions. These cell groups were chosen because of their roles in regulation of respiratory and sympathetic activity, integration of multiple afferent inputs and coordination of visceral and somatic outputs. Average values of pHi were measured from images such as shown in Figure 3. The panel demonstrates the potential resolution of the used method. Note the pH scale is given on the right of the panel, with the darker gray at the bottom indicating pH 6.5 and the lighter at the top indicating pH 7.5. The histogram distribution of pHi values in the brainstem is shown in Figure 4.

During oxygen deprivation, at the time point when oxygen deprivation caused apnea, measured values of brain stem regional pHi proportionally decreased and were significantly lower than in control animals. In addition, hypoxic loading reduced pHi variations within the regions studied.

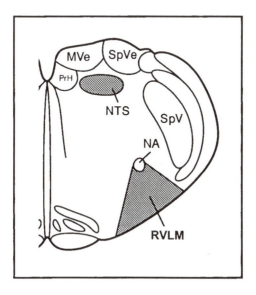

Figure 2. Cross sectional diagram of the level (-12.3 mm from the bregma) of the brain stem analyzed. The two regions studied are indicated. RVL and NA, rostral ventrolateral medulla and the nucleus ambiguus; NTS, nucleus tractus solitarius.

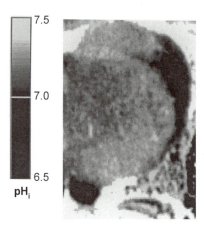

Figure 3. Gray scale intracellular pH image of a section through the brainstem of rat under normoxic conditions. The calibrated pH scale is shown on the right.

3.2. The Levels of Metabolites during Oxygen Deprivation Induced Respiratory Depression

The frozen section from the block face was photographed and then lyophilized. The same region of interest was dissected and assayed for lactate, PCr and ATP. The results are also presented in Table 1. In the control rats the lactate and the PCr values were as expected within studied regions. However, ATP concentrations were lower than those from cortical and hippocampal levels. Thus, the brainstem regions that we measured had increased PCr/ATP ratios. These did not represent artifact from freezing since PCr levels were in the expected range, indicating that fixation was adequate. The lactate levels in all studied regions in rats exposed to hypoxic loading were higher than measured levels in control animals, while PCr and ATP levels were lower than in control animals. However, PCr/ATP ratio was significantly lower in hypoxic than in control animals (1.23 ± 0.04 vs 2.85 ± 0.13; $p < 0.05$), suggesting disproportional depletion of PCr and ATP. While ATP levels were $36 \pm 6\%$ (mean $\pm$ sd) lower than in control animals, measured PCr concentrations were only $29 \pm 2\%$ of values found in control rats. Regional changes in PCr and ATP were not significantly different.

4. DISCUSSION

In anesthetized animals, exposure to hypoxia results in typical changes in the pattern of breathing, characterized by initial increase in frequency and amplitude, followed within minutes by a decrease in respiratory output. The decline is more pronounced and has faster dynamics in vagotomized animals if arterial oxygen partial pressure is below 40 mmHg. In the studies reported here we examined the effects of reduction in oxygen availability on regional metabolic changes within medulla oblongata at the time point when hypoxia caused respiratory depression.

The result showed for the first time that respiratory depression induced by hypoxia is associated with regional changes in intracellular pH. A comparable degree of intracellular acidosis occurred in both regions which contain neuronal elements of importance in

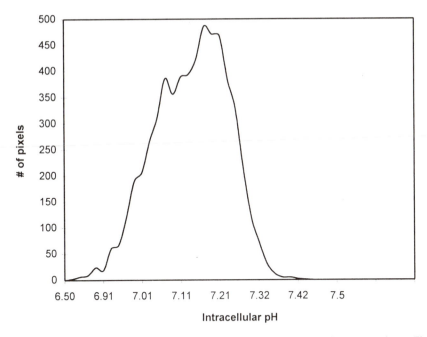

Figure 4. The histogram distribution of intracellular pH values in the brainstem of the normoxic rat. The graph was constructed from the image of figure 3 with one-half of the brainstem chosen as the region of interest analyzed. Intracellular pH was 7.13 ± 0.11.

regulation of respiratory activity and sympathetic outflow. Furthermore, we found that the increase in lactate levels in any of studied nuclei paralleled changes in intracellular pH, suggesting that reduction in oxygen promoted production of lactic acid and intracellular acidosis. There are no data to suggest that mild intracellular acidosis, comparable to that reported here within brainstem nuclei may cause membrane hyperpolarization and apnea. However, Neubauer et al. [1] demonstrated that in anesthetized animals, prevention of brain acidosis by treatment with dichloroacetate, which inhibits production of lactic acid, abolishes the depression of breathing activity during progressive mild to moderate hypoxia. Furthermore, it has been shown that hypoxia is also associated with extracellular acidosis.[23] It was reported that moderate increase in H^+ concentration in extracellular fluid (pH 6.5) markedly reduces NMDA receptor activation.[4] Hence, hypoxia-induced acidosis by various pathways may reduce cell activity.

Measurements of the PCr and ATP, in the same medullary regions in which the intracellular pH and the lactate levels were determined, revealed significantly lower PCr and ATP concentrations in hypoxic rats than in control animals.

In animals exposed to a steady state level of hypoxic stress, at the time point when respiratory depression occurred, fall of PCr was more accentuated than the decrease of ATP. This suggests that the decline in ATP level is "buffered" and delayed by the operation of the creatine phosphate system . Because the concentration of PCr in the brain is greater than of the adenine nucleotides and the equilibrium in PCr reaction is shifted toward ATP synthesis, the initial hydrolysis of PCr during oxygen deprivation is not followed by a proportional decline in ATP concentration. However, as duration and severity of hypoxia increases, demonstrable decreases in cellular ATP concentrations can be measured. In these studies, when complete cessation of breathing activity occurred, ATP concentrations were for 36% lower than in a control animals, while PCr concentrations were only 29% of expected values.

In summary, systemic hypoxia in anesthetized, vagotomized and mechanically ventilated rats, at the time point when respiratory depression occurs, as the physiological response to systemic oxygen deprivation, is associated with comparable decrease in intracellular pH, PCr and ATP in brain stem nuclei involved in regulation of breathing activity. However, the relative contribution of each metabolic component on initiation of hypoxia-induced respiratory depression and the time course of metabolic events associated with the respiratory output changes, from the moment of exposure to the occurrence of apnea, need to be examined.

REFERENCES

1. Neubauer JA, JE Melton, and NH Edelman: Modulation of respiration during brain hypoxia. *J Appl Physiol* **68**:441–451 (1990).
2. LaManna JC, JK Griffith, BR Cordisco, C-W Lin, and WD Lust: Intracellular pH in rat brain in vivo and in brain slices. *Can J Physiol Pharmacol* **70**:S269-S277 (1992).
3. Tombaugh GC and RM Sapolsky: Mild acidosis protects hippocampal neurons from injury induced by oxygen and glucose deprivation. *Brain Res* **506**:343–345 (1990).
4. Giffard RG, H Monyer, CW Christine, and DW Choi: Acidosis reduces NMDA receptor activation, glutamate neurotoxicity, and oxygen-glucose deprivation neuronal injury in cortical cultures. *Brain Res* **506**:339–342 (1990).
5. Monaghan DT and CW Cotman: Distribution of N-methyl-D-aspartate-sensitive L-[^{3}H]glutamate-binding sites in rat brain. *J Neurosci* **5**:2909–2919 (1985).
6. Bianchi AL, M Denavit-Saubié, and J Champagnat: Central control of breathing in mammals: Neuronal circuitry, membrane properties, and neurotransmitters. *Physiol Rev* **75**:1–45 (1995).
7. Jiang C, FJ Sigworth, and GG Haddad: Oxygen deprivation activates an ATP-inhibitable K$^+$ channel in substantia nigra neurons. *J Neurosci* **14**:5590–5602 (1994).
8. Jiang C and GG Haddad: A direct mechanism for sensing low oxygen levels by central neurons. *Proc Natl Acad Sci USA* **91**:7198–7201 (1994).
9. Davies NW, NB Standen, and PR Stanfield: The effect of intracellular pH on ATP-dependent potassium channels of frog skeletal muscles. *J Physiol (Lond)* **445**:549–568 (1992).
10. Petroff OAC, JW Prichard, KL Behar, JR Alger, JA den Hollander, and RG Shulman: Cerebral intracellular pH by ^{31}P nuclear magnetic resonance spectroscopy. *Neurol* **35**:781–788 (1985).
11. Chesler M and RP Kraig: Intracellular pH of astrocytes increases rapidly with cortical stimulation. *Am J Physiol* **253**:R666-R670 (1987).
12. LaManna JC and KA McCracken: The use of neutral red as an intracellular pH indicator in rat brain cortex *in vivo. Anal Biochem* **142**:117–125 (1984).
13. Csiba L, W Paschen, and K-A Hossmann: A topographic quantitative method for measuring brain tissue pH under physiological and pathological conditions. *Brain Res* **289**:334–337 (1983).
14. Anderson RE, FB Meyer, and FH Tomlinson: Focal cortical distribution of blood flow and brain pH$_i$ determined by in vivo fluorescent imaging. *Am J Physiol* **263**:H565-H575 (1992).
15. LaManna JC: Intracellular pH determination by absorption spectrophotometry of neutral red. *Met Br Dis* **2**:167–182 (1987).
16. Griffith JK, BR Cordisco, C-W Lin, and JC LaManna: Distribution of intracellular pH in the rat brain cortex after global ischemia as measured by color film histophotometry of neutral red. *Brain Res* **573**:1–7 (1992).
17. LaManna JC, JK Griffith, BR Cordisco, HE Bell, C-W Lin, S Pundik, and WD Lust: Rapid recovery of rat brain intracellular pH after cardiac arrest and resuscitation. *Brain Res* **687**:175–181 (1995).
18. Sick TJ, TS Whittingham, and JC LaManna: Determination of intracellular pH in the in vitro hippocampal slice preparation by transillumination spectrophotometry of neutral red. *J Neurosci Meth* **27**:25–34 (1989).
19. Haxhiu MA, J Mitra, E van Lunteren, EN Bruce, and NS Cherniack: Hypoglossal and phrenic responses to cholinergic agents applied to ventral medullary surface. *Am J Physiol* **247**:R939-R944 (1984).

20. Pontén U, RA Ratcheson, LG Salford, and BK Siesjö: Optimal freezing conditions for cerebral metabolites in rats. *J Neurochem* **21**:1127–1138 (1973).
21. Lowry OH and JV Passonneau: A Flexible System of Enzymatic Analysis. Academic Press, New York, (1972).
22. Lust WD, GK Feussner, EK Barbehenn, and JV Passonneau: The enzymatic measurement of adenine nucleotides and P-creatine in picomole amounts. *Anal Biochem* **110**:258–266 (1981).
23. Xu F, M Sato, MJJ Spellman, RA Mitchell, and JW Severinghaus: Topography of cat medullary ventral surface hypoxic acidification. *J Appl Physiol* **73**:2631–2637 (1992).

5

EFFECT OF ANESTHESIA ON CEREBRAL TISSUE OXYGEN AND CARDIOPULMONARY PARAMETERS IN RATS

Ke Jian Liu,[1] P. Jack Hoopes,[2] Ellis L. Rolett,[2] Brion J. Beerle,[3] A. Azzawi,[1] Fuminori Goda,[1] Jeff F. Dunn,[1] and Harold M. Swartz[1]

[1]Departments of Radiology
[2]Medicine
[3]Anesthesiology
Dartmouth Medical School
Hanover, New Hampshire 03755

1. INTRODUCTION

General anesthesia is known to alter cardiopulmonary and hematological parameters which affect tissue oxygenation. However, the effect of various types of anesthetics on the relationship between brain tissue pO_2 and these physiologic parameters is still largely unknown.

Electron paramagnetic resonance (EPR) oximetry is a technique which measures pO_2 levels in tissues noninvasively through the interaction of molecular oxygen with some paramagnetic materials, including measurements of oxygen *in vivo* in conscious animals [1]. This has been possible because of the development of low frequency EPR instruments (1 GHz or lower) suitable for use in viable tissue [2,3] and the development of new stable paramagnetic particles (fusinite, India ink, lithium phthalocyanine) with oxygen sensitive EPR spectra [4,5,6]. These particles combine several desirable properties as probes of the pO_2 including high sensitivity to the pO_2, resistance to chemical reactions, and a high degree of inertness in biological systems. After the implantation of the paramagnetic materials the technique can be entirely non-invasive and the measurements can be done without anesthesia. This makes it possible to study the effect of anesthesia on tissue pO_2. Another advantage of the technique is that the exact location of the paramagnetic particles in tissues can be determined by magnetic resonance imaging (MRI) [7,8], therefore providing precise spatial information on where the pO_2 is being measured.

In this report, we describe our preliminary results on the effect of injectable and inhalation anesthetics on cerebral pO_2 and cardiopulmonary parameters. The aims of this study are to determine the relationship of brain tissue pO_2 and arterial pO_2 in rats receiving four commonly used anesthetics with different effects on cardiopulmonary parameters

Oxygen Transport to Tissue XVIII, edited by Nemoto and LaManna
Plenum Press, New York, 1997

and cerebral oxygenation. These data should lead to a better understanding of the physiology associated with changes of cerebral pO_2 due to anesthesia.

2. MATERIALS AND METHODS

2.1. Material

Lithium phthalocyanine crystals were obtained from Dr. M. Moussavi (LETI, Grenoble, France). Details concerning synthesis, characterization and calibration of LiPc for pO_2 measurements have been reported [4,9]. The line width of the EPR signal is a linear function of pO_2 (see Figure 2), and is independent of the type of tissue being measured, local metabolic processes, the presence of other paramagnetic species, or pH. The high density of unpaired spins combined with a narrow intrinsic line width of LiPc allows measurements of pO_2 in the brain using one or more crystals with a diameter of ~ 200 μm.

2.2. Animal Preparation

Male Wistar rats weighing 200–250 g were obtained from Charles River Laboratories (Wilmington, MA). Twenty-four hours prior to pO_2 measurements the animals were anesthetized with ketamine/xylazine (100/10 mg/kg, i.m.), and LiPc crystals were implanted in the cerebral cortex through a small hole (500 μm in diameter) in the cranium using specific land marks for consistent implantation (depth, 4 mm). The spatial localization of the crystals in the cerebral cortex was verified by MRI and by examination of a gross section of the brain [8].

2.3. Anesthesia

Four representative anesthetic agents were selected for this study. Two injectable anesthetics, pentobarbital (60 mg/kg, i.m.) and ketamine/xylazine (100/10 mg/kg i.m.), and two inhalation anesthetics, isoflurane (2%) and halothane (1.5%) were used. These doses/concentrations were chosen based on literature and personal experience in order to produce a consistent level of depth of anesthesia. The anesthetic level was determined by lack of movement and pain response. Animals were allowed to breathe spontaneously.

2.4. Electron Paramagnetic Resonance

The spectra of LiPc were obtained using an EPR spectrometer constructed in our laboratory with a low frequency (1.2 GHz, L-band) microwave bridge [2]. An extended loop resonator was positioned over the brain of the animal. Typical settings for the spectrometer were: incident microwave power, 10 mW; magnetic field center, 425 gauss; scan range, 1 gauss; modulation frequency, 27 kHz. Modulation amplitude was set at less than one-third of the EPR line width, typically around 20–50 mG. Scan time was 1 minute. Usually 5 scans were averaged to achieve better signal to noise ratio of the spectra. The total EPR scan time for any measurement was less than 10 minutes including positioning of the animal, adjustment of the spectrometer, and accumulation of 5 scans. The EPR line widths were converted to pO_2 using a calibration curve determined for each batch of LiPc crystals.

2.5. Assessment of Cerebral pO_2 with EPR

The EPR spectra of the oximetry probe LiPc were measured to obtain cerebral pO_2 values in both anesthetized and unanesthetized animals using a low frequency EPR spectrometer. Unanesthetized animals were restrained in a specially constructed device which held the animals in a comfortable but non-movable position. A total of 8 rats were studied. Cerebral pO_2 in each animal was measured before and during the administration of the four different anesthetic agents, during a period of 4–6 weeks. There was at least a one-week interval between each treatment to assure that the previous anesthetic was metabolized completely. Rats were divided into two groups of 4 each, and the anesthetic agents were delivered in a different sequence for each group in order to minimize non-random effects.

2.6. Cardiopulmonary Assessments Techniques

Blood samples were obtained using a sterile cut-down procedure on the carotid artery. Arterial blood (0.3–0.4 ml) was drawn into a 1 cc dry heparin coated syringe and blood gases were assessed immediately on a standard clinical blood gas analyzer (Ciba-Corning 238 pH/Blood Gas Analyzer). Mean systemic blood pressure, heart and respiration rate, and ECG measurements were obtained using standard noninvasive techniques. Core body temperature was measured rectally with a thermister and body temperature was held constant at 37.5±0.5°C.

2.7. Statistical Analysis

ANOVA statistic methods were applied to the experimental data to test statistical significance. Values were considered statistically significant if the p-value was ^{2} 0.05.

3. RESULTS

The paramagnetic material LiPc was chosen for this study because of its high oxygen sensitivity and high spin density. LiPc crystals (size, ~ 200 μm) implanted in the cerebral cortex result in minimal tissue disturbance. Figure 1 demonstrates the EPR spectra of LiPc in air (21% oxygen, or 159 mmHg) and in nitrogen (0% oxygen). The line width of the EPR signal of LiPc is a linear function of pO_2 throughout the experimental region (Figure 2). Since LiPc responds to partial pressure of oxygen (pO_2) rather than concentration of oxygen ([O2]), LiPc can be used to measure cerebral pO_2 using the calibration curve in Figure 2 without having to obtain the information on the solubility of oxygen in the brain tissue [4].

Compared to the control rats (unanesthetized rats), all four anesthetics used in this study reduced the cerebral pO_2 to varying degrees. As expected, ketamine/xylazine and pentobarbital had the greatest depressant effect on pO_2 (almost 50%), while the gas anesthetics had the least effects (Figure 3).

Because of the design of the experiment, certain factors, such as long post-implantation latent periods, surgery associated with blood drawing, and previous use of other anesthetics, could potentially affect the following measurement in the same rat. Control pO_2 values were obtained in each animal in an unanesthetized state before and after the use of anesthetics (minimum of 72 hours following the anesthetic experiment). Figure 4 shows

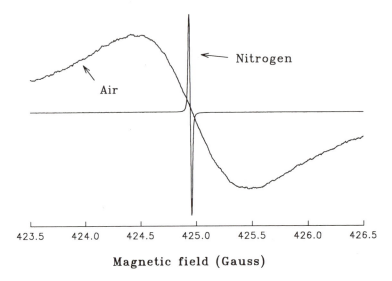

Figure 1. EPR spectra of LiPc in air and nitrogen. The line width of the spectrum is 15 mG and 1024 mG in air and nitrogen, respectively. The line width is defined as the difference in magnetic field between maximum and minimum of the EPR signal.

that cerebral pO_2 remains constant over the 30 day time span of the experiment, suggesting that LiPc retains its oxygen sensitivity over a relatively long time and that repeated anesthetic procedures in the same animal produce valid results if the animals are fully recovered from the previous anesthetic procedure. Figure 4 also shows that since cerebral pO_2 responded to anesthesia treatment, sensitivity of the response of the LiPc to oxygen is not changed, and LiPc is capable of reporting cerebral pO_2 accurately and correctly.

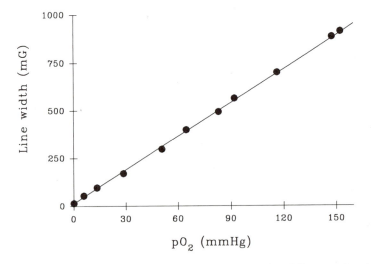

Figure 2. Calibration of the line width of the EPR spectra of LiPc to pO_2. Since LiPc responds to the partial pressure of oxygen (pO_2), this calibration curve is independent of the surrounding environment around the crystal, where oxygen solubility could be very different.

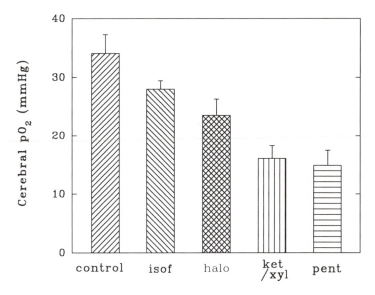

Figure 3. Effect of anesthesia on cerebral pO_2. Ketamine/xylazine mixture (100/10 mg/kg) and sodium pentobarbital (60 mg/kg) were injected into the rats intramuscularly. Isoflurane (2%) and halothane (1.5%) were delivered to the animal through a nose cone using room air (21% O2). The pO_2 values, expressed as mean ± SEM (n=8 animals), were taken 20 minutes after the start of anesthesia. All animals breathed room air spontaneously.

The effect of different anesthetics on the cardiopulmonary parameters is summarized in Table 1. Ketamine/xylazine differed from the other agents in terms of causing a higher blood pressure and lower heart rate. Ketamine/xylazine and pentobarbital depressed respiration (higher arterial pCO2 and lower arterial pO_2) to a greater extent than isoflurane and halothane.

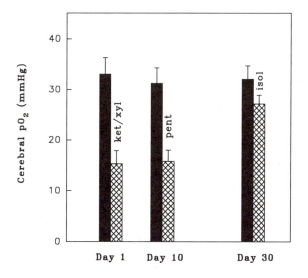

Figure 4. The relationship of cerebral pO_2 with time in the same animals using different anesthetics administered over a period of one month. Awake animals were measured in a restraining device.

Table 1. Effect of anesthetics on the cardiovascular parameters of rats (mean±SD; n=4)

	isoflurane	halothane	ket/xyl	pentobarbital
Blood pressure (mmHg)	68 ± 16[*]	65 ± 23[*]	119 ± 17	65 ± 21[*]
Heart rate (BPM)	321 ± 26[*]	332 ± 20[*]	244 ± 20	335 ± 31[*]
pCO_2 (mmHg)[†]	43.5 ± 3.5[*]	46.4 ± 4.4[*]	56.4 ± 2.7	50.8 ± 4.0
pO_2 (mmHg)[†]	87.1 ± 10.7[*]	80.6 ± 6.4	63.6 ± 4.1	69.8 ± 12.1
pHa[†]	7.44 ± 0.03[*#]	7.41± 0.02	7.35± 0.02	7.38 ± 0.03
O_2 sat (%)[†]	96.5 ± 1.2[*]	95.4 ± 1.2	90.5 ± 1.2	92.8 ± 4.9

[†]These are values for arterial blood, which were obtained 20 minutes after the start of the anesthesia.
[*]Significantly different from ketamine/xylazine ($p<0.05$).
[#]Significantly different from ketamine/xylazine and pentobarbital ($p<0.05$).

4. DISCUSSION

These results demonstrate that anesthetic agents altered the cerebral tissue pO_2 and arterial blood gas pO_2 in a reproducible manner which was dependent on the type of anesthetic and its route of administration. These changes in arterial blood pO_2 are most likely related to respiratory depression and alterations in metabolism [10]. All four anesthetics tested reduced the cerebral tissue pO_2 compared with similar measurement in unanesthetized animal, however the decrease was much larger for the injectable anesthetics (Figure 3).

Pentobarbital produced the greatest decrease in cerebral tissue compared to pO_2 values from unanesthetized animals. Pentobarbital anesthesia, administered intraperitoneally, resulted in the largest variations in pO_2 and cardiopulmonary parameters.

Compared to the unanesthetized state ketamine/xylazine resulted in a marked reduction in heart rate but maintained relatively normal blood pressure [11]. Tissue and blood pO_2 values for ketamine/xylazine anesthesia were similar to pentobarbital, but were significantly lower than with the gas anesthetics.

Inhalation anesthetics produced the most consistent anesthetic depth over time with the smallest deviation in cerebral tissue pO_2 values despite significant reductions in blood pressure [11]. Inhalation anesthetics yielded higher blood pO_2 and higher tissue pO_2 compared with injectable anesthestics, although the values were not significantly different between isoflurane and halothane anesthesia.

Cerebral tissue pO_2 values were, as expected, lower than blood pO_2 levels for all four anesthetics studied.

While the general trend was similar for all four anesthetics (i.e., lower cerebral pO_2 values were found with lower arterial pO_2 values), there was not a quantitative relationship between these two parameters. For example, pentobarbital anesthesia resulted in the lowest cerebral pO_2 levels but the blood pO_2 value was slightly higher than that of ketamine/xylazine. Therefore it appears that direct measurement of cerebral pO_2 will provide information that cannot be inferred quantitatively from arterial blood pO_2.

The relationships between cerebral pO_2 and blood pressure and heart rate were less regular than with blood pO_2. Except for ketamine/xylazine the values of the blood pressure and heart rate were the same for the various anesthetics. Ketamine/xylazine decreased the heart rate while maintaining normal blood pressure, but resulted in a cerebral pO_2 similar to that observed with pentobarbital.

We conclude that general anesthesia reduce both cerebral pO_2 and arterial blood pO_2 compared with unanesthetized animals. Inhalation anesthetics, despite their hypotension effects, are the preferred agents for optimizing cerebral tissue and blood pO_2 in spontaneously ventilating experiments requiring anesthesia. This study demonstrates the correlation between cerebral tissue and blood gas pO_2 levels during standard anesthetic procedures with common anesthetics. In general, tissue pO_2 values are less than blood pO_2 levels during controlled anesthesia and inhalation agents provide a significantly higher tissue and blood gas pO_2 than do injectable agents.

ACKNOWLEDGMENTS

This work was supported by NIH grant 34250, and used the facilities of the IERC at Dartmouth supported by NIH grant RR 01811.

REFERENCES

1. Swartz, H.M., and Walczak, T., *In vivo* EPR: prospects for the 90's, *Phys. Med.*, 9 (1993) 41–48.
2. Nilges, M.J., Walczak, T., and Swartz, H.M., 1 GHz *in vivo* ESR spectrometer operating with a surface probe, *Phys. Med.* 5 (1989) 195–201.
3. Colacicchi, S., Alecci, M., Gualtieri, G., Quaresima, V., Ursini, C.L., Ferrari, M., and Sotgiu, A., New experimental procedures for *in vivo* L-band and radio frequency EPR spectroscopy/imaging. *J. Chem. Soc. Perkin Trans.* 2 (1993) 2077–82.
4. Liu, K.J., Gast, P., Moussavi, M., Norby, S.W., Vahidi, N., Walczak, T., Wu, M., and Swartz, H.M., Lithium phthalocyanine: A probe for electron paramagnetic resonance oximetry in viable biological systems, *Proc. Natl. Acad. Sci. USA*, 90 (1993) 5438–5442.
5. Vahidi, N., Clarkson, R.B., Liu, K.J., Norby, S.W., Wu, M., and Swartz, H.M., *In vivo* and *in vitro* EPR oximetry with fusinite: a new coal-derived, particulate EPR probe, *Magn. Reson. Med.*, 31 (1994) 139–146.
6. Swartz, H.M., Liu, K.J., Goda, F., and Walczak, T., India ink: A potential clinically applicable EPR oximetry probe, *Magn. Reson. Med.*, 31 (1994) 229–232.
7. Bacic, G., Liu, K.J., O'Hara, J.A., Harris, R.D., Szybinski, K., Goda, F., and Swartz, H.M., Oxygen tension in a murine tumor: A combined EPR and MRI study, *Magn. Reson. Med.*, 30 (1993) 568–572.
8. Liu, K.J., Bacic, B., Hoopes, P.J., Jiang, J., Du, H., Ou, L.C., Dunn, J.F., Swartz, H.M., Assessment of cerebral pO_2 by EPR oximetry in rodents: effects of anesthesia, ischemia, and breathing gas. *Brain Res.*, 685 (1995) 91–98.
9. Turek, P., Andre, J.J., Giraudeau, A., and Simon, J., Preparation and study of a lithium phthalocyanine radical: optical and magnetic properties, *Chem. Phys. Lett.* 134 (1986) 471–476.
10. Pavlin, E.G., and Hornbein, T.F., Anesthesia and the control of ventilation. In: Handbook of physiology, Section 3, Vol II, Control of breathing , Part 1. Chapter 25, pp. 793–813.
11. Baker, H.J., Lindsey, J.R., and Weisbroth. The Laboratory Rat, Vol 1, Appendix 1. pp411–412. 1979 (Academic Press).

6

THE FUNCTIONING GERBIL BRAIN *IN VIVO*

Correlation between ^{31}P NMR Spectroscopy and the Multiparametric Monitoring Approach

A. Mayevsky,[1] S. Nioka,[2] D. J. Wang,[2] and B. Chance[2]

[1]Department of Life Sciences
Bar-Ilan University
Ramat Gan 52900, Israel
[2]Department of Biochemistry and Biophysics
Medical School
University of Pennsylvania
Philadelphia, Pennsylvania 19104–6089

1. INTRODUCTION

The normal brain consumes about 20% of the total body O_2 uptake although it weighs only
1–2% of the total body weight. One of the main reasons for this high oxygen consumption is the need for maintaining continuous ionic homeostasis. Ionic homeostasis is achieved by the active pumping of ions and is dependent upon ATP availability (Ericinska and Silver, 1989). These ionic activities are responsible for more than 50% of the total brain energy consumption and they are inhibited under conditions of restricted oxygen supply, such as ischemia. For this reason the interrelation between CBF (oxygen supply), mitochondrial activity, energy stores and physiological functions such as ion homeostasis and electrical activity under ischemia and reperfusion is a key factor in understanding the pathogenesis and treatment of stroke.

Various approaches have been used for studying the effects of ischemia on various parameters in the gerbil brain (Breuer and Mayevsky, 1992, for review see Mayevsky and Breuer, 1990). Several studies have used the Mongolian gerbil as a model for ischemia due to the incompleteness of its circle of Willis (Levine and Payan, 1966; Mayevsky and Breuer, 1990). Magnetic resonance spectroscopy (MRS) of ^{31}P has been used as a noninvasive tool for continuous monitoring of brain energetics under various conditions (Younkin et al., 1984; Mayevsky et al., 1988; Hilberman et al., 1984).

We developed a new multiprobe assembly, which can be used inside the magnet, such that the hemodynamic, metabolic, electrical and ionic activities could be monitored continuously and simultaneously with ^{31}P-MRS. Relative CBF was measured by a Laser Doppler flowmeter using a fiber optic probe (Wadhwani and Rapoport, 1990). Mitochondrial activity was evaluated by monitoring the NADH redox state using surface fluorometry (Chance et al., 1962; Mayevsky and Chance, 1982; Mayevsky, 1984). Ionic homeostasis was evaluated by the extracellular levels of K^+ and Ca^{2+} measured by surface ion-selective minielectrodes (Crowe et al., 1977; Yoles et al., 1991). The electrical activities were assessed by the DC steady potential as well as by the electrocorticogram (ECoG).

This study was carried out in order to determine whether it is possible to measure, simultaneously and in real time, parameters that are measurable by the multiprobe assembly with parameters that are measurable using NMR spectroscopy so as to more precisely determine injury during pathological interventions or conditions.

2. METHODS

2.1. NADH Surface Fluorometry

The intramitochondrial NADH redox state was monitored by using a Y-shaped light guide (made of optical fibers) connected to a DC fluorometer/reflectometer (Mayevsky and Chance, 1982; Mayevsky, 1984). This technique is based upon the fact that NADH when illuminated by 366 nm light may fluorescence, and blue 450 nm light (410–480 nm) is emitted. The source for the 366 nm light was a 100 watt air-cooled mercury arc lamp. The light passed through the excitation bundle of the light guide towards the brain. The emitted light, transmitted through the other bundle of the light guide, was split in a 90:10 ratio and transmitted to photomultipliers for the measurement of NADH fluorescence (450 nm) and reflectance
(366 nm), respectively. A standard signal (0.5 V), used to calibrate the system, was set to give a half scale deflection on the recorder. The calibration of the fluorescence and reflectance signals was accomplished under normoxic conditions and the changes in these signals were calculated relative to the calibrated signals. This type of calibration is not absolute, but provides reliable and reproducible results from various laboratory animals (Mayevsky, 1984). In order to correct the fluorescence signal for changes in tissue hemodynamics and in absorbance properties, we used a correction technique suggested by several groups, which has been discussed previously in detail (Jobsis et al., 1971; Harbig et al., 1976; Mayevsky and Chance, 1982). The reflectance signal was subtracted from the fluorescence signal at a 1:1 ratio as described previously (Mayevsky, 1984).

2.2. Laser Doppler Flowmetry

In order to obtain real-time measurements of the CBF and the MPA from the same cortical area, we used the Laser Doppler flow meter (LDF) technique (Stern et al., 1977; Habert et al., 1989; Dirnagl et al., 1989). During the past few years this technique has been calibrated against the H_2 clearance probe or against (^{14}C) iodoantipyrine autoradiography which are both well established methods for quantitative monitoring of CBF. The LDF apparently measures relative changes demonstrating a significant correlation to the relative changes in the CBF measured by the two other quantitative approaches (for review, see Wadhwani and Rapoport, 1990).

The principle of the Laser Doppler flowmetry is to utilize the Doppler shift, namely, the frequency change that light undergoes when reflected by moving red blood cells. A beam of low power laser or diode laser light is transmitted by an optical fiber to the tissue. After the multiple scattering of the light, another optical fiber will pick up the reflected light and put it into the photodetector. The run signal is analyzed by a complicated algorithm developed by each of the manufacturers and the results are presented as percent of a full scale (0–100%) providing relative flow values. The change in the total back-scattered light is an indirect indicator for the blood volume in the tested tissue volume. In the present study, we have used the LDF made by TSI Inc., USA (for details, see Borgos, 1990).

2.3. Multiprobe Assembly (MPA)

The K$^+$ and Ca^{2+} electrodes (WPI Inc., USA), DC electrodes, ECoG electrodes as well as the light guide were held in a multiprobe assembly as described previously in detail (Friedli et al., 1982; Mayevsky, 1983; Mayevsky, 1993). The probes were mounted in a lucite holder (cannula) which can be cemented directly to the skull (Fig. 1) and can be

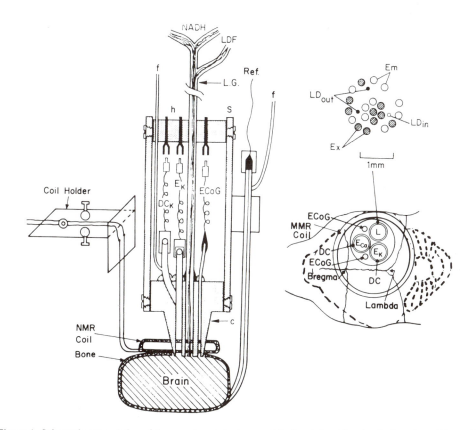

Figure 1. Schematic presentation of the experimental set up used in the study. A longitudinal section of the multiprobe assembly connected to the NMR coil and the gerbil brain is shown on the left side. The relative locations of the various probes on the brain are shown on the right side. ECoG - Electrocorticographic electrodes. E$_k$, E$_{ca}$, DC$_k$ - potassium, calcium and DC electrode. c - plexiglass multiprobe holder. h - connection holder. s - plexiglass sleeve. Ref - reference electrode. f - feeling tube of DC or reference electrode. L.G. - light guide Ex, Em - excitation and emission fibers for NADH monitoring. LDin LDout - fibers for CBF monitoring by Laser Doppler flowmeter.

removed very easily from the skull at the end of the experiment without any damage, so that the same electrodes can be used for performing repetitive experiments within a short period of time.

2.4. ^{31}P MRS Data Acquisition

An Otsuka Electronics (USA), Inc. magnetic resonance spectrometer was used with a 2.1 Tesla superconducting 30 cm bore Oxford magnet. A 35.8 MHz radio frequency pulse with a 20–30 µsec pulse width was transmitted through a 2.5 cm two-turn double tuned copper surface coil placed directly on the skull to give approximately a 90° flip angle. This pulse was preceded by a long, low power pulse to saturate a very broad bone peak (Cerdan et al., 1986). Each free induction decay (FID) was collected for 80 msec. The pulse interval was 4 sec, so that data were accumulated at a rate of 15 FID per min with a total of 60 FID for each 4 min data collection period. For the final analysis a 10 Hz line broadening was applied and baseline correction was achieved by a 600 Hz convolution difference. These manipulations gave a flat baseline and a signal to noise level of 6 at the β-ATP peak. The data were Fourier transformed, phased and fitted (Fig. 2). Details of this method have been published previously (Nioka et al., 1990). Quantitation of the metabolite values was determined from the areas of the peak obtained by MRS as described previously (Nioka et al., 1991).

2.5. Animal Preparation

The gerbils were anesthetized by an IP injection (0.3 ml/100 gr) of Equithesin (each ml contained 9.72 mg pentobarbital, 42.51 mg chloral hydrate, 21.25 mg magnesium sulfate, 44.34% w/v propylene glycol, 11.5% alcohol and water). Equithesin was also given 1 hour after the initial dose in 30 min intervals (0.1 ml/100gr). The animals were placed in a head holder and the skin was removed above the dorsal area of the skull. A 6 mm hole was drilled in the parietal bone arc to accommodate the lower part of the MPA's cannula. The dura mater was removed gently and the MPA was placed on the brain using a micromanipulator attached to the operating table. During this procedure, the two-turn copper surface coil (15 mm diameter) was located on the exposed skull (Fig. 1). The MPA and the coil were cemented to the skull by dental acrylic held with 4 plastic screws inserted into the skull. The two common carotid arteries were isolated and 4–0 silk sutures were placed around them for later occlusion. Body temperature was maintained by wrapping the gerbil in a water heating mantle. The animal was released from the head holder and transferred into the center of the 2.1 Tesla magnet together with the cemented MPA and MRS coil.

All the parameters were monitored via the long fibers and wires connected to the measuring devices located out of the range of the magnetic field. The various parameters were recorded on a Grass multichannel pen recorder.

3. RESULTS

Each of the gerbils used in the present study was exposed to a short term (5 min) as well as long term (20 min) bilateral carotid artery occlusion (complete ischemia). At least 60 minutes were allowed for recovery or until the ECoG showed a completely recovered

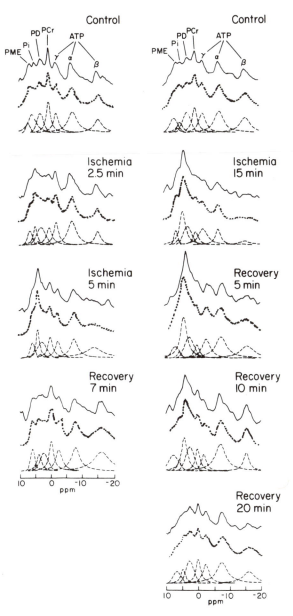

Figure 2. ^{31}P MRS spectra and Fourier transformations of two gerbils exposed to 5 or 15 min of ischemia. Raw (top trace), fitted (middle trace) and component (bottom trace curves are shown). Peak identifications shown from right to left are three ATP resonance peaks, PCr phosphodiester (PDE), Pi, and phosphomonoester (PME). The abscissa is frequency in ppm referenced to the PCr resonance at 0 ppm and the ordinate is relative intensity.

pattern. Fig. 3 presents typical MPA measurements following 5 minute of ischemia (induced by bilateral carotid artery occlusion).

It can be seen that the occlusion of both arteries led to severe ischemia as indicated by the decrease in CBF (LDF) and the increase in the NADH redox state (CF). Two minutes after inducing ischemia an ischemic depolarization (ID) event was recorded in the

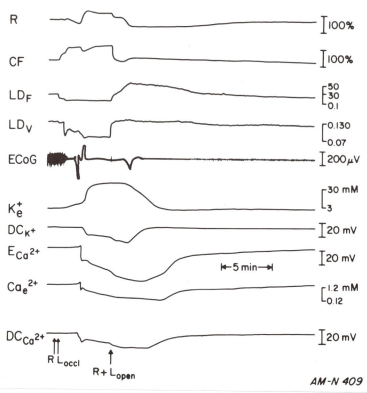

Figure 3. Effect of bilateral carotid artery occlusion (R, Loccl) on hemodynamic, metabolic, ionic and electrical activities in the gerbil brain. R, CF - 366 nm reflectance and 450 nm corrected NADH fluorescence. LDF, LDV - cerebral blood flow and volume measured by the Laser Doppler flowmeter. ECoG - electrocortigram. K^+e, $Ca^{2+}e$, DC K^+, DC Ca^{2+} - extracellular levels of potassium, calcium and DC potential around each of the electrodes. ECa^{2+} - electrical potential measured by the calcium electrode.

various parameters monitored. A massive decrease in blood volume was recorded by the Laser Doppler flowmeter (LDV) as well as by a large increase recorded in the reflectance trace (R) indicating a decrease in the amount of blood in the area being measured by the probe. Extracellular K^+ levels exhibited two increase steps during the ischemic episode. Initial leakage began simultaneously with the occlusion and a steep slope appeared during the ID event, characterized by a negative shift in the DC potential and a decrease in extracellular calcium. The ECoG became isoelectric immediately after the occlusion, recovering gradually after reperfusion.

Upon the reopening of the carotid arteries, the energy state and blood volume exhibited a rapid return to their preischemic levels. The CBF exhibited a hyperemic response during the initial 5–8 minutes of recovery. The effects of 5 minutes ischemia on the MRS spectra in two gerbils are shown in Fig. 2. The changes in the PCr and ATP peaks during ischemia as well as the recovery are very clear.

In order to compare the data accumulated by the MPA and the MRS, quantitative analysis of all measured parameters was performed at 5 minute intervals. Fig. 4 shows typical effects of 20 minute bilateral carotid artery occlusion on the various parameters as calculated. Part A exhibits the hemodynamic changes occurring in the three major parameters, i.e., CBF, CBV (volume) and NADH redox state. After 4 control points (total 15

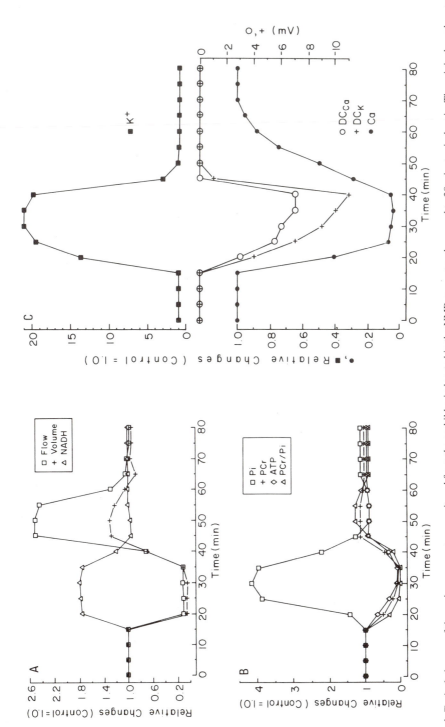

Figure 4. Typical changes of the various parameters monitored from the gerbil brain located in the NMR magnet and exposed to 20 minutes ischemia. The original numbers measured were normalized in order to present a few of them on the same ordinate scale. Only the DC potential is presented in absolute units (mv). a: cerebral blood flow and volume, NaDH redox state; b: Pi, PCr, ATP PCr/Pi; C: K^+, DCa^{2+}, DCK^+, Ca^{2+}.

minutes) ischemia was induced and CBF as well as CBV decreased to the minimal levels within 5 minutes. Concomitantly, the intramitochondrial NADH redox state reached maximal levels. The low CBF and high NADH remained unchanged until the reopening of the two carotid arteries. NADH returned to its preischemic levels within 10 minutes, while CBF showed a large hyperemic response during the recovery phase. The CBV showed a small overshoot response.

The energy state of the gerbil brain during the ischemia is shown in Fig. 4B. PCr and ATP levels decreased gradually during the ischemic episode and reached minimal levels 15 minutes after the occlusion. Ten minutes elapsed following reopening of the vessels, before the high energy compounds returned to their preischemic levels.

The typical disturbances in ionic homeostasis caused by the ischemic event are shown in Fig. 4C. The major changes in extracellular K^+ and Ca^{2+} occurred during the first 10 minutes of ischemia followed by small changes during the remaining 10 minutes. In this specific gerbil, recovery of the two ions did not exhibit identical kinetics. Most of the K^+ recovered within 10 minutes (after a slow initial phase) while the recovery of Ca^{2+} was much slower and was complete only after 30 minutes. The DC steady potential demonstrated a negative shift when measured concentric to the K^+ and Ca^{2+} electrodes. Return of the DC potential to baseline levels occurred after 5–10 minutes of reperfusion whereas during the initial 5 minutes changes were minimal.

A total of 9 gerbils were used. However, not all the results were adequate for statistical evaluation. In some of the experiments, only part of the results were recorded due to technical difficulties. All gerbils demonstrated similar qualitative responses to ischemia. The effect of ischemia and 2 steps of recovery on the various parameters measured during 4 ischemic episodes of 20 min ischemia each was examined by analysis of variance. The results are presented in Table 1. It can be seen that during ischemia, the levels of all parameters were significantly different from the control values.

The initial recovery period was divided into two stages according to the rate of K^+ recovery. During the first phase of recovery (the first 5 min), the energy levels as well as the CBF demonstrated a partial return to their preischemic levels. CBF and high energy phosphate compounds did recover to the preischemic level. CBF at this phase exhibited a hyperemic state as shown also in Fig. 4B. K^+ and Ca^{2+} at the second recovery phase did not yet reach their preischemic levels and a longer period of time was necessary for regaining normal ionic homeostasis.

In order to test the homogeneity of the responses at various brain locations under the MPA, the DC steady potential changes (negative shift during ischemia) measured in the areas of the K^+ and Ca^{2+} electrodes were compared. Figure 5 demonstrates a significant correlation between the 2 DC measurements, suggesting similar responses at the two measuring sites.

The interrelation between the hemodynamic, metabolic and ionic homeostasis was evaluated by correlation analyses. The effect of flow on the PCr/Pi or the extracellular K^+ levels demonstrated a threshold-like connection although linear regression demonstrated a significant correlation (Fig. 6A and 6B). A more distinct correlation was calculated between the direct measure of energy availability (PCr/Pi) and the extracellular K^+ representing ionic homeostasis (Fig. 6C).

During the ID event, an uncorrectable artifact was introduced to the NADH signal. Therefore, the NADH results from the various gerbils was not included in the quantitative

Table 1. Relative blood flow, ions and phosphagens concentration in normal, ischemic and recovery conditions

	Flow	K (mM)	Ca (mM)	[Pi]	[PCr]	[ATP]	PCr/Pi
Normal	2.7 ± 2.0	2.7 ± 0.5	1.07 ± 0.15	2.1 ± 0.5	2.9 ± 0.3	2.4 ± 0.1	1.6 ± 0.4
Ischemia	0.0 ± 0.0*	62.0 ± 5.3*	0.11 ± 0.07*	9.1 ± 1.4*	0.4 ± 0.3*	0.5 ± 0.3*	0.1 ± 0.0*
Recovery 1	1.5 ± 1.3	58.0 ± 5.2*	0.10 ± 0.05*	6.0 ± 0.6*	1.2 ± 0.9[6]	1.2 ± 0.8*	0.5 ± 0.3*
Recovery 2	3.5 ± 1.5[6]	25.8 ± 14.7[7,6]	0.30 ± 0.20*	2.7 ± 1.2[7,6]	3.1 ± 0.8[7]	2.2 ± 0.4[7,6]	1.4 ± 0.8[7,6]

Recovery 1: potassium recovery begins

Recovery 2: potassium recovers at maximum rate

Analysis of variance test: different from normal *P 0.05

different from ischemia [6]P 0.05

Recovery 2 is different from Recovery 1 [7]P 0.05

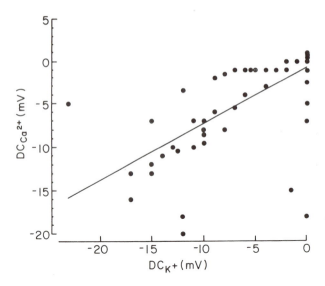

Figure 5. The correlation between the DC potential measured by the two electrodes located concentric to the K[+] and Ca electrodes. The baseline values in all four gerbils used were set to 0.

analysis. In principle, ischemia led to a quick maximal increase in NADH (as shown in Fig. 3 and 4A) followed by a fast recovery within 5–10 minutes after the reperfusion.

4. DISCUSSION

^{31}P-MRS is the sole available tool for noninvasive direct *in vivo* monitoring of the human brain's energy state. Several investigators have applied this technique to various experimental and clinical situations. For example, Thurlborn et al. (1982) have used this method for discovering a correlation between the ^{31}P NMR spectra and edema one hour following carotid ligation in the Mongolian gerbil while Wyatt et al. (1989) and Azzopardi et al. (1989) used this method for the assessment of perinatal hypoxic-ischemic brain injury. Reviews on the uses of this method have been published by Shulman et al. (1993) and Prichard and Rosen (1994).

However, in order to enable the complete interpretation of data measured by the ^{31}P-MRS, correlation of these data with other physiological and biochemical parameters must be possible (Mayevsky et al., 1988; Wyatt et al. 1989; Chance, 1993). One such attempt has been made by Gyulai et al. (1988) who correlated ^{31}P-NMR and NADH fluorometry measurements in the *in vivo* gerbil brain. Mayevsky et al. (1988) studied this correlation in newborn puppies. Since more than 50% of the energy produced in the brain is used by various active transport mechanisms (such as Na^+-K^+-ATPase) it is important to be able to correlate all these activities in the same animal model.

For this study we adopted the gerbil brain, which is a convenient model for inducing cerebral ischemia, while monitoring MPA and NMR signals in real-time. We have also reported the successful use of a multiprobe assembly for measuring various physiological and metabolic parameter in the *in vivo* brain in the gerbil (Mayevsky et al., 1990a), the rat (Mayevsky et al., 1990b) as well as intraoperatively in patients (Mayevsky et al., 1991).

The special developed MPA for NMR studies enabled the correlation of hemody-namic (CBF), metabolic (NADH), ionic (K$^+$, Ca^{2+}) and electrical (ECoG, DC potential) activities with the ^{31}P-NMR parameters (PCr/Pi, ATP, Pi). The combination of the various probes and the NMR coil enabled the overlapping of data points such that the kinetics of the ischemic process as well as the recovery could be investigated.

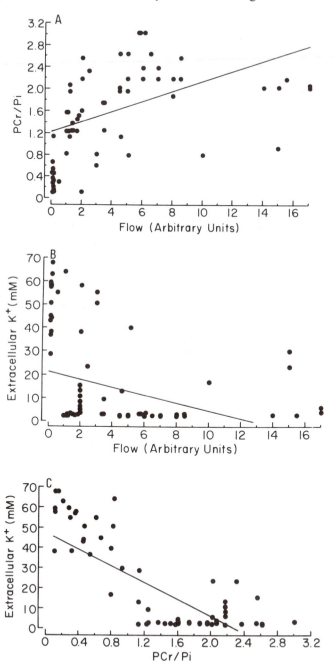

Figure 6. Correlation between CBF, PCr/Pi and extracellular K$^+$ measured in 4 gerbils exposed to ischemia in the NMR magnet. a: CBF vs OCr/Pi; b: CBF vs extracellular K$^+$; c: PCr/Pi vs extracellular K$^+$.

In the present study it was possible to monitor the extracellular K^+ and Ca^{2+} inside the magnet for the first time. This enabled the correlation between the energy state of the brain (PCr/Pi) and the active pumping of ions during ischemia and after reperfusion. Under bilateral carotid occlusion, the CBF parameter showed that the brain reached a state of complete ischemia. This was corroborated by the maximal level of intramitochondrial NADH indicating very low tissue oxygen levels. In the present study, the number of parameters correlated with ^{31}P-NMR values was greater than in previously reported studies (Gyulai et al., 1988; Mayevsky et al., 1988). Figure 4A,B and C demonstrate a clear correlation between the ^{31}P-NMR values and the multiparametric values. During the 20 minutes of ischemia, the brain was depleted of energy and the ionic homeostasis was completely disturbed. It was found that the kinetics of the changes in CBF and NADH were very fast while the kinetics of changes in K^+ and Ca^{2+} were slower and were recorded after the appearance of the ischemic depolarization (Fig. 3). The decrease in energy reserves was slower and reached minimal levels 15–20 minutes after the occlusion of the two carotid arteries.

The initial 5 minutes of recovery led to return to almost normal values of CBF and NADH. At this point, recovery of the energy stores was less than 50%, suggesting that pumping activity of ions was also slow. The main recovery processes took place 5–10 min after reperfusion as seen by the levels of K^+. The recovery of Ca^{2+} was even slower than the K^+. This sequence of changes shows the direct coupling between CBF and mitochondrial oxidative phosphorylation, leading to the recovery of PCr and ATP, and the ability of the brain to recover and restore its ion homeostasis.

The results presented in this study demonstrate that it is possible to compare the numerous parameters measured simultaneously by the multiprobe assembly (MPA) and the measurement of energy stores (PCr/Pi, ATP) as measured by the NMR technique during bilateral carotid occlusion in the gerbil. However, since the energy state and the ionic homeostasis of the brain are of utmost importance in preserving the physiological function of the brain (and therefore of the entire body) this dual technique could be used for the assessment of the state of the brain under various physiological and pathological conditions for a better understanding and perhaps also for the better treatment of pathological conditions of the brain.

5. REFERENCES

Azzopardi D, Wyatt JS, Cady B, Delpy DT, Baudin J, Stewart AL, Hope PL, Hamilton PA, Reynolds EOR. (1989) Prognosis of newborn infants with hypoxic-ischemic brain injury assessed by phosphorous magnetic resonance spectroscopy. *Pediat Res* 25:445–451

Borgos JA. (1990) TSI's LDV blood flowmeter. In: *Laser Doppler Blood Flowmetry* (Shepherd AP, Oberg PA, eds), Kluwer Academic Pub., Boston, pp 73–92

Breuer Z, Mayevsky A. (1992) Brain vasculature and mitochondrial responses to ischemia in Gerbils: II. Strain differences and statistical evaluation. *Brain Res* 598:251–256

Cerdan S, Harihara Subramanian V, Hilberman M, Cone J, Egan J, Chance B, Williamson JR. (1986) ^{31}P NMR detection of mobile dog brain phospholipids. *Mag Reson Med* 3: 432–439,.

Chance B, Cohen P, Jobsis F, Schoener B. (1962) Intracellular oxidation-reduction states *in vivo*. *Science* 137:499–508

Chance B. (1993) NMR and time-resolved optical studies of brain imaging, optical imaging of brain function and metabolism. U. Dirnagl et al. (Eds.), Plenum Press, New York.

Crowe W, Mayevsky A, Mela L. (1977) Application of a solid membrane ion selective electrode to *in vivo* measurements. *Am J Physiol* 233:C56-C60

Dirnagl U, Kaplan B, Jacewicz M, Pulsinelli W. (1989) Continuous measurement of cerebral cortical blood flow by Laser Doppler Flowmetry with a rat stroke model. *J Cereb Blood Flow Metab* 9:589–596

Erecinska M, Silver IA. (1989) ATP and brain function. *J Cereb Blood Flow Metab* 9:2–19

Friedli CM, Sclarsky DS, Mayevsky A. (1982) Multiprobe monitoring of ionic, metabolic and electrical activities in the awake brain. Am J Physiol 243:R462-R469

Gyulai L, Chance B, Ligeti L, McDonald G, Cone J. (1988) Correlated in vivo 31P-NMR and NADH fluorometric studies on gerbil brain in graded hypoxia and hyperoxia. *Am J Physiol* 254:C699-C708

Haberl RL, Heizer ML, Marmarou A, Ellis EF. (1989) Laser Doppler assessment of brain microcirculation: Effect of systemic alterations. *Am J Physiol* 256:H1247-H1254

Harbig K, Chance B, Kovach AGB, Reivich M. (1976) *In vivo* measurement of pyridine nucleotide fluorescence from cat brain cortex. *J Appl Physiol* 41:480–488

Hilberman M, Subramanian VH, Haselgrove J, Cone J, Egan JW, Gyulai L, Chance B. (1984) *In vivo* time-re-solved brain phosphorous nuclear magnetic resonance. *J Cereb Blood Flow Metab* 4:334–342

Jobsis FF, O'Conner MJ, Rosenthal M, VanBuren JM. (1971) Fluorometric monitoring of metabolic activity in the intact cerebral cortex. In: *Neurophysiology studied in man* Excerpta Medica, pp 18–26: 253

Levine S, Payan H. (1966) Effects of ischemia and other procedures on the brain and retina of the Gerbil (*Merio-nes unguiculatus*). *Exp Neurol* 16:255–262

Mayevsky A, Breuer Z. (1990) The Mongolian gerbil as a model for cerebral ischemia. In: *Cerebral Ischemia and Cerebral Resuscitation* (Schurr A, Rigor BM, eds), CRC Press, pp 27–46.

Mayevsky A, Chance B. (1982) Intracellular oxidation reduction state measured *in situ* by a multichannel fiber-op-tic-surface fluorometer. *Science* 217:537–540

Mayevsky A, Duckrow RB, Yoles E, Zarchin N, Kanshansky D. (1990b) Brain mitochondrial redox state, tissue hemodynamic and extracellular ion responses to four-vessel occlusion and spreading depression in the rat. *Neurological Res* 12:243–248

Mayevsky A, Flamm ES, Pennie W, Chance B. (1991) A fiber optic based multiprobe system for intraoperative monitoring of brain functions. *SPIE Proc* 1431:303–313

Mayevsky A, Subramanian VH, Chance B. (1988) Brain oxidative metabolism of the newborn dog: Correlation between ^{31}P NMR spectroscopy and pyridine nucleotides redox state. *J Cereb Blood Flow Metab* 8:201–207

Mayevsky A, Yoles E, Zarchin N, Kaushansky D. (1990a) Brain vascular ionic and metabolic responses to is-chemia in the Mongolian gerbil. *J Basic & Clinical Physiol & Pharmacol* 1:207–220

Mayevsky A. (1983) Multiparameter monitoring of the awake brain under hyperbaric oxygenation. *J Appl Physiol* 54:740–748

Mayevsky A. (1984) Brain NADH redox state monitored *in vivo* by fiber optic surface fluorometry. *Brain Res Rev* 7:49–68

Mayevsky A. (1993) Biochemical and physiological activities of the brain as *in vivo* markers of brain pathology. In: *Cerebral, Revascularization* (Bernstein EF, Callow AD, et al, eds), Med-Orion Pub. pp 51–69

Nioka S, Chance B, Smith DS, Mayevsky A, Reilly MP, Alter C, Asakura T. (1990) Cerebral energy metabolism and oxygen state during hypoxia in neonate and adult dogs. *Pediat Res* 28:54–62

Nioka S, Smith DS, Mayevsky A, Dobson G, Veech RL, Subramanian H, Chance B. (1991) Age dependence steady state mitochondrial oxidative metabolism during brain hypoxia in dogs. *Neurological Res* 13:25–32

Prichard J.W. and Rosen B.R. (1994) Functional study of the brain by NMR. *J Cereb Blood Flow and Metabol* 14: 365–372

Shulman R.G., Blamire A.M., Rothman D.L. and McCarthy G. (1993) Nuclear magnetic resonance imaging and spectroscopy of human brain function. *Proc. Natl. Acad. Sci.* 90:3127–3133

Stern MD, Lappe DL, Bowen PD, Chimosky JE, Holoway GA, Keiser HR. (1977) Continuous measurement of tissue blood flow by Laser Doppler spectroscopy. *Am J Physiol* 232:H441-H448

Thulborn KR, Du Bouley GH, Duchen LW, Radda G. (1982) A ^{31}P nuclear magnetic resonance *in vivo* study of cerebral ischemia in the gerbil. *J Cereb Blood Flow Metab* 2:299–306

Wadhwani KC, Rapoport SI. (1990) Blood flow in the central and peripheral nervous systems. In: *Laser-Doppler Blood Flowmetry* (Shephard AP, Oberg PA, eds), Kluwer Academic Pub. pp 265–304

Wyatt JS, Edwards AD, Azzopardi D, Reynolds EOR. (1989) Magnetic resonance and near infrared spectroscopy for investigation of perinatal hypoxic-ischemic brain injury. *Arch Dis. in Childhood* 64: 953–963

Yoles E, Zarchin N, Mayevsky A. (1991) Effects of age on brain metabolic ionic and electrical responses to anoxia in the newborn dog *in vivo*. *J Basic & Clinical Physiol & Pharmacol* 2:297–313

Younkin DP, Delivoria-Papadopoulos M, Leonard CJ, Subramanian VH, Eleff S, Leigh JS, Chance B. (1984) Unique aspects of human newborn cerebral metabolism evaluated with phosphorus nuclear magnetic reso-nance spectroscopy. *Ann Neurol* 16:581–586

7

DETERMINATION OF THE PCO$_2$-DEPENDENT COMPONENT OF THE H$^+$ CONCENTRATION IN VENOUS AND ARTERIAL BLOOD PLASMA

Masaji Mochizuki

Geriatric Respiratory Research Center
Nishimaruyama Hospital
4–7–25 Maruyama Nishimachi, Chuo-Ku
Sapporo 064, Japan

ABSTRACT

In normal venous blood plasma, the regression line of [H$^+$] plotted against the PCO$_2$ was linear against the square root of PCO$_2$. Sequential measurements in venous and arterial blood of PCO$_2$ and [H$^+$] showed that the venous-arterial (V-A) difference in [H$^+$] was linearly related to the V-A difference in the square root of PCO$_2$, the regression line having the same slope as that of the venous [H$^+$] plotted against the square root of PCO$_2$. These findings suggested that the venous [H$^+$] on the regression line represents the PCO$_2$-dependent component, of [H$^+$], [H$^+$]*. The PCO$_2$-independent component, Δ[H$^+$], can then be given by subtracting [H$^+$]* from the measured [H$^+$]. The Δ[H$^+$] in venous blood agreed well with that in arterial blood with a correlation coefficient of 0.99, supporting the validity of the value of [H$^+$]*.

INTRODUCTION

The H$^+$ concentration, [H$^+$], in blood plasma is closely correlated with that of bicarbonate, [HCO$_3^-$], as given by the Henderson equation (1). The [HCO$_3^-$] is influenced not only by changes in PCO$_2$, but also by ionic shifts across the plasma boundary (2, 3). When the PCO$_2$, changes, [H$^+$] in the plasma changes approximately in parallel with [HCO$_3^-$], as shown by the CO$_2$ dissociation curve (4,5). However, when the change in [HCO$_3^-$] is caused by ionic shifts without a change in PCO$_2$, [H$^+$] changes inversely with [HCO$_3^-$] (1). Thus, when a change in [HCO$_3^-$] occurs in the absence of a change in PCO$_2$, the ratio (M) of [H$^+$] to [HCO$_3^-$] changes in accordance with an excess or a deficit of strong ions, fixed acids or bases in the plasma. This PCO$_2$-independent component remains almost unchanged despite changes in PCO$_2$, thus the M ratio also remains constant.

We found that in normal individuals, the value of M in venous blood was distributed within a narrow range around the mean. This suggested that the PCO_2-dependent component of $[H^+]$ was proportional to that of $[HCO_3^-]$. In addition, since the M ratio and the PCO_2-independent component were maintained at almost constant levels during transit of blood through the lung capillaries, the PCO_2-dependent component of $[H^+]$ could be determined from the relationship between the venous-arterial difference of $[H^+]$ and that of PCO_2. Furthermore, the PCO_2-independent component of $[H^+]$ and $[HCO_3^-]$ could be evaluated by subtracting the PCO_2- dependent H^+ and HCO_3^- components from the respective measured values.

METHODS

In the first series of experiments the pH, PCO_2, PO_2 and hemoglobin concentration, Hb, were measured in venous blood from 122 normal volunteers of both sexes, with M ratios between 1.33 and 1.73 x 10^{-6}. The blood was sampled from the medial arm vein at rest in normocapnia. The ages of the subjects ranged from 21 to 80 years with a mean of 60.4 ± 20.3 years. To demonstrate the influence of age upon the relationship between PCO_2 and $[H^+]$, the measured data were subdivided into two groups according to the age of the donors. In the young group (n = 47) the age range was from 21 to 57 years with a mean of 36.6 ± 11.1 years; in the elderly group (n = 75) the age range was from 62 to 80 years with a mean of 75.1 ± 4.5 years. The mean Hb concentration in the young group was 14.1 ± 1.5 g/100 ml; that in the elderly group was 11.9 ± 1.8 g/100 ml. In a second series, sequential measurements were made in venous and arterial blood samples (n = 79) from 48 patients of both sexes ranging in age from 69 to 94 years (mean age 82.8 ± 6.8 years). The arterial and venous blood samples from any one patient were obtained within about one minute of each other. Venous blood was sampled from the medial arm vein, and arterial blood from the femoral artery. A combined blood gas analyzer (Ciba Corning 188) was used to measure pH, PCO_2, PO_2 and Hb concentration, all the measurements were performed in duplicate.

The $[H^+]$ was obtained from pH, and the $[HCO_3^-]$ value was calculated from the PCO_2 and $[H^+]$, using the Henderson equation as given by

$$[HCO_3^-] = K' \bullet s \bullet PCO_2/[H^+]. \qquad (1)$$

The dissociation constant (K') in Eq. (1) was 7.943 x 10^{-7} eq/liter and s (CO_2 solubility), 3.08 x 10^{-5} eq/liter/mmHg. To obtain the M ratio $[H^+]$ was divided by $[HCO_3^-]$.

RESULTS

The M ratio plotted against PCO_2 in venous plasma is shown in Fig. 1. The measured ratios for the young group are shown by filled circles and those for the elderly group, by open circles. Since there was no significant difference in M ratio between the two groups, statistical analysis was done on the values as a whole (n = 122), without separation into two groups. The interrupted and dashed lines show respectively the mean and SD of the M ratio. The ratio was distributed in parallel with PCO_2 over the range of 32 to 58 mmHg. The mean value of M, M*, was (1.527 ± 0.075) x 10^{-6}. If, when M = M*, $[H^+]$ =

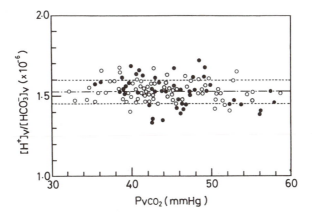

Figure 1. The distribution of the ratio, [H⁺]/[HCO₃⁻], plotted against PCO₂ in venous blood plasma from normal young (filled circles) and elderly (open circles) volunteers. The interrupted and dashed lines show, respectively, the mean and SD of the ratio.

[H⁺]* and [HCO₃⁻] = [HCO₃⁻]*, then setting M* into Eq. (1), gives the following values on the respective regression lines:

$$[H^+]^* = 6.112 \bullet \sqrt{PCO_2}, \text{ neg/liter,} \tag{2}$$

and

$$[HCO_3^-]^* = 4.003 \bullet \sqrt{PCO_2}, \text{ meq/liter.} \tag{3}$$

In Fig. 2, [H⁺] in venous plasma is plotted against the square root of PCO_2. The correlation coefficient was 0.925. The regression line shown by the interrupted line, was linear and numerically given by

$$[H^+]^* = 2.35 + 5.76 \bullet \sqrt{PCO_2}, \text{ neq/liter.} \tag{4}$$

In practice, Eq. (4) was fairly closely approximated by Eq. (2). The SD of the deviation of the measured [H⁺] values from the regression line was 1.00 neq/liter. The solid lines show the regression of [H⁺] in oxygenated and in deoxygenated blood equilibrated in a tonometer (5). In accordance with the Haldane effect (6), the [H⁺] in the oxygenated blood was about 3.6 neq higher than that in the deoxygenated blood; this indicates the lack of a Haldane effect in venous blood plasma. In addition, the slope of the regression lines of the tonometer blood was about 30% higher than that of venous blood, suggesting that a HCO₃⁻ shift normally occurs across the capillary wall in the peripheral tissue (7).

Figure 3 shows the relationship between venous ([H⁺]$_v$) and arterial (H⁺]$_a$) [H⁺]. The correlation coefficient between [H⁺]$_v$ and [H⁺]$_a$ was 0.785, and the regression line was given by

$$[H^+]_a = 9.6 + 0.67 \bullet [H^+]_v, \text{ neq/liter.} \tag{5}$$

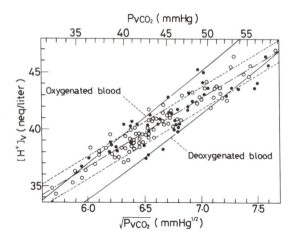

Figure 2. The distribution of [H$^+$] plotted against PCO$_2$ values obtained from the same young (filled circles) and elderly (open circles) volunteers as shown in Fig. 1. The interrupted line shows the regression line, and the dashed lines show the SD of the differences in individual [H$^+$] from the regression line. The solid lines show the regression lines of [H$^+$] obtained in the sampled blood oxygenated and deoxygenated in a tonometer.

In contrast to [H$^+$], the M ratios in venous and arterial blood were closely correlated, as shown in Fig. 4. The correlation coefficient between M$_v$ and M$_a$ was 0.989, and the regression line was given by

$$M_a = 1.01 \bullet M_v - 0.04 \times 10^{-6}. \tag{6}$$

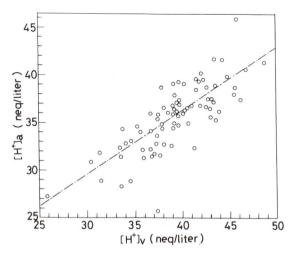

Figure 3. The relationship between [H$^+$] in venous (v) and arterial (a) blood samples (n = 79) taken sequentially from 48 elderly patients.

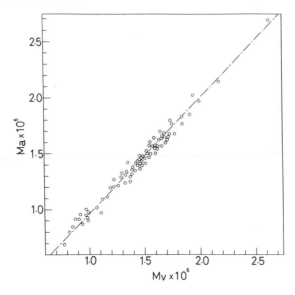

Figure 4. The $[H^+]/[HCO_3^-]$ ratio, (M) obtained in arterial blood (M_a) plotted against that in venous blood (M_v) from the same patients shown in Fig. 3.

The mean difference, ($M_v = M_a$), was $(0.027 \,''' \, 0.049) \times 10^{-6}$, suggesting that the PCO_2-independent components of $[H^+]$ and $[HCO_3^-]$ remained unchanged during the mixing process in the venous system and despite the change in PCO_2 in the lung capillary.

Figure 5 shows the venous-arterial difference in $[H^+]$, $([H^+]_v - [H^+]_a)$, plotted against that in $\sqrt{PCO_2}$, $(\sqrt{P_vCO_2} - \sqrt{P_aCO_2})$. The relationship between these two differences was linear, the correlation coefficient being 0.972. The SD of the deviation of the individual values of $([H^+]_v - [H^+]_a)$ from the regression line was 0.59 neq, being much smaller than that of $[H^+]_v$ plotted against $\sqrt{P_vCO_2}$ (1.00 neq/liter) shown in Fig. 2. The regression line was given by the following equation:

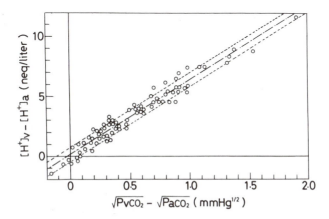

Figure 5. The venous-arterial difference in $[H^+]$ plotted against that of the square root of PCO_2 obtained in the same patients shown in Fig. 3. The interrupted line shows the regression line, and the dashed line, the SD of the deviation of individual $[H^+]$ values from the regression line.

$$[H^+]_v - [H^+]_a = 0.155 + 6.23 \bullet (\sqrt{P_vCO_2} - \sqrt{P_aCO_2}), \text{ neq/liter.} \tag{7}$$

The slope of the regression line (Eq. 7) was fairly close to that of Fig. 2 (Eq. 2), suggesting that the PCO_2-independent component of $[H^+]$ was removed by subtracting $[H^+]_a$ from $[H^+]_v$, that is, $[H^+]_v - [H^+]_a = [H^+]_v* - [H^+]_a*$. This supported the finding that the $[H^+]*$ given by Eq. (2) represented the PCO_2-dependent component of $[H^+]$ in venous blood.

Subtracting $[H^+]*$ (Eq. 2) and $[HCO_3^-]*$ (Eq. 3) from the measured values of $[H^+]$ and $[HCO_3]$, respectively, the PCO_2-independent components, $\Delta[H^+]$ and $\Delta[HCO_3^-]$, can easily be obtained. Thus, to demonstrate the validity of the value of $[H^+]*$, venous and arterial values of $\Delta[H^+]$ and $\Delta[HCO_3^-]$ were compared. The relationship between $\Delta[H^+]_v$ and $\Delta[H^+]_a$ is shown in Fig. 6, where the correlation coefficient was 0.992 and the regression line was given by

$$\Delta[H^+]_a = 0.947 \bullet \Delta[H^+]_v - 0.29, \text{ neq/liter.} \tag{8}$$

The mean difference, $(\Delta[H^+]_v - \Delta[H^+])_a$, was 0.21 ± 0.61 neq/liter. Figure 7 shows the

$\Delta[HCO_{3\,a}^-]$ plotted against $\Delta[HCO_3^-]_v$, where the correlation coefficient was 0.989 and the regression line was given by

$$\Delta[HCO_3^-]_a = 0.98 \bullet \Delta[HCO_3^-]_v + 0.18, \text{ meq/liter.} \tag{9}$$

The mean difference, $\Delta[HCO_3^-]_v - \Delta[HCO_3^-]_a)$, was -0.18 ± 0.46 meq/liter.

The factors on the right side of Eqs. (2) and (3) are respectively given by $\sqrt{M^*} \bullet K' \bullet s$ and $\sqrt{K'} \bullet s/M^*$.. Therefore, $[H^+]*$ (Eq. 2) increases and $[HCO_3^-]*$ (Eq. 3) decreases, as $M*$

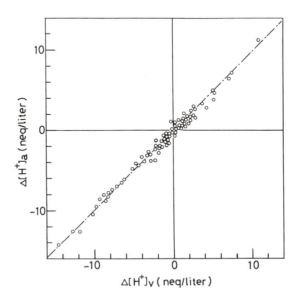

Figure 6. The PCO_2 independent H^+ component, $\Delta[H^+]_a$, in arterial blood plotted against that in venous blood, $\Delta[H^+]_v$, obtained from the same patients shown in Fig. 3.

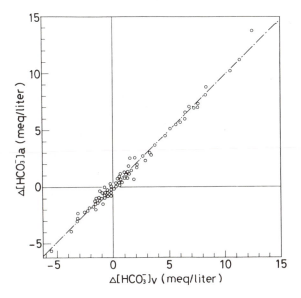

Figure 7. The PCO_2-independent HCO_3^- component, $\Delta[HCO_3^-]_a$, in arterial blood plotted against that in venous blood, $\Delta[HCO_3^-]_v$, obtained from the same patients shown in Fig. 3.

increases. Thus, reciprocal changes appear between $\Delta[H^+]$ and $\Delta[HCO_3^-]$, when M^* is varied. When M^* in arterial blood, M_a^*, was 1.527×10^{-6}, the mean $\Delta[H^+]$ difference, $(\Delta[H^+]_v - \Delta[H^+]_a)$ had a plus value (0.21 neq/liter) and the mean $\Delta[HCO_3^-]$, $(\Delta[HCO_3^-]_v - \Delta[HCO^-]_a)$, a minus value ($-0.18$ meq/liter). This suggested the M_a^* differs from M_v^* To confirm this, the mean differences, $(\Delta[H^+]_v - \Delta[H^+]_a)$ and $(\Delta[HCO_3^-]_v - \Delta[HCO^-]_a)$, were calculated by varying M_a^*, while keeping M_v^* constant at 1.527×10^{-6}. The result is shown in Fig. 8. When $M_a^* = 1.507 \times 10^{-6}$, $(\Delta[H^+]_v - \Delta[H^+]_a)$ (open circles) closely ap-

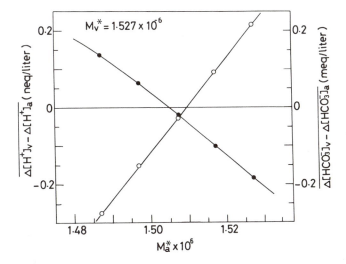

Figure 8. The mean venous-arterial difference of the PCO_2-independent components, $(\Delta[H^+]_v - \Delta[H^+]_a)$ (open circles) and $\Delta[HCO_3^-]_v - \Delta[HCO_3^-]_a$ (filled circles), plotted against the M^* in arterial blood (M_a^*), where the M^* in venous blood (M_v^*) was maintained at 1.527×10^{-6}.

proached ($\Delta[HCO_3^-]_v$ - $\Delta[HCO^-]_a$) (filled circles). This means that M_a^* is about 0.02 smaller than M_v^*, as shown in Fig. 4 and thus, the $[H^+]^*$ ($[H^+]_a^*$) in arterial blood is given by

$$[H^+]_a^* = \sqrt{M_a^*} \bullet K^{'} \bullet s \bullet PCO_2 = 6.072 \bullet \sqrt{PCO_2}, \text{ (neq/liter)}. \tag{10}$$

DISCUSSION

As shown in Figs 2 and 5, it is justifiable to assume that the $[H^+]^*$ given by Eq. (2) represents the PCO_2-dependent H^+ component in venous plasma. Designating $[H^+]^*$ and $[HCO_3^-]^*$ at two different values of PCO_2, P_1 and P_2, by the subscripts 1 and 2, the ratios $[H^+]^*_1/[H^+]^*_2$ and $[HCO_3^-]^*_1/[HCO_3^-]^*_2$ are equally given from Eq. (2) and Eq. (3) by

$$[H^+]^*_1/[H^+]^*_2 = [HCO_3^-]^*_1/[HCO_3^-]^*_2 = \sqrt{P_1/P_2}. \tag{11}$$

Taking the natural logarithms of Eq. (11), the following relationship is derived:

$$\Delta \ln [H^+]^* = \Delta \ln [HCO_3^-]^* = 0.5 \bullet \Delta \ln PCO_2, \tag{12}$$

where $\Delta \ln [H^+]^* = \ln [H^+]^*_1 - \ln [H^+]^*_2$, $\Delta \ln [HCO_3^-]^* \ln [HCO_3^-]^*_1 - \ln [HCO_3^-]^*_2$ and $\Delta \ln PCO_2 = \ln P_1 - \ln P_2$. Equation (12) indicates that the changes in chemical potential of $[H^+]^*$ and $[HCO_3^-]^*$ are both equal to the half that of PCO_2. Such an equilibrium state is considered to result from a HCO_3^- or Cl^- shift across the capillary wall (7), because it is not observed in blood in a tonometer.

Figure 6 suggests that the PCO_2-independent H^+ component in arterial blood is approximately equal to that in venous blood. Theoretically, however, $\Delta[H^+]$ is slightly dependent upon the PCO_2. The measured $[H^+]$ and $[HCO_3^-]$ values are given by the sum of their respective PCO_2-dependent and PCO_2-independent components. Moreover, when $M = M^*$, the measured values of $[H^+]$ and $[HCO_3^-]$ are equal to $[H^+]^*$ and $[HCO_3^-]^*$ at any PCO_2, and $\Delta[H^+] = \Delta[HCO_3^-] = 0$. Thus, by setting these values into the Henderson equation, the following expression is derived:

$$\{[H^+]^* + \Delta[H^+]\}\{[HCO_3^-]^* + \Delta[HCO_3^-]\} = [H^+]^* \bullet [HCO_3^-]^*. \tag{13}$$

Rearranging Eq. (13), the PCO_2-independent H^+ component is expressed by:

$$\Delta[H^+] = - \Delta[HCO_3^-] \bullet [H^+]^*/\{[HCO_3^-]^* + \Delta[HCO_3^-]\}. \tag{14}$$

When $\Delta[HCO_3^-] \ll [HCO_3^-]^*$, $\Delta[H^+]$ will be entirely independent of PCO_2. However, as $\Delta[HCO_3^-]$ increases, $\Delta[H^+]$ will become affected by PCO_2. Figure 9 shows the relationship between $\Delta[HCO_3^-]$ and $\Delta[H^+]$ in a PCO_2, range of 30 to 60 mmHg. When $\Delta[HCO_3^-] = 10$ meq/liter, at 30 mmHg PCO_2, whereas at 60 mmHg PCO_2 it is - 11.5 neq/liter. Thus, in this case, the change in $\Delta[H^+]$ caused by changing PCO_2 from 30 to 60 mmHg is equal to about 10% of $\Delta[H^+]$.

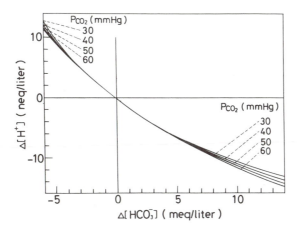

Figure 9. Theoretical relationship between $\Delta[H^+]$ and $\Delta[HCO_3^-]$ obtained from the Henderson equation, where the measured $[H^+]$ and $[HCO_3^-]$ were respectively taken to be $[H^+]^* + \Delta[H^+]$) and ($[HCO_3^-]^* + \Delta[HCO_3^-]$) and when $M = M^*$, $\Delta[H^+] = \Delta[HCO_3^-] = O$.

The acid-base imbalance has hitherto been expressed by an excess or a deficit of $[HCO_3^-]$ from normal, that is, the base excess, BE (3). The BE value can be calculated from pH, PCO_2 and the Hb concentration using the equation as follows (8):

$$BE = (1 - 0.0143 \bullet Hb) \{[HCO_3^-] - 24.5 + (8 + 1.4 \bullet Hb)(pH - 7.4)\}, \qquad (15)$$

where Hb is the Hb concentration in blood, (g/100ml). The factor of the last term of Eq. (15), (8 + 1.4 Hb), represents the slope, $\Delta[HCO_3^-]/\Delta pH$, that is, the buffer value of blood plasma equilibrated in vitro. This becomes about 30 meq/liter/pH, when Hb = 15 g/100 ml, as shown in our measured data (5). Since $\Delta[HCO_3^-]$ is calculated from pH and PCO_2, $\Delta[HCO_3^-]$ is closely correlated with the BE of Eq. (15). Comparing BE with $\Delta[HCO_3^-]$ obtained from the same pH and PCO_2, the relationship between the two parameters was numerically obtained. Figure 10 shows the BE depicted against $\Delta[HCO_3^-]_a$ in a PCO_2 range of 20 to 60 mmHg. The Hb was taken from the mean Hb value in normal volunteers to be 13.5 g/100 ml. The $\Delta[HCO_3^-]_a$ was calculated using $M_a^* = 1.507 \times 10^{-6}$ (Eq. 10). As shown in Fig. 10, the BE was generally given by the non-linear equation of $\Delta[HCO_3^-]$ and PCO_2. In normal venous blood shown in Fig. 1, $\Delta[HCO_3^-]_v$ was distributed within ± 2 meq/liter, and therefore, the BE was approximated by the following linear equation of $\Delta[HCO_3^-]_v$, P_vCO_2 and the Hb:

$$BE = 0.144 \bullet (P_vCO_2 - 33.6) + 1.16 \bullet \Delta[HCO_3^-]_v - 0.04 \bullet (Hb - 12.9). \qquad (16)$$

The SD of the deviation of the individual BE values from those of Eq. (16) was as small as 0.09 meq/liter, demonstrating that the BE was dependent on $\Delta[HCO_3^-]$. In general, the effect of the Hb concentration on the BE is very small and, in addition, PCO_2 has nothing to do with the acid-base imbalance. Therefore, it is clear for Eq. (16) and the computed data of Fig. 10 that the determinant factor of the acid-base imbalance is $\Delta[HCO_3^-]$.

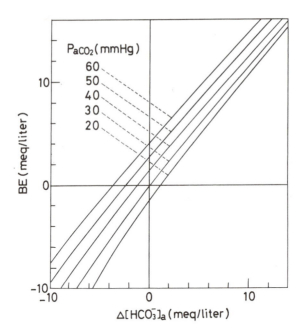

Figure 10. The relationship between $\Delta[HCO_3^-]_a$ and BE calculated from the same P_aCO_2 and pH. The BE was obtained at a constant Hb of 13.5 g/100 ml. The $\Delta[HCO_3^-]_a$ was computed by taking M^* to be M_a^* (= 1.507 x 10^{-6}).

ACKNOWLEDGMENTS

The author wishes to thank the late Dr. T. Morioka and Dr. K. Kawachi for their valuable assistance in the gas analysis and their critique of the analytical methods. He is also indebted to Dr. Johannes Piiper, Göttingen, Germany and Dr. Ann Silver, Cambridge, UK, for their helpful comments and for revising the manuscript.

REFERENCES

1. Henderson, L.J. 1909. Das Gleichgewicht zwischen Basen und Säuren im tierischen Organismus. Ergeb. Physiol. *8*: 254–325.
2. Van Slyke, D.D., and G. E. Cullen. 1917. Studies of acidosis. I. The bicarbonate concentration of the blood plasma; its significance and its determination as a measure of acidosis. J. Biol. Chem. *30*: 289–346.
3. Siggaard Andersen, O., and K. Engel. 1960. A new acid-base nomogram. An improved method for the calculation of the relevant blood acid-base data. Scand. J. Clin. & Lab. Invest. *12*: 177–186.
4. Harms, H., and H. Bartels. 1961. CO_2-Dissoziationskurven des menschlichen Blutes bei Temperaturen von 5 - 37°C und unterschiedlicher O_2-Sättigung. Pflügers Arch. *272*: 384–392.
5. Tazawa, H., M. Mochizuki, M. Tamura, and T. Kagawa. 1983. Quantitative analyses of CO_2 dissociation curve of oxygenated blood and Haldane effect in human blood. Jpn. J. Physiol. *33*: 601–618.
6. Christiansen, J., C.G. Douglas, and J.S. Haldane. 1914. The absorption and dissociation of carbon dioxide by human blood. J. Physiol *48*: 244–271.
7. Shaw, L.A., and A.C. Messer. 1932. The transfer of bicarbonate between the blood and tissue caused by alterations of the carbon dioxide concentration in the lungs. Am. J. Physiol. *100*: 122–136.
8. Siggaard Andersen, O. 1966. Titratable acid or base of body fluids. *In*: Symposium of current concept of acid-base measurement. Ann. N.Y. Acad. Sci. *133*: 41–58.

8

ACTIVATION OF TYROSINE HYDROXYLASE IN STRIATUM OF NEWBORN PIGLETS IN RESPONSE TO HYPOCAPNIC ISCHEMIA AND RECOVERY

Piotr Pastuszko and David F. Wilson

Department of Biochemistry and Biophysics
Medical School, University of Pennsylvania
Philadelphia, Pennsylvania 19104

ABSTRACT

The present study describes the effect of hypocapnic ischemia caused by hyperventilation on striatal levels of dopamine, DOPAC, HVA and activity of tyrosine hydroxylase in striatal synaptosomes isolated from the brain of newborn piglets. Hyperventilation did not result in statistically significant changes in the striatal level of dopamine and its major metabolites; however, it was observed that after 20 min of recovery the levels of striatal tissue dopamine , DOPAC and HVA increase by 195%, 110% and 205%, respectively. The level of DOPA (3,4-dihydroxyphenylalanine), which was used as an index of tyrosine hydroxylase activity, also increased after recovery. The rate of dopamine synthesis was 32 pmoles/mg protein/10 min in control piglets and after recovery this increased to 132 pmoles/mg protein/10 min. Measurement of the tyrosine hydroxylase activity in Triton X-100 treated synaptosomes showed that, after 20 min of recovery, there was an increase in Vmax with no change in Km for pteridine cofactor, compared to control. This is consistant with the enzyme having been covalently modified (activated) during tissue ischemia caused by hyperventilation and remaining activated well into the recovery period. We postulate that ischemia can induce long lasting alterations in dopamine synthesis, which may play some role in mediation of hypoxic cell injury in immature brain.

INTRODUCTION

Tyrosine hydroxylase [L-tyrosine, tetrahydropterdine: oxygen oxidoreductase, EC 1.14.16.2] catalyzes the conversion of L-tyrosine to L-3,4-dihydroxyphenylalanine (DOPA), which is the initial and rate limiting step in the biosynthetic pathway of catecho-

Oxygen Transport to Tissue XVIII, edited by Nemoto and LaManna
Plenum Press, New York, 1997

lamines such as dopamine, norepinephrine and epinephrine in the central nervous system (Nagatsu et al., 1964; Levitt et al., 1965). Alteration in the activity or level of this enzyme can therefore have physiological consequences for the neuronal function. There are several possible mechanisms for altering the activity of tyrosine hydroxylase in the brain. Activation of this enzyme, which is often expressed as an increased affinity of tyrosine hydroxylase for its pterine cofactor, has been reported to occur after electrical stimulation (Alousi and Weiner,1966), potassium stimulated depolarization (Harris and Roth, 1971; Greene and Rein, 1978), short term increases in catecholamines release, etc. The activation of tyrosine hydroxylase *in vivo* by electrical stimulation and *in vitro* by depolarization by high potassium has been proposed to involve phosphorylation of enzyme by calcium and calmodulin dependent protein kinases. Tyrosine hydroxylase can also be activated by protein phosphorylation by the cyclic AMP dependent and c-AMP independent protein kinases (Lovenberg et al., 1975; Goldstein et al., 1976; Pollock et al., 1981; El Mestikawy et al., 1983, 1985). Long term regulation has been reported to occur through alterations in the amount of enzyme present in the tissue (Mueller et al., 1969; Thoenen et al., 1969; Tank et al., 1985).

Synthesis of monoamine neurotransmitters in the brain has been reported to be altered by exposure of the animal to hypoxic conditions. Hypoxic episodes cause increased release of catecholamines from intracellular stores (Obrenovich et al., 1990; Globus et al., 1988; Slivka et al., 1988; Damsma et al., 1990; Baker et al., 1991) which can result in increase in the activity of tyrosine hydroxylase by relieving the inhibition by product (see above). During hypoxia the tissue level of oxygen is decreased, however, and since oxygen is a substrate for tyrosine hydroxylase the oxygen pressure may become limiting in the rate of catecholamine synthesis.

Our previous study showed that during recovery after hyperventilation extracellular level of DOPA, which is an index of activity of tyrosine hydroxylase, increased in extracellular medium as measured by *in vivo* microdialysis. To characterize this effect we have investigated the effect of hyperventilation and recovery on the activity of tyrosine hydroxylase in the striatal synaptosomes isolated from the brain of newborn piglets.

MATERIALS AND METHODS

Newborn piglets, 2–4 days of age were used throughout the study. This animal model has been chosen because the level of maturation of the brain of animals is approximately equal to term newborn. Anesthesia was induced by halothane (4% mixed with 100% oxygen) and 1.5% lidocaine was used as local anesthetic. A tracheotomy was performed and the femoral artery and vein were cannulated. Fentanyl 30 µg/kg was injected intravenously at approximately 1 hr intervals throughout the experiment. The animals were then paralyzed with tubocurarine and ventilated mechanically with 22% O_2/78% N_2O. The control ventilatory rate was 25/min and during the experiments was increased to 95/min for a period of 20 min., then returned to the control rate for the 20 min recovery period.

Preparation of Crude Synaptosomal Fraction (P2)

At the indicated time, the animals were decapitated and the striatum were rapidly removed. The P2 fraction was prepared by homogenizing the striatum in the isotonic medium containing 0.32 M sucrose, 10 mM Tris-HCl and 1 mM EDTA, final pH 7.4. The homogenate was centrifuged for 3 minutes at 1,000 g and then the supernatant fraction centrifuged for 20 minutes at 20,000 g. The synaptosomes were resuspended in Krebs-Henseleit buffer (140 mM NaCl, 5 mM KCl, 5 mM NaHCO$_3$, 1.3 mM MgSO$_4$, 1 mM Tris-Phosphate and 10 mM Tris-Hepes, pH 7.2) supplemented with 10 mM glucose and 1 mM CaCl$_2$. The medium also contained 100 µM m-hydroxybenzylhydrazine, an inhibitor of aromatic L-amino acid decarboxylase.

Incubations

All incubations were carried out at 37ºC while shaking with air as the gas phase. The synaptosomes prepared from three groups of animals (control, hyperventilation, recovery) were incubated for 5 to 40 minutes. The appropriately incubated synaptosomes were used either directly to measure dopamine synthesis or were treated with Triton X-100 (final concentration 0.2%) and then used to assay tyrosine hydroxylase activity.

Measurements of Dopamine, DOPAC, and HVA Levels

The striatal tissue was homogenized in 1% cold trichloroacetic acid and concentration of dopamine and its metabolites were measured directly in the TCA extracts by HPLC using a Whatman Parastil 10 SCX column. The elution was carried out with 25 mM monochloracetic acid, pH 2.85, containing 100 µM EDTA. The retention times for DOPAC, dopamine and HVA were 6.5 min, 8.5 min, and 11 min, respectively.

Measurement of the Rate of Dopamine Synthesis by Dihydroxyphenylalanine (DOPA) Formation

Samples (250 µl) containing 2 mg of protein were incubated for 5–40 min with substrate, 40 µM L-tyrosine. The reaction was terminated at the indicated time intervals by adding cold trichloroacetic acid (final concentration 1% by weight) to quench the enzymatic activity. Samples were centrifuged to remove precipitated materials and then analyzed by HPLC for level of DOPA. The HPLC analysis of DOPA was carried out using an Alltech Associates Adsorbosphere catecholamines column 100 mm in length x 4.6 mm in diameter, with 3 µm particle size C18 packing. The mobile phase consisted of 0.1 M citric acid, 0.32 mM sodium cetyl sulfate, 0.1 mM EDTA and 10% acetonitrile, pH 2.7. The electrochemical detector was polarized to 800 mV. A standard solution of DOPA was injected at the beginning and the end of each experiment. A flow rate of 0.7 ml/min gave retention time for DOPA of 3.3 min.

Measurement of Tyrosine Hydroxylase Activity in Detergent Treated Samples

Tyrosine hydroxylase activity was measured by HPLC by a modified method of Hirata et al. (1983). The incubation mixture contained: 0.25 M Tris-Hepes at pH 7.2, 800 units catalase, 800 units sheep liver pteridine reductase, 1 mM NADPH, 100 µM L-tyrosine, 100 µM L-tyrosine, 100 µM m-hydroxybenzylhydrazine, 1–2 mg of Triton broken synaptosomes and different concentration of pteridine cofactor, 6-methyl-5,6,7,8-tetrahydropteridin, dissolved in 1 M 2-mercaptoethanol. The final concentration of 6-MPH$_4$ was from 50 µM to 2000 µM. The assay mixture was incubated for 20 min at 37°C and the reaction was terminated by adding perchloric acid (0.2 M final concentration) containing α-methyl DOPA as the internal standard and, 0.25% EDTA as the reducing agent. The samples were centrifuged and Tris-HCl, pH 9.0 (0.7 M final concentration) was added to the clear supernatant in order to adjust the pH to 8.0–8.5. Alumina (100 mg) was then added to adsorb the catechols and the liquid removed by aspiration. The alumina was washed 3 times with 5 ml volumes of distilled water. The catechols were extracted from the alumina with 250 μl of 0.5 M HCl. Aliquots (20 μl) of the acid extract was injected into HPLC and levels of DOPA and α-methyl-DOPA were measured. The DOPA formed by tyrosine hydroxylase was calculated by the ratio of peaks of DOPA and α-methyl-DOPA.

Measurement of Protein

Protein was measured according to the method of Lowry et al. (1951) using bovine serum albumin as the standards.

Statistical Analysis

The data are presented as the mean values ± SD. The statistical significance was determined using the paired t-test.

RESULTS

Effect of Hyperventilation and Recovery on Striatal Concentration of Dopamine, DOPAC, and HVA

The studies were carried out on three groups of animals: control; subjected to an increase ventilatory rate from 25/min (control) to 95/min. for 20 min; hyperventilated animals followed by recovery. period of 20 min. We previously showed that during these conditions cortical oxygen pressure decreased from 35–40 Torr (control) to about 16 Torr (hyperventilation) and during recovery return to control values (Wilson et al. 1991). The effects of hyperventilation and recovery on striatal concentration of dopamine and its major metabolites DOPAC and HVA are presented in Figure 1. Hyperventilation did not cause statistically significant changes in the tissue levels of dopamine, DOPAC and HVA. However, the levels of all three compounds increased during the recovery period. The level of dopamine increased from about 230 pmoles/mg protein to about 680 pmoles/mg protein; the levels of DOPAC and HVA increased by about 110% and 205%, respectively.

Effect of Hyperventilation and Recovery on Rate of Dopamine Synthesis

The rate of dopamine synthesis was investigated in synaptosomes prepared from piglets which were controls, hyperventilated, and recovered from hyperventilation. Figure 2 shows hyperventilation resulted in an increase in the rate of dopamine synthesis, particularly in the recovery group. In synaptosomes from controls, the rate of dopamine synthesis was 32.5 pmoles/mg protein/10 min and this increased due to hyperventilation and recovery to 63 pmoles/mg protein/10 min and 132 pmoles/ mg protein/ 10 min, respectively. The increase in the rate of dopamine synthesis in response to recovery from hyperventila-

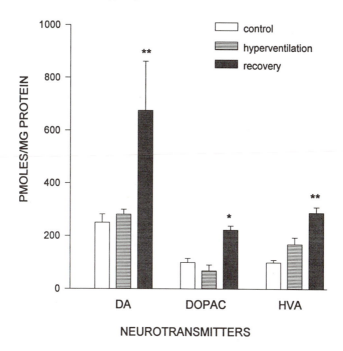

Figure 1. Effect of hyperventilation and recovery on the striatal level of dopamine (DA), DOPAC and HVA in newborn piglets. The striatum from three grup of animals (control, hyperventilation and recovery) were homogenized in 1% TCA , centrifuged and the levels of DA, DOPAC and HVA were measured in supernatant by HPLC as described in Materials and Methods. Data are means ± SD for 4 experiments. * p< 0.01; **p< 0.005

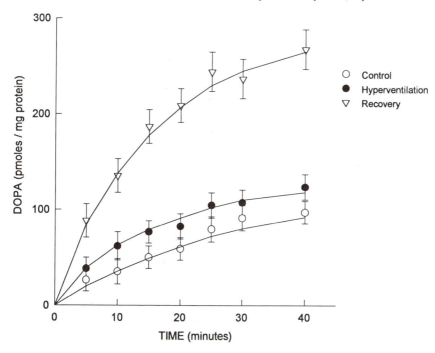

Figure 2. Effect of hyperventilation and recovery on rate of dopamine synthesis in synaptosomes from striatum of newborn piglets. Synaptosomal fraction from tree grup of animals were incubated for 5–40 minutes at 37°C and then level of DOPA was measured as described in Materials and Methods. Data are means ± SD for 4 experiments.

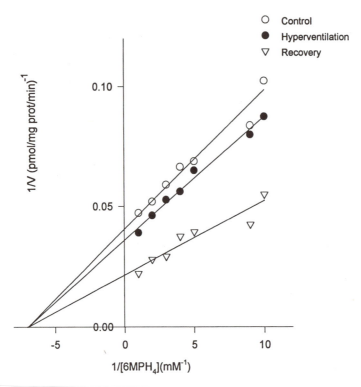

Figure 3. Dependence of the tyrosine hydroxylase activity on concentration of 6-MPH$_4$ in synaptosomes from control animals, and after hyperventilation and recovery. The synaptosomes were treated with Triton X-100 and the tyrosine activity measured as described in Materials and Methods. The results are for representative experiment. Summary of results are presented in Table 1.

tion was statistically significant at all of the measured time points.($p < 0.01$ for 5 min and $p < 0.005$ for the remaining time points). The data also show that increasing the ventilatory rate to 65/min follow by 20 min recovery caused an increase in the rate of dopamine synthesis by about 95% (results from two experiments).

Effect of Hyperventilation and Recovery on Kinetic Parameters of Tyrosine Hydroxylase

The tyrosine hydroxylase activity was measured in synaptosomal fractions treated with Triton X-100 to destroy the integrity of the synaptosomal membranes. Analysis of the cofactor, 6-MPH$_4$, dependence of tyrosine hydroxylase activity was carried out in the presence of 100 μM tyrosine and different concentrations of 6-MPH$_4$. As can be seen, activation of tyrosine hydroxylase by hyperventilation, and particulary by recovery, was associated with a statistically significant increase in Vmax and a small, not significant, decrease in Km for 6-MPH$_4$. In control synaptosomes the Km for pteridine cofactor was 208 ± 23 μM and the Vmax was 37.1 ± 3.9 pmoles/mg protein/min. In synaptosomes from piglets which were hyperventilated and hyperventilated followed by recovery, Vmax increased to 44 ± 4.8 pmoles/mg protein/min and 56.9 ± 5.9 pmoles/mg protein/min, respectively.

Table 1. Effect of hyperventilation and recovery on the K_M and V_{max} of tyrosine hydroxylase for 6-MPH$_4$

Conditions	K_M (μM)	V_{max} (pmoles/min/mg protein)
Control	160 ± 23	25.6 ± 1.2
Hyperventilation	172 ± 39	29.1 ± 2.3
Recovery	136 ± 31	46.9 ± 2.9 *

The kinetics parameters of tyrosine hydroxylase were measured in broken synaptosomes prepared from striatum of newborn piglets (control, hyperventilation, recovery) as described in Materials and Methods. The values are means ± SD for four experiments. * $p < 0.005$.

DISCUSSION

In the present study, we have examined the effect of hyperventilation and recovery on the striatal level of dopamine and its major metabolites, DOPAC and HVA; and also the effect of these conditions on the activity of tyrosine hydroxylase, the rate limiting enzyme in synthesis of catecholamines. We observed that in piglets recovering from a period of hyperventilation the levels of dopamine, DOPAC and HVA increased significantly compared to control levels. The increased levels of dopamine and its major metabolites could reflect either an increase in activity of tyrosine hydroxylase and/or changes in the activity of monoamine oxidase, a key enzyme in catabolism of dopamine. Measurements of the kinetic constants of tyrosine hydroxylase indicated that the enzyme is activated during recovery and that this activation was associated with an increase in Vmax, with no significant change in the apparent affinity (Km) of the enzyme for pteridine cofactor. The exact mechanism(s) involved in the changes in activity of tyrosine hydroxylase observed in this study is not known. The data are consistent with the enzyme having been covalently modified (activated) during tissue hypoxia and remaining activated well into the recovery period. One possibility is that the hypoxia-induced increase in tyrosine hydroxylase activity was secondary to depolarization of synaptosomal membranes. El Mestikawy et al. (1983; 1985) and Bustos et al. (1976) showed that tyrosine hydroxylase activation resulting from depolarization using high potassium was associated with an increase in intrasynaptosomal calcium and in the increased Vmax of the enzyme. The authors concluded that calmodulin-dependent protein phosphorylation was involved in this activation. Chowdhury and Fillenz (1988) suggested that in synaptosomes stimulation of dopamine synthesis by addition of 50 mM potasium is mediated by protein kinase C. We have also observed that treatment of synaptosomes with hypoxia induces an activation of tyrosine hydroxylase (Pastuszko et al., 1985). The data suggest that hypoxia caused an increase in intracellular calcium, activating calcium dependent protein kinases that phosphorylated tyrosine hydroxylase. The rapidity with which tyrosine hydroxylase activity is affected by hyperventilation suggested that *de novo* protein synthesis is not involved in this response.

Our unpublished results showed that after 20 min recovery from hyperventilation, the activity of monoamine oxidase increases only about 20% compared to control activity of this enzyme. This increase was not large enough to be significantly different from control. We suggested that in striatum of newborn piglets the increases in levels of dopamine, DOPAC and HVA observed after hyperventilation are caused, at least in part, by activation of tyrosine hydroxylase by the resulting ischemia.

The changes in the activity of tyrosine hydroxylase induced when the newborns are subjected to a period of hyperventilation can have physiological consequences. Several studies have provided evidence for a role of dopamine in the mediation of ischemic cell injury (Globus et al., 1987; Clemens and Phebus, 1988; Marie et al., 1992). Dopamine can activate the D1 receptors, which can caused activation of cAMP cascade. In striatum, dopamine can also modulate glutamate release through its effect on D2 receptors. Administration of D2 receptor agonist into striatum is reported to inhibit the depolarization induced release of dopamine in the striatum (Yamamoto and Davy, 1992). Oxidation of the excess of dopamine coud also be partially responsible for the production of free radicals during reperfusion (Slivka and Cohen, 1985). Zhang and Piantadosi (1991) postulated that H_2O_2 generation from catabolism of dopamine during reoxygenation after hypoxia is very important to the pathogenesis of CNS oxygen toxicity. Through such mechanisms, dopamine can increase the level of this neurotransmitter (by activation of tyrosine hydroxylase) which could contribute to the maturation of hypoxic/ischemic cell damage in striatum.

Our results indicated that hyperventilation, by decreasing the oxygen pressure in the brain, can cause major alteration in the metabolism of catecholamines, and can contribute to immature brain injury.

ACKNOWLEDGMENTS

This work was supported in part by a grant NS-31465 from NIH.

REFERENCES

Alousi A. and Weiner N. (1966) The regulation of norepinephrine synthesis in sympathetic nerves: effect of nerve stimulation, cocaine, and catecholamine-releasing agents. *Proc. Natl. Acad. Sci. USA* 56, 1491–1496.

Baker A.J., Zornow M.H., Scheller M.S., Yaksh T.L., Skilling S.R., Smullin D.H., Larson A.A., and Kuczenski R. (1991) Changes in extracellular concentration of glutamate, aspartate, glycine, dopamine, serotonin, and dopamine metabolites after transient global ischemia in the rabbit brain. *J. Neurochem.* 57, 1370–1379.

Bustos G., Roth R.H., and Morgenroth V.H. (1976) Activation of tyrosine hydroxylase in rat striatal slices by K^+-depolarization-effect of ethanol. *Biochem. Pharmacol.* 25, 2493–2497

Chowdhury M. and Fillenz M. (1988) K^+-dependent stimulation of dopamine synthesis in striatal synaptosomes is mediated by protein kinase C. *J. Neurochem.* 50, 624–629

Clemens J.A. and Phebus L.A. (1988) Dopamine depletion protects striatal neurones from ischemia-induced cell death. *Life Science,* 42, 707–713.

Damsma G., Boisvert D.P., Mudrick L.A., Wenkstern D., and Fibiger H.C. (1990) Effects of transient forebrain ischemia and pargyline on extracellular concentrations of dopamine, serotonin and their metabolites in the rat striatum as determined by in vivo microdialysis. *J. Neurochem.* 54, 801–808.

El Mestikawy S., Glowinski J., and Hamon M. (1983) Tyrosine hydroxylase activation in depolarized dopaminergic terminals-involvement of Ca^{2+}- dependent phosphorylation. *Nature* 302, 830–832.

El Mestikawy S., Gozlan H., Glowinski J., and Hamon M. (1985) Characteristics of tyrosine hydroxylase activation by K^+- induced depolarization and/or forskolin in rat striatal slices. *J. Neurochem.* 45, 173–184

Globus M.Y-T., Ginsberg M.D., Dietrich W.D., Busto R., and Scheinberg P. (1987) Substantia nigra lesion protects against ischemic damage in the striatum. *Neurosci. Letters* 80, 251–256.

Globus M.Y-T., Busto R., Dietrich W.D., Martinez E., Valdes I., and Ginsberg M.D. (1988) Effect on ischemia on the in vivo release of striatal dopamine, glutamate, and γ-aminobutyric acid studied by intracerebral microdialysis. *J. Neurochem.* 51, 1455–1464.

Goldstein M., Bronaugh R. L., Ebstein B., and Roberge C. (1976) Stimulation of tyrosine hydroxylase activity by cyclic AMP in synaptosomes and in soluble striatal enzyme preparations. *Brain Res.* 109, 563–574.

Greene L.A. and Rein G. (1978) Short-term regulation of catecholamine biosynthesis in a nerve growth factor responsive clonal line of rat pheochromocytoma cells. *J. Neurochem.* 30, 549–555.

Harris J.E. and Roth R.H. (1971) Potassium-induced acceleration of catecholamine biosynthesis in brain slices. I.Study on the mechanism of action. *Mol. Pharmacol.* 7, 593–604.

Hirata, Y., Togari, A., and Nagatsu, T. (1983) Studies on tyrosine hydroxylase system in rat brain slices using high performance liquid chromatography with electochemical detection. *J. Neurochem.* 40, 1585–1589.

Levitt M., Spector S., Sjoerdsma A., and Udenfriend S. (1965) Elucidation of the rate-limiting step in norepinephrine biosynthesis in the perfused guinea pig heart. *J. Pharmacol. Exp. Ther.* 148, 1–8.

Lovenberg W., Bruck E.A., and Hanbauer I. (1975) ATP, cyclic AMP and magnesium increase the affinity of rat striatal tyrosine hydroxylase for its cofactors. *Proc. Natl. Acad. Sci. USA* 72, 2955–2958.

Lowry O.H., Rosebrough N.J., Farr A.L., and Randall R.J. (1951) Protein measurement with the Folin phenol reagent. *J. Biol. Chem.* 193, 1268–1274.

Marie C., Mossiat C., Beley A. and Bralet J. (1992) Alpha-Methyl-para-tyrosine pretreatment protects from striatal neuronal death induced by four-vessel occlusion in the rat. *Neurochem. Research*, 17, 961–965.

Mueller R.A., Thoenen H., and Axelrod J. (1969) Increase in tyrosine hydroxilase activity after resperine administration. *J. Pharmacol. Exp. Ther.* 169, 74–79.

Nagatsu T., Levitt M., and Udenfriend S. (1964) Tyrosine hydroxylase. The initial step in norepinephrine biosynthesis. *J. Biol. Chem.* 239, 2910–2917.

Obrenovitch T.P., Sarna G.S., Matsumoto T., and Symon L. (1990) Extracellular striatal dopamine and its metabolites during transient cerebral ischaemia. *J. Neurochem.* 54, 1526–1532.

Pollock R.J., Kapatos G., and Kaufman S. (1981) Effect of cyclic AMP-dependent protein phosphorylating conditions on the pH- dependent activity of tyrosine hydroxylase from beef and rat striata. *J. Neurochem.* 37, 855–860.

Slivka, A., and Cohen, G. (1985) Hydroxyl radical attack on dopamine. *J. Biol. Chem.* 260, 15466–15472.

Slivka, A., Brannan, T.T., Weinberger, J., Knott, P.J., and Cohen, G. (1988) Increase in extracellular dopamine in the striatum during cerebral ischemia: A study utilizing cerebral microdialysis. *J. Neurochem.* 50, 1714–1718.

Tank A.W., Lewis E.J., Chikaraishi D.M., and Weiner N. (1985) Elevation of RNA coding for tyrosine hydroxilase in rat adrenal gland by resperine treatment and exposure to cold. *J. Neurochem.* 45, 1030–1033.

Thoenen H., Mueller R.A., and Axelrod J. (1969) Trans-synaptic induction of tyrosine hydroxylase. *J. Pharmacol. Exp. Ther.* 169, 249–254.

Wilson D.F., Pastuszko A., DiGiacomo J.E., Pawlowski M., Schneiderman R., and Delivoria-Papadopoulos, M. (1991) Effect of hyperventilation on oxygenation of the brain cortex of newborn piglets. *J. App. Physiol.* 70(6), 2691–2696.

Yamamoto B.K., and Davy S. (1992) Dopaminergic modulation of glutamate release in striatum as measured by microdialysis. *J. Neurochem.* 58, 1736–1742.

Zhang J. and Piantadosi C.A. (1991) Preventation of H_2O_2 generation by monoamine oxidase protects against CNS O_2 toxicity. *J. Appl. Physiol.* 71(3),1056–1061.

9

METABOLIC MECHANISMS OF ANOXIA TOLERANCE IN THE TURTLE BRAIN

Miguel A. Pérez-Pinzón,[1] Peter L. Lutz,[2] Thomas J. Sick,[1] and Myron Rosenthal[1]

[1]Department of Neurology
School of Medicine
University of Miami
[2]Department of Biological Sciences
Florida Atlantic University
Miami, Florida 33101

INTRODUCTION

Turtle brain survives anoxia by maintaining ATP levels necessary to avoid the loss of ion homeostasis and the uncontrolled release of excitotoxic neurotransmitters [1–6]. A central question toward defining anoxic tolerance in turtle brain is how do ATP production and ATP use remain matched despite complete inhibition of oxidative metabolism. Indirect evidence of both a Pasteur effect and a hypometabolic state have been proposed previously. For example, calculations based on creatine phosphate depletion and lactate accumulation during anoxia suggested that ATP production was markedly reduced (by approx 88%) [1, 2]. Also, enzymatic studies of turtle brain suggested the presence of an initial Pasteur effect followed by a decrease in the glycolytic rate[7]. Depression of electrical activity in the turtle brain further strengthened the proposal of the presence of a hypometabolic state [5, 8–10].

The present research was designed to test two hypotheses: (a) that a reactive increase in anaerobic glycolysis ('Pasteur effect') provides an initial compensation for inhibition of oxidative phosphorylation during the early stages of anoxia; and (b) that after prolonged anoxia, the metabolic rate of turtle brain becomes markedly depressed. Calorimetry and oxygen consumption techniques were used to determine metabolic rates in isolated turtle cerebellum during the transition to anoxia, anoxia and re-oxygenation. We conclude that oxidative and glycolytic rates vary sensitively with turtle brain tissue oxygenation, and that increased anaerobic glycolysis contributes to maintaining ATP production at aerobic levels during the early phase of anoxia. Subsequently, a hypometabolic state is reached, yet ATP is still maintained indicating that decreased ATP use must occur. A preliminary report of these findings has been presented [11].

MATERIALS AND METHODS

Isolation and handling of the turtle cerebellum has been described previously [5]. In brief, freshwater turtles (*Trachemys scripta elegans*) of either sex weighing 600–900 g were quickly decapitated. After retraction of the skin and muscle overlying the skull, the brain was isolated and immersed in turtle artificial cerebrospinal fluid (ACSF) of composition: 100 mM NaCl, 3.5 mM KCl, 26 mM NaHCO$_3$, 1.25 mM NaH$_2$PO$_4$, 2.0 mM CaCl$_2$, 2.0 mM MgSO$_4$, 20 mM glucose. This solution was equilibrated with 95% O$_2$ and 5% CO$_2$ at room temperature. The cerebellum (50–80 mg wet wt) was dissected from the brain and kept in the ACSF for at least 30 min since this delay was greater than the time required for evoked potential recovery [5]. The isolated tissues were then placed in ACSF-containing chambers specific either for flow-through microcalorimetry or for the measurement of oxygen consumption.

After a 2 hr equilibration period in the closed chamber, heat output of isolated cerebellum was measured with an LKB 10700–1 Flow-through microcalorimeter during normoxia (ACSF, flowing through the cell at 1 ml/min, was bubbled with 95% O$_2$, 5% CO$_2$) and during anoxia produced by substituting N$_2$ for O$_2$ in the gas mixture bubbling the ACSF. The temperature of the calorimeter was set to 25°C. Heat output from a reference chamber, through which ACSF flowed in parallel to that of the sample chamber, was subtracted from heat output of the sample chamber to account for ambient influences [12]. ACSF oxygenation was periodically sampled with a Radiometer-Copenhagen blood gas analyzer.

To measure oxygen consumption, the cerebellum was placed on a nylon mesh held by an O-ring in a chamber with volume either 1.8 or 2.1 ml (Gilson). This chamber was equipped with a Clark-type platinum electrode and was filled with oxygenated ACSF at ambient temperature. The electrode was positioned at the side of the chamber, approx 5 mm from the cerebellum. Oxygen was uniformly distributed in the ACSF with a magnetic stirring rod positioned under the mesh. Oxygen consumption was calculated from the decline in oxygen tension vs time (approx 10 min per interval) by linear interpolation of a chart recording. This measurement was made with reference to the maximal change in the oxygen tension of the ACSF in the chamber recorded prior to placing the cerebellum in the chamber. This maximal oxygen shift was produced by maximally oxygenating the ACSF with 95% O$_2$, 5% CO$_2$ and then by substituting N$_2$ for O$_2$ in this gas mixture. The oxygen shift was calculated from the equation defined by Larrabee [13] (see also Martin et al. [14]).

For metabolite measurements, the isolated turtle cerebellum was quickly extracted from ACSF-containing recording chambers, immersed in liquid nitrogen until frozen, placed in cryotubes and stored at -70° C. Subsequently, the frozen tissue was placed in a glove box at -30° C, weighed and homogenized in 5 vol 0.1 N HCl in methanol for 6 min. The homogenate was removed from the glove box, homogenized in 30 vol of 0.3 N perchloric acid containing 1 mM EDTA in ice with a glass homogenizer, and centrifuged for 10 min at 10,000 g. The supernatant was neutralized with 2 N KOH in 0.4 mM imidazole. Metabolites were determined by enzyme-linked assays [15].

The statistical significance among different groups was estimated using one-way analysis of variance. A Dunnet's post-hoc test was used to determine significance differences within groups.

RESULTS

Oxygen Consumption

Mean bath oxygenation (bpO_2) was 1.66 ± 0.09 mM (n = 7) (in this and subsequent sections, data is presented relative to standard error of the mean) and mean oxygen consumption (VO_2) was 0.408 ± 0.05 mM/g/sec (n = 7). To assure constancy over time, VO_2 was measured for 5 hrs in three control tissues in which bpO_2 was kept close to control by intermittent re-bubbling with 95% O_2 and 5% CO_2. Initial oxygen consumption values were similar to those reported above and were unchanged during 5 hrs.

VO_2 declined with bpO_2 (Figure 1, n = 7, r = 0.911). For this figure, VO_2 values were grouped into bpO_2 ranges which were each 10% of the control bpO_2 for each animal. Whenever multiple VO_2 values were calculated within a bpO_2 range for each tissue, the mean of these VO_2 rates was first calculated and then this value was plotted in Figure 1. In four of the tissues from which Figure 1 was derived, VO_2 was recorded during prolonged periods in which bpO_2 was reduced only by oxygen consumption itself (i.e. closed system). In three other tissues, ACSF oxygenation was decreased between each VO_2 recording by transiently bubbling the ACSF with 95% N_2 (balance CO_2). Since plots of oxygen consumption vs ACSF oxygenation were similar when ACSF oxygenation was decreased by either protocol, data from all tissues are plotted in Figure 1.

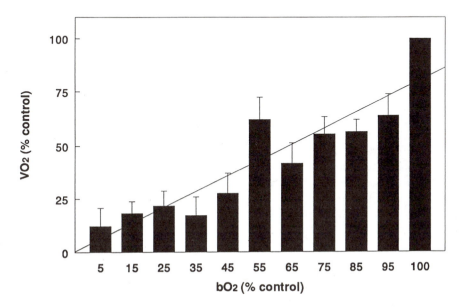

Figure 1. Oxygen consumption (VO_2) vs bath oxygen partial pressure (bpO_2) (both as percentage from control baseline) in the isolated turtle cerebellum. Decline of VO_2 was linear (r = 0.911, n = 7).

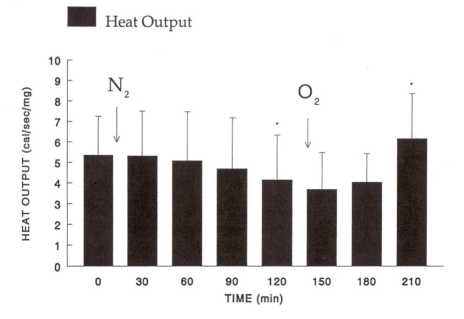

Figure 2. Heat output of the isolated turtle cerebellum during normoxia, 2 h of anoxia and re-oxygenation. A significant declined in heat output was registered at 120 min of anoxia (P = 0.05, n = 5). Recovery occurred within 90 min.

Heat Production

Heat output of isolated turtle cerebellum was determined continuously under control conditions and subsequently during 120 minutes of anoxia and 90 minutes of recovery. This data is shown in Figure 2. Prior to experimental manipulation, pO_2 in the ACSF bathing the isolated tissue averaged 630±35 Torr (n = 5), and tissue heat output was 0.032±0.01 cal/g/min (n = 5). At time zero in this experiment, the oxygenated gas mixture in the ACSF was replaced with 95% N_2 (5% CO_2). For statistical purposes, this time was considered the onset of anoxia, but the pO_2 decline in the ACSF was not immediate. Rather, bath pO_2 declined to approx 0–3 torr within 15 min and no ACSF oxygen tension was recordable after that time. Although mean heat output appeared to decline, there was no significant difference from control until 120 minutes following onset of anoxia. At this time, mean heat output was 0.025±0.01 cal/g/min (n = 5; P = 0.05), which was approx 78% of the control value.

Despite restoration of oxygen to the ACSF at 120 minutes of anoxia, the heat output continued to decline for 30 min afterward (150 min from time zero). At 210 minutes, heat output increased to 0.037±0.008 cal/g/min (n = 4) which was higher (but not significantly) than control values.

Levels of ATP, phosphocreatine and lactate were measured at specific times following onset of anoxia (Figure 3). These were not significantly altered during anoxia (1.15±0.15 and 1.40±0.29 mM/g wet weight; n = 4 during normoxia and 2 hrs of anoxia, respectively). Similar results were shown previously [5].

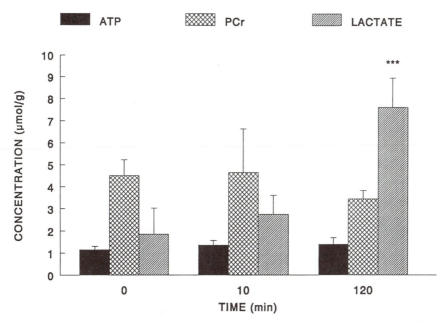

Figure 3. Levels of ATP, phosphocreatine and lacatate obtained at increasing times after onset of anoxia. ATP levels were not significantly changed despite 2 h of anoxia (n = 4) but PCr declined significantly (p < 0.05, n = 4). Lactate increased significantly (p < 0.01, n = 4), after 2 h of anoxia.

DISCUSSION

Calorimetric measurements of heat production yielded the first direct evidence that anoxia produced a reversible, hypometabolic state in isolated turtle cerebellum. A hypometabolic state was suggested by the general depression in metabolic rate observed in the diving turtle [16]. Such a hypometabolic state in intact turtle brain had also been suggested by calculations of ATP production [1, 2]. However, calculated decreases in ATP production were larger (80% vs 22%) in intact turtle brain compared to isolated turtle cerebellum. This difference is likely due, at least in part, to the fact that the intrinsic metabolic rate of *in vitro* brain tissues was much lower (perhaps by 50%) than that found *in vivo*. Deafferentation and depression of spontaneous neural activity have been suggested as possible causes for the lower metabolic rate of *in vitro* preparations [17, 18].

From thermodynamic estimates, comparisons can be made between the oxygen consumption and heat production data presented here. Specifically, the 0.408 mmol/g/min of O_2 consumed by isolated turtle cerebellum (c.f. Figure 1) should represent 0.184 joules/g/min [5]. Likewise, the 0.032 cal/g/min heat production of normoxic turtle brain should represent 0.135 joules/g/min. These values are not statistically different, although they were obtained by different techniques in separate tissues (see Gnaiger [12]). This further supports the conclusion that the turtle brain in normoxia depends predominately upon oxidative phosphorylation for energy production.

Other reports support a higher contribution of aerobic glycolysis in brain slices from rat [17] or turtle [19]. Lipton and Wittingham [17] suggested that such a high glycolytic rate may reflect a decreased mitochondrial capacity of *in vitro* preparations. The high glycolytic rate of some *in vitro* models may also result from an anoxic core [17] or from a decrease in intracellular pH during the isolation procedure which may activate glycolytic pathways [20]. However, no evidence of an anoxic core was found by polarographic measurements in isolated turtle cerebellum [5]. It is also possible that the turtle brain may not suffer a large decrease in intracellular pH during the isolation procedure.

The calorimetry data indicates a substantial Pasteur effect during anoxia in isolated turtle cerebellum. A Pasteur effect has been controversial since it was not observed in earlier studies of anoxia in turtle brain slices [19]. However, Kelly and Storey [7] suggested that these was an increase in the glycolytic flux during the transition to anoxia but a decrease after 1 hour of anoxia. Our data supports that during the transition to anoxia, ATP-generating pathways (i.e. glycolysis) are more efficiently coupled with ATP-utilizing pathways [21]. We found that heat production was initially unchanged by anoxia, indicating that the glycolytic rate was increased by as much as 19 fold if approx 36 of 38 ATP molecules were produced by oxidative phosphorylation during normoxia. While this increase seems excessive compared to the known 4–5 fold increase in glycolysis of intact mammalian brain during the transition to anoxia [22], it may be explained by *in vitro* differences (i.e. the depressed metabolic rate of the *in vitro* preparation may allow for a greater increase in glycolysis during anoxia) and by an intrinsically higher glycolytic capacity of turtle brain [7, 23]. One possible reason why Robin et al. [19] reported no Pasteur effect during anoxia could be that their preparations (brain slices) were bathed with only 5 mM glucose. We recently reported that 5 mM glucose was insufficient to maintain ion homeostasis and ATP levels during anoxia and that the isolated turtle cerebellum required approx 20 mM glucose [5].

Mechanisms to promote anoxia tolerance in the turtle brain likely include adaptations that are sensitive to oxygen availability (e.g. [24, 25]). We show here that the isolated turtle brain functions as an 'oxygen conformer' (i.e. a tissue whose oxygen consumption varies with oxygen supply over broad ranges). The contrasting term, 'oxygen regulator', is applied to systems whose oxygen consumption is independent of oxygen availability down to very low values. Isolated mitochondria fit the oxygen regulator pattern which may apply also to mammalian brain and contribute to its vulnerability.

Since oxygen consumption declined with even small decreases in bpO_2 in the isolated turtle cerebellum, this suggests that an oxygen-sensitive mechanism controlled the glycolytic rate. The identity of a putative oxygen-sensor during the transition to anoxia in turtle brain remains unknown. One possible sensor is cytochrome oxidase (cytochrome a,a$_3$) as has been proposed in mammalian carotid body [26]. Since, the redox state of this cytochrome varied more sensitively to changes in tissue oxygenation in turtle than rat brain [27], we suggest that the *in situ* O_2 affinity of the turtle brain cytochrome a,a$_3$ is less than that of rat brain. In intact turtle brain also, lactate increased before full reduction of cytochrome a,a$_3$ during hypoxia [2]. These data indicate that the full reduction of cytochrome oxidase (or anoxia itself) is not the signal for anaerobic glycolysis. Rather, glycolysis may be closely linked to shifts in the cytochrome redox state which could account for the apparent higher sensitivity of glycolysis to hypoxia in turtle than rat brain.

ACKNOWLEDGMENTS

We are grateful to Elena Martinez and Raul Busto for their technical support. These studies were supported in part by PHS Grant NS 14325.

REFERENCES

1. Chih, C.P., Z.C. Feng, M. Rosenthal, P.L. Lutz, and T.J. Sick, Energy metabolism, ion homeostasis, and evoked potentials in anoxic turtle brain. *Am J Physiol*, **257**(4 Pt 2): p. R854–60. 1989.
2. Lutz, P.L., P. McMahon, M. Rosenthal, and T.J. Sick, Relationships between aerobic and anaerobic energy production in turtle brain in situ. *Am J Physiol*, **247**(4 Pt 2): p. R740–4. 1984.
3. Lutz, P., G. Nilsson, and M. Perez-Pinzon, Anoxia tolerant animals, from a neurobiological perspective. *Comp. Biochem. Physiol.*, : p. In press. 1995.
4. Nilsson, G.E. and P.L. Lutz, Release of inhibitory neurotransmitters in response to anoxia in turtle brain. *Am J Physiol*, **261**(1 Pt 2): p. R32–7. 1991.
5. Perez-Pinzon, M.A., M. Rosenthal, P.L. Lutz, and T.J. Sick, Anoxic survival of the isolated cerebellum of the turtle Pseudemis scripta elegans. *J Comp Physiol [b]*, **162**(1): p. 68–73. 1992.
6. Sick, T.J., M. Rosenthal, J.C. LaManna, and P.L. Lutz, Brain potassium ion homeostasis, anoxia, and metabolic inhibition in turtles and rats. *Am J Physiol*, **243**(3): p. R281–8. 1982.
7. Kelly, D.A. and K.B. Storey, Organ-specific control of glycolysis in anoxic turtles. *Am J Physiol*, **255**(5 Pt 2): p. R774–9. 1988.
8. Feng, Z.C., M. Rosenthal, and T.J. Sick, Suppression of evoked potentials with continued ion transport during anoxia in turtle brain. *Am J Physiol*, **255**(3 Pt 2): p. R478–84. 1988.
9. Perez-Pinzon, M.A., M. Rosenthal, T.J. Sick, P.L. Lutz, J. Pablo, and D. Mash, Downregulation of sodium channels during anoxia: a putative survival strategy of turtle brain. *Am J Physiol*, **262**(4 Pt 2): p. R712–5. 1992.
10. Perez-Pinzon, M.A., C.Y. Chan, M. Rosenthal, and T.J. Sick, Membrane and synaptic activity during anoxia in the isolated turtle cerebellum. *Am J Physiol*, **263**(5 Pt 2): p. R1057–63. 1992.
11. Perez-Pinzon, M., J. Bedford, M. Rosenthal, P. Lutz, and T. Sick. *Metabolic adaptations to anoxia in the isolated turtle cerebellum.* in *Soc. for Neuroscience.* 1991.
12. Gnaiger, E., Heat dissipation and energetic efficiency in animal anoxibiosis: Economy contra power. *J. Exp. Zool.*, **228**: p. 471–490. 1983.
13. Larrabee, M.G., Oxygen consumption of excised sympathetic ganglia at rest and in activity. *J. Neurochem.*, **2**(81–101). 1958.
14. Martin, F.R., J. Sanchez-Ramos, and M. Rosenthal, Selective and nonselective effects of 1-methyl-4-phenylpyridinium on oxygen consumption in rat striatal and hippocampal slices. *J Neurochem*, **57**(4): p. 1340–6. 1991.
15. Lowry, O.H. and J. Passonneau, *A flexible system of enzyme analysis.* 1972, New York: Academic Press.
16. Jackson, D.C., Metabolic depression and oxygen depletion in the diving turtle. *J. Applied Physiol.*, **24**: p. 503–509. 1968.
17. Lipton, P. and T. Wittingham, Energy metabolism and brain slice function, in *Brain Slices*, R. Dingledine, Editor. 1984, Plenum Press: New York and London. p. 113–153.
18. McIlwain, H. and H. Bachelard, *Biochemistry and the Central Nervous System.* 1971, Edinburgh: Churchill Livingston.
19. Robin, E.D., N. Lewiston, A. Newman, L. Simon, and J. Theodore, Bioenergetic pattern of turtle brain and resistance to profound loss of mitochondrial ATP generation. *Proc. Natl. Acad. Sci.*, **76**: p. 3922–3926. 1979.
20. Wu, T. and E. Davies, Regulation of glycolytic flux in energetically controlled free system. *Arch. Biochem.Biophys.*, **209**: p. 85–99. 1981.
21. Duncan, J.A. and K.B. Storey, Subcellular enzyme binding and the regulation of glycolysis in anoxic turtle brain. *Am J Physiol*, **262**(3 Pt 2): p. R517–23. 1992.
22. Siesjo, B., *Brain energy metabolism.* 1978, New York: Wiley.
23. Brooks, S.P. and K.B. Storey, Regulation of glycolytic enzymes during anoxia in the turtle Pseudemys scripta. *Am J Physiol*, **257**(2 Pt 2): p. R278–83. 1989.
24. Hochachka, P.W., Defense strategies against hypoxia and hypothermia. *Science*, **231**(4735): p. 234–41. 1986.
25. Lutz, P., M. Rosenthal, and T. Sick, Living without oxygen: Turtle brain as a model of anaerobic metabolism. *Mol. Physiol.*, **8**: p. 411–425. 1985.
26. Mills, E. and F. Jobsis, Mitochondrial respiratory chain carotid body and chemoreceptor response to changes in oxygen tension. *J. Neurophysiol.*, **35**: p. 405–428. 1972.
27. Sick, T.J., E.P. Chasnoff, and M. Rosenthal, Potassium ion homeostasis and mitochondrial redox status of turtle brain during and after ischemia. *Am J Physiol*, **248**(5 Pt 2): p. R531–40. 1985.

10

AGE-RELATED CHANGES IN BRAIN METABOLISM AND VULNERABILITY TO ANOXIA

Eugene L. Roberts, Jr.,[1,2] Ching-Ping Chih,[2] and Myron Rosenthal[1]

[1]Department of Neurology
University of Miami School of Medicine
Miami, Florida 33136
[2]Geriatric Research, Education, and Clinical Center
Miami VA Medical Center
Miami, Florida 33125

1. INTRODUCTION

Aged brain tissue suffers more histopathological damage following ischemia[1] and greater electrophysiological dysfunction following anoxia[2]. In this short review, we consider the hypothesis that alterations in brain energy metabolism underlie age-related increases in brain vulnerability to anoxia, hypoxia, or ischemia (see also refs. 3–8). Investigations from our laboratories suggest that age-related decreases in the capacity of brain tissue to meet energy demand may limit recovery of ion homeostasis and excitability following large ion shifts or anoxia. These findings are consistent with earlier reports that glycolytic fluxes in rat brain during ischemia[6] and glucose utilization during hyperthermia[9] increased less with age and that resynthesis of depleted metabolic intermediates was slower in aged brains[10]. Such studies further suggest the hypothesis that age-related decreases in the capacity of brain tissue to match energy production to demand may limit recovery after metabolic insults.

2. BRAIN AGING AND RESPONSES TO ION SHIFTS

Aging did not affect the reduction/oxidation (redox) state of cytochrome a,a_3 of 'resting', intact brains[11]. However, when large ion shifts (increased intracellular Na^+ and extracellular K^+) occurred because of cortical spreading depression (CSD), the reduction/oxidation (redox) state of cytochrome a,a_3 transiently shifted toward oxidation in young rats, but toward reduction in aged rats[12]. This suggested that oxidative phosphorylation was adequate for 'resting' but not intensely active conditions in the aged cerebral cortex since reductive shifts of mitochondrial components usually indicate that oxygen use is insufficient to meet heightened electron input to the mitochondrial respiratory chain[13].

The shift toward reduction of cytochrome a,a$_3$ in the aged brain during CSD may be due to limited oxygen delivery (e.g., ref. 14) or to intracellular derangements limiting oxygen use. We tested this latter possibility while eliminating the former possibility by examining oxygen consumption in rat hippocampal slices, which have no cerebrovasculature[15]. As in the intact 'resting' brain (e.g., refs. 7,16–19), oxygen consumption was unchanged by age in the slices. However, when the K$^+$ activity (K^+_o) of the bathing medium was raised, oxygen consumption increased significantly more in young adult slices than in slices from aged rats[15] (Fig. 1).

Activity-induced reductive shifts of cytochrome a,a$_3$ in the intact aged brain, and the smaller, K$^+$-induced increases in oxygen consumption in aged adult slices, demonstrate that aging acts intracellularly to limit the brain's capacity to increase oxidative phosphorylation to meet heightened ATP demand. In a related study of intact rat brains[20], aging prolonged the re-reduction of cytochrome oxidase after oxidative shifts of this cytochrome were evoked by electrocortical stimulation. Since mitochondrial electron transport is tightly coupled to ATP production, slowed re-reduction of cytochrome a,a$_3$ in the aged brain suggested slowed ATP recovery due to prolonged ATP use (i.e., slower or less efficient energy use after stimulation) or to a decreased capacity of cortical tissue to recover metabolically after increased energy demand. We speculate that the derangement underlying these effects of age may limit compensatory processes during anoxia or ischemia and recovery afterward.

3. BRAIN AGING AND ANOXIA

Aging impairs brain tissue survival of anoxia. Evidence for this includes observations that hippocampal slices from aged Fischer 344 rats lost ion homeostasis sooner during anoxia, and recovered K^+_o homeostasis more slowly and synaptic transmission less completely, than slices from younger rats[2]. Age-related alterations in glucose metabolism may have played a major role in these findings. This possibility was examined by manipulating the glucose concentration surrounding slices exposed to short (one minute of anoxic depolarization) anoxia. Increasing the glucose concentration in the artificial cerebrospinal fluid (ACSF) from 5 to 10 mM delayed anoxic depolarization (defined as the sudden loss

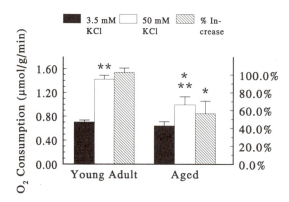

Figure 1. Oxygen consumption in hippocampal slices from young adult (6 mon. old) and aged (26 mon. old) Fischer 344 rats (all males; data and statistical analysis from ref. 15.). Oxygen consumption increased in both age groups when KCl in the artificial cerebrospinal fluid (ACSF) was increased to 50 mM (**- P<0.01 (Duncan's test) for both age groups compared with their respective controls). However, oxygen consumption in 50 mM KCl and the percent increase in oxygen consumption were less in the aged group (*- P<0.05 (Duncan's test)). Error bars in this and subsequent figures are standard errors. For all data bars, n=4 animals.

Figure 2. The effects of age, glucose concentration, and substrate type (glucose or lactate) on the onset of anoxic depolarization (determined from recordings of extracellular K^+ (K^+_o) changes in stratum pyramidale; K^+_o was recorded with double-barrel K^+-sensitive microelectrodes (see ref. 21 for methods). All data and analyses are from ref. 21. 0 mM glucose ACSF used 20 mM sodium lactate as the metabolic substrate instead of glucose. *- in 10 mM glucose, time to anoxic depolarization was greater in the young adult group compared with the other two age groups (P<0.05). **- time to anoxic depolarization was shorter in lactate-containing ACSF compared with ACSF containing 10 or 20 mM glucose (no effect of age) (P<0.01). +- time to anoxic depolarization increased faster between 5 and 10 mM glucose in the young adult group compared with the middle-aged group.

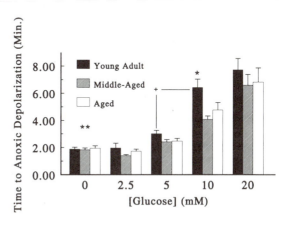

of ion homeostasis during anoxia) in slices (see ref. 21). However, this increase in glucose concentration delayed anoxic depolarization more in slices from young adult (6–9 months old) Fischer 344 rats compared with middle-aged (16–19 months old) rats[21] (Fig. 2). Also, recovery of K^+_o homeostasis following anoxia was fastest at a lower glucose concentration (10 mM) in the young adult group than in the other two age groups (note though that this difference was statistically significant only between the young and middle-aged groups[21]) (Fig. 3). Finally, increasing concentrations of glucose enhanced postanoxic recovery of synaptic transmission least in aged rats compared with young and middle-aged rats[21] (Fig.

Figure 3. The time needed for K^+_o to return to preanoxic levels following anoxia (t_{base}) reached its minimum at a lower glucose concentration in young adult rats compared with the other two age groups. All data and analyses are from ref. 21. *- t_{base} for the young adult group was significantly less than for the other two age groups (P<0.05). **- t_{base} was significantly less in the young adult group compared with the middle-aged group. ++- t_{base} declined faster between 10 and 20 mM glucose in middle-aged rats compared with young adult rats (P<0.05) due to t_{base} already reaching its minimum in 10 mM glucose in the young adult group. ##- t_{base} was longer in 20 mM lactate ACSF than in 10 or 20 mM glucose (no effect of age) (P<0.01).

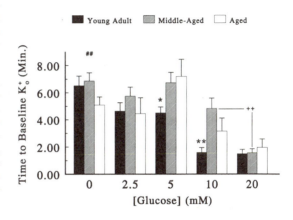

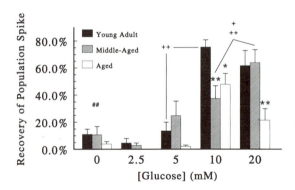

Figure 4. Age-related differences in the influence of glucose concentration on recovery of synaptic transmission from anoxia. 'Recovery of Population Spike' refers to the percent recovery of the orthodromic population spike recorded in hippocampal subfield CA1 one hour after cessation of anoxia. Recordings of the orthodromic population spike were made from the reference barrel of the K_o^+-sensitive microelectrode. All data and analyses are from ref. 21. The absence of a data bar for the aged group in 2.5 mM glucose indicates that none of the aged slices recovered synaptic transmission. 10 mM glucose:*- lower than the young adult group (P<0.05); **- lower than the young adult group (P<0.01). 20 mM glucose: **- lower than other two age groups (P<0.01). ##- Recovery of synaptic transmission was significantly less in lactate-containing ACSF compared with ACSF containing 10 or 20 mM glucose (no effect of age) (P<0.05). Increasing glucose from 5 to 10 mM: ++- Recovery of the orthodromic population spike rose faster in young adults than in middle-aged adults (P<0.01). Increasing glucose from 10 to 20 mM: Recovery increased in this interval in the middle-aged group compared with the young adult (+- P<0.05) and aged adult (++- P<0.01) groups.

4). These results suggest that aging diminished the ability of brain tissue to increase glucose metabolism to meet energy demands during and after anoxia.

Age-related declines in glycolytic capacity may have been one way that aging altered the brain's metabolic response to anoxia. This possibility was studied by comparing the responses of slices from different age groups to anoxia when glycolysis was eliminated in slices by substituting 20 mM lactate for glucose. In all age groups, age-related differences in responses to anoxia (i.e., times to anoxic depolarization and postanoxic recovery of K_o^+ homeostasis and synaptic transmission) reported earlier[2] were not seen in the absence of glycolysis[21] (Figs. 2–4). Also, all responses resembled those in 2.5 or 5 mM glucose, and were significantly different from those in 10 or 20 mM glucose[21] (Figs. 2–4).

While age-related alterations in anaerobic glycolysis may be one explanation for earlier anoxic depolarization in middle-aged and aged hippocampal slices, other possible explanations include lower ATP or phosphocreatine (PCr) levels before anoxia, or inefficient use of ATP or PCr during anoxia. Loss of ion homeostasis during anoxia in the brain has been tied to ATP levels (e.g., ref. 22 (review)). However, earlier anoxic depolarization with aging could not have been due to lower ATP or PCr levels before anoxia since the levels of these high energy phosphates were unchanged by age, as well as by glucose concentration or substrate[21] (glucose compared with 20 mM lactate) (Fig. 5A). Also, aging did not alter energy demand or efficiency of energy use during anoxia since anoxic depolarization occurred at similar times in all age groups when lactate was used as the metabolic substrate[21] (Fig. 2).

After anoxia, lower ATP or PCr levels might have contributed to decreased post-anoxic recovery of synaptic transmission, particularly in the aged group, since successful synaptic transmission needs sufficient ATP levels (e.g., ref. 23). However, like the

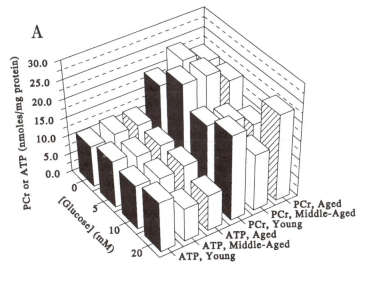

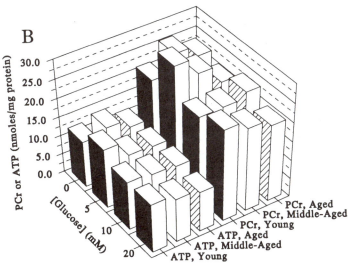

Figure 5. Aging did not affect ATP or PCr levels before or one hour after anoxia. A. Before Anoxia: For each bar, the number of slices used was equal to 1–3. Data are from ref. 21, where data were presented with respect to age only. B: One hour after anoxia, ATP ($P<0.05$, $F_{1,33}=6.67$) and PCr ($P<0.01$, $F_{1,33}=7.69$) increased compared with preanoxic values. For each ATP or PCr data bar, the number of slices used per glucose concentration was (1) 0 mM glucose (20 mM lactate): 3 (all age groups); (2) 5 mM glucose: 2 (young adult) and 3 (middle-aged and aged); (3) 10 mM glucose: 3 (young adult and middle-aged) and 2 (aged); and (4) 20 mM glucose: 5 (young adult), 2 (middle-aged), and 1 (aged). A three-way analysis of variance was used to analyze all data in this figure. Only one slice was used per rat.

preanoxic period, ATP and PCr levels were unchanged by age, glucose concentration, or substrate (Fig. 5B). In fact, ATP and PCr levels were higher after anoxia than before anoxia (Fig. 5B). Thus, age-related differences in post-anoxic recovery of synaptic transmission could not have been due to lack of recovery of ATP or PCr levels from anoxia.

4. DISCUSSION

Aging compromises the ability of brain tissue to meet metabolic challenges imposed by spreading depression, elevated K^+_o, or anoxia[12,15,21]. These age-related limitations were not apparent in 'resting' conditions, where the redox state of cytochrome a,a_3[12], oxygen consumption[15], and tissue levels of ATP and PCr[21] were unchanged by age. The influence of aging on energy metabolism in the brain may be analogous to a failing heart, which may function adequately under a normal work load, but not when challenged with increased activity or metabolic insults.

Our studies suggest at least two potential loci for age-related alterations in energy metabolism that may reduce the brain's capacity to respond to metabolic challenges. First, aging may decrease the availability of electrons for reducing molecular oxygen, perhaps via age-related changes in the cytochrome oxidase complex. A reduced availability of electrons could explain smaller peak oxygen consumption in hippocampal slices from aged rats[15]. Findings that cortical spreading depression caused greater reduction of cytochrome a,a_3 in aged brains[12] support altered electron transfer.

Second, aging may decrease the brain's capacity to increase glycolytic ATP production in response to metabolic challenges. This possibility is suggested from the responses of hippocampal slices to anoxia. With glucose available as the metabolic substrate, slices from aged rats were more vulnerable to anoxia. However, with lactate as the substrate, age-related differences in responses to anoxia disappeared. Since glucose (but not lactate) metabolism requires glycolysis, these results suggest that aging may decrease the brain's capacity to augment glycolytic ATP production in response to anoxia. Such a limitation on glycolysis could also underlie a limitation on the aging brain's ability to increase oxygen consumption.

Either of the putative age-related derangements described above could diminish the capacity of aged brain to withstand anoxia or ischemia. Additional studies will be required to define the mechanism(s) underlying these derangements to determine whether links exist between these changes and the aging brain's susceptibility to anoxic or ischemic insults.

5. ACKNOWLEDGMENTS

Work reported here was supported in part by PHS grant AG08710 (ELR), and by a grant from the American Federation for Aging Research (AFAR) (ELR).

6. REFERENCES

1. Yao H, Sadoshima S, Ooboshi H, Sato Y, Uchimura H, Fujishima M. Age-related vulnerability to cerebral ischemia in spontaneously hypertensive rats. Stroke 1991;22(11):1414–8.
2. Roberts EL Jr, Rosenthal M, Sick TJ. Age-related modifications of potassium homeostasis and synaptic transmission during and after anoxia in rat hippocampal slices. Brain Res 1990;514(1):111–8.
3. Benzi G, Arrigoni E, Agnoli A, et al. Influence of age upon the cerebral metabolic changes induced by acute hypoxia on the synaptosomes from dog brain. Exp Gerontol 1982;17(1):19–31.
4. Benzi G, Agnoli A, Giuffrida AM. Influence of aging on cerebral derangement by acute severe hypoxia during hypovolemic hypotension. Neurobiol Aging 1984;5(3):213–20.
5. Hoffman WE, Albrecht RF, Miletich DJ. Cerebrovascular response to hypoxia in young vs aged rats. Stroke 1984;15(1):129–33.

6. Hoyer S, Krier C. Ischemia and aging brain. Studies on glucose and energy metabolism in rat cerebral cortex. Neurobiol Aging 1986;7(1):23–9.
7. Benzi G, Giuffrida AM. Changes of synaptosomal energy metabolism induced by hypoxia during aging. Neurochem Res 1987;12:149–57.
8. Benzi G, Pastoris O, Vercesi L, Gorini A, Viganotti C, Villa RF. Energetic state of aged brain during hypoxia. Gerontol 1987;33(3–4):207–12.
9. Parmacek MS, Fox JH, Harrison WH, Garron DC, Swenie D. Effect of aging on brain respiration and carbohydrate metabolism of CBF1 mice. Gerontol 1979;25(4):185–91.
10. McNamara M, Miller A, Shen A, Wood J. Restitution of ATP and creatine phosphate after experimental depletion in young, adult, and old rats. Gerontol 1978;24:95–103.
11. Sylvia AL, Rosenthal M. The effect of age and lung pathology on cytochrome a,a_3 redox levels in rat cerebral cortex. Brain Res 1978;146(1):109–22.
12. Sylvia AL, Rosenthal M. Effects of age on brain oxidative metabolism in vivo. Brain Res 1979;165(2):235–48.
13. Chance B, Williams GR. The respiratory chain and oxidative phosphorylation. Adv Enzymol 1956;17:65–134.
14. Milito SJ, Raffin CN, Rosenthal M, Sick TJ. Potassium ion homeostasis and mitochondrial redox activity in brain: relative changes as indicators of hypoxia. J Cereb Blood Flow Metab 1988;8(2):155–62.
15. Martin FR, Roberts EL Jr, Rosenthal M. Potassium-induced increases in oxygen consumption are diminished by age in rat hippocampal slices [published erratum appears in Brain Res 1989 Sep 11;497(1):204]. Brain Res 1989;492(1–2):392–6.
16. Garbus J. Respiration of brain homogenates of old and young rats. Am J Physiol 1955;183:618–9.
17. Lassen NA, Feinberg I, Lane MH. Bilateral studies of cerebral oxygen uptake in aged and normal subjects and in patients with organic dementia. J Clin Invest 1960;39:491–500.
18. Fox JH, Parmacek MS, Patel-Mandlik K. Effect of aging on brain respiration and carbohydrate metabolism of Syrian hamsters. Gerontologia 1975;21(4):224–30.
19. Buchweitz-Milton E, Weiss HR. Cerebral oxygen consumption and blood flow in Fischer-344 rats of different ages. Neurobiol Aging 1987;8:55–60.
20. Sylvia AL, Harik SL, LaManna JC, Wilkerson T, Rosenthal M. Abnormalities of cerebral oxidative metabolism with aging and their relation to the central noradrenergic system. Gerontol 1983;29:248–61.
21. Roberts EL, Chih CP. Age-related alterations in energy metabolism contribute to the increased vulnerability of the aging brain to anoxic damage. Brain Res 1995;678(1–2):83–90.
22. Hansen AJ. Effect of anoxia on ion distribution in the brain. Physiol Rev 1985;65:101–47.
23. Yamamoto C, Kurokawa M. Synaptic potentials recorded in brain slices and their modification by changes in the level of tissue ATP. Exp Brain Res 1970;10:159–70.

11

[BASE EXCESS] VS [STRONG ION DIFFERENCE]

Which Is More Helpful?

Robert Schlichtig

Departments of Anesthesiology and Critical Care Medicine; Medicine; and
    Surgery
University of Pittsburgh
V.A. Medical Center
Pittsburgh, Pennsylvania 15240

ABSTRACT

Blood [base excess] ([BE]) is defined as the change in [strong acid] or [strong base] needed to restore pH to normal at normal PCO_2. Some believe that [BE] is unhelpful because [BE] may be elevated with a "normal" [strong ion difference] ([SID]), where a strong ion is one that is always dissociated in physiological solution, and where [SID] = [strong cations] - [strong anions]. Using a computer simulation, the hypothesis was tested that [SID] = [SID Excess] ([SIDEx]), where [SIDEx] is the change in [SID] needed to restore pH to normal at normal PCO_2. The most current version of the plasma [SID] ($[SID]_p$) equation was used as a template, and an [SIDEx] formula, of the Siggaard-Andersen form, derived: $[SIDEx]_p = [HCO_3^-]_p - 24.72 + (pH_p - 7.4) \times (1.159 \times [alb]_p + 0.423 \times [Pi]_p)$. [SID] was compared to [SIDEx] over the physiologic range of plasma buffering, and it was found that [SIDEx] varied by ~ 15 mM at any given [SID], thereby faulting the hypothesis. It is concluded that [SID] can be "normal" with an elevated [SIDEx], the latter being an expression of the [BE] concept, and a more helpful quantity in physiology.

The "metabolic" component of a given acid-base disturbance is usually estimated as whole blood [base excess] ($[BE]_{WB}$), where $[BE]_{WB}$ is defined as the change in [strong acid] or [strong base] needed to restore plasma pH (pH_p) to 7.4 at PCO_2 of 40 Torr [1-3]. However, the [BE] approach has been criticized as "inadequate for interpretation of complex acid-base derangements such as those seen in critically ill patients [4-5]." The proposed alternative is the strong ion difference (SID) method, where a strong ion is one that is always dissociated in solution, and where [SID] = [strong cations] - [strong anions] [4-8].

On the one hand, it does not seem possible, by the definitions of these entities, to change [SID] without also changing [BE]. On the other hand, a selected group of critically ill patients with hypoproteinemia has been reported in whom [SID] was "normal" (i.e. ~

40 mEq·l^{-1}) but [BE]$_{WB}$ clearly increased [4,5,9]. The idea was that hypoproteinemia caused the alkalosis, due to a deficiency of plasma weak acid buffer, necessitating increased [HCO$_3$$^-$]$_p$ to maintain electrical neutrality. How could [SID] be "normal," but [BE] increased? The purpose of the current exercise was to address this question. An [SID excess] ([SIDEx]) formula was developed, conceptually identical to Siggaard-Andersen's [BE], and [SID] was compared to [SIDEx] over the physiological range of plasma [albumin] ([alb]$_p$), plasma [phosphate] ([Pi]$_p$), and plasma pH (pH$_p$).

METHODS

The unabridged SID formula of Figge et al. [8] was used. On a computer spread sheet, pH was varied between 7.6 and 6.8, in 0.0055 pH unit decrements. [SID]$_p$ was held constant at 40 mEq·l^{-1}, so that plasma [albumin] ([alb]$_p$), and [Pi]$_p$ could be treated as independent variables. PCO$_2$ was solved using the Figge formula:

$$PCO_2 = \{[SID]_p + 1000 \times ([H^+]_p - K_w/[H^+]_p) - [Pi]_p \times Z + 10E4 \times [alb]_p \times X/66500\}/1000$$
$$\times (K_{c1}/[H^+]_p - K_{c1} \times K_{c2}/[H^+]_p^2) \tag{1}$$

where $Z = (K_1 \times [H^+]_p^2 + 2 \times K_1 \times K_2 \times [H^+]_p + 3 \times K_1 \times K_2 \times K_3)/([H^+]_p^3 + K_1 \times [H^+]_p^2 + K_1 \times K_2 \times [H^+]_p + K_1 \times K_2 \times K_3)$

where all quantities are plasma quantities; where K$_w$; K$_{c1}$ and K$_{c2}$; and K$_1$, K$_2$, K$_3$ are equilibrium constants for water; the carbonic acid system; and phosphoric acid systems, respectively; where X is the net negative electrical charge per albumin molecule at pH$_p$, and where [alb]$_p$ and [Pi]$_p$ are in mg·dl^{-1} and mEq·l^{-1}, respectively. Correct input of Eq. 1 onto the computer spread sheet was checked by comparing [SID]$_p$ to [SID]$_p$ given by the abridged formula of Figge et al., i.e.

$$[SID]_p = 1000 \times K_{c1} \times PCO_2/(10^{-pHp}) + 10 \times [alb]_p \times (0.123 \times pH_p - 0.631) + [Pi]_p \times (0.309$$
$$\times pH_p - 0.469). \tag{2}$$

Development of Siggaard-Andersen [SID]$_p$ and [SIDEx]$_p$ Formulae from the Figge Formula

With [SID]$_p$ set constant at 40 mM, the relation of [HCO$_3$$^-$]$_p$ vs pH$_p$ was analyzed by linear regression over the pH$_p$ range of 6.8 to 7.6 for each possible combination of [Pi]$_p$ and [alb]$_p$, where [Pi]$_p$ = 0, 1, 2, or 3 mEq·l^{-1}; and where [alb]$_p$ = 1, 2, 3, 4, 5, or 6 mg·dl^{-1}. The slope and y-intercept of each [HCO$_3$$^-$]$_p$ vs pH$_p$ relation was expressed as a linear function of [alb]$_p$ at each [Pi]$_p$. The change in slope and y-intercept per change in [Pi]$_p$ was computed iteratively.

The overall relation between [BE]$_p$, [alb]$_p$, and [Pi]$_p$ was expressed in the Siggaard-Andersen form, [SID]$_p$ = [HCO$_3$$^-$]$_p$ + [A$^-$]$_p$, where A$^-$ is negatively charged, non-volatile, weak acid buffer. The accuracy of the resulting formula was compared to the Figge formula (Eq. 1) over the range of [SID]$_p$ from 10 to 50 mEq·l^{-1}, with [alb]$_p$ and [Pi]$_p$ changing over the above range, totalling 483 data points.

[SIDEx]$_p$ for any given ([alb]$_p$, [Pi]$_p$, pH$_p$, PCO$_2$) data set was computed by solving Eq. 2 for the [alb]$_p$ and [Pi]$_p$, at pH$_p$ = 7.40, PCO$_2$ = 40 Torr. The [SIDEx]$_p$ formula was expressed in the Siggaard-Andersen format [1-3], i.e. [SIDEx]$_p$ = [HCO$_3$$^-$]$_p$ - normal [HCO$_3$$^-$]$_p$

+ (pH$_p$ - 7.4) × B. The accuracy of this formula was verified by comparing [SIDEx]$_p$ to [SIDEx]$_p$ computed directly from the Figge formula.

Comparison of [SID]$_P$ to [SIDEx]$_P$

To test the hypothesis that [SID]$_p$ = [SIDEx]$_p$, the difference between maximum and minimum [SIDEx]$_p$ was computed at each [SID]$_p$ (n = 483 data sets).

RESULTS

At constant [SID]$_p$, all [HCO$_3^-$]$_p$ vs pH$_p$ relations were linear ($r^2 \geq 0.999$). At [Pi]$_p$ = 0 mM, the relation between [HCO$_3^-$]$_p$, pH$_p$, and [alb]$_p$ was:

$$[HCO_3^-]_p = (-1.159 \times [alb]_p - 0.00166) \times pH + 5.827293 \times [alb]_p + 40 \qquad (3)$$

To correct this relation for variable [Pi]$_p$, it was found that 0.42326 × [Pi]$_p$ could be subtracted from the slope of this relation; while adding 1.277 × [Pi]$_p$, to the y-intercept of this relation. The overall relation between pH$_p$, [HCO$_3^-$]$_p$, [alb]$_p$, and [Pi]$_p$, in the Siggaard-Andersen (OSA) form [1-3], was:

$$[SID]_p = [HCO_3^-]_p + pH_p \times [(1.159 \times [alb]_p + 0.00166) + (0.42326 \times [Pi]_p)] - 5.827293 \times$$
$$[alb]_p - 1.277 \times [Pi]_p \qquad (4)$$

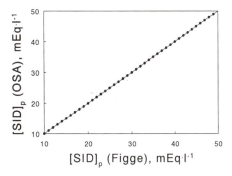

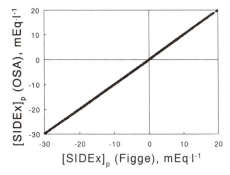

Figure 1. (top panel) shows the relation between [SID]$_p$ calculated directly, using Figge's formula; and [SID]$_p$, calculated using Eq. 4, which is written in the Siggaard-Andersen (OSA) format. The slope of the relation was 1.0; the y-intercept 0.0, and r^2 was 1.0. Fig. 1 (bottom panel) shows the relation between [SIDEx]$_p$, calculated using Figge's formula, and [SIDEx]$_p$, calculated using Eq. 5. The slope of this relation was 1.0; the y-intercept 0.06, and r^2 was 1.0.

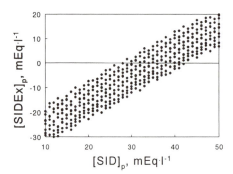

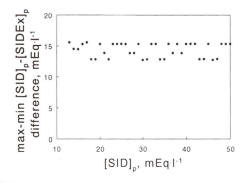

Figure 2. (top panel) shows the relation between $[SID]_p$ and $[SIDEx]_p$, which is analagous to comparing $[SID]_p$ to $[BE]_p$. At any given $[SID]_p$, $[SIDEx]_p$ was widely variable. Even though $[SID]_p$ might be "normal" at ~ 40 $mEq \cdot l^{-1}$, the change in [strong acid or base] (i.e. the change in $[SID]$) needed to restore pH to normal at normal PCO_2 may be large. Fig. 2 (bottom panel) shows that the maximum-minimum difference between $[SID]_p$ and $[SIDEx]_p$ at any given $[SIDE]_p$ averaged about 15 $mEq \cdot l^{-1}$.

The Siggaard-Andersen form of the $[SIDEx]_p$ equation was:

$$[SIDEx]_p = [HCO_3^-]_p - 24.72 + (pH_p - 7.4) \times (1.159 \times [alb]_p + 0.423 \times [Pi]_p) \qquad (5)$$

DISCUSSION

[SIDEx] is idéntical to Siggaard-Andersen's [BE] approach to acid-base. [SIDEx] = [BE]. $[SIDEx]_p$ is simple to compute (Eq. 5), accurately (Fig. 1). This analysis further shows that [SID] is not the same as [SIDEx] (Fig. 2). It is therefore incorrect to conclude [4,5,9] that hypoalbuminemia is the cause of an alkalosis, on the basis that $[SID]_p$ is "normal," because an $[SID]_p$ of 40 mM is not normal for a patient with decreased $[alb]_p$ and/or $[Pi]_p$ (Fig. 2). In order to restore pH_p to normal, it would be necessary for kidneys to remove strong base from plasma, which would cause $[SID]_p$ to be less, and this smaller $[SID]_p$ would then be "normal."

At the heart of this controversy is the question, "in physiology, which independent variable is regulated to restore pH_p to normal: [SID] or [non-volatile weak acid buffer]?" In a test tube, either [SID] or [albumin] may be varied [6,7,10]. In physiology, however, kidneys regulate [SID], and liver regulates [albumin]. Kidneys are primarily responsible for retaining or excreting strong cations or strong anions, and can generally do so within a day or so of a change in acid-base status. Liver synthesizes albumin, the most important non-volatile plasma weak acid buffer, but is not generally considered a modulator of acid-base status. In fact, $[alb]_p$ changes very slowly in patients [11], by about 0.1 $mg \cdot dl^{-1} day^{-1}$, including those who have recently been very severely traumatized [12], i.e. those who are truly critically ill. Therefore, a patient with a "normal" $[SID]_p$; decreased $[albumin]_p$; and increased [BE] (or [SIDEx]) does not have a "primary hypoproteinemic alkalosis" [9], but rather has a "metabolic alkalosis" (Fig. 2), because kidneys have not, for whatever reason (usually dehydration or zealous use of diuretics), compensated for the (slowly) decreasing $[alb]_p$. The concept of a "normal" [SID] is flawed, and [BE] remains the most appropriate conceptual approach to acid-base [13].

REFERENCES

1. Siggaard-Andersen, O. *The acid-base status of blood* (Fourth Edition), Copenhagen, Munksgaard, 1974, pp. 80–83.
2. Siggaard-Andersen O. The Van Slyke equation. *Scand. J. Clin. Lab. Invest.* 37; 15–20, Suppl. 146, 1977.
3. Siggaard-Andersen O, Wimberley PD, Fogh-Andersen N, Gøthgen IH. Measured and derived quantities with modern pH and blood gas equipment: calculation algorithms with 54 equations. Scand. J. Clin. Lab. Invest. 48, Supp. 198, 7–15, 1988.
4. Fencl V, Leith DE. Stewart's quantitative acid-base chemistry: applications in biology and medicine. Resp. Physiol. 91: 1–16, 1994.
5. Fencl V, Rossing TH. Acid-base disorders in critical care medicine. Ann. Rev. Med. 40: 17–29, 1989.
6. Stewart, P.A. *How to Understand Acid-Base: A Quantitative Acid-Base Primer for Biology and Medicine.* New York: Elsevier/North-Holland, 1981, Table 7.3.
7. Stewart, P.A. Modern quantitative acid-base chemistry. *Can. J. Physiol. Pharmacol.* 61: 1444–1461, 1983.
8. Figge, J., T. Mydosh, and V. Fencl. Serum proteins and acid-base equilibria: a follow-up. *J. Lab. Clin. Med.* 120: 713–719, 1992.
9. McAuliffe JJ, Lind LJ, Leith DE, Fencl V. Hyproproteinemic alkalosis. Am. J. Med.81: 86–90, 1986.
10. Rossing TH, Maffeo N, Fencl V. Acid-base effects of altering plasma protein concentration in human blood in vitro. *J. Appl. Physiol.* 61: 2260–2265, 1986
11. Courtney ME, Greene HL, Folk CC, Helinek GL, Dmitruk A. Rapidly declining serum albumin values in newly hospitalized patients: prevalence, severity, and contributory factors. JPEN 6: 143–145, 1982.
12. Sganga G,Siegel JH, Brown G, Coleman B, Wiles CE, Belzberg H, Wedel S. Reprioritization of hepatic plasma protein release in trauma and sepsis. Arch Surg 120: 187–199, 1985.
13. Schlichtig R. Base excess - a powerful clinical tool in the ICU. *Critical Care State of the Art*, Society of Critical Care Medicine, volume 17, 1996 (in press).

12

[BASE EXCESS] AND [STRONG ION DIFFERENCE] DURING O_2-CO_2 EXCHANGE

Robert Schlichtig

Departments of Anesthesiology and Critical Care Medicine; Medicine; and
  Surgery
University of Pittsburgh
V.A. Medical Center
Pittsburgh, Pennsylvania 15240

ABSTRACT

Detecting uptake or production of "metabolic acid" by a given tissue is often of interest. [Base excess] ([BE]) is the change in [strong acid] or [strong base] needed to restore pH to normal at normal PCO_2. However, [BE] seems to have the potential for minor inaccuracy during hypercarbia, and venous blood is hypercarbic relative to arterial. Another approach is [strong ion difference] ([SID]), where a strong ion is one that is always dissociated in solution, and where [SID] = [strong cation] - [strong anion]. The hypothesis was tested that a-v $[SID]_p$ might be used to detect metabolic acid uptake or production by tissue. A computer simulation of O_2-CO_2 exchange was performed, using the Siggaard-Andersen [BE] equations, which provide an existing conceptual template. It was assumed that a change in [BE] = a change in [SID] (Adv. Exp. Med. Biol., in press). (A-v) $[SID]_p$ decreased linearly with decreasing $[HbO_2]$ during equimolar O_2-CO_2 exchange (Δ mEq $[SID]_p \cdot l^{-1}$ per Δ $gHbO_2 \cdot dl^{-1}$ = 0.6, r^2 = 1.0), and erythrocyte [BE] ($[BE]_e$) and $[SID]_e$ decreased commensurately, such that $[BE]_{WB}$ remained constant. These changes represent ion exchanges between erythrocyte and plasma, governed by the Gibbs-Donnan equilibrium. It is concluded that a-v $[SID]_p$ may be used to examine a-v differences in [metabolic acid], based on [BE] concepts.

The concentration of "metabolic acid" ([metabolic acid]) in blood increases during endotoxemia [1], exercise [2,3,4] and shock [5]. To identify organ(s) responsible, it is necessary to measure arteriovenous [strong acid]. Two methods are available.

Whole blood base excess ($[BE]_{WB}$), is the change in [strong acid]$_{WB}$ or [strong base]$_{WB}$ needed to restore plasma pH (pH_p) to 7.4 at PCO_2 of 40 torr, and is an excellent method for distinguishing "respiratory," from "metabolic" acidosis in arterial blood [6,7,8]. However, while [BE] is most helpful conceptually [9], use of [BE] in venous blood presents two problems. First, $[BE]_{WB}$ may employ *in vitro* assumptions that are slightly inaccurate during hypercarbia *in vivo* [8,10,11], and venous blood is hypercarbic relative to arterial. The problem seems to be that [BE] assumes greater [hemoglobin] ([Hb]) than is actually effective *in vivo*, where Hb is diluted in the extracellular volume. The "Van Slyke" version [7] of the $[BE]_{WB}$ equation is:

$$BE]_{WB} = \{[HCO_3^-]_p - 24.4 + (2.3 \times [Hb] + 7.7) \times (pH_p - 7.4)\} \times (1-0.023 \times [Hb]) \quad (1)$$

This equation may be thought of conceptually as:

$$[BE] = ([HCO_3^-] + [A^-]) - (normal\ [HCO_3^-] + normal\ [A^-]) \quad (2)$$

where A^- is negatively charged non-volatile weak acid. Missing or excess charges are attributed to abnormal [strong acid] or [strong base], and $[A^-]_{WB}$ is computed using actual, as opposed to effective, [Hb]. This problem has been adequately addressed in arterial blood by standard $[BE]_{WB}$ ($[SBE]_{WB}$) [12], by assuming that effective [Hb] *in vivo* is approximately one third of that *in vitro*. However, it is not clear whether this assumption is sufficiently accurate to examine arteriovenous differences.

A second and related problem with using [BE] to detect (a-v) differences is the magnitude of change in Hb buffering *in vivo* during O_2 desaturation. Desaturation renders Hb a stronger weak acid buffer, i.e. increases its effective pK value. Consequently, $[HCO_3^-]_p$ is greater at any given PCO_2, creating the appearance of a larger $[BE]_{WB}$, whereas [strong acid] or [strong base] has not changed. This artifact can be corrected using the "O_2 desaturation transform factor," [4] which is $0.19\ mM\cdot \Delta\ g\ [HbO_2]\cdot dl^{-1}$ *in vitro* [6]. *In vivo*, however, the magnitude of the O_2 desaturation transform factor might be different.

An alternative approach to acid-base analysis is strong ion difference (SID) [13,14,15], where a strong ion is one that is always dissociated in physiologic solution. [SID] can usually be approximated as: $[Na^+] + [K^+] - [Cl^-] - [La^-]$. Although [BE] does not equal [SID], a change in [BE] must always accompany a change in [SID], and vice-versa [9]. While the [SID] approach is tedious, and often unnecessarily so, [SID] can be measured directly, free of assumptions regarding buffering. Using the [BE] conceptual approach to hypercarbia and desaturation, perhaps $[SID]_p$ might be used to assess arteriovenous (a-v) differences. The purpose of the present exercise is to use the [BE] concept to quantify (a-v) $[SID]_p$ during simulated O_2-CO_2 exchange, to see how (a-v) $[SID]_p$ might be used to measure tissue metabolic acid uptake or production.

METHODS

The Van Slyke equations of Siggaard-Andersen [7,16] were used to model $[BE]_p$, $[BE]_e$, and $[BE]_{WB}$ during hypercarbia and desaturation:

$$[HCO_3^-]_e = [HCO_3^-]_p \times 0.835 \times antilog\ (1.492 - 0.23 \times pH_p) \quad (3)$$

$$pH_e = 7.19 + 0.77 \times (pH_p - 7.4) + 0.035 \times (1-sO_2) \quad (4)$$

$$[BE]_e = [HCO_3^-]_e - 12.6 + 63 \times (pH_e - 7.19) \quad (5)$$

$$[BE]_{WB} = (1 - Ht) \times [BE]_p + Ht \times [BE]_e \quad (6)$$

where equations 2 and 3 represent expressions of the Gibbs-Donnan equilibrium between plasma and erythrocyte, i.e. $[H^+]_p/[H^+]_e = [Cl^-]_e/[Cl^-]_p = [HCO_3^-]_e/[HCO_3^-]_p$, these ratios depending on pH [17]. This requirement causes HCO_3^- formed within erythrocyte to exchange with plasma Cl^- [18,19,20].

Simulation of Respiratory Acidosis, without O_2 Exchange

The condition simulated was $[BE]_{WB} = 0$ mM, $[Hb] = 12$ g·dl^{-1}, $\%HbO_2 = 100\%$. $[HCO_3^-]_p$ was calculated using Eq. 1, starting with pH = 7.40. PCO_2 was calculated using pH_p, $[HCO_3^-]_p$ and the Henderson-Hasselbalch equation. pH_p was then progressively decreased from 7.40 to 7.21 in arbitrary 0.01 unit decrements. For each $(pH_p, [HCO_3^-]_p, PCO_2)$ data triplet, $[BE]_e$ and $[HCO_3^-]_e$ were calculated using Eqs. 2 - 4. The change in [BE] (Δ [BE]) in whole blood, erythrocyte, and plasma was assumed equal to Δ [SID] [9]. Δ [SID] was expressed as the change from the starting value, i.e. the value calculated at pH_p = 7.4, PCO_2 = 40 Torr.

Simulation of O_2-CO_2 Exchange

The condition studied was RQ = 1.0, $[Hb] = 12$ g·dl^{-1} %, $HbO_2a = 100$, $pH_pa = 7.40$, $PaCO_2 = 40$ Torr. O_2-CO_2 exchange for this condition was simulated over the HbO_2v range of 100% to 0%, using a previously described [21] method that gives pH_pv and $[HCO_3^-]_pv$ for any given $\%HbO_2v$. For each $(\%HbO_2v, pH_pv, [HCO_3^-]_pv)$ data triplet, venous $[BE]_{WB}$ ($[BE]_{WB}v$) was taken as:

$$[BE]_{WB}v = \{[HCO_3^-]_pv - 24.4 + (2.3 \times [Hb]v + 7.7) \times (pH_pv - 7.4)\} \times (1-0.023 \text{ x } [Hb]v) - 0.19 \text{ mM·}\Delta [HbO_2]^{-1} \tag{7}$$

where $[HbO_2]$ is in g·dl^{-1}, and 0.19 mM·$\Delta [HbO_2]^{-1}$ is the "O_2 saturation transform factor" [4], representing the apparant, as opposed to actual, change in $[BE]_{WB}$ during desaturation. This O_2 desaturation transform factor corrects $[BE]_{WB}$ only for the increment in $[HCO_3^-]_p$ due to the changed pK of desaturated hemoglobin. Venous $[BE]_e$ ($[BE]_ev$) was calculated by solving Eq. 5 for $[BE]_e$.

RESULTS

Figure 1 shows the relation between [BE] (top panel) and $[HCO_3^-]$ (bottom panel) predicted by the Siggaard-Andersen formulae in whole blood, plasma, and erythrocyte as PCO_2 increased from 40 to 75 Torr in fully saturated blood. While $[BE]_{WB}$, by definition, remained constant, $[BE]_p$ increased progressively, whereas $[BE]_e$ decreased progressively. $[SID]_p$, like $[BE]_p$ was not constant as PCO_2 varied, because of plasma-erythrocyte ion exchanges governed by the Gibbs-Donnan equilibrium.

Figure 2 simulates blood transit from artery ($\%HbO_2 = 100$) to vein ($\%HbO_2$ varying from 100 to 0). The top panel shows the changes in $[BE]_p$ and $[BE]_e$, which were qualitatively the same as the changes occurring during hypercarbia alone (Fig. 1). However, the magnitude of change was greater, because Hb becomes a "stronger" weak acid buffer when desaturated. Again, $[BE]_{WB}$ remained constant. The bottom panel of Fig. 2 shows (a-v) differences in $[SID]_p$ and $[HCO_3^-]_p$ as a function of (a-v) $[HbO_2]$, showing how a-v $[SID]_p$ or $[HCO_3^-]_p$ might be used to detect metabolic acid production or uptake. During O_2

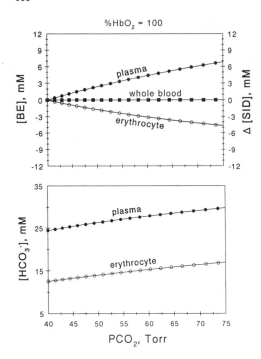

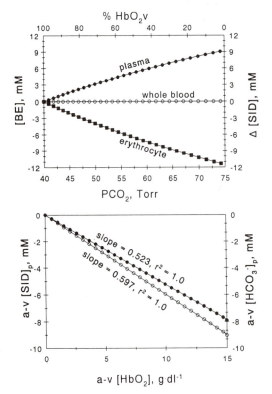

Figure 1. Behavior of [base excess] (top panel) and [HCO₃⁻] (bottom panel) as a function of PCO₂, predicted by the Siggaard-Andersen equations *in vitro*. In this simulation, [Hb] is 15 g·dl⁻¹, and %HbO₂ is 100. Δ [SID] is the change in [SID] relative to [SID] at PCO₂ of 40 torr, and is assumed equal to [BE] [9] in this simulation.

Figure 2. Behavior of [BE], [SID], and [HCO₃⁻] during progressive O₂-CO₂ exchange, [Hb] = 15 g·dl⁻¹, respiratory quotient = 1.0. Top panel shows actual changes in [BE] and Δ [SID] predicted by the Siggaard-Andersen equations as blood is progressively desaturated and replaced with CO₂. Bottom panel shows data of top panel expressed as (a-v) [SID]ₚ (open circles) and (a-v) [HCO₃⁻]ₚ (closed circles) vs (a-v) [HbO₂].

- CO_2 exchange, with no change in whole blood [strong acid] or [strong base], the relation of (a-v) $[SID]_p$ vs (a-v) $[HbO_2]$ was linear (slope = 0.597, y-intercept = 0, r^2 = 1.0). The relation of (a-v) $[HCO_3^-]_p$ and (a-v) $[HbO_2]$ was also linear (slope = 0.523, y-intercept = 0, r^2 = 1.0).

DISCUSSION

This simulation indicates that reciprocal changes in [BE] or [SID] occur in plasma and erythrocyte during hypercarbia alone (Fig. 1), and during O_2-CO_2 exchange (Fig. 2). Use of these [BE] formulae in this *in vitro* simulation was justified on the basis that they predicted acid-base variables nearly identically as did the independently-derived *in vitro* Dill nomogram [21].

Using the Siggaard-Andersen concepts, a-v $[SID]_p$ can be employed *in vivo* to examine a-v differences in [metabolic acid], free of assumptions regarding buffering (Fig. 2). $[BE]_p$ changes linearly with O_2-CO_2 exchange, due to the Gibbs-Donnan equilibrium (Eqs. 2 and 3). However, whereas the magnitude of change *in vivo* might be influenced by assumptions regarding buffering, [BE] cannot change without a change in [SID] [9]. A-v $[SID]_p$, in turn, can be measured directly, and a-v $[SID]_p$ must still change in proportion to a-v $[HbO_2]$ *in vivo*, as *in vitro*.

Accurate measurement of [SID] is tedious, because a slight inaccuracy in each individual [strong ion] can compound the accuracy of any given [SID] measurement. If a large number of observations can be obtained, however, it would seem better to employ a-v $[SID]_p$ than a-v $[BE]_{WB}$, because a-v $[SID]_p$ can be measured, whereas a-v $[BE]_{WB}$ must be estimated from pH_p and $[HCO_3^-]_p$, using assumptions about buffering that may potentially be inaccurate *in vivo*. The potential for unmeasured [strong ion] is another potential problem when using the [SID] approach. However, $[SID]_p$ can also be estimated from $[alb]_p$, $[Pi]_p$, pH_p, and PCO_2 [15], and [unmeasured strong ion]$_p$ quantified [1]. A-v [SID] might also be measured in lysed whole blood [2,4]. However, accurate equations for detecting [unmeasured strong ions] in whole blood, unlike plasma [15] do not seem to exist.

In summary, when attempting to determine whether or not a given tissue is taking up or producing "metabolic acid," a linear relation between a-v $[SID]_p$ and a-v $[HbO_2]$, or between a-v $[HCO_3^-]_p$ and a-v $[HbO_2]$ indicates that tissue is not producing metabolic acid.

REFERENCES

1. Kellum JA, Bellomo R, Kramer DJ, Pinsky MR. Hepatic anion flux during acute endotoxemia. J. Appl. Physiol. 78: 2212–2217, 1995.
2. Lindinger MI, McKelvie RS, Heigenhauser GJF. K^+ and Lac^- distribution in humans during and after high-intensity exercise: role in muscle fatigue attenuation? J. Appl. Physiol. 78: 765–777, 1995.
3. Lindinger MI, Heigenhauser GJF, McKelvie RS, Jones NL. Blood ion regulation during repeated maximal exercise and recovery in humans. Am J Physiol 262: R126-R136, 1992.
4. Stainsby WN, Eitzman PD. Roles of CO_2, O_2, and acid in arteriovenous $[H^+]$ difference during muscle contractions. J. Appl. Physiol. 65: 1803–1810, 1988.
5. Schlichtig R., and Bowles SA. Distinguishing between aerobic and anaerobic appearance of dissolved CO_2 in intestine during low flow. J. Appl. Physiol. 76: 2443–2451, 1994.
6. Siggaard-Andersen O. *The acid-base status of blood* (Fourth Edition), Copenhagen, Munksgaard, 1974, pp. 80–83.
7. Siggaard-Andersen O. The Van Slyke equation. Scand. J. Clin. Lab. Invest. 37; 15–20, Suppl. 146, 1977.

8. Schlichtig R. Base excess - a powerful clinical tool in the ICU. Critical Care Symposium, Society of Critical Care Medicine, 1: 1–32, 1996.

9. Schlichtig R. [Base excess] vs [strong ion difference]: which is more helpful? Adv. Exp. Med. & Biol. (this volume).

10. Prys-Roberts C., G.R. Kelman, J.F. Nunn. Determination of the in vivo carbon dioxide titration curve of anaesthetized man. *Br. J. Anaesth.* 38: 500–509, 1966.

11. Roos A., L.J. Thomas. In-vitro and in-vivo carbon dioxide dissociation curves of true plasma. *Anesthesiology* 28: 1048–1063, 1967.

12. Severinghaus J.W. Acid-base balance nomogram - a Boston-Copenhagen detante. *Anesthesiology* 45: 539–541, 1976.

13. Stewart PA. *How to Understand Acid-Base: A Quantitative Acid-Base Primer for Biology and Medicine.* New York: Elsevier/North-Holland, 1981, Table 7.3.

14. Stewart PA. Modern quantitative acid-base chemistry. *Can. J. Physiol. Pharmacol.* 61: 1444–1461, 1983.

15. Figge J, Mydosh T, Fencl V. Serum proteins and acid-base equilibria: a follow-up. J. Lab. Clin. Med. 120: 713–719, 1992

16. Siggaard-Andersen O, Wimberley PD, Fogh-Andersen N, Gøthgen IH. Measured and derived quantities with modern pH and blood gas equipment: calculation algorithms with 54 equations. Scand. J. Clin. Lab. Invest. 48, Supp. 198,

17. Funder J, Wieth JO. Chloride and hydrogen ion distribution between human red cells and plasma. Acta Physiol. Scand. 68: 234–245, 1966. 7–15, 1988.

18. Chow EI, Crandall ED, Forster RE. Kinetics of bicarbonate-chloride exchange across the human red blood cell membrane. J. Gen. Physiol. 68: 633–652, 1976.

19. Crandall ED, Bidani A. Effects of red blood cell HCO_3^-/Cl^- exchange kinetics on lung CO_2 transfer: theory. J. Appl. Physiol. 50: 265–271, 1981.

20. Klocke RA. Rate of bicarbonate-chloride exchange in human red cells at 37° C. J. Appl. Physiol. 40: 707–714, 1976.

21. Schlichtig R. Simulation of respiratory venous PCO_2 *in vitro. Acta Anaesthesiologica Scandinavica* 39: Suppl. 107, 143–149.

13

RESPONSE OF CORTICAL OXYGEN AND STRIATAL EXTRACELLULAR DOPAMINE TO METABOLIC ACIDOSIS IN NEWBORN PIGLETS

Outi Tammela, Dekun Song, Marta Olano, Maria Delivoria-Papadopoulos, David F. Wilson, and Anna Pastuszko

Departments of Biochemistry and Biophysics, of Physiology, and of
    Pediatrics
Medical School, University of Pennsylvania
Philadelphia, Pennsylvania 19104

ABSTRACT

This study determined the relationships of metabolic acidosis, cortical oxygen pressure, and striatal extracellular dopamine in the brain of newborn piglets. After a baseline period of 120 minutes, a 0.6 N HCl solution was infused intravenously to decrease the blood pH to about 7.0–7.05. The metabolic acidosis was then corrected by injecting sodium bicarbonate and measurements were continued for one hour. The results show that decreased blood pH to about 7.2–7.15 does not cause a statistically significant change in mean blood pressure, cortical oxygen pressure or striatal extracellular dopamine. Further decrease in pH caused significant decrease in both blood pressure and cortical oxygen pressure. By the end of the period of acidosis the cortical oxygen pressure decreased from the control value of 43 ± 4 Torr to 22 ± 8 Torr. Changes in the extracellular level of striatal dopamine were parallel to changes in cortical oxygen pressure. The extracellular dopamine increased to 1270 % of the control on the end of HCl injection. Infusion of bicarbonate to correct the acidosis resulted in an increase of cortical oxygen and progressive decline of dopamine in the extracellular medium. It is suggested that the level of extracellular dopamine in the striatum of newborn piglets was not directly affected by decrease in pH but was dependent on changes in tissue oxygen pressure during metabolic acidosis.

INTRODUCTION

Metabolic acidosis is common in both preterm and term infants. The stress of vaginal birth (Comline and Silver, 1972; Vannucci and Duffy, 1974), hypotension (Siesjo and Zwetnow, 1970), ischemia (Yashon et al. 1970) or anoxia (Drewes and Gilboe, 1973) may

Oxygen Transport to Tissue XVIII, edited by Nemoto and LaManna
Plenum Press, New York, 1997

be accompanied by metabolic acidosis in the newborn. Several studies have suggested that there is a coupling between acidosis and brain cell damage, particularly during the posthypoxic/postischemic period. The physiological mechanisms of metabolic acidosis are not fully understood, but it has been reported that severe acidosis is associated with disturbances in cerebral blood flow, periventricular hemorrhage, leucomalacia, increased vascular resistance and decreased myocardial function (see review, Walter, 1992). Siesjo and coworkers (1985, 1988, 1993) showed that acidosis causes damage to inhibitory GABAergic cells, inhibition of Na^+/H^+ exchange, decrease in lactate oxidation, inhibition of mitochondrial respiration, acceleration of coupled Na^+/H^+ and Cl^-/HCO_3^- exchange, and rise of intracellular calcium. Disturbance of these cellular and molecular mechanisms can be a trigger of observed cell damage or necrosis.

The purpose of this study was to determine the relationships of metabolic acidosis, cortical oxygen pressure, and extracellular dopamine in the brain of newborn piglets. The results show that decrease in blood pH to about 7.2–7.15 does not cause significant changes in cortical oxygen pressure or extracellular dopamine in the striatum. Further decrease in blood pH resulted in decreased cortical oxygen pressure and consequently increased extracellular levels of dopamine.

MATERIALS AND METHODS

Animal Model

Newborn piglets, age 3–5 days, were used for the study. Anesthesia was induced with 4% halothane mixed with 96% oxygen and 1.5% lidocaine-HCl was used as a local anesthetic. A tracheotomy was performed and thereafter the halothane was reduced to 0.6–0.8%. Two femoral arteries (one for blood sampling and the other for continuous heart rate and blood pressure monitoring) and one femoral vein were cannulated. The piglets were then paralyzed with tubocurarine and ventilated mechanically with a mixture of nitrous oxide (78–79%) and oxygen (21–22%); halothane was completely withdrawn. Fentanyl citrate was injected intravenously at approximately one-hour intervals throughout experiments. The animal was wrapped in a thermal blanket and its head was placed in a Kopf stereotaxic frame. The scalp was removed to expose the skull. Two holes (with diameters of approximately 6 mm and 4 mm) were opened in the skull over the left parietal hemisphere for measurement of cortical capillary oxygen pressure and cerebral blood flow. A third hole about 4 mm in diameter was drilled over the right parietal hemisphere and a microdialysis probe was implanted into the caudate nucleus (coordinates A- 5 mm, L-8 mm and V- 15 mm from brema).

Measurement of Cortical Oxygen Pressure

The cortical oxygen pressure was measured optically by the oxygen dependent quenching of phosphorescence as described by Wilson et al (1991).

Microdialysis and Biochemical Measurements

An unbuffered Ringer solution (140 mM NaCl, 2.5 mM KCL, 1.3 mM $CaCl_2$ and 0.9 mM $MgCl_2$) was infused through the microdialysis probe at 2 μl/min. The microdialysis probes used during the present study had an outside diameter of 0.4 mm and dialysis length at the tip of 3 mm (CMA 12 probes, Bioanalytical System, Inc). The dialysis samples were collected at 5 min intervals following a two hour stabilization period and analyzed immediately for dopamine content using a BAS Liquid Chromatography system with electrochemical detection. The BAS microbore ODS column (100 x 1mm, 3 μm particle diameter) was equilibrated with a mobile phase of 0.1 M monochloroacetic acid (final pH 2.8), containing 0.5 mM EDTA, 0.15 g/l sodium octyl sulfate and 2% acetonitrile. Ten μl of the dialysate was directly injected into the microbore column. The detection limit of the assays was 1–5 fmole/sample. Identification and quantification of dopamine was conducted by comparison with chromatogram of standard solution. The retention time for dopamine was 8 minutes. In each experiment, the efficacy of the microdialysis probe was determined *in vitro* at 37°C for all of the compounds measured.

Hemodynamical and Laboratory Data

Arterial blood pressure and heart rate were continuously monitored from the femoral artery (Blood pressure analyzer Micro-Med, Inc., 707 Lyndon Lane, Louisville, Kentucky). Cerebral blood flow was measured by means of a laser Doppler system (MPM3S, Oxford Optronix Microvascular perfusion monitor, U.K.). The 400 micron diameter laser probe was positioned in a direct upright position so that the tip of the probe was touching the dura. The hematocrit of each animal was measured in the beginning of experiment. Blood pH, $PaCO_2$ and PaO_2 were measured using a Model 178 pH/Blood Gas Analyzer (Corning).

Experimental Protocol

After a baseline period of 120 minutes with stable hemodynamics, cerebral blood flow, cortical oxygen pressure, normal blood gas and acid-base status, a 0.6 N HCl solution was infused intravenously at 0.20–1.03 ml/min to achieve the rate of decrease in blood pH. Infusion of acid was stopped when a pH of 7.0–7.05 was reached and the acidotic condition was held for 10 minutes. The metabolic acidosis was then corrected by injecting intravenously a 0.5 mM sodium bicarbonate solution (2 ml/kg). After the injection of bicarbonate measurements were continued for a recovery period of one hour. The cortical oxygen pressure, cerebral blood flow, mean arterial blood pressure and heart rate were registered every five minutes. The blood gas analysis was performed at 10 minute intervals during baseline conditions and at 5 minute intervals during the rest of the experiment.

To follow the effects of milder metabolic acidosis on the measured parameters, in a second group of animals the acid solution was infused only until a pH of about 7.20 was reached. The same experimental protocol was then followed as described above.

In a third group of animals, a 0.6 N NaCl solution was infused intravenously in the same volume as the HCl. All the measurements of cortical oxygen pressure, hemodynamics and blood gases were made according to the protocol described above.

The ventilator settings were adjusted to maintain the PaO_2 and $PaCO_2$ levels constant throughout the experiments. At the end of each experiment, the anesthetized animals were euthanized by intravenous administration of saturated KCl solution.

Statistical Analysis

The significance of the difference between control, acidosis and recovery and between bicarbonate vs physiological saline groups was determined using the Student's t test and $p < 0.05$ was considered significant.

RESULTS

Effect of HCl Infusion on Arterial pH and Blood Gases

There were no significant differences in blood gases between the groups of animals under control conditions, at the end of HCl injection or at the end of recovery from metabolic acidosis. The PaO_2 values were 126 ± 12 Torr, 96 ± 26 Torr and 111 ± 20 Torr, respectively while the $PaCO_2$ values were 39 ± 4 Torr, 41 ± 8 Torr and 39 ± 4 Torr, respectively. The latter was maintained essentially constant throughout the study by adjusting the ventilatory rate after bicarbonate infusion. There were also no significant differences in heart rate between the groups of animals; the mean heart rates were 180 ± 45, 225 ± 32 and 225 ± 38 beats per minute, respectively.

The effect of the HCl infusion on arterial pH is shown in Figure 1. The data are the means for three representative experiments. The duration of acid infusion, as the means for 11 experiments was 38 ± 14 minutes and the volume of acid infused was 10 ± 4.5 ml. The arterial pH decreased steadily during infusion of acid from 7.43 ± 0.04 to 7.04 ± 0.05 ($n = 11$; $p < 0.001$). Infusion of bicarbonate solution on the end of the period of acidosis caused an increase of arterial pH to 7.21 ± 0.08 (statistically different from control value, $p < 0.05$) whereas when the infusion consisted of the same volume of saline there was a progressive decrease of pH (Figure 2). By 30 min after the end of the period of acidosis, the pH in bicarbonate group was 7.18 ± 0.05 compared to 6.97 ± 0.05 in saline group and by 1 hr the arterial pH in saline group of animals further decreased to 6.77 ± 0.05. The difference between the saline and bicarbonate treated groups was already statistically significant by 20 min of recovery.

During the mild HCl induced acidosis protocol, pH decreased to 7.22 ± 0.06 ($n = 5$, statistically significantly different from control, $p < 0.05$) with a volume of infused acid of 5 ± 1.2 ml ($n = 5$). The mean time of acid infusion was 32 ± 8 min. Infusion of bicarbon-

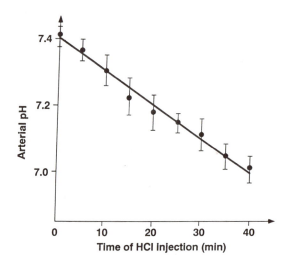

Figure 1. Effect of HCl infusion on arterial pH in newborn piglets: time dependence. The 0.6 N HCl was infused intravenously at a rate designed to achieve a decrease in arterial pH to about 7.0 in about 30 minutes. The measured values of arterial pH are presented as the means ± SEM for 3 representative experiments.

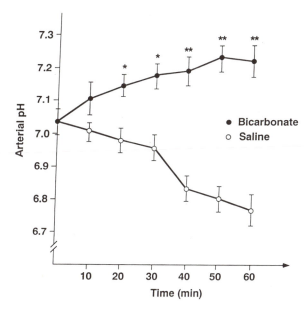

Figure 2. Effect of injection of sodium bicarbonate solution on the physiological parameters of acidotic newborn piglets. At the end of the period of infusion of HCl, equal volumes of either sodium bicarbonate or physiological saline solutions were infused and the measurements continued for a 1 hr period. The results are presented as the means ± SEM for 8 experiments (sodium bicarbonate) or 5 experiments (physiological saline). * $p < 0.05$; ** $p < 0.001$ for difference between the saline treated group and the bicarbonate treated group.

ate after the period of acidosis increased pH to 7.37 ± 0.05, a value which was not statistically significantly different from the control value.

Effect of Metabolic Acidosis on Mean Arterial Blood Pressure and Blood Flow in Newborn Piglets

The effect of acid infusion on blood pressure is presented on Figure 3A. As can be seen, decrease in arterial pH below about 7.15 ± 0.07 resulted in a significant decrease in mean arterial blood pressure from 90 ± 11 Torr (control) to 61 ± 9 Torr. By the end of acid infusion the blood pressure decreased to 53 ± 9 Torr. Infusion of bicarbonate increased blood pressure to 71 ± 7 Torr, which is not significantly different from the control. Injection of saline after the end of acidosis resulted in a constant value of blood pressure during the first 30 min of recovery and then blood pressure began to progressively decrease. It decreased to 35 Torr by the end of the 60 min period ($p < 0.001$ for a difference between the bicarbonate vs saline treated groups).

Mild acidosis, in which the pH was decreased to about 7.2, caused a decrease in blood pressure to 67 ± 12 Torr which was not statistically different from control. After injection of saline solution blood pressure stayed at the same slightly lower level for much of the recovery period (up to 45 min). It then fell progressively and by the end of experiment the blood pressure had decreased to below 45 Torr. Injection of bicarbonate completely reversed the pH induced decrease in blood pressure; during 15 min it increased to 88 ± 9 Torr and stayed at this level to the end of experiment.

Decrease in pH by infusion of HCl had only a slight effect on blood flow in the surface of the cortex as measured by laser Doppler. By the end of the period of metabolic aci-

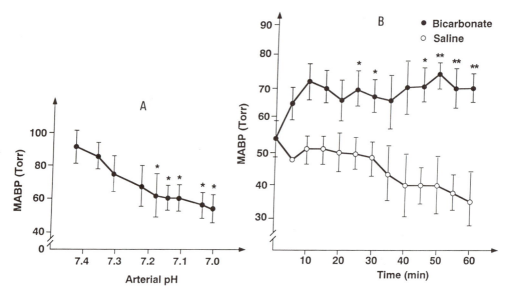

Figure 3. Changes in blood pressure during metabolic acidosis (A) and during bicarbonate treatment after infusion of HCl (B). The results in Figure 3A are means ± SEM for 8 experiments. * p < 0.05. The results in Figure 3B are means ± SEM for 8 experiments (sodium bicarbonate) or 5 experiments (physiological saline). * p < 0.05 ; ** p < 0.001 for difference between the saline treated and bicarbonate treated groups.

dosis, blood flow tended to be lower than the control by about 17 ± 8 % but this change was not statistically significant. Injection of bicarbonate increased blood flow again by about 10% and within 10 minutes it was not different from control.

Effect of Metabolic Acidosis on Cortical Oxygen Pressure

Figure 4A shows the response of cortical oxygen pressure to changes in arterial pH. It can be seen that cortical oxygen pressure decreased significantly from the control value of 43 ± 4 Torr to 30.5 ± 3.5 Torr when pH decreased to 7.15 (p < 0.05). Further decrease in pH was paralleled by a decrease in cortical oxygen pressure. By the end of the period of acidosis the cortical oxygen pressure was 22 ± 8 Torr. Infusion of bicarbonate resulted in a rise in cortical oxygen pressure to about 27 ± 7 Torr which was, however, still significantly below the control level (p < 0.05). Infusion of saline resulted in progressive decrease in cortical oxygen pressure, to about 7 ± 5 Torr by the last measurement, values much lower than in the bicarbonate treated group (Figure 4B).

During mild acidosis cortical oxygen decreased to 35 ± 4 Torr (n = 5) and this change was not significantly different from control values. The bicarbonate infusion at the end of acidosis caused an increase of cortical oxygen to 39 ± 4 Torr.

Effect of Metabolic Acidosis on Extracellular Level of Dopamine in Striatum of Newborn Piglets

Changes in extracellular level of striatal dopamine during metabolic acidosis are presented in Figure 5A. A statistically significant rise in extracellular level of this neurotransmitter by about 140% was observed when arterial pH was decreased to about 7.15.

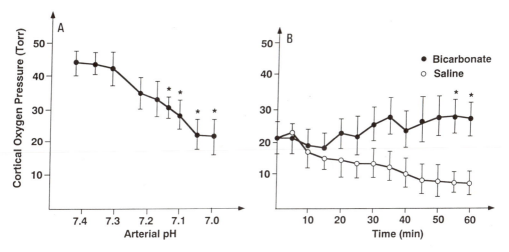

Figure 4. Response of cortical oxygen pressure to metabolic acidosis (A) and during bicarbonate treatment after acid infusion (B) in newborn piglets. The results in Figure 4A are means ± SEM for 8 experiments. * $p < 0.05$. The results in Figure 4B are means ± SEM for 8 experiments (sodium bicarbonate) or 5 experiments (physiological saline). * $p < 0.05$ for difference between the saline treated and bicarbonate treated groups.

By the end of metabolic acidosis, the extracellular dopamine reached a level of 1270% of control. Infusion of bicarbonate to correct the acidosis resulted in progressive decline dopamine levels in the extracellular medium. By 30 min after the end of the period of acidosis, the level of extracellular dopamine was down to about 400% of control and remained at this level, significant higher than control level ($p < 0.01$), to the end of experiment. In the group of animals in which saline was injected instead of bicarbonate after metabolic acidosis, the extracellular dopamine rose steadily to about 3,000% of control by the last measurement.

During mild acidosis the slight rise in extracellular dopamine was not statistically significant.

DISCUSSION

The purpose of this study was to determine the response of the dopaminergic system in striatum of newborn piglets to metabolic acidosis. In an earlier study we characterized the response of dopaminergic system to alterations in oxygen pressure in different pathological models: a hypocapnic ischemia model with low blood flow and alkalization of blood (Pastuszko et al, 1993), a hypoxic hypoxia model with high blood flow and a pH more acidic than control (Huang et al, 1994; Pastuszko, 1994) and hemorragic hypotension (Yonetani et al, 1994). In these models, the changes in extracellular dopamine in striatum of newborn piglets were similarly dependent on the oxygen concentration in the tissue. The dopamine levels were essentially independent of other parameters such as blood flow and blood pH.

The present data are consistent with our hypothesis that during mild hypoxic/ischemic conditions the extracellular dopamine level is predominantly dependent on the tissue oxygen pressure. Decrease in blood pH to about 7.2–7.25, which was defined as mild acidosis, did not significantly alter cortical oxygen pressure or the extracellular level of

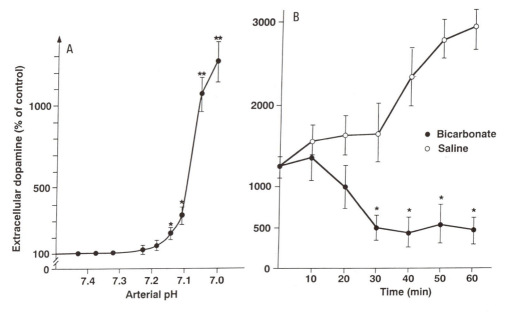

Figure 5. Extracellular levels of dopamine in the striatum during metabolic acidosis (A) and during bicarbonate treatment after HCl infusion (B). The results in Figure 5A are means ± SEM for 6 experiments. * p < 0.01; ** p < 0.001. The results in Figure 5B are means ± SEM for 6 experiments (sodium bicarbonate) or 4 experiments (physiological saline). * p < 0.001 for difference between the saline treated and the bicarbonate treated groups.

dopamine. In addition, this decrease in pH caused no significant changes in blood flow or blood pressure. Further decrease in pH to less that 7.2 -7.15 resulted in decrease in blood pressure and cortical oxygen pressure, with consequent increase in extracellular dopamine. The observed statistically significant decrease in blood pressure for these conditions is in agreement with earlier observations from our laboratory (Wagerle et al, 1988). The difference in magnitude of these changes could be the result of the different anesthetics used and somewhat different design of the experiments.

The infusion of HCl caused a small, not statistically significant, decrease in blood flow as monitored by laser Doppler. As was proposed earlier by Wagerle et al (1988), this small decrease of cerebral blood flow during the acute stage of metabolic acidosis in newborn piglets can be mediated by alteration of tissue oxygenation or possibly via sympathetic activation.

In the present study, after metabolic acidosis, the pH of the blood was realkalinized by injection of sodium bicarbonate. The use of sodium bicarbonate for this purpose has been questioned by several authors, primarily because addition of bicarbonate generates CO_2 and raises arterial PCO_2. This can result in a paradoxical intracellular acidification (Kucera et al.1989; Shapiro et al, 1989; Ilberti et al, 1988; Bersin et al, 1989, Makisalo et al, 1989).

Studies on newborn animals, however, have shown that, in contrast to adults, bicarbonate improves the intracellular cerebral pH in spite of increasing the PCO_2, improves oxygenation and reduces the metabolic acidosis (Wheeler et al, 1979; Sessler et al, 1987). Additional, a recent study of Fanconi et al (1993) showed that correction of metabolic acidosis, by sodium bicarbonate, in newborn infants with normal cardiovascular function improves pH and base deficit. The results presented in this paper are in agreement with the above data. In our experimental model of metabolic acidosis in newborn piglets injection of sodium bicarbonate causes a statistically significant rise blood pH, blood pressure and cortical oxygen pressure. As a result of the increase in cortical oxygen pressure, the level of extracellular dopamine in striatum decreased. Although these parameters did not fully reach control levels by 1 hour after the bicarbonate infusion, the beneficial effect of bicarbonate is readily observed in the comparison with data of saline injection. Injection of saline, in volume equal to the bicarbonate solution after metabolic acidosis, leads to further decrease of blood pH, blood pressure and cortical oxygen pressure. In consequence, there was major re-accumulation of extracellular striatal dopamine.

Our data show that in newborn piglets metabolic acidosis decreased cortical oxygen pressure and consequently increased the level of striatal extracellular dopamine. The effect of the decrease in pH was small until below 7.2, after which further decrease led to serious disturbances in brain metabolism. Administration of sodium bicarbonate after metabolic acidosis significantly improved all of the measured parameters.

In conclusion, the present data are consistent with the suggestion that during mild acidosis the changes in blood pH *per se* do not determine the changes in extracellular dopamine in the striatum. In addition, it is postulated that the level of extracellular dopamine in striatum of newborn piglets was dependent on changes in tissue oxygen pressure secondary to the metabolic acidosis.

ACKNOWLEDGMENTS

This work was supported in part by a grant NS-31465 from NIH.

REFERENCES

Bersin R.M., Chatterjee K., and Arieff A.I. (1989) Metabolic and hemodynamic consequences of sodium bicarbonate administration in patients with heart disease. *Am. J. Med.* **87**, 7–14.

Comline R.S., and Silver M. (1972) The composition of foetal and maternal blood during parturition in the ewe. *J. Physiol.* **222**, 233–256.

Drewes L.R., and Gilboe D.G. (1973) Glycolysis and the permeation of glucose and lactate in the isolated perfused dog brain during anoxia and postanoxia recovery. *J. Biol. Chem.* **218**, 2489–2496.

Fanconi S., Burger R., Ghelfi D., Uehlinger J., and Arbenz U. (1993) Hemodynamic effects of sodium bicarbonate in critiacally ill neonates. *Int. Care Med.* **19**, 65–69.

Huang C., Lajevardi N., Tammela O., Pastuszko A., Delivoria-Papadopoulos M., and Wilson D.F. (1993) Relationship of extracellular dopamine in striatum of newborn piglets to cortical oxygen pressure. *Neuroch. Res.* **19**, 649–655.

Iberti T.J., Kelly K.M., Gentil D.R., Rosen M., Katz D.P., Premus G., and Benjamin M. (1988) Effects of sodium bicarbonate in canine hemorrhagic shock. *Crit. Care Med.* **16**, 779–782.

Kucera R.R., Shapiro J.I., Whalen M.A., Kindig N.B., Filley G.F., and Chan L. (1989) Brain pH effects of NaHCO$_3$ and Carbicarb in lactic acidosis. *Crit. Care Med.* **17**, 1320–1323.

Makisalo H.J., Soini H.O., Nordin A.J., and Hoeckersted K.A.V. (1989) Effects of bicarbonate therapy on tissue oxygenation during resuscitation of hemorrhagic shock. *Crit. Care Med.* **17**, 1170–1174.

Pastuszko A. (1994) Metabolic response of dopaminergic system during hypoxia-ischemia and reoxygenation in the immature brain. *Biochem. Med. Metab. Biol.* **51**, 1–15

Pastuszko A., Lajevardi N., Chen J., Tammela O., Wilson D.F., and Delivoria-Papadopoulos M. (1993) Effects of graded levels of tissue oxygen pressure on dopamine metabolism in the striatum of newborn piglets. *J. Neurochem.* **60**, 161–166.

Sessler D., Mills P., Gregory G., Litt L., and James T. (1987) Effects of bicarbonate on arterial and brain intracellular pH in neonatal rabbits recovering from hypoxic lactic acidosis. *J. Pediatr.* **111**, 817–823.

Shapiro J.I., Whalen M.A., Kucera R.R., Kindig N.B., Filley G.F., and Chan L. (1989) Brain pH responses to sodium bicarbonate and carbicarb during systemic acidosis. *Am. J. Physiol.* **256,** H1316-H1321.

Siesjo B.K. (1985) Acid-base homeostasis in the brain: Physiology, chemistry and neurochemical pathology. *Progress in Brain Res.* **63,** 121–154.

Siesjo B.K. (1988) Acidosis and ischemic brain damage. *Neurochem. Patholog.* **9,** 31–88.

Siesjo B.K., Katsura K-I., Mellergard P., Ekholm A., Lundgren J., and Smith M-L. (1993) Acidosis-related brain damage. *Progress in Brain Res.* **96,** 23–48.

Siesjo B.K., and Zwetnow N. (1970) The effect of hypovol hypotension on extra and intracellular acid-base parameters and energy metabolites in the rat brain. *Acta Physiol. Scand.* **79,** 114–124.

Vannucci R.C., and Duffy T.E. (1974) Influence of birth on carbohydrate and energy metabolism in rat brain. *Am. Physiol.* **226,** 933–940.

Wagerle C. L., Kumar P.K., Belik J., and Delivoria-Papadopoulos M. (1988) Blood-brain barrier to hydrogen ion during acute metabolic acidosis in piglets. *J. Appl. Physiol.* **65,** 776–781.

Walter J.H. (1992) Metabolic acidosis in newborn infants. *Arch. Dis. Child* **67,** 767–769.

Wheeler A.S., Sadri S., Gutsche B.B., Devore J.S., David-Mian Z., and Latisevsky H. (1979) Intracraneal hemorrhage following intravenous administration of sodium bicarbonate or saline solution in the newborn lamb asphyxiated in utero. *Anaesth.* **51,** 517–521.

Wilson D.F., Pastuszko A., DiGiacomo J.E., Pawlowski M., Schneiderman R., and Delivoria-Papadopoulos M. (1991) Effect of hyperventilation on oxygenation of the brain cortex of newborn piglets. *J. Appl. Physiol.* **70,** 2691–2696.

Yashon D., Wagner C.F., Demian Y.K., and White R. (1970) Cerebral lactate accumulation and glucose exhaust during circulatory arrest. *Pro. Soc. Exp. Biol. Med.* **133,** 728–730.

Yonetani M., Huang C., Lajevardi N., Pastuszko A., Delivoria-Papadopoulos M., and Wilson D.F (1994) Effect of hemorrhagic hypotension on extracellular level of dopamine, cortical oxygen pressure and blood flow in brain of newborn piglets. *Neurosci. Lett.* **180,** 247–252.

14

CLINICAL VALUE OF TRANSCUTANEOUS PO$_2$ ASSESSMENT DURING HYPERBARIC OXYGEN THERAPY

A. J. van der Kleij, R. Kooyman, and D. J. Bakker

Department of Surgery
Academic Medical Center
University of Amsterdam
PO Box 22700, 1100 DE Amsterdam
The Netherlands

INTRODUCTION

The reason that transcutaneous PO$_2$ electrodes (TcPO$_2$) are more frequently used during clinical normobaric conditions to assess tissue oxygenation is because the method is non-invasive and relatively simple. Also in hyperbaric medicine TcPO$_2$ measurements are more frequently used e.g. to predict the final outcome of woundhealing enhancement [10,16] or to adjust the administered oxygen in order to keep the TcPO$_2$ values within or above certain limits [21]. During normobaric conditions TcPO$_2$ values are age related according to the linear regression line TcPO$_2$ = 96.6 - 0.47 x age (in years) [4]. However, it has been reported that TcPO$_2$ values during normobaric conditions may differ [4] or not [17] between age groups. Variations and differences between the measurement site, shoulder [20], forearm [7], anterior chest [6] has also been investigated. During normobaric conditions only TcPO$_2$ values at the forehead, cheek, medial site of the leg and the scapular region are sites differing from other sites of the body [17].

Most of all these studies report their TcPO$_2$ results as a single value (mean ± s.d.) registered after a certain time interval (e.g. 10 minutes) or after the total period of exposure to (hyper)oxygenation, suggesting that the registrated TcPO$_2$ values are not subjected to changes in time. Therefore, we analysed our TcPO$_2$ results obtained during HBO (3 ATA) therapy in a clinical routine session. These TcPO$_2$ values were registered at 15-minute intervals at the subclavicular region and/or in the region of interest (e.g. irradiated skin or wound edge).

Oxygen Transport to Tissue XVIII, edited by Nemoto and LaManna
Plenum Press, New York, 1997

PATIENTS AND METHOD

TcPO$_2$ measurements of 231 patient session were analysed. These patients had been daily treated with HBO therapy. Each hyperbaric session consisted of pressurising the multi-place chamber (98 m^3) with compressed air from 1 ATA to 3 ATA in 12 minutes, followed by a period of 75 minutes at 3 ATA. Oxygen (8 l.min^{-1}) was administered by a nose/mouth mask. Twenty minutes before pressurisation a polarographic transcutaneous pO$_2$ (PtcO$_2$, TINA^{TM}, Radiometer) sensor was applied in the subclavicular region and/or a second sensor in the region of interest (e.g. irradiated skin or wound edge). Skin was prepared with an alcohol swab and calibration of the transcutaneous PO$_2$ electrode was performed at normobaric conditions. In children the skin was heated to 44°C and in adults to 45°C. While breathing oxygen TcPO$_2$ values were recorded at 1 ATA (T0), at each 0.1 ATA increase and at 3 ATA after 15' (T1), 30' (T2), 45' (T3),and 60' (T4) minutes. The percent change from baseline values (T0) of the subclavicular region was calculated at all 4 time points (T1-T4). Subclavicular TcPO$_2$ values at 0.1 ATA not higher than 90 mm Hg were considered to be from patients not yet properly wearing the oxygen mask or too late started with oxygen, and excluded from statistical analysis. Nonparametric tests (Mann-Whitney U test; Kruskal-Wallis U test) were used to compare patients groups and time intervals.

RESULTS

During hyperoxygenation increasing age was overall associated with lower measured subclavicular TcPO$_2$ values (Figure 1). However, dividing the patients into a group older and younger than 35 years no decreasing subclavicular TcPO$_2$ values with increasing age was found during hyperbaric oxygenation (Figures 2, 3).

The median and the mean of the subclavicular TcPO$_2$ values of the two age groups were statistically significant different (Mann-Whitney U test, $p \ll 0.05$, Table 1). In order to evaluate the effect of duration of exposure to hyperoxygenation on the results of subclavicular TcPO$_2$ values the Wilcoxon Matched-pairs test was used. This revealed statistically significant differences between related time points T2 and T1, T3 and T1 and T4 and T1 for both age groups (Table 1). The percent change (Figures 4, 5) of the baseline (normobaric while breathing oxygen 8l/mmin) values at T1, T2, T3 and T4 was for the young group of patients ($\ll$35 years) higher and only at time point T2 statistically significant higher compared with the older group of patients ($\gg$35 years). Also the differences between time points T2, T3 and T4 compared with T1 were statistically significant different (Table 2). The percent change of baseline values in the older group of patients showed an increase with increasing age (Figure 6).

DISCUSSION

Our transcutaneous PO$_2$ data were obtained during routine clinical hyperbaric oxygen settings and not during standardized experimental conditions. This may be one cause of the wide range of our results. Another contributing factor to the wide range of the results, especially in the younger group of patients, was most likely a partly dislodged or not used oxygen mask caused by the child himself. Furthermore, during the hyperbaric oxy-

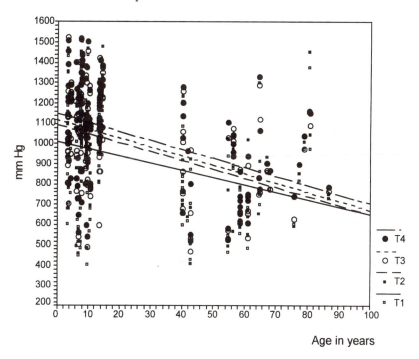

Figure 1. Linear regression line of subclavicular TcpO₂ values in mmHg for all ages.

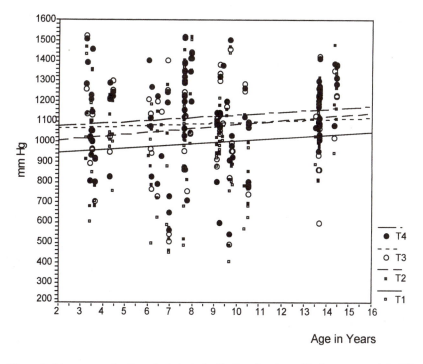

Figure 2. Linear regression line of subclavicular TcpO₂ values in mmHg for age group 1 (n=96).

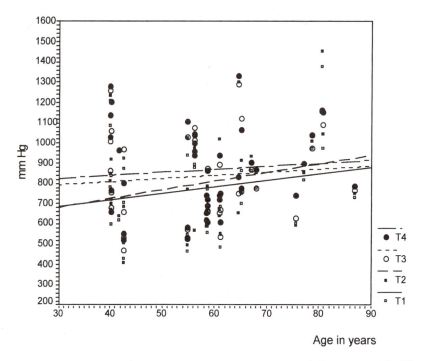

Figure 3. Linear regression line of subclavicular TcpO₂ values in mmHg for age group 2 (n=41).

gen sessions it was noticed that hyperactivity of a child, e.g. crying, resulted in much lower TcPO₂ values, a third additional factor.

One important indication to apply hyperbaric oxygen in general is tissue ischaemia and tissue hypoxia. For ischaemic wounds hyperbaric oxygen therapy is used to enhance woundhealing [2,8,9,18] and for hypoxia hyperbaric oxygen therapy is used to treat radiation induced proctitis or cystitis [1,3].

The rationale for this treatment is based on three fundamental observations. First, fibroblast triggered by lactate can not synthesize collagen without enough available oxygen[12]. Secondly, experimental data have shown a positive effect of HBO on capillary-neoangiogenesis in chronic hypoxic tissue [13,14,15]. Finally, neoangiogenesis is accelerated by a steep oxygen gradient [19]. The ischaemic skin wounds require tissue oxygenation pre-assessment which is performed with transcutaneous PO₂ electrodes.

It has been described [5] that variations in TcPO₂ measurements over a period of time are approximately 10% from the mean for an individual and start to play a role below 35 mm Hg reflecting skin ischaemia. In clinical practice the regional perfusion index (= TcPO₂ value of region of interest/subclavicular TcPO₂ value, RPI) is a parameter used to express skin ischaemia in order to predict the final outcome of hyperbaric oxygen therapy[16]. For example, assume and using our results, a periwound TcPO₂ at time point T1 is increased from 35 mm Hg to 210 mm Hg and the mean subclavicular TcPO₂ is 775.5 mm Hg (Table 1). The RPI at T1 is at that moment 0.27. Let us assume that 0.25 is regarded as cut-off value not to treat a patient. In the worst case the periwound TcPO₂ is not increased at T4 while the subclavicular TcPO₂ is 867.7 mm Hg changing the RPI into 0.24. It is obvious that the lowest RPI value has to be used in clinical studies to derive cut-off values for routine protocols. Therefore, the duration of exposure to hyperoxygenation has

Table 1. Subclavicular transcutaneous pO2 values registered after 15 (T1), 30 (T2), 45 (T3), and 60 minutes (T4) hyperbaric oxygen therapy (3 ATA) while patients breathing 8 l/min. oxygen by mask. Data are expressed in mean values ± standard error of the means (SEM) and the coëfficient of variation (CV=SEM/mean). The non-parametric Mann-Whitney U test was used to evaluate statistical differences between the two age groups. The Wilcoxon Matched-Pairs Signed-Ranks test was used to evaluate statistical differences between related results T2 and T1, T3 and T1, T4 and T1

| | Age group 1 | | | Age group 2 | | | p value | |
	Median (mm Hg)	Mean (mm Hg) ± SEM	CV	Median (mm Hg)	Mean (mm Hg) ± SEM	CV	Mann-Whitney U test	Wilcoxon Matched-Pairs test Group I and II
T1	1007.0	994.7 ± 25.5	0.0256	724.0	775.5 ± 34.0	0.044	<< 0.001	-
T2	1106.0	1072.6 ± 23.6	0.0220	750.0	802.1 ± 35.2	0.044	<< 0.001	<< 0.001
T3	1110.0	1090.5 ± 22.3	0.0204	780.0	836.4 ± 35.5	0.042	<< 0.001	<< 0.001
T4	1148.0	1123.7 ± 22.6	0.0201	836.0	867.7 ± 33.0	0.038	<< 0.001	<< 0.001

Table 2. Percent change of baseline values, (normobaric, 8 l/min. oxygen by mask) after 15 (T1) 30 (T2) 45 (T3) 60 (T4) minutes hyperbaric oxygenation. Subclavicular transcutaneous pO2 values registered after 15 (T1), 30 (T2), 45 (T3), and 60 minutes (T4) hyperbaric oxygen therapy (3 ATA) while patients breathing 8 l/min. oxygen by mask. Data are expressed in mean values ± standard error of the means (SEM) and the coëfficient of variation (CV=SEM/mean). The non-parametric Mann-Whitney U test was used to evaluate statistical differences between the two age groups. The Wilcoxon Matched- Pairs Signed-Ranks test was used to evaluate statistical differences between related results T2 and T1, T3 and T1, T4 and T1

| | Age group 1 | | | Age group 2 | | | p value | |
	Median (mm Hg)	Mean (mm Hg) ± SEM	CV	Median (mm Hg)	Mean (mm Hg) ± SEM	CV	Mann-Whitney U test	Wilcoxon Matched-Pairs test Group I and II
% change at T1	360.7	406.7 ± 23.6	0.0581	316.4	331.6 ± 20.0	0.060	p = 0.122	-
% change at T2	392.2	446.8 ± 24.5	0.0548	323.9	350.3 ± 22.6	0.065	p = 0.041	<< 0.001
% change at T3	399.9	464.4 ± 27.0	0.0582	348.5	366.2 ± 20.6	0.056	p = 0.150	<< 0.001
% change at T4	412.7	473.9 ± 24.7	0.0522	353.7	382.2 ± 20.2	0.053	p = 0.081	<< 0.001

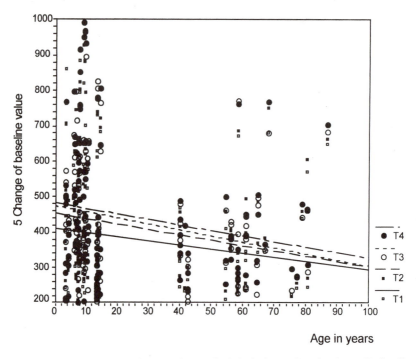

Figure 4. Linear regression line of percent change of subclavicular TcpO$_2$ values in mmHg for all ages.

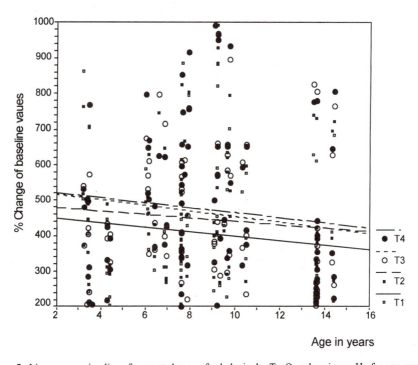

Figure 5. Linear regression line of percent change of subclavicular TcpO$_2$ values in mmHg for age group 1.

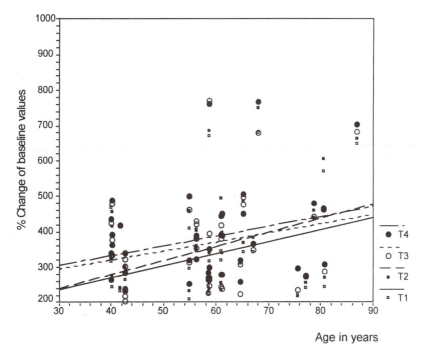

Figure 6. Linear regression line of percent change of subclavicular TcpO$_2$ values in mmHg for age group 2.

to be taken into account when TcPO$_2$ results are interpreted. The ratio between TcPO$_2$ and arterial PO$_2$ is extremely constant. Other factors influencing TcPO$_2$ measurements like oxygen consumption of the skin, skin thickness are overruled by extreme high arterial PO$_2$ values [11].

This explains that during hyperbaric oxygenation the age related decrease can not be observed. On the other hand the influence of skin thickness is expressed by the differences of height of the absolute TcPO$_2$ values in the young group compared with the old group of patients.

Our findings indicate that results of TcPO$_2$ measurements obtained during hyperbaric oxygenation are subject to the duration of exposure to hyperbaric oxygen and must be taken into account in clinical situations. In addition, the age related decrease of subclavicular TcPO$_2$ with increasing age can not be found during hyperbaric oxygenation.

REFERENCES

1. Bevers R.F.M., Bakker D-J., Kurth K.H. Hyperbaric oxygen treatment for haemorrhagic radiation cystitis. Lancet; 346: 803–805,1995.
2. Campagnoli, P. Oriani, G., Sala, G., Meazza, D., Sacchi, C., Ronzio, A. Montino, O., Michael, M. Prognostic value of TcPO$_2$ during hyperbaric oxygen therapy. J Hyperbaric Medicine. Vol.7: No. 4:223–227,1992.
3. Charneau J., Bouachour G., Personn B., Burtin P., Rongeray J., Boyer J. Severe hemorrhagic radiation proctitis advancing to gradual cessation with hyperbaric oxygen. Digest.Dis.Sci. 36: 373–375, 1991.
4. Cina C., Katsamouris A., Megerman J., Brewster D.C., Strayhorn E.C., Robinson J.G., Abbott W.M. Utility of transcutaneous oxygen tension measurements in peripheral arterial occlusive disease. J. Vasc. Surg. Vol.1: No.2: 362–371, 1984.

5. Coleman L.C., Dowd G.S.E., Bentley G. Reproduciblity of TcPO$_2$ measurements in normal volunteers. Clin. Phys Physiol. Meas. 7: 259–263, 1986.
6. Dowd G.S.E., Linge K., Bentley G. Measurement of transcutaneous oxygen pressure in normal and ischemic skin. J. Bone Joint Surg. 65-B: 79, 1983.
7. Glenski J.A., Cucchiari R.F. Transcutaneous O$_2$ and CO$_2$ monitoring of neurosurgical patients: detection of air embolism. Anesthesiology. 64: 546, 1986.
8. Hammarlund C., Sundberg T. Hyperbaric oxygen reduced size of chronic leg ulcers: A randomized double-blind study. Plas Reconstr Surg ; 93:829–833; 1994.
9. Hart G.B., Meyer G.W., Strauss M.B., Messina V.J. Transcutaneous partial pressure of oxygen measured in a monoplace hyperbaric chamber at 1, 1,5 and 2 atm abs oxygen. J. Hyperbaric Medicine. Vol. 5: No. 4: 223–229, 1990.
10. Harvard, T.R.S., Volny, J., Golbranson, F. , Bernstein, E.F., Fronek, A. Oxygen inhalation-induced transcutaneous PO$_2$ changes as a predictor of amputation level. J Vasc Surg.; 2: 220–227, 1985.
11. Huch A., Huch R. Hollmann G., Hockerts T., Keller H.P., Seiler D., Sadzek J., Lübbers D.W. Transcutaneous pO$_2$ of volunteers during hyperbaric oxygenation. Biotelemetry 4: 88–100, 1977.
12. Hunt, T. K., Dai, M. P. The effect of varying ambient oxygen tensions on wound metabolism and collagen synthesis. Surg Gynaecol Obstet. 135:561 - 567, 1972.
13. Knighton, D.R., Silver, I.A., Hunt, T.K. Regulation of wound healing angiogenesis: Effect of oxygen and inspired oxygen concentrations. Surg. 90: 262–270, 1981.
14. Marx R.E., Ehler W.J., Tayapongsak P.T., Pierce L.W. Relationship of oxygen dose to angiogenesis induction in irradiated tissue. Am. J. Surg. 160: 519–524, 1990.
15. Marx R.E., Johson R.P. Problem wounds in oral and maxillofacial surgery. In: Problem wounds; The Role of Oxygen. Davis J.C., Hunt T.K. (Eds). Elsevier Science Publishing, New York. pp. 65–123,1988
16. Mathieu D., Wattel, F., Bouachour, G., Billard, V., Defoin J.F. Post-traumatic limb ischemia: Prediction of final outcome by transcutaneous oxygen measurement in hyperbaric oxygen. J. Trauma. 30: 307–314, 1990
17. Orenstein A., Mazkereth R., Tsur H. Mapping of the human body skin with the transcutaneous oxygen pressure method. Ann. Plast. Surg. Vol. 20: No. 5: 419–425, 1988
18. Oriani G., Lewis D., Favales F. et al. Hyperbaric oxygen therapy in diabetic gangrene. J of Hyperbaric Med. ;5(3): 171–175,1990.
19. Sheffield, P. J. Tissue oxygen measurements. In: Problem wounds; The Role of Oxygen. Davis J.C., Hunt T.K. (Eds). Elsevier Science Publishing, New York.: 17–51, 1988.
20. Tremper K.K., Shoemaker W.C. Continuous CPR monitoring with transcutaneous oxygen and carbon dioxide sensors. Crit. Care Med. 9:417, 1981
21. Voûte P. A., Kleij van der A. J., Kraker de J., Hoefnagel C.A., Tiel-van Buul M. M. C. , Gennip. van H. Clinical experience with radiation enhancement by hyperbaric oxygen in children with recurrent neuroblastoma stage IV. Eur J Cancer. Vol. 31A: No. 4: 596–600, 1995

15

CORONARY FLOW RESPONSE AFTER MYOCARDIAL ISCHEMIA MAY PREDICT LEVEL OF FUNCTIONAL RECOVERY

R. J. F. Houston,[1] S. H. Skotnicki,[2] A. Heerschap,[3] and B. Oeseburg[1]

[1]Physiology Department
[2]Cardiothoracic Surgery Institute
[3]Radiodiagnostic Institute
Faculty of Medical Sciences
University of Nijmegen, Post Box 9101
NL-6500 HB Nijmegen
The Netherlands

1. INTRODUCTION

After its widespread introduction in the 1970s, cold crystalloid cardioplegia rapidly became standard practice in cardiac surgery. A changing patient population, with more elderly patients, patients requiring reoperation, and undergoing more complex procedures, is creating a demand for more sophisticated cardioprotective protocols. Continuous blood cardioplegia has been used, conferring the advantages of blood perfusion, including greater oxygen-carrying and buffering capacity, and avoiding ischemia and thus reperfusion injury, but creating the problem of an obscured operating field. The most recent proposal, intermittent warm blood cardioplegia, offers a still, clear operating field, with ischemic intervals short enough to prevent serious damage. Buckberg *et al* (1995) review the history of cardioprotection, detail the various options now available, and plead for the introduction of integrated myocardial management, in which the surgeon adapts the cardioprotective strategy to the needs of each patient, rather than adopting an adversarial position. Buckberg (1994) also observes that new cardioprotective techniques are being introduced without an adequate scientific basis.

In order to conduct fundamental research into cardioprotective techniques, we have modified our blood-perfused working isolated rat heart set-up (Olders *et al* 1990) for use inside the vertical bore of an NMR magnet. This allows continuous metabolic monitoring using phosphorus NMR to measure high-energy phosphates, and extensive hemodynamic control and monitoring. To provide baseline hemodynamic and metabolic data, we subjected a series of hearts to episodes of normothermic total ischemia of varying duration. A

Oxygen Transport to Tissue XVIII, edited by Nemoto and LaManna
Plenum Press, New York, 1997

full description of the model, and full analysis of the NMR results are being published elsewhere.

While analyzing the data from these experiments, we looked particularly for quantities which might predict rapid recovery of function once the heart was restarted. Such information could be of value to the cardiac surgeon, to assess how easy it will be to wean a patient off circulatory support. Recovery of function as a yardstick for myocardial protection contrasts with the protection of hearts with compromised circulation, where minimization of infarct size is the goal.

2. METHOD

The animal procedures were approved by the Faculty Ethical Committee on Animal Research. An adult male Wistar (WS) rat, weight 400–500g, is anesthetized with diethyl ether. Its heart is removed as quickly as possible and rapidly cooled in ice-cold buffer to achieve arrest. After trimming, the ascending aorta is cannulated, and the heart is suspended inside the NMR coil. Immediately the cannula is in place, Langendorff perfusion with buffer is started to minimize ischemic damage. Perfusion begins within 10 minutes of removal of the heart. The left atrium is then cannulated, and the system is switched to working configuration. The sutures are also used to attach stainless steel pacing wires. The heart is slightly overpaced, typically at 360 beats per minute. (The heart is paced to synchronize it with the NMR system, to minimize movement artefacts.) The perfusion system allows either a working or Langendorff configuration, using either an erythrocyte suspension or a buffer solution both as perfusate and pumped fluid. The buffer is a modified, phosphate-free Krebs-Henseleit solution with added glucose and albumin. The erythrocyte suspension consists of the same solution to which are added bovine erythrocytes which have been centrifuged out of whole blood and washed three times to avoid problems of clotting or immune responses. The hematocrit is typically 25%. Phosphate is omitted from the solution to avoid interference with the NMR signal of intracellular inorganic phosphate. For the same reason, bovine erythrocytes, which do not contain 2,3-diphosphoglycerate, are used instead of porcine, which do. Pressures are maintained by fluid columns (preload 2 kPa, afterload 13 kPa). The working heart is loaded by a specially designed air chamber ('windkessel') to simulate vascular compliance. Roller pumps circulate the solutions through filters and membrane oxygenators supplied with carbogen (95% O_2, 5% CO_2). Temperature is maintained by warm water jackets on all vessels and round the two meter long tubing leading to and from the heart, and by a stream of warm, humid air flowing around the heart. Aortic output is measured using an ultrasonic flow probe (T206, Transonic Inc., Ithaca, NY, USA). Coronary flow is measured continuously by collecting and weighing the perfusate dripping from the heart. The scale has a digital interface to allow the data to be collected automatically. The collected fluid is discarded as it has perfused the heart, and may be contaminated. Pressures and flow rates are recorded on a personal computer using the Poly physiological data collection program (Inspektor Systems BV, Amsterdam, The Netherlands). The perfusate is switched to erythrocyte suspension, the heart is installed inside the magnet, and the NMR system is set up and adjusted. At the end of the experiment, the dry weight of the heart is determined to allow normalization of results.

In the series of experiments described here, baseline readings (preload and afterload pressures, aortic and coronary flow rates, and NMR spectra) from the working heart were recorded for 30 minutes. Then the heart was made globally ischemic by clamping off both tubes (aortic and atrial) leading to and from the heart. Normothermia was maintained for a given time between 5 and 43 minutes (NMR spectra being recorded throughout), then the heart was reperfused in Langendorff mode with the erythrocyte suspension, at a pressure of 13 kPa, for 10 minutes. The perfusion system was then switched to working configuration, and hemodynamic and NMR data were recorded for a further 30 minutes. Data from hearts which could not develop a positive aortic flow (more than enough to supply their own coronary flow, which leaves the aorta prior to the flow sensor) into a pressure of 13 kPa, are not included here.

3. RESULTS AND ANALYSIS

We were interested to see whether there was a hemodynamic quantity, potentially measurable in the operating theater, which was predictive of functional recovery. The quantity we chose to assess functional recovery was power output recovery. This was calculated by taking the ratio of power after restart, expressed as the product of aortic flow and pressure, to that before arrest. As these hearts have reserve coronary flow (they are not fully vasodilated, as is seen with buffer perfusate), reactive hyperemia on reperfusion could occur. There appeared to be a relationship between the characteristics of this coronary flow response and power output recovery. In relatively undamaged hearts, coronary flow rapidly increased to a peak typically three or four times the normal value within one to two minutes after reperfusion, then declined gradually to normal. A typical recording is shown as a solid line in fig. 1. In more severely damaged hearts, the rate of increase was much lower, and the peak smaller, perhaps twice normal flow rate, and only reached after several minutes. See the lowest (broken) trace in fig. 1.

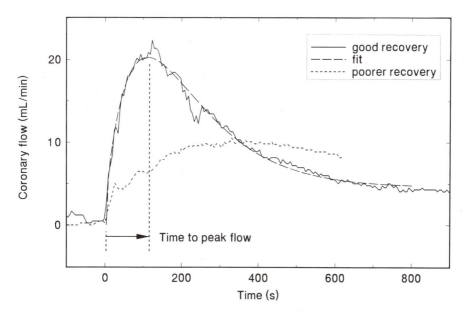

Figure 1. Coronary flow response on reperfusion. The solid line shows coronary flow rate plotted against time for one experiment, in which the heart showed good recovery of function after 21 min ischemia. The data were filtered with a 5-term moving average filter. The result of fitting these data to the mathematical model described is shown (long dashes). The lowest curve (short dashes) shows coronary flow after a longer period of ischemia (43 min), when functional recovery was poorer. The coronary flow peak is less pronounced and is reached less quickly. This trace stops after 10 min: interventions to improve output caused flow alterations not relevant to this discussion.

As these data were collected by pumping the perfusate dripping from the heart and weighing it, the curves are rather noisy. To analyze the data, a mathematical model of the coronary flow response was developed. First, a simple, discrete-time simulation was written, based on the following assumptions:

1. there is a backlog of demand, in other words an oxygen debt to be repaid
2. there is a constant demand for oxygen
3. coronary flow changes based on the total demand, the sum of (1) and (2)
4. a share of the coronary flow is used to clear the backlog.

The initial simulation rapidly gave curves of the required shape, but assumption (4) introduces a non-linear differential equation, so it was replaced by:

4a. the backlog declines exponentially to zero.

This gave curves of very similar shape, with only a slight change in the shape of the peak. The data are too noisy for this to be of relevance. The above definitions can be stated as differential equations:

$$f' = k_1 (b + d - f)$$

$$b' = -k_2 b$$

where f is coronary flow, b is backlog or oxygen debt, d is constant demand, k_1 and k_2 are constants, and f' and b' are time derivatives. k_1 and k_2 are made equal (k), which means that the flow peak, the asymptote which approaches steady flow, and the decline of the backlog all have the same time constant. The last two of these items are completely overshadowed by the flow peak, and differences in the time constants could not in any case be determined from the data recorded. This simplification reduces the number of parameters, simplifies the solution, and improve curve fitting. Knowing that b tends to zero and f tends to d with increasing time, an appropriate solution is:

$$f = kB_0 t e^{-kt} + d (1 - e^{-kt})$$

$$b = B_0 e^{-kt}$$

where B_0 is backlog at time 0, and t is time.

The data from each of 15 experiments were fitted to this model on a PC using the Marquardt-Levenberg nonlinear least squares algorithm, as implemented in Axum 3.0 (Trimetrix Inc., Seattle WA, USA). To eliminate the effect of heart size, power output recovery, R, is defined as power output 10 minutes after reperfusion divided by power output before ischemia. Correlations were sought between power output recovery and the parameters derived from the fitted curves. A significant correlation was found with the rate constant k, but this quantity is not readily measurable. The time to peak coronary flow, t_p, which is easy to comprehend, can be derived from the flow equation above:

$$t_p = (B_0 + d) / kB_0$$

In each experiment, d was much smaller than B_0, so as an approximation

$$t_p \approx 1 / k$$

Power output recovery, R, is plotted against time to peak coronary flow, t_p, in fig. 2. To distribute the points more evenly, a logarithmic scale was used for the horizontal axis. The equation of the correlation line as fitted using Axum is

$$R = -0.45 \text{ (SE 0.14)} \log_{10} t_p + 1.74 \text{ (SE 0.28)}$$

with t_p in seconds. The 90% data confidence limits from this line are also shown. Using Instat 2.04+ (GraphPad Software, San Diego CA, USA), the correlation coefficient between power output recovery and log of time to peak coronary flow was calculated to be r = -0.68, which is very significantly different from zero (Pearson linear correlation, 2-tailed p value = 0.005). With a linear horizontal scale, many of the data points clustered together to the left of the horizontal axis. This exaggerated the contribution of a small number of hearts with long times to peak flow, and gave a less significant correlation (r = -0.57, p = 0.027).

4. DISCUSSION

From the correlation line it can be seen that a time to peak flow of 30s predicts a 100% recovery of power output, while a time to peak flow of 300s (5 min) predicts only 60% recovery. With the small number of experiments (15), there is of course a wide margin of error on these predictions. This type of information could be of clinical use during reperfusion in the operating theater, to give an early prediction of whether to expect rapid recovery of ventricular function in a given patient, or whether that patient might be diffi-

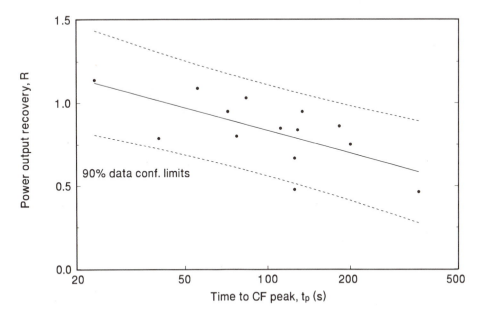

Figure 2. Power output recovery, expressed as power output (aortic flow rate times afterload pressure) 10 minutes after reperfusion divided by power output before ischemia, plotted against time to peak coronary flow, for 15 experiments (note: two data points coincide). The equation of the fitted line is $R = -0.45 \log_{10} t_p + 1.74$, and 90% data confidence intervals from this line are shown.

cult to wean off cardiopulmonary bypass, or require postoperative support, either with drugs or mechanical support. Suryapranata *et al* (1994) studied vasodilatory reserve in the reperfused myocardium using computer-assisted digital subtraction cine-angiography, and concluded that "coronary flow reserve measurement on reperfusion ... correlated significantly with regional myocardial function". Note that in this context, reperfusion means restoration of blood flow by angioplasty after acute myocardial infarct. A more appropriate measurement methodology for the operating theater may be the intracoronary Doppler catheter, as reviewed by Hartley (1989).

Little has been published to date on coronary flow patterns during reperfusion in the sense of restoring coronary flow after ischemia. Yanagida *et al* (1994) observed that 100% recovery of coronary flow on reperfusion was necessary for good functional recovery, which supports our observations, but that was in a buffer-perfused model, with no coronary flow reserve, and thus no possibility of reactive hyperemia. A model such as ours permits assessment at a functional level, rather than low-level investigation of the reasons for observed characteristics. Obviously, a rapid increase in coronary flow causes a corresponding rapid resumption of oxygen supply and thus aerobic metabolism. We may speculate however that the connection between coronary flow response and functional recovery is to do with the fact that vasomotor response and ventricular contraction are both muscle functions, and may both be disrupted in a similar way by an excessively long period of ischemia.

5. CONCLUSION

Coronary flow response on reperfusion could be of use in the operating theater to make an early prediction of rapid recovery of heart function.

6. SUMMARY

Is there a quantity, potentially measurable in the operating theater, which predicts rapid recovery of heart power output after surgical intervention with ischemia? We have enhanced our blood-perfused, ejecting, isolated rat heart model for use inside the magnet of an NMR spectrometer, in order to conduct fundamental research into cardioprotective techniques. To provide a baseline, we investigated the effect of normothermic ischemic insults of varying duration. Hemodynamic and metabolic data were collected, and analyzed to seek measures predictive of rapid recovery of aortic power output, which was selected as the most important measure of function. The presence of erythrocytes in the perfusate ensures that oxygen supply is sufficient to support a physiological workload, and that there is reserve coronary flow. On reperfusion, reactive hyperemia occurs: coronary flow increases to a peak, then declines to a steady value. This response was mathematically modeled, and the data for each of fifteen experiments were fitted to the model. Correlating power output recovery against time to reach peak coronary flow yielded the following equation:

$$R = -0.45 \log_{10} t_p + 1.74$$

where R is the ratio of power output ten minutes after reperfusion to that before the ischemic insult, and t_p is the time taken to reach peak coronary flow, in seconds. The correlation is very significant (p = 0.005). In the clinic, coronary flow response on reperfusion could be used to predict the patient's need for post-operative support.

7. ACKNOWLEDGMENTS

We acknowledge the invaluable technical support of J. Evers and Ir H.J. van den Boogert, the surgical preparation by Drs T. Klinkenberg and Drs M. Oude Ophuis, and the important contribution of Dr Z. Turek to this work, which was supported by Dutch Heart Foundation investment subsidy 902–19–115.

8. REFERENCES

Buckberg, G.D., 1994, Normothermic blood cardioplegia. Alternative or adjunct? J Thorac Cardiovasc Surg 107(3): 860–867

Buckberg, G.D., Beyersdorf, F., Allen, B.S., and Robertson, J.M., 1995, Integrated Myocardial Management: Background and Initial Application, Journal of Cardiac Surgery 10(1): 68–89

Hartley, C.J., 1989, Review of intracoronary Doppler catheters, Int J Card Imaging 4(2–4): 159–68

Olders, J., Boumans, T., Evers, J., and Turek, Z., 1990, An experimental set-up for the blood perfused working isolated rat heart, Adv Exp Med Biol 277: 151–160

Suryapranata, H., Zijlstra, F., MacLeod, D.C., van den Brand, M., de Feyter, P.J., Serruys, P.W., 1994, Predictive value of reactive hyperemic response on reperfusion on recovery of regional myocardial function after coronary angioplasty in acute myocardial infarction, Circulation 89(3): 1109–17

Yanagida, S., Ohsuzu, F., Sakata, N., Maie, S., Akanuma, M., Takayama, E., Hayashi, K., Aosaki, N., and Nakamura, H., 1994, Protective Effects of Verapamil and Adenosine Treatment on High Energy Phosphate Metabolism in Ischemic and Reperfused Myocardium, Japanese Heart Journal 35(4): 455–465

16

MYOCARDIAL ADAPTATION TO ACUTE OXYGEN SHORTAGE

A Kinetic Analysis

Giampiero Merati,[1] Sonia Allibardi,[2] Giovanna Marrazza,[3] Marco Mascini,[3] and Michele Samaja[1]

[1]Dipartimento di Scienze e Tecnologie Biomediche, Università di Milano
[2]Istituto Scientifico San Raffaele, Milano
[3]Dipartimento di Sanità Pubblica, Firenze
Italy

1. INTRODUCTION

In this study, we examined the bioenergetic mechanisms underlying myocardial adaptation to O_2-limited perfusion. Shortened O_2 supply to contracting tissue results in nearly immediate metabolic and performance decline due to fast turnover rate of high-energy phosphates compared to their intracellular concentration.[1] Thus, to maintain adequate ATP production, tissue is forced to divert from aerobic to anaerobic pathways: although less efficient than aerobic ones, glycolytic ATP production under hypoxic, high-flow conditions may account for up to half of total energy requirements.[2] However, if low O_2 supply is associated with reduced flow, the heart preferentially downregulates energy demand to meet supply.[3] Whereas these processes were verified during *sustained* ischemia or hypoxia, it appears important to assess the mechanisms underlying *acute* regulation of performance. The main reason for this is the need to understand to a greater extent reperfusion injury and the generation of endogenous myocardial protection, both of which may be strictly linked to bioenergetic processes.

In the past, several studies of metabolic and biochemical processes were accelerated by kinetic analysis of data, where the role of single components of a reaction or chain of reactions is assessed free of the effects of products. By analogy, we tested the hypothesis that the kinetic approach is useful to understand the mechanism of heart adaptation to O_2 supply limitation. Although the heart response to O_2 shortage is complicated by several overlapping phenomena (changes of lactate production, O_2 consumption, glycolysis activity, coronary reactivity and others), we believe that kinetic analysis may provide clues both to identify those paths that, although plausible, are not synchronous with the observed phenomena, and to give a deeper insight into relevance and importance of various paths of regulation of contractile systems under conditions of O_2 limitation.

Comparing the response to low-flow ischemia (LFI) and to hypoxemia (Hyp) at the same degree of O_2 deprivation provided a tool to characterize the role of free radicals in determining reperfusion injury,[4] of lactate in downregulating myocardial function [2,3] and of coronary flow in preserving the ATP pool.[5] In this study, we report the time course of myocardial adaptation to LFI or Hyp at the same degree of O_2 deprivation. We show that metabolic pathways, and especially the changes in glycogen and lactate metabolisms, play a primary role in developing acute myocardial response to stress.

2. MATERIALS AND METHODS

Ad libitum fed Sprague-Dawley male rats (250–280 g, n=13/group) were anesthetized by i.p. heparinized sodium thiopental (100 mg/kg body weight), hearts were excised and perfused (Langendorff mode) with Krebs-Henseleit buffer (2.0 mM free Ca^{++}, 11 mM glucose, pH 7.4, 37°C). The medium was equilibrated at the desired PO_2 (670 or 67 mmHg) and PCO_2 (43 mmHg) in membrane oxygenators. The volume of the intraventricular balloon was adjusted to achieve end-diastolic pressure (EDP) ~10 mmHg and was kept constant throughout. Measurements also included heart rate (HR), left ventricle developed pressure (LVDP), coronary perfusion pressure (CPP), venous PO_2 (cannula in the pulmonary artery and Clark-type electrode) and venous [lactate] (n=4/group, lactate oxidase-based electrochemical biosensors, Mascini and Marrazza, personal communication). To account for different flows, this parameter is expressed as net lactate release (J_{Lac}=[lactate]·flow). Hearts (n=4/group) were finally freeze-clamped for tissue glycogen determination after digestion with amyloglucosidase.[6]

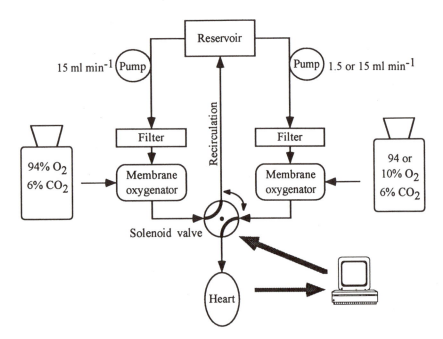

Figure 1. Scheme of the apparatus used in this study.

To synchronize the rapid change of one condition with fast data acquisition, two circuits were devised (Fig.1), each consisting of a Minipuls 2 roller pump (Gilson, France), a filter (8 μm pore size, 47 mm diameter, Nuclepore Corp., Pleasanton, CA) and an oxygenator (Dideco, Mirandola, Italy). One of the circuits was normally set for baseline perfusion (Table 1) whereas the other was set for either LFI or Hyp. The flow of the circuits was diverted either to the aortic cannula (dead volume=0.35 ml) or through recirculation under the control of a computer-activated solenoid electric valve (Sirai, Pioltello, Italy). A back pressure of 80–100 mmHg was applied to recirculation to prevent undesired adjustments of flow secondary to changes of perfusion pressure and resistance.

Data were acquired and the solenoid valve was operated by LabView 3.0 software and NB-MIO-16 Multifunction I/O Board (National Instruments, Austin, Texas) running on an Apple Macintosh Quadra 700 (Cupertino, California). We employed one output (solenoid valve) and three input channels (two pressure transducers and PO_2 electrode). The application acquires default and calibration values, controls valve switching, monitors myocardial performance, performs automatic background calculations and stores data in worksheets. Data were normally sampled at 30 s intervals, but the sampling rate was 5 s for 2 min in the correspondence of valve switching.

3. RESULTS

The described system was suitable to monitor the desired kinetics. The response time for all parameters except PO_2 was <1 ms and ~1.4 s for LFI and Hyp, respectively. The response time for PO_2 was ~17 s due to the intrinsic characteristics of the electrode. The reader is cautioned of this problem when dealing with the PO_2-time curves.

As expected, myocardial performance decreased by a larger extent during LFI than during Hyp.[4] Figure 2 shows typical patterns of contraction at different times after the onset of O_2 shortage. Whereas the immediate (t≤20 s) responses to LFI and Hyp were essentially similar, performance declined steadily during LFI, but remained sustained for several minutes in Hyp hearts (Fig.3, p<0.0001). It appears that at the onset of LFI the decline of LVDP approached an exponential decay of the type $y=0.035^x$ (Fig.4). Whereas EDP increased steadily in Hyp hearts *vs* decrease in LFI hearts (Fig.3, p<0.0001), HR remained essentially constant for several minutes after onset of LFI and Hyp (p=NS, not shown). Figure 3 also shows that at the onset of LFI, CPP fell within the time required for the first sampling, i.e., ≤5 s, whereas it remained essentially stable at the onset of Hyp. Whereas during LFI J_{Lac} reached a steady value within 120 s, during Hyp it overshooted up to 7 μmoles/min ~120 s after beginning of O_2 shortage and then stabilized at 4.4±0.4 μmoles/min (p<0.0001 *vs* LFI). The adaptation of PO_2 was faster at the onset of Hyp

Table 1. Experimental protocol

Parameter	Baseline	O_2 shortage	
		Low-flow ischemia	Hypoxemia
Time duration, min	20	10	10
Flow, ml/min	15	1.5	15
PO_2, mmHg	670	670	67
O_2 supply, μmoles/min/heart	14.1	1.41	1.41

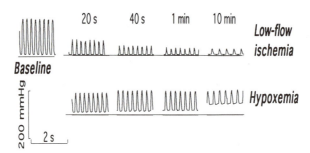

Figure 2. Typical examples of ventricular pressures during baseline and at selected times after the onset of either low-flow ischemia or hypoxemia.

($t_{50\%}$=36±12 s) than of LFI ($t_{50\%}$=85±30 s, p<0.05 since t=20 s). Tissue glycogen content was 107±19, 51±9 and 21±5 μmoles/g dry weight at the end of baseline, LFI and Hyp, respectively.

4. DISCUSSION

Even when matched for O_2 supply, LFI and Hyp elicit different steady-state responses because of a chain of events originating from flow: different flows induce different lactate washout rates and hence intracellular [lactate] levels, thereby causing different degrees of depression of glycolysis and hence different ATP production and performance.[2,3] The kinetics of adaptation to LFI and Hyp were essentially similar for t≤20 s suggesting that the factors that acutely regulate myocardial performance are related to O_2 availability, in agreement with previous studies in working dog gastrocnemius.[7] For t20 s, however, the adaptations to LFI and Hyp are different indicating that flow-related factors overtake control of myocardial performance. Explaining such differences may help to identify the mechanisms underlying myocardial response to O_2 shortage.

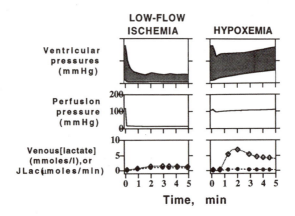

Figure 3. Kinetic adaptation of systolic and end-diastolic pressures (top panels), perfusion pressure (central panels), and venous [lactate] (circles) and net lactate release (diamonds). Error bars omitted for clarity.

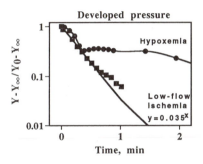

Figure 4. The adaptation of developed pressure to low-flow ischemia approximates an exponential equation.

The features of the employed model and comparative analysis of the observed kinetics help to exclude some paths of regulation. For example, control by neurohormonal factors is ruled out in isolated perfused hearts. Changes of intracellular Ca^{++} transients do not provide satisfactory explanation as they occur on a time scale longer than that observed here [8] and therefore appear to be a consequence, not the cause, of the new heart metabolic status. The changes in coronary perfusion inhomogeneities and the garden hose effect,[9] although likely to occur in this model, do not appear primarily involved in short-term myocardial regulation as they depend on CPP changes, which are not synchronous with the observed ventricular pressures changes. Adaptations of aerobic metabolism are also unlikely as the changes of PO_2 were slower than those of performance. Although this should be taken with care as the response time of the PO_2 electrode may be misleading, it was already shown that the contribution of aerobic metabolism is essentially similar during LFI and Hyp.[3]

If venous [lactate] is considered a reliable index of cell [lactate], then the higher [lactate] during LFI reflects low washout. Lactate-induced acidosis inhibits glycolysis and depresses contractility [10,11] thus explaining depressed performance in LFI hearts. Downregulation is blunted in Hyp hearts due to high flow that increases washout of lactate. The glycolytic source of the extra-ATP required to maintain sustained performance in Hyp hearts is indicated by the higher J_{Lac} observed during sustained Hyp. It was calculated that under the selected experimental conditions, glycolytic ATP production may account for up to half of the total energy requested by Hyp hearts.[3]

The J_{Lac} peak observed at the onset of Hyp appeared to be synchronous with the phase of sustained myocardial activity. It is thus tempting to speculate that the activity outbreak observed in Hyp, but not in LFI hearts is due to transient increase of anaerobic ATP production. Indeed, J_{Lac} bursts indicate O_2-limited ATP production.[12] In dog gracilis muscles subjected to rest-work transition, the burst of glycolysis can occur in times as short as 5 s, and glycolysis can be activated to its maximal rate within 30 s indicating that glycolysis may function effectively in support of mitochondrial oxidative phosphorylation.[13] Computer simulation studies have predicted that the early J_{Lac} peak that occurs in hearts subjected to work-jump is due to rapid activation of phosphofructokinase and phosphorylase *b*.[14]

Despite the high glucose concentration in the medium that should have saturated the glucose transport system,[15] our hearts used relevant amounts of glycogen when exposed to Hyp. In contrast, tissue glycogen decreased by a lesser extent in hearts exposed to LFI. The fast utilization rate of glycogen is supported by the acceleration of glycogenolysis when fatty acids are omitted from the perfusate.[16] Our data are consistent with the computer simulation prediction that the acute increase of energy demand is first met by glycogen breakdown followed by increased glucose uptake from the perfusate.[14]

In conclusion, kinetic analysis of the phenomena that occur during acute exposure to LFI or Hyp may allow to assess in detail relevance and sequence of some of the metabolic events that originate functional changes (lactate and glycogen). Noticeably, this role was documented in the past by theoretical computer-assisted extrapolations only.[14] We believe that kinetic analysis of properly selected protocols represents an approach that allows understanding microcirculation and the effects of morphological and metabolic recruitments secondary to external stresses.

5. ACKNOWLEDGMENTS

Supported by BTBS Target Project, CNR, Roma, Italy.

6. REFERENCES

1. P.W. Hochachka and G.O. Matheson, Regulating ATP turnover rates over broad dynamic work ranges in skeletal muscles. *J. Appl. Physiol.* 73:1697, (1992).
2. M. Samaja, S. Casalini, S. Allibardi and A. Corno, Effects of energy demand in ischemic and in hypoxemic isolated rat hearts, in: "Oxygen Transport to Tissue XVI," M.C. Hogan, O. Mathieu-Costello, D.C. Poole and P.D. Wagner, eds., Plenum Press, New York (1994) p.393.
3. M. Samaja, S. Casalini, S. Allibardi, A. Corno and S.L. Chierchia, Regulation of bioenergetics in O_2-limited isolated rat hearts. *J. Appl. Physiol.* 77:2530, (1994).
4. M. Samaja, R. Motterlini, F. Santoro, G. Dell'Antonio and A. Corno, Oxidative injury in reoxygenated and reperfused hearts. *Free Rad. Biol. Med.* 16:255, (1994).
5. M. Samaja, R. Motterlini, S. Allibardi, S. Casalini, G. Merati, A. Corno and S.L. Chierchia, Myocardial metabolism and function in acutely ischemic and hypoxemic isolated rat hearts. *J. Mol. Cell. Cardiol.* 27:1213, (1995).
6. R.S. Carr and J.M. Neff, Quantitative semi-automated enzymatic assay for tissue glycogen. *Comp. Bioch. Physiol.* 77B•:447, (1984).
7. M.C. Hogan, R.S. Richardson and S.S. Kurdak, Initial fall in skeletal muscle force development during ischemia is related to oxygen availability. *J. Appl. Physiol.* (1995).(In Press)
8. J.A. Lee and D.G. Allen, The effects of repeated exposure to anoxia on intracellular calcium, glycogen and lactate in isolated ferret heart muscle. *Pflug. Arch.* 413:83, (1988).
9. W.M. Vogel, C.S. Apstein, L.L. Briggs, W.H. Gaasch and J. Ahn, Acute alterations in left ventricular diastolic chamber stiffness. Role of the "erectile" affect of coronary arterial pressure and flow in normal and damaged hearts. *Circ. Res.* 51:465, (1982).
10. P.M. Matthews, D.J. Taylor and G.K. Radda, Biochemical mechanisms of acute contracture failure in the hypoxic rat heart. *Cardiovasc. Res.* 20:13, (1986).
11. H.Z. Zhou, D. Malhotra and J.I. Shapiro, Contractile dysfunction during metabolic acidosis: role of impaired energy metabolism. *Am. J. Physiol.* 261:H1481, (1991).
12. J.B. Hak, J.H.G.M. Van Beek, M.H. Van Wijhe and N. Westerhof, Dynamics of myocardial lactate efflux after a step in heart rate in isolated rabbit hearts. *Am. J. Physiol.* 265:H2081, (1993).
13. R.J. Connett, T.E.J. Gayeski and C.R. Honig, Energy sources in fully aerobic rest-work transitions: a new role for glycolysis. *Am. J. Physiol.* 248:H922, (1985).
14. M.J. Achs, D. Garfinkel and L.H. Opie, Computer simulation of metabolism of glucose-perfused rat heart in a work-jump. *Am. J. Physiol.* 243:R389, (1982).
15. J.L. Zweier and W.E. Jacobus, Substrate-induced alterations of high energy phosphate metabolism and contractile function in the perfused heart. *J. Biol. Chem.* 262:8015, (1987).
16. J.R. Neely, C.F. Whitfield and H.E. Morgan, Regulation of glycogenolysis in hearts: effects of pressure development, glucose and FFA. *Am. J. Physiol.* 219:1083, (1970).

17

A METHOD TO DETERMINE RED BLOOD CELL SPACING IN CAPILLARIES OF RAT HEART

David A. Silverman and Karel Rakusan

Department of Physiology
University of Ottawa
Ottawa, Ontario, K1H 8M5
Canada

INTRODUCTION

Researchers have traditionally focused on blood capillaries as the primary site of diffusive oxygen transfer to tissue. Many theoretical studies assume that capillary blood is continuous and homogeneous with respect to its oxygen supply. However, this "continuum assumption" ignores the particulate nature of blood, whereby erythrocytes are discrete O_2 sources.

In capillaries, red blood cells (RBCs) flow in single file, separated by plasma gaps of variable lengths. A modelling study in skeletal muscle has shown that oxygen flux from these plasma gaps becomes negligible with increasing distance from the erythrocyte (Federspiel and Popel 1986). In addition, other authors have determined that there is a decrease in tissue pO_2 caused by wider spacing of RBCs (Hoofd et al. 1994). Thus, capillary geometry alone may not be adequate in modelling oxygen supply to tissue, as portions of the capillary network may be non-functional with respect to oxygen supply.

Despite the importance of RBC spacing for O_2 supply, as indicated by the theoretical studies, our knowledge of realistic values for capillary hematocrit (Hct) and related RBC spacing in coronary capillaries is lacking. The primary reason for this is the lack of proper methodology for visualization of RBCs within coronary capillaries. While *in vivo* observations are appropriate and useful in skeletal muscle, only superficial layers of the heart may be observed in such a fashion. Even so, the beating heart poses technical difficulties for such observations.

Vetterlein and coworkers (1989) determined the red cell content of coronary capillaries using fluorescent microscopy. These authors determined the fraction of plasma gaps per capillary length, but no values for individual cell spacing were presented. The first observations of RBC spacing in coronary capillaries were made in the rat by Honig et al. (1989). However, RBC-free capillaries were not visualized, and the sample size was

Oxygen Transport to Tissue XVIII, edited by Nemoto and LaManna
Plenum Press, New York, 1997

small. In both of the above studies, hearts were frozen irrespective of the phase of the cardiac cycle, and capillaries were not categorized according to their location in the terminal vascular bed. Inspired by these reports, this study was designed to develop a method to systematically visualize RBCs in a large number of coronary capillaries. In addition, the method would allow visualization of RBCs as a function of capillary type (capillaries located *proximal* or *distal* to their feeding arterioles).

In this paper, we describe the method we developed which allows for simultaneous visualization and identification of proximal capillaries, distal capillaries and the RBCs within them, in frozen heart tissue. In addition, preliminary results are presented from the application of the technique to the midmyocardium of rat hearts arrested in diastole.

METHODS

This study required the development of two novel experimental techniques: (i) an efficient method to rapidly freeze the heart *in situ*, minimizing changes in RBC distribution, and (ii) a method to visualize RBCs within capillaries as a function of capillary type in the same tissue sample.

Development of Freezing Technique

Various techniques for rapid freezing of the heart were attempted. Here, we report the two most favourable approaches. The heart could be frozen: (i) by direct contact with liquid nitrogen by submersion or (ii) by use of a heat sink. As a heat sink, we specifically designed copper clamps to match the shape of rat hearts, and precooled them in liquid N_2. In order to determine the most rapid transmural freezing method, a wire connected to a thermocouple digital thermometer (Cole Parmer) was inserted into the left ventricular cavity of an excised heart, via the aorta. The large vessels of the heart were clamped shut, closing any opening to the cavity and securing the thermistor wire. The heart was warmed in normal saline (37°C) and then either (i) submerged in liquid N_2 or (ii) clamped with precooled clamps; cavity temperature was recorded every 5 seconds.

Freezing of tissue occurred most rapidly with precooled clamps (see Results and Discussion).

Development of Staining Technique

The staining procedure includes a modified version of a method previously developed, whereby capillaries in frozen tissue can be identified as either proximal or distal to their feeding arterioles. This method was first introduced by Lojda (1979) and first applied to cardiac tissue in our laboratory (Batra et al., 1989, 1991). Briefly, portions of the capillary network which are proximal to their feeding arterioles can be distinguished from those capillaries located more distal to these arterioles, based on the differential localization of enzymes along the length of capillaries. Alkaline Phosphatase (AP) activity has been demonstrated in the endothelial cells of arteriolar capillaries by use of the azo-coupling method. Dipeptidyl Peptidase IV (DPP IV) activity has been demonstrated in the endothelial cells of venular capillaries. Together, enzymatic differentiation of capillaries is possible; proximal (arteriolar) capillaries stain blue via AP and distal (venular) capillaries stain red via DPP IV.

The difficulty was combining this enzymatic stain with a stain to visualize RBCs. Various histological stains and staining methods exist which allow for RBC visualization in paraffin sections (eg. Sheehan and Hrapchak 1980, Garvey et al. 1987), as well as in plastic sections (eg. Dupont 1979). However, these methods were incompatible with our dual staining of capillary walls. White (1950) has shown that the globin of erythrocytes and intranuclear histones retain Orange G. We found Papanicolaou OG-6 (OG6) to be compatible with the enzymatic stain, and to efficiently stain RBCs orange, in frozen tissue sections.

Modifications involving reagent temperatures and concentrations, as well as incubation times and sequence were made. Finally, a staining procedure which sequentially stains RBCs, distal capillaries, then proximal capillaries was developed, hereafter referred to as the 'triple stain'. Cryostat sections (16 μm) were prefixed by floating the tissue in a solution of chloroform-acetone (1:1 vol/vol, -20°C) for 15 minutes. The sections were put onto slides and sequentially incubated for 40 minutes in OG6, 110 minutes in a medium sensitive to DPP IV, and 25 minutes in a medium sensitive to AP. Sections were rinsed with distilled water between incubations. Finally, sections were postfixed for 15 minutes in 4% formalin and mounted with glycerol gelatin.

Microscopy

From stained sections, representative tracings of capillaries and RBCs were made from the midmyocardium (longitudinal orientation) of the left ventricle. Regions were selected randomly using a 40X objective, based on the following criteria; (i) staining in the field of view was regular and consistent, and (ii) the tissue was not damaged. Following selection of the field, the objective was increased to 63X and tracings were made by the use of a drawing arm (Olympus Drawing Attachment Model BH2-DA, NFK 5X eyepiece) connected to a microscope (Olympus BH-2). The overall drawing magnification was 625X.

From these tracings, morphometric measurements (described below) could be obtained. These measurements were digitized with the aid of a graphic tablet (Bioquant Hipad™ Tablet) connected to a software package (Bioquant IV, R&M Biometrics Inc., TN).

Parameter Definitions

Various morphometric parameters were defined (Fig. 1), as described below.

1. Capillary Hematocrit

$$\frac{\text{aggregate RBC length}}{\text{total capillary length}}$$

This parameter represents a one dimensional, *linear capillary hematocrit*, which can be taken to represent the actual capillary hematocrit. For each capillary type, the sum of all RBC lengths, measured along the direction of the capillary, is determined (=aggregate RBC length). Total capillary length is determined as the sum of all capillary portions of each capillary type from all tracings. Thus, each heart will have one capillary Hct value per capillary type, based on all tracings from that heart. Since all capillaries are traced, this parameter does account for plasma perfused capillaries (no RBCs), which effectively decrease capillary Hct.

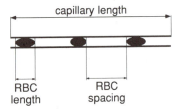

Figure 1. Schematic representation of tracings made from triple stained tissue. See text for description of parameters.

2. Normalized Capillary Hematocrit

$$\frac{\text{capillary Hct}}{\text{large vessel Hct}}$$

Capillary Hct is normalized to determine whether variability in large vessel Hct between animals affects Hct at the capillary level. The parameter is calculated from the measured capillary Hct (above) and Hct of blood taken from the femoral vein, determined using micro-capillary tubes (Micro-capillary centrifuge and reader, International Equipment Company, Mass.). Each heart will have one value for normalized capillary Hct per capillary type.

3. RBC spacing

In capillary portions with two or more RBCs, the edge-to-edge distance between two adjacent RBCs is determined for each capillary type. This length measurement is taken along the path of the capillary. From each heart, a mean RBC spacing value can be determined for each capillary type, based on at least 100 individual measurements. A spacing value is not included in the data if a capillary branch exists between two RBCs or a RBC exists within a branch point.

Application of Developed Techniques

Young male Sprague-Dawley rats (BW: 130–155g) were used to apply the above techniques. Following anaesthesia (sodium pentobarbitol: 52mg/kg), a blood sample was taken from the femoral vein for large vessel Hct determination. A tracheotomy was performed and the animal was artificially ventilated (Harvard Apparatus Rodent Respirator). The chest cavity was opened, and the heart was kept moist with warm saline (37°C). A bolus injection of KCl, into the apex of the left ventricle, was used to arrest the heart in diastole. Immediately, the heart was frozen with precooled freezing clamps, excised while still in contact with the clamps, and placed in liquid N_2. Hearts were stored at -86°C until cryostat sectioning.

Tissue sections (16μm) of longitudinal midmyocardium were subjected to the triple staining procedure. Representative tracings were made and length measurements of capillary Hct and RBC spacing were then taken.

Statistical Analyses

Student's paired t-tests were used to determine if there were significant differences between proximal and distal capillaries at $P \leq 0.05$.

RESULTS

Development of Techniques

Transmural freezing of the heart was achieved most rapidly using precooled copper freezing clamps (Fig. 2). Cavity temperature reached 0°C within 3.75sec. when precooled clamps were used, but not until 10.75sec. when submerged in liquid N_2.

The thermistor wire alone reached 0°C in 0.2sec., and its full response time from 37°C to -175°C was less than 2sec.

Application of Techniques

From stained tissue, representative tracings of the midmyocardium were made. The mean total lengths of capillaries traced were 22.9 ± 3.6 mm and 15.5 ± 1.3 mm for proximal and distal capillaries, respectively.

Both capillary Hct and normalized capillary Hct were greater in distal portions of capillaries compared to proximal (Fig. 3). These increases are significant for both capillary Hct (p=0.0003) and normalized capillary Hct (p=0.0019). Interestingly, capillary Hct was only 14% in distal capillary portions, approximately 40% of large vessel Hct.

A related trend was seen in RBC spacing, which was smaller in distal portions of the capillary network (Fig. 4). However, this difference did not reach significance (p=0.0989).

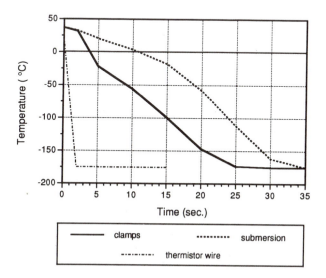

Figure 2. Cavity temperature of rat hearts submerged in liquid nitrogen (n=5) or frozen with precooled freezing clamps (n=5), as a function of time. Hearts were warmed to 37°C and exposed to liquid nitrogen or freezing clamps at time=0sec. Temperature was taken at t=0, 2, 5sec., and every 5sec. following.

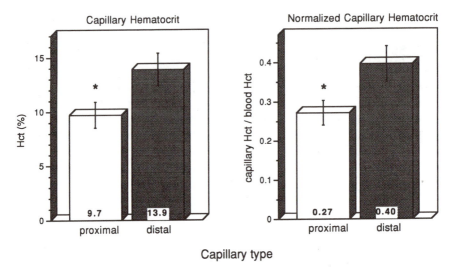

Figure 3. Capillary Hct (n=6) and normalized capillary Hct (n=5) in the left ventricular midmyocardium of rat hearts arrested in diastole as a function of capillary type. Values represent mean ± SEM. *P≤0.05 vs. distal capillaries.

DISCUSSION

A novel histological procedure whereby RBCs can be visualized within capillaries as a function of capillary type has been developed. This is the result of many trials of various freezing and staining methods. Morphometric determination of capillary hematocrit,

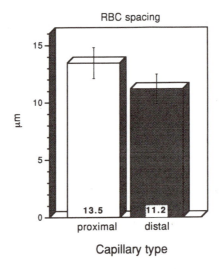

Figure 4. RBC spacing in the left ventricular midmyocardium of rat hearts arrested in diastole as a function of capillary type. Values represent mean ± SEM. n=6.

RBC spacing, as well as variability in RBC spacing is now possible. The results for the midmyocardium of hearts arrested in diastole are the first of their kind.

Development of Freezing Technique

In any morphometric study, the characteristics of the objects being measured in tissue sections should reflect those characteristics seen *in vivo*. Thus, it was extremely important that the positions of erythrocytes (which determine RBC spacing) were preserved during the experimental protocol. To do so, two requirements needed to be satisfied: (i) the freezing of the heart must be as rapid as possible, and (ii) the freezing method itself should not affect the position of RBCs.

To determine a rapid freezing method, we compared direct submersion of tissue in liquid N_2, with tissue frozen by precooled clamps. The hearts used in these trials were similar in size to those used in our diastolic study. As can be seen in Figure 2, the freezing point inside the ventricular cavity was reached within 3.75sec. following contact with the clamps, less than half the time taken if submerged in liquid N_2. Not only is freezing slower with submersion, but arrest of the heart and subsequent submersion in liquid N_2 could potentially alter RBC geometry (eg. due to physical movement of the heart and the time taken to transfer to liquid N_2). It should be noted that subsequent analyses were performed in the midmyocardial region, which would be frozen even sooner than the inner regions.

Thus, the use of clamps is advantageous for two main reasons: (i) manipulation is minimized by *in situ* freezing and (ii) transmural freezing is quickest. However, it is important to consider possible alterations in RBC geometry due to the clamps themselves, as maintenance of cardiac structure is important. Thus, the clamps were specifically designed to match the contours of rat hearts. The contoured clamps serve to encase the entire heart and prevent squeezing of the heart which would occur if copper "plates" were used. According to Vetterlein and coworkers (1991), who used flat, precooled clamps to freeze hearts, only vessels >100μm appeared flattened. Thus, in the event of minor squeezing by our contoured clamps, presumably only larger vessels in the epicardial layer would be affected.

An alternative to the introduction of clamps into the chest cavity would be direct application of liquid N_2 (eg. pouring). This technique was abandoned due to several potential complications: (i) freezing with liquid N_2 was determined to be slower, (ii) the heart was often frozen to other tissues in the region (eg. liver, lungs), (iii) the entire surface of the heart was not exposed to liquid N_2 and (iv) the rate of application could be variable, thus affecting equal transmural freezing across the heart.

Finally, young animals (i.e. small hearts) were used to minimize transmural freezing distances. Clark and Clark (1983) determined that after 1sec. exposure to liquid N_2, the depth of freezing in tissue was at least 1mm. In addition, Judd and Levy (1991) suggest that blood viscosity increases greatly when temperature decreases (from 37°C to 10°C). Taken together, blood redistribution is probably negligible during the freezing process of rat heart. We believe that (i) *in situ* freezing, (ii) the use of contoured copper freezing clamps, and (iii) the use of smaller animals, and thus smaller hearts, will result in morphometric observations which accurately reflect those seen *in vivo*.

Development of Staining Technique

It was also necessary to develop a method to visualize RBCs within the capillary network. The major obstacles were (i) combining RBC staining procedures with the existing method for dual staining of capillary walls, and (ii) fixing the RBCs to prevent lysis upon thawing. Papanicolaou Orange G-6 was found to be compatible with the AP/DPP IV staining procedure. It has been used to stain erythrocyte globins and intranuclear histones (White 1950). Since mammalian RBCs are not nucleated, presumably only globins are being stained. The chloroform/acetone incubation served to fix the RBCs during thawing, preventing lysis. Other reagents (eg. ethanol) were not as effective, or could not be used in conjunction with the AP/DPP IV stain.

Application of Techniques - Preliminary Results

In tissue exposed to the triple stain procedure, there was a prevalence of proximal (blue) capillary portions compared to distal (red). In fact, proximal capillaries accounted for 60% of the total capillary length drawn. This proportion is in the range of the blue/red distribution found previously (Batra et al. 1991).

Preliminary results in the midmyocardium of rat hearts arrested in diastole suggest that capillary Hct is greater in distal portions of capillaries (approximately 43% greater than proximal). PO_2 in distal portions is lower, and therefore this arrangement represents an improved geometrical condition for oxygen transfer to tissue. Capillary Hct and RBC spacing are related; however, capillary Hct also incorporates plasma perfused (no RBCs) capillaries. Thus, changes in capillary Hct may be due to changes in both RBC spacing and the number of plasma perfused capillaries. Although RBC spacing decreased in distal capillary portions, significance was not reached. Therefore, decreases in RBC spacing may contribute to changes in Hct, but the increase seen in Hct may not be explained by decreased RBC spacing alone.

CONCLUSION

The combination of freezing and staining techniques result in a method that can be used to examine capillary Hct and related RBC spacing, important determinants of O_2 supply to tissue. In principle, this technique will be useful not only in the heart, but in other tissues. Limitations of this method should be noted: (i) only frozen tissue can be used, (ii) the staining does not allow for exact determination of capillary diameters, since the enzymatic stain is relatively diffuse, and (iii) exact RBC dimensions cannot be determined, since the cutting angle may affect RBC dimensions.

We plan to examine different phases of the cardiac cycle (eg. systole), as well as different regions of the heart, to determine differences in these important O_2 determinants.

ACKNOWLEDGMENTS

The authors wish to thank Mrs. Ching Kuo and Mrs. Barbara Hebert for their valuable technical assistance.

REFERENCES

Batra, S., Kuo, C., and Rakusan, K., 1989, Spatial distribution of coronary capillaries: A-V segment staggering, in: "Oxygen Transport to Tissue-XI", K. Rakusan, G.P. Biro, T.K. Goldstick, Z. Turek, eds., Plenum Press, New York and London, pp. 241–247.

Batra, S., Rakusan, K., and Campbell, S.E., 1991, Geometry of capillary networks in hypertrophied rat heart, *Microvasc.Res.* 41:29–40.

Clark, A. and Clark, P.A.A., 1983, Capture of spatially homogeneous chemical reactions in tissue by freezing, *Biophys.J.* 42:25–30.

Dupont Company, 1979, Instruction manual: staining procedures for plastic embedded tissue, Newtown, Connecticut, pp. 28.

Federspiel, W.J. and Popel, A.S., 1986, A theoretical analysis of the effect of the particulate nature of blood on oxygen release in capillaries, *Microvasc.Res.* 32:164–189.

Garvey, W., Fathi, A., Bigelow, F., Carpenter, B., and Jimenez, C., 1987, A combined elastic, fibrin, and collagen stain, *Stain Technol.* 62:365–368.

Honig, C.R., Frierson, J.L., and Gayeski, T.E.J., 1989, Anatomical determinants of O_2 flux density at coronary capillaries, *Am.J.Physiol.* 256:H375-H382.

Hoofd, L., Bos, C., and Turek, Z., 1994, Modelling erythrocytes as point-like O_2 sources in a Kroghian cylinder model, *in*: "Oxygen Transport to Tissue-XV", P. Vaupel, R. Zander, D.F.Bruley, eds., Plenum Press, New York and London, pp. 893–900.

Judd, R.M., and Levy, B.I., 1991, Effects of barium-induced cardiac contraction on large- and small-vessel intramyocardial blood volume, *Circ.Res.* 68:217–225.

Lojda, Z., 1979, Studies on Dipeptidyl(Amino)Peptidase IV (Glycl-Proline Naphthylamidase), *Histochemistry.* 59:153–166.

Sheehan, D.C. and Hrapchak, B.B., 1980, Mallory's aniline blue collagen stain, *in*: "Theory and practice of histotechnology 2nd Edit.", Battelle Press, Detroit, pp. 191.

Vetterlein, F., Hemeling, H., Sammler, J., Pethö, A., and Schmidt, G., 1989, Hypoxia-induced acute changes in capillary and fiber density and capillary red cell distribution in the rat heart, *Circ.Res.* 64:742–752.

Vetterlein, F., Menzel, F., Kreuzer, H., and Schmidt, G., 1991, Acute changes in microvascular blood flow distribution in the myocardium of the rat during partial occlusion of the right coronary artery; effects of dihydroergotamine, *Int.J.Microcirc.:Clin.Exp.* 10:289–302.

White, J.C., 1950, Investigations on some cellular stain reactions, *Proc.Biochem.Soc.Biochem.,J.* 46:24–25.

18

OXYGEN TRANSPORT TO ISCHEMIC CARDIAC MYOCYTES

Eiji Takahashi and Katsuhiko Doi

Department of Physiology
Yamagata University School of Medicine
Yamagata 990–23, Japan

INTRODUCTION

Po$_2$ at mitochondrial innermembrane is determined by capillary blood Po$_2$ and Po$_2$ gradients between these two sites. The Po$_2$ gradient of actively metabolizing tissue such as beating heart is considerably higher. Consequently, intracellular Po$_2$ of the normal heart in situ may be as low as P$_{50}$ of cytosolic myoglobin (2 ~ 5 Torr) (Coburn et al., 1973; Gayeski and Honig, 1991; Wittenberg, 1989). This cytosolic Po$_2$ is still considerably higher than the apparent K$_m$ of cytochrome a,a$_3$ and unlikely to interfere with the mitochondrial oxidative phosphorylation. In contrast to the normal state, the oxygen pressure gradient must be precisely regulated in the case of hypoxia, because, if oxygen pressure gradients remain constant, a decrease of capillary blood Po$_2$ of a small magnitude (even 2 ~ 5 Torr) would deplete intracellular oxygen.

Several mechanisms may alter Po$_2$ gradients. Recruitment of closed capillary vessels in hypoxia considerably decreases the diffusion resistance and oxygen flux density, thus decreasing oxygen pressure gradients. Myoglobin facilitated diffusion of oxygen from plasma membrane to mitochondrial membrane may reduce intracellular Po$_2$ gradients (Honig and Gayeski, 1993). In the present study, we propose another mechanism that significantly reduces Po$_2$ gradients both of intracellular and extracellular so that minimum oxygen supply to mitochondria is maintained even in very severe hypoxia.

METHODS

We used single individual cardiac myocytes isolated from the ventricles of the Sprague-Dawley rat. Details of enzymatic isolation of the myocyte were reported elsewhere (Takahashi and Doi, 1995). The use of single cardiomyocytes gave us an opportunity to specifically examine changes in diffusional oxygen transport during hypoxia. To assess changes in intracellular Po$_2$ during hypoxic challenge, we continuously monitored the light

Oxygen Transport to Tissue XVIII, edited by Nemoto and LaManna
Plenum Press, New York, 1997

absorption of a single individual cardiac myocyte using a newly developed microspectro-photometric technique (Takahashi and Doi, 1995). The technique measures the fractional binding of oxygen to myoglobin thus reporting cytosolic Po_2 with maximum sensitivity of $2 \sim 5$ Torr.

Firstly, we conducted an experiment to see whether the Po_2 gradients change (decrease) when the cell was made hypoxic. 10 µl cell suspension containing 10^5 cells/ml was placed in a measuring cuvette (volume 120 µl). Humidified gas of various oxygen concentrations flowed over the surface of the suspension. Due to very thin liquid layer and relatively high gas flow (3 ml/min), equilibrium between the gas phase and liquid phase was established within 5 min. Magnitude of Po_2 gradients is proportional to oxygen consumption rate. Therefore, we assessed the Po_2 gradients by comparing the intracellular oxygenation of a myocyte in the presence and in the absence of oxygen flux into the cell, while extracellular Po_2 was changed from 70.6 Torr to 0.6 Torr. Cellular oxygen consumption was abolished by 2 mM NaCN. Measurements were conducted at room temperature.

Secondly, to examine physiological effects of changes in the Po_2 gradient, we conducted a simulation of ischemia in a single cardiomyocyte. The cell was placed in an airtight measuring cuvette (dead space 120 µl) and perfused with a HEPES buffer solution at 3 ml/min at 36 ± 0.5 °C. The cell was firstly perfused with the buffer solution equilibrated to 1.01% O_2 gas. The Po_2 of the extracellular medium at this time may be comparable with that in vivo (Wittenberg, 1989). Then, the perfusion pump was suddenly turned off and inlet and outlet tubings of the cuvette were clamped so that oxygen supply to the cuvette was completely discontinued. This was continued for 60 min and was followed by perfusion with the HEPES buffer solution equilibrated to 99.999% N_2 gas added with 0.2 mM $Na_2S_2O_4$. We continuously measured intracellular oxygenation during simulated ischemia and anoxic perfusion.

RESULTS

Measurement of Oxygen Pressure Gradients

Abolition of oxygen flux into the cell by 2 mM NaCN significantly increased intracellular Po_2 for extracellular Po_2 of 4.4 Torr and 2.4 Torr (Table 1), thus demonstrating Po_2 gradients for 2.1 Torr and 1.6 Torr, respectively. We did not detect significant Po_2 gradients for extracellular Po_2 of 0.6 Torr.

Simulated Ischemia

Due to consumption of oxygen inside the measuring cuvette by myocytes, intracellular Po_2 dropped from 7.3 Torr (control perfusion) to 1.8 Torr within 5 min following the stop flow (simulated ischemia) (Fig. 1). The rate of fall was quite high (1.1 Torr/min) so that one might have expected that the intracellular space was completely depleted of oxygen within 10 min after the onset of simulated ischemia. However, the speed of decrease in intracellular Po_2 reduced significantly when intracellular $Po_2 < 2$ Torr. Finally, intracellular Po_2 30 min after onset of the stop flow was still significantly higher than the Po_2 during anoxic perfusion (0.9 ± 0.6 Torr, $p<0.05$). Slight drop of the cuvette temperature following stop flow did not account for these changes in intracellular Po_2.

Table 1. Measurement of oxygen pressure gradients in single individual cardiomyocytes

Extracellular Po_2 (Torr)	Intracellular Po_2 (Torr)	ΔPo_2 (Torr)	n
4.4	2.3 (+1.8/-1.3)	2.1*	11
2.4	0.76 (+0.6/-0.6)	1.6*	14
0.6	-0.009 (+0.6/-0.5)	0.6	21

Average intracellular Po_2 is indicated with + and - SD; ΔPo_2, oxygen pressure gradients; *, $p<0.05$.

DISCUSSION

Recent in vivo measurements in the blood perfused beating heart have demonstrated quite low intracellular Po_2; around P_{50} of myoglobin (2 ~ 5 Torr) (Coburn et al., 1973; Gayeski and Honig, 1991). Though low in the absolute level, this intracellular Po_2 is high enough to support oxidative ATP production by mitochondria, because of extremely high oxygen affinity of cytochrome a,a_3 (K_m = 0.05 ~ 0.1 Torr, Hoshi, Hazeki, and Tamura, 1993). However, if we assume an unchanged Po_2 gradient, it is presumable that a decrease of capillary blood Po_2 of a small magnitude could easily deplete oxygen at mitochondria.

In the present study, we have demonstrated in single cardiac myocytes that oxygen pressure gradients in fact reduced when the cell was made hypoxic. Furthermore, in the simulated ischemia, we have demonstrated significant decrement of the rate of fall of intracellular Po_2 when cytosolic Po_2 became very low. Thus, we conclude that severe hypoxia decreases both oxygen consumption rate and oxygen pressure gradients thereby significantly retarding deoxygenation of the intracellular space in ischemia.

The present mechanism to maintain minimum intracellular Po_2 may be regarded as the final defense mechanism of cellular oxygen transport against ischemia. As speculated by Piper, Noll and Siegmund (1994), this mechanism may ensure the intracellular Po_2 just sufficient to maintain the minimum electron flux in the respiratory chain so that the mitochondrial membrane potential is maintained. Thus, although mitochondria are unable to supply enough ATP for cardiac contraction, irreversible cell damage caused by Ca^{2+} release from mitochondria may be significantly retarded.

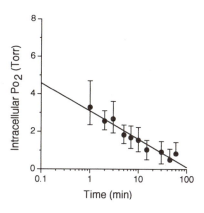

Figure 1. Changes in intracellular (cytosolic) Po_2 during simulated ischemia. Note that the data were plotted in logarithmic scale.

Opposite to that decreases in oxygen consumption augment the oxygen transport through decrease in the Po_2 gradient, increases in oxygen consumption could increase Po_2 gradients and relatively reduce intracellular Po_2. The heart can vary its oxygen consumption 20-fold (Wittenberg, 1989). Therefore, to maintain relatively constant Po_2 gradients and intracellular Po_2, oxygen diffusion resistance between capillary blood and mitochondria must decrease exactly reciprocally. Recent measurements of oxygen saturation of myoglobin in the heart by cryospectrophotometry (Gayeski and Honig, 1991) and ^{1}H NMR (Jelicks and Wittenberg, 1995) have demonstrated that intracellular oxygenation is quite stable even when oxygen consumption was significantly altered. These results, together with the present study, suggest the presence of precise regulatory mechanisms of the Po_2 gradients in the heart.

ACKNOWLEDGMENT

Part of this study was supported by grants provided by the Ministry of Education, Science, and Culture of Japan (#07670048) and by the Ichiro Kanehara Foundation.

REFERENCES

Coburn, R. F., Ploegmakers, F., Gondrie, P., and Abboud, R. (1973) Myocardial myoglobin oxygen tension. *Am. J. Physiol.* 224:870–876.

Gayeski, T. E. J. and Honig, C. R. (1991) Intracellular Po_2 in individual cardiac myocytes in dogs, cats, rabbits, ferrets, and rats. *Am. J. Physiol.* 260:H522-H531.

Honig, C. R. and Gayeski, T. E. J. (1993) Resistance to O_2 diffusion in anemic red muscle: roles of flux density and cell Po_2. *Am. J. Physiol.* 265:H868-H875.

Hoshi, Y., Hazeki, O., and Tamura, M. (1993) Oxygen dependence of redox state of copper in cytochrome oxidase in vitro. *J. Appl. Physiol.* 74:1622–1627.

Jelicks, L. A. and Wittenberg, B. A. (1995) ^{1}H nuclear magnetic resonance studies of sarcoplasmic oxygenation in the red cell-perfused rat heart. *Biophys. J.* 68:2129–2136.

Piper, H. M., Noll, T., and Siegmund, B. (1994) Mitochondrial function in the oxygen depleted and reoxygenated myocardial cell. *Cardiovas. Res.* 28:1–15.

Takahashi, E. and Doi, K. (1995) Visualization of oxygen level inside a single cardiac myocyte. *Am. J. Physiol.* 268: H2561-H2568.

Wittenberg, B. A. and Wittenberg, J. B. (1989) Transport of oxygen in muscle. *Ann. Rev. Physiol.* 51:857–878.

19

THE S FACTOR—A NEW DERIVED HEMODYNAMIC OXYGENATION PARAMETER—A USEFUL TOOL FOR SIMPLIFIED MATHEMATICAL MODELING OF GLOBAL PROBLEMS OF OXYGEN TRANSPORT

Kevin Farrell and Thomas Wasser

Lehigh Valley Hospital
Allentown, Pennsylvania 18103

ABSTRACT

We describe a new derived hemodynamic oxygenation parameter, the S factor (S). The factor is based on oxygen delivery and oxygen consumption and can range from -3 to 1. It allows simplified mathematical modeling of clinical problems of oxygen transport and can be applied to many clinical situations.

A new hemodynamic oxygenation parameter, the S factor (S), is introduced as an aid to mathematical modeling. It is defined as follows:

$$S = \frac{\dot{D}O_2 - 4\dot{V}O_2}{\dot{D}O_2} \qquad (1)$$

($\dot{D}O_2$ = oxygen delivery, $\dot{V}O_2$ = oxygen consumption)

S can theoretically vary from -3 ($\dot{D}O_2 = \dot{V}O_2$) to +1 ($\dot{V}O_2 = 0$). When $\dot{D}O_2/\dot{V}O_2 = 4$ (ie. OER = 0.25), S = 0. An S < 0 implies utilization of reserve oxygen transport capacity. An S > 0 implies increased oxygen delivery in relation to oxygen consumption (ie. "shunted oxygen delivery"). By algebraic manipulation and substitution of the components of $\dot{D}O_2$ into Equation 1:

$$\dot{D}O_2 = \dot{Q} \times Ca \times 10$$

$$\dot{D}O_2 = \dot{Q}\,[(Hb)(Sat)(1.36) + PaO_2(.0031)]\,10 \qquad (2)$$

Oxygen Transport to Tissue XVIII, edited by Nemoto and LaManna
Plenum Press, New York, 1997

the following equations can be derived:

$$\dot{Q} = \frac{4\dot{V}O_2}{(1-S)[1.36Hb\,(Sat) = (.0031\,PaO_2)]\,10} \tag{3}$$

$$Hb = \frac{[4\dot{V}O_2/10\dot{Q}\,(1-S)] - (.0031PaO_2)}{1.36(Sat)} \tag{4}$$

Ca - Cv (Ca = arterial content, Cv = venous content) can be determined by substituting components of oxygen consumption:

$$\dot{V}O_2 = \dot{Q}\,(Ca - Cv)\,x\,10 \tag{5}$$

into equation 1 and solving for Ca - Cv.

$$Ca - Cv = \frac{\dot{D}O_2 - (1-S)}{4\dot{Q}\,x\,10} \tag{6}$$

Equation 6 can be simplified to:

$$Ca - Cv = \frac{Ca\,(1-S)}{4} \tag{7}$$

A previously defined relationship[1] between mixed venous PO_2 (PvO_2) and $\dot{D}O_2/\dot{V}O_2$ (where calculated P_{50} is 26.6 ± 1.0) can be used to modify S in a clinically relevant manner.

$$PvO_2 = 5.44\dot{D}\,O_2/\dot{V}O_2 + 18.16 \tag{8}$$

The relationship between S and PvO_2 can be defined by substituting Equation 4 into Equation 1 and solving for PvO_2.

$$PvO_2 = [21.76/(1-S)] + 18.16 \tag{9}$$

As an example, at a PvO_2 of 28 torr (anaerobic threshold), S = -1.2. The relationship between PvO_2 and S is shown in Figure 1. S, which can also be defined as $1 - 4(\dot{V}O_2/\dot{D}O_2)$ or 1 - 4(OER), is a useful tool for mathematical modeling of global problems of oxygen transport because the previously derived equations with the S value allow the components of oxygen transport to be interrelated in a clinically relevant manner. Additional advantages of using S in mathematical modeling are:

1. Conceptually it 'fits' in that in regards to the sign (+ or -), as a -S implies utilization of reserve oxygen transport capacity and a +S implies wasted or excess oxygen delivery (shunted).
2. These concepts are easily quantified using the S factor.

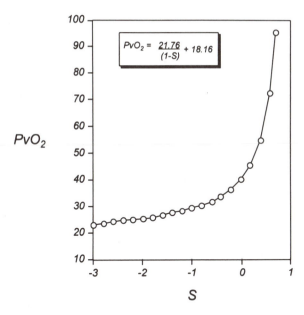

$$PvO_2 = \frac{21.76}{(1-S)} + 18.16$$

Figure 1. Relationship between PvO_2 and S.

3. It 'spreads out' the difference between values for parameters (OER or S) integrating components of oxygen transport, ie. in the 'normal state' regarding oxygen transport, OER = 0.25 and S = 0. At the anaerobic threshhold (PvO_2 = 28 torr), OER = 0.55 and S = -1.2. Thus, the change in OER from 'normal state' to anaerobic threshold is 0.3 (0.55 - 0.25) and the change in S is 1.2. This represents a four-fold increase.

Four examples of mathematical modeling of global problems of oxygen transport using the S factor are described below.

1. PROGRESSIVE NORMO-VOLEMIC ANEMIA WITH NORMAL METABOLIC RATE AND NORMOXIA

* VO_2 is fixed at 125 mils/min/m^2, SaO_2 = 0.99. S cannot become more negative than -.8 (this corresponds to a PvO_2 of 30.2 torr). Equation 3 is used to determine cardiac output as hemoglobin decreases (Figure 2). This cardiac output response to normo-volemic anemia is very similar to prior clinical observations.[2] The change in Ca - Cv can be determined by using Equation 7 and these changes (in A - V difference) are shown in Figure 3. This model predicts increase in cardiac output and decrease in Ca - Cv starting at 7 grams% of hemoglobin.

2. A JEHOVAH'S WITNESS OXYGEN TRANSPORT PLOT

• *Prediction of Hemoglobin that Would Predict the Anaerobic Threshold*

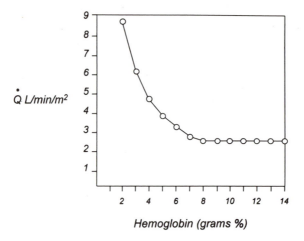

Figure 2. Relationship of cardiac output to hemoglobin in progressive normo-volemic anemia.

- *Determination of Hemoglobin at which Neuromuscular Paralysis Should Be Instituted to Decrease Oxygen Consumption*

Equation 4 is used to plot VO_2 vs hemoglobin where maximum sustainable cardiac output is fixed at 3.5 L/min/m² (mimicking a patient with hemodynamically significant aortic stenosis) and 8.0 L/min/m² (mimicking an untrained young to middle-aged person without heart disease). For both of these levels of maximum sustainable cardiac output, plots are done at S = -1.2 (anaerobic threshhold) and S = -.34 (corresponding to PvO_2 about 34 torr), a proposed point at which to initiate neuromuscular paralysis when there is still some reserve oxygen transport available. In addition, the influence of hypoxia (SaO_2 = 0.85) is shown for both the anaerobic threshhold plots (Figure 4)

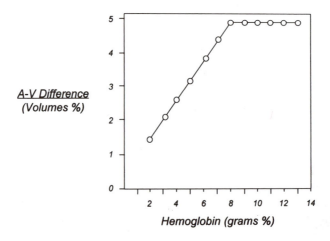

Figure 3. Relationship of hemoglobin and Ca - Cv (A-V difference) in progressive normo-volemic anemia.

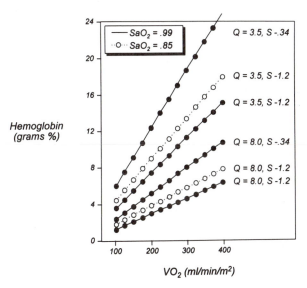

Figure 4. Relationships of hemoglobin levels to oxygen consumption. A Jehovah's witness oxygen transport plot.

3. CARDIAC OUTPUT IN RESPONSE TO HYPOXIA

Equation 3 is used to model the cardiac output response to hypoxia (SaO_2 changing from 0.99 to 0.8) with: 1) varying oxygen consumptions and a value of hemoglobin fixed at 10 grams% (Figure 5); and 2) at $\dot{V}O_2$ levels of 100 ml/min/m^2 and 250 ml/min/m^2 with varying concentrations of hemoglobin (7, 10 and 14 grams%, see Figure 6). These models show a progressive rise in cardiac output, with decreasing hemoglobin and increasing oxygen consumption. These effects are additive. For a given hemoglobin and oxygen con-

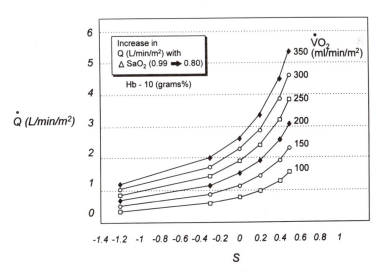

Figure 5. Cardiac output responses to hypoxia at varying oxygen consumptions and hemoglobin level fixed at 10 grams%.

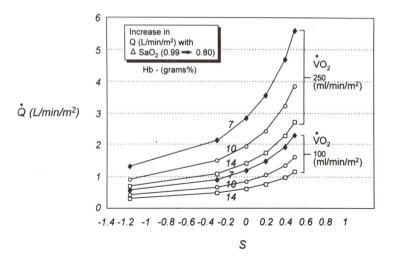

Figure 6. Cardiac output responses to hypoxia at oxygen consumptions of 100 ml/min/m² and 250 ml/min/m², with varying levels of hemoglobin concentration.

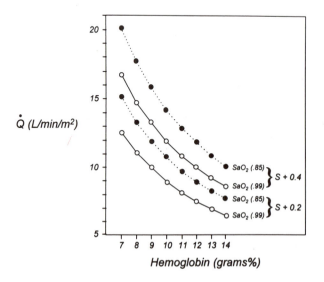

Figure 7. The influence of hypoxia on the relationship of cardiac output and hemoglobin concentration in a model of thermal injury.

sumption, the higher the S value the greater the increase in cardiac output in response to hypoxia.

4. THE INFLUENCE OF HYPOXIA ON THE RELATIONSHIP BETWEEN CARDIAC OUTPUT AND HEMOGLOBIN IN A MODEL OF THERMAL INJURY

Thermal injury is modeled using Equation 3 where oxygen consumption is fixed at 250 ml/min/m^2 (approximately twice normal). S is positive (+ 0.2 and + 0.4 in this model) which mimics a wasted or 'shunted' oxygen delivery (Figure 7). The influence of hypoxia is shown in two different plots (SaO$_2$ 0.99 and SaO$_2$ 0.85) at both levels of S. This model predicts an astronomical level of cardiac output (approximating 20 L/min/m^2 for a patient with a major thermal injury with hypoxia and hemoglobin of 7 grams%).

CONCLUSION

A new derived hemodynamic oxygenation parameter, the S factor (S), has been described. Its use allows simplified mathematical modeling of clinical problems of oxygen transport. The wide variety of problems modeled above exemplifies its usefulness.

REFERENCES

1. Farrell K, Reed JF. Integrated metabolic and circulatory responses to oxygen demand - Analysis of oxygenation-hemodynamic data in critically ill burn patients. *Crit Care Med* 1994;22:A62.
2. Watkins GM, Rabelo A, Bevilacqua RG, et al. Bodily changes in repeated hemorrhage. *Surg Gynecol Obstet* 1974;139:161–175.

EVALUATION OF MYOGLOBIN FUNCTION IN THE PRESENCE OF AXIAL DIFFUSION

Jason D. Gardner and Roy W. Schubert

Biomedical Engineering Department
Louisiana Tech University
711 S. Vienna, Ruston, Louisiana 71272

ABSTRACT[*]

Facilitation of oxygen transport by myoglobin has been assessed by many researchers. Yet, the models used in these studies often assume that radial diffusion is the primary transport mechanism in tissue. Axial diffusion is typically neglected. In this study, oxygen transport by myoglobin facilitation is added to a proven cardiac tissue model which contains axial diffusion in the tissue and capillary regions, the Radially-Averaged, Axially-Distributed (RAAD) model. Previous research has shown that the axial diffusion in the capillary and tissue regions becomes coupled, causing a reduction in the pO_2 at the capillary inlet. The objective is to determine if this coupling effect increases the facilitation of oxygen transport by myoglobin. The RAAD model consists of non-interacting cylinders of tissue (Krogh cylinders), with each perfused by a central capillary. Derivation of the equations describing the RAAD model yields a stiff, fourth-order, non-linear, ODE, BVP. The equation set is solved numerically. Parameters for myoglobin concentration and diffusion coefficient are chosen to maximize myoglobin facilitation. The effect of myoglobin is assessed by observing changes in the pO_2 profiles for the model with and without myoglobin. Also, the RAAD model is compared to experimental pO_2 data to determine if the inclusion of myoglobin improves the model prediction. The computer simulations show that myoglobin does facilitate diffusion, but only to a small extent. The changes in the capillary pO_2 profiles for the model with and without myoglobin are not significant, pO_2 reductions are 0.8% at the inlet and 2% at the outlet. The model prediction is not substantially improved with the addition of myoglobin. The sum of squared error is reduced by 0.1%, from 5.6834 without myoglobin, to 5.6779 with myoglobin. The steady state solution of the RAAD model with myoglobin suggests that, in the presence of axial diffusion, facilitation of oxygen diffusion to tissue is not myoglo-

---

[*] For list of parameters, see p. 168.

Oxygen Transport to Tissue XVIII, edited by Nemoto and LaManna
Plenum Press, New York, 1997

bin's primary function. No conclusion can be made about the transient function of myoglobin.

1. INTRODUCTION

Several researchers have modeled oxygen transport to tissue. Many of these models describe oxygen transport in tissue as simple radial diffusion, meaning that oxygen is believed to exit the capillary and enter the tissue in the radial direction. Often axial, or lengthwise, diffusion is neglected. An example of such a model is the Krogh cylinder model, which consists of a central capillary surrounded by a concentric cylinder of metabolizing tissue. In the Krogh model, oxygen is delivered to the tissue by passive radial diffusion, and axial diffusion is neglected. However, modeling of experimental data has suggested that axial diffusion may be important in the delivery of oxygen to tissue.[1] Through pO_2 measurements taken from an isolated perfused cat heart using the Whalen-Nair microelectrode, Schubert discovered that pO_2 predictions from the Krogh cylinder model did not match experimental data.[2,3] Schubert has proposed a radially-averaged, axially-distributed model. The model retains the Kroghian geometry, but replaces the radial gradients with a mass transfer coefficient, and adds diffusive axial transport in the tissue region.[1] The original radially-averaged model did not include axial diffusion in the capillary. He found that to have the radially-averaged model adequately predict the experimental pO_2 distributions, the tissue axial diffusion coefficient for oxygen ($D_{Z,O2}$) had to be increased to ten times what was accepted as normal. This phenomenon could be explained by an enhancement of diffusion in the heart preparation, or perhaps an oversimplification in the model.

Napper added to the radially-averaged model by addressing the assumption of zero-order oxygen consumption in the model tissue region. He replaced the zero-order kinetics with Michaelis-Menten kinetics, which more accurately represents tissue oxygen consumption. Napper found that including Michaelis-Menten kinetics in the model slightly reduced the need for a high value of axial oxygen diffusion coefficient. By replacing zero-order oxygen consumption in the RAAD model with Michaelis-Menten consumption the magnitude of $D_{Z,O2}$ was reduced to eight times normal.[4] Clearly the exclusion of Michaelis-Menten kinetics did not entirely explain the enhanced diffusion implied in Schubert's experimental data.

Fletcher observed that including axial diffusion in the capillary region smoothed oscillations in the radial-averaged model solution.[6] Also, as was discovered later, including axial diffusion in the capillary caused a coupled diffusion effect between the tissue and capillary regions.[6] The radially-averaged model with capillary axial diffusion is called the Radially-Averaged, Axially-Distributed (RAAD) model.

The use of a mass transfer coefficient for radial oxygen transport was questioned. Zhang performed a mathematical comparison between the original Krogh model, the RAAD model, and a two-dimensional model (axial and radial diffusion in the tissue, and axial diffusion in the capillary).[5,7] He concluded that the Krogh model was inadequate for predicting pO_2 distributions in the heart. Zhang also discovered that the RAAD model could be used instead of the two-dimensional model to accurately predict pO_2 distributions. Recall that, for accurate RAAD model predictions, the $D_{Z,O2}$ must be elevated to eight to ten times normal. Still there has been no explanation for the enhanced diffusion exhibited in the experimental data. The explanation clearly did not reside within the replacement of radial diffusion by a mass transfer coefficient.

Another RAAD model simplification was the exclusion of myoglobin kinetics. In addition to acting as a buffer for oxygen in tissue, myoglobin (Mb) facilitates oxygen transport. Myoglobin binds reversibly with oxygen in a 1:1 reaction to form oxymyoglobin (MbO_2). Myoglobin is believed to facilitate oxygen diffusion by binding to oxygen in areas of high oxygen concentration, diffusing as MbO_2 to areas of lower oxygen concentration, and then releasing the bound oxygen. Myoglobin was initially excluded from the RAAD model because the then current literature suggested that myoglobin did not diffuse in tissue. However, more recent findings suggest that myoglobin does diffuse in tissue.[8] Therefore myoglobin facilitated oxygen diffusion may significantly contribute to oxygen transport and may account for the enhanced diffusion implied by Schubert's pO_2 data.

The magnitude of myoglobin's facilitative effect is questionable. Myoglobin-facilitated oxygen transport has been assessed by many researchers, but they have not validated modeling results with a comparison to experimental data.[9,10,11,12,13] Often, model-to-model comparisons are made. The problem with many evaluations of myoglobin facilitation in tissue is that the basic model used was faulty in that it cannot mimic experimental results at the tissue level. Researchers often use models that reproduce whole organ results, but these models cannot predict tissue level data. As shown by Schubert and Zhang, the RAAD model more closely predicts tissue level pO_2 distributions in an isolated cat heart preparation than other models.[5,7] Yet, the model requires an elevation of diffusion to match the data. The discovery of a coupling between axial diffusion in the capillary and in the tissue suggests that myoglobin's facilitative effect may be more pronounced in the presence of axial diffusion. Evaluation of myoglobin function using the RAAD model will determine if myoglobin facilitation is significant in the presence of axial oxygen transport. The model results are compared to experimental data to determine whether myoglobin is the explanation for enhanced oxygen diffusion in the isolated cat heart preparation.

2. METHODS

The tissue model used in this simulation is the RAAD model, Fig. 1. The model is based upon the Krogh cylinder concept. The RAAD tissue model consists of non-interacting cylinders of tissue; each cylinder perfused by a central capillary. This basic cylinder tissue unit is then repeated to represent a larger portion of tissue. In the tissue region there

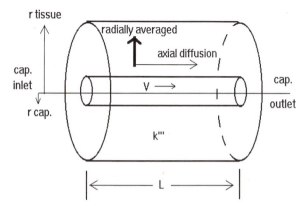

Figure 1. RAAD model.

is axial diffusion of oxygen, zero-order consumption, and myoglobin kinetics. Michaelis-Menten kinetics has been excluded in this simulation so that the independent action of myoglobin facilitation can be determined. Oxygen flux leaving the capillary is represented by a concentration difference times a mass transport coefficient, meaning that the tissue is space-averaged radially. The capillary region includes axial diffusion of oxygen. The assumption of a radially-averaged tissue region has been critically evaluated and appears legitimate.[5,7]

To include myoglobin facilitation in the RAAD model, a reaction term is added which will represent the oxygen-myoglobin reaction, as well as diffusion of oxymyoglobin. The myoglobin reaction is assumed to be at equilibrium. This assumption will lead to a slight underestimate of facilitation.[14] This assumption also greatly simplifies the resulting differential equations, from sixth to fourth order, making numerical solution tolerable. The formulation of the myoglobin reaction term follows the development by Fletcher.[14]

The RAAD model assumptions are: (1) steady state, (2) straight-parallel-concurrent-homogeneously-distributed capillaries (Krogh cylinders), (3) constant perfusate velocity, (4) slight solubility of oxygen in perfusate, (5) radially uniform capillary, (6) axial diffusion in capillary, (7) zero-order homogeneous oxygen consumption, (8) radially uniform tissue, (9) axial diffusion in tissue, and (10) oxygen-myoglobin reaction at equilibrium. The model is subject to the following boundary conditions: (1) no diffusion flux at the venous end of the capillary, (2) no flux condition at all outer tissue surfaces, and (3) tissue oxygen concentration is zero at the venous end of the capillary. Condition 3 requires that myoglobin release all of its bound oxygen. This will maximize the facilitative effect of myoglobin. The use of condition 3 causes the format of the model output to differ from previous modeling efforts. When determining the facilitative effect of myoglobin, many researchers will compare the end tissue oxygen with and without myoglobin reaction; the difference caused by myoglobin facilitation. In this case the end tissue pO_2 is specified and the amount of diffusion facilitation by myoglobin is estimated by observing changes in inlet capillary pO_2.

Formulation of the mathematical problem describing the RAAD model yields a stiff, fourth-order, nonlinear, ordinary-differential equation, boundary-value problem. The inclusion of myoglobin transport introduces a nonlinear reaction term which complicates the problem and makes analytic solution impossible.

The following equations describe the transport of species in the RAAD model (overbar denotes normalization).

Equations describing tissue region :

transport of oxygen,

$$\frac{d^2 \overline{C}_{O2,TIS}}{d\overline{Z}^2} + \alpha \cdot \left[\overline{C}_{O2,CAP} - \overline{C}_{O2,TIS} \right] - K = 0 \tag{1}$$

transport of oxymyoglobin,

$$D_{MbO2,TIS} \frac{d^2 C_{MbO2,TIS}}{dZ^2} = 0 \tag{2}$$

where,

$$[\alpha = \frac{2\,r_{CAP}\,Z_O^{\,2}\,P}{\left(r^2_{TIS} - r^2_{CAP}\right)\cdot D_{Z,TIS}} \qquad\qquad K = \frac{k\,Z_O^{\,2}}{D_{Z,TIS}\,C_O}$$

Eq. 2 can also be represented by:

$$D_{MbO2,TIS}\,C_{Mb,TOT}\,\frac{d^2 Y}{d\,Z^2} = 0 \tag{3}$$

where, Y is the fraction of myoglobin saturated with oxygen and is described by,

$$Y = \frac{\overline{C}_{O2,TIS}\,k_1}{\overline{C}_{O2,TIS}\,k_1 + k_2}$$

Eqs. 1 and 3 can be combined to form one equation describing the tissue region:

$$\frac{d^2\overline{C}_{O2,TIS}}{d\,\overline{Z}^{\,2}} + \alpha\cdot\left[\overline{C}_{O2,CAP} - \overline{C}_{O2,TIS}\right] - K + \overline{S}_{MbO_2} = 0 \tag{4}$$

with,

$$\overline{S}_{MbO_2} = \frac{D_{MbO2,TIS}\,C_{Mb,TOT}\,Z_o^{\,2}}{D_{O2,TIS}\,C_o}\,\frac{d^2 Y}{d\,\overline{Z}^{\,2}}$$

Including diffusion in the capillary eases the mathematical solution.[6] Generally, the diffusion of oxygen in the capillary is thought to contribute little to oxygen transport relative to convection. But, when coupled to axial diffusion in the tissue, capillary axial diffusion can produce significant effects on the tissue pO_2 distribution and significantly lowers the inlet pO_2 needed for adequate oxygenation.[6] This coupling may enhance the effects of myoglobin facilitation.

Equations describing capillary region: transport of oxygen,

$$\frac{d^2\overline{C}_{O2,CAP}}{d\,\overline{Z}^{\,2}} - \omega\cdot\frac{d\,\overline{C}_{O2,CAP}}{d\,\overline{Z}} - \beta\cdot\left[\overline{C}_{O2,CAP} - \overline{C}_{O2,TIS}\right] = 0 \tag{5}$$

where,

$$\omega = \frac{v_{CAP}\,Z_O}{D_{Z,CAP}} \qquad\qquad \beta = \frac{2\,Z_O^{\,2}\,P}{r_{CAP}\,D_{Z,CAP}}$$

In the literature there is no general agreement about a myoglobin concentration in tissue, or a myoglobin diffusion coefficient.[8,15,16,17] Therefore the highest possible values of C_{Mb} and D_{Mb} were used, to provide a maximal facilitation estimate. These values were $C_{Mb} = 1.0 \times 10^{-6}$ mol/cm^3 and $D_{Mb} = 2.97 \times 10^{-6}$ cm^2/s, the absolute maximum diffusion coefficient as predicted by Stokes-Einstein formula.[14] Parameters used for the RAAD model are found in Fletcher.[6] Parameters describing the oxygen-myoglobin reaction were taken from Fletcher.[14]

The equation set was solved numerically using a finite-difference routine called PASVA. The PASVA routine is a variable order, variable step, finite-differencing routine for nonlinear systems with two-point boundary conditions and is well suited for this problem.[18] Simulations were performed on a mainframe computer using the FORTRAN programming language.

Schubert's experimental pO_2 measurements were taken in a randomized experiment. There was no information regarding microeletrode tip position relative to blood vessels, other than the fact that the tip was not within a blood vessel. The experimental data is in a histogram format (%volume of tissue vs. bins of pO_2). Therefore to compare the RAAD model solution to the experimental data, the results will be put into a histogram format. This is done by dividing the cylinder of tissue into a set of curved regions equivalent to the sampling region of an oxygen microelectrode. The average pO_2 in each of these regions is found and the volume is noted. The volumes are totaled for a given range of pO_2. With this information, a histogram can then be constructed.[3,6] In the limit, the histogram is a probability density of pO_2 in the tissue region.

3. RESULTS

The finite-difference routine required 240 nodes to solve with an execution time of about two minutes on a mainframe computer. Numerical convergence was ensured by adjusting the user-specified error criteria until the desired accuracy was achieved.

3.1. RAAD Model with Myoglobin

Figures 2–4 are plots of output from the RAAD model with myoglobin facilitation. Figure 2 shows the experimental data and RAAD model output in histogram form. The ex-

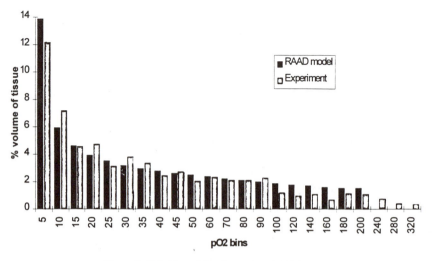

Figure 2. RAAD model and experimental histograms.

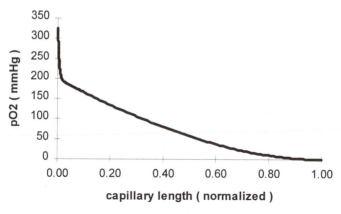

Figure 3. Axial profile of capillary pO_2 from RAAD model with myoglobin.

perimental data represents 1800 random pO_2 samples.[2] The model prediction follows the trend of the experimental distribution. Notice the leftward shift toward lower pO_2 values of the histograms for both the RAAD model and the experimental data.

Figures 3 and 4 show the axial profiles of pO_2 in the capillary and tissue, respectively.

The steep drop in pO_2 at the inlet is due to a strong axial component of diffusion, and the coupling of diffusion between the capillary and tissue regions. Both of these effects tend to flatten the axial profile and bring much of the tissue to a lower, yet more uniform pO_2. Except for the first 5% of the inlet, the pO_2 gradient between the capillary and tissue regions in the RAAD model solution is small. The difference is below 5 mmHg for most of the capillary length. Values for the pO_2 difference between the regions for the RAAD model with myoglobin are given in Table 1.

The saturation of myoglobin in the tissue versus capillary length is plotted in Fig. 5. Myoglobin remains saturated for most of the capillary length, and does not release much bound oxygen until the end of the capillary.

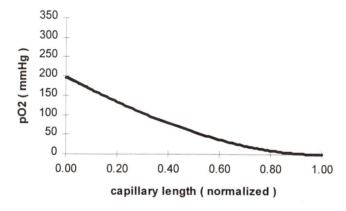

Figure 4. Axial profile of tissue pO_2 from RAAD model with myoglobin.

Table 1. pO$_2$ driving force for oxygen
transport between the capillary and tissue
regions in the RAAD model with myoglobin

Capillary length (normalized)	pO$_2$ difference (mmHg) [capillary minus tissue]
0.00	129.67
0.25	3.37
0.50	2.50
0.75	1.39
1.00	0.01

3.2. Comparison between RAAD Model Output with and without Myoglobin

As shown in Fig. 6, the change in inlet capillary pO$_2$ went from 328.8 mmHg without myoglobin, to 326.3 mmHg with myoglobin, which is a difference of 2.5 mmHg or 0.8%. This means that with myoglobin, the tissue required 2.5 mmHg less oxygen at the capillary inlet for the same amount of oxygen delivery.

The addition of myoglobin to the RAAD model changes the output pO$_2$ profiles very little. This similarity in the profiles prevents clear plotting on the same axes because the profiles seem to overlap. A plot of the difference in the capillary pO$_2$ profiles between the Mb and no Mb RAAD solutions is given in Fig. 7. The difference ranges from 2.5 mmHg at the capillary inlet, to 0.0003 mmHg at the outlet.

Figure 8 shows a close-up of the capillary exit for the RAAD model output with and without myoglobin. The exit pO$_2$ difference between the two solutions is very small, 0.0003. The outlet pO$_2$ was 0.0146 mmHg without myoglobin, and 0.0143 mmHg with myoglobin, a change of 2%.

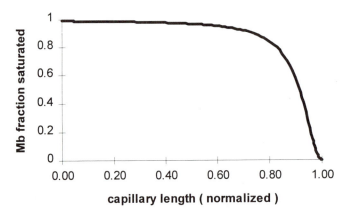

Figure 5. Axial profile of myoglobin oxygen-saturation in tissue. The fraction saturated represents the amount of MbO$_2$, i.e. saturated Mb, divided by the total amount of Mb, both saturated and unsaturated. A value of 1 means that 100% of the Mb is saturated with O$_2$.

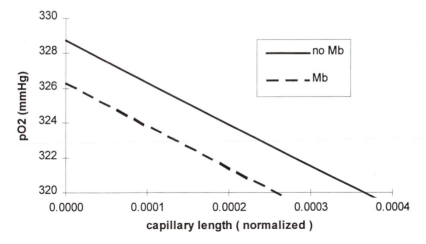

Figure 6. Close-up of inlet for capillary pO_2 profiles with and without Mb.

3.3. RAAD Model versus Experimental Data

The RAAD model histogram can be fitted to the experimental data. This is done by varying the axial diffusion coefficient for oxygen ($D_{Z,O2}$) in the model in an attempt to reduce the sum squared error (SSE) between the experimental and predicted histograms. Without myoglobin in the model, $D_{Z,O2}$ must be elevated to approximately ten times literature values for the RAAD model to closely predict the experimental pO_2 measurements. The $D_{Z,O2}$ required for the RAAD model to match the experimental data before the addition of myoglobin was 10.48 times normal. After adding myoglobin, the model required a $D_{Z,O2}$ of 10.22 times normal, which is a reduction of about 3%. The SSE between model

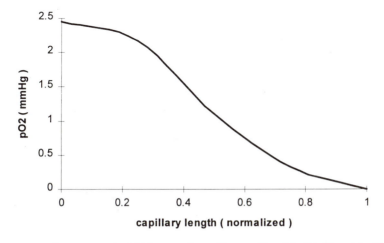

Figure 7. Plot of the difference (no Mb - Mb) between the capillary profiles of the RAAD model with and without Mb.

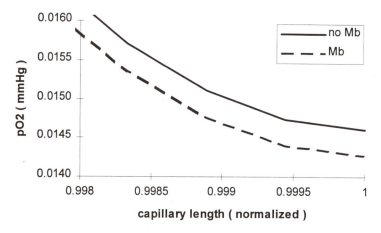

Figure 8. Close up of capillary exit showing the difference between the capillary pO_2 profiles for the RAAD model with and without Mb.

and experimental was reduced with the addition of myoglobin, meaning that the model with myoglobin provided a better prediction of the experimental data. The SSE without myoglobin was 5.6834, and the SSE with myoglobin was 5.6779, a reduction of 0.1%.

4. DISCUSSION

4.1. Output of RAAD Model with Myoglobin

From Figs. 3 and 4, it is obvious that the inlet and exit values for capillary pO_2 are not typical physiological values. The high capillary inlet pO_2 and extremely low outlet pO_2 are characteristic of an artificial linear perfusate. The parameters used in these simulations reflect the experimental conditions of the isolated perfused cat heart.

The addition of myoglobin to the RAAD model did little to change the pO_2 profiles and histogram predicted by the model. Capillary profiles for the Mb and no Mb case were very similar (Fig. 7); so much so that they could not be plotted in their entirety on the same graph without the semblance of overlap. The capillary inlet pO_2 changed only 0.8% with the addition of myoglobin, and the outlet changed 2% (Figs. 6,8). The inclusion of myoglobin did not improve the RAAD model prediction significantly. The SSE between model and experiment was reduced by only 0.1%. The effects of adding myoglobin to the model were minuscule, even though parameter values for myoglobin diffusivity and concentration used in the simulations were quite high. For example, the diffusivity of myoglobin in skeletal muscle was recently measured to be 1.2×10^{-7} cm^2/s, roughly 25 times lower than the value used in this simulation.[16] From this it is clear that myoglobin facilitation does not contribute greatly to the RAAD model.

4.2. Myoglobin and the Need for Elevated Diffusion Coefficient

The elevated $D_{z,O2}$ required for the model to match the experiment was reduced by only 3%. In contrast, Napper found that the inclusion of Michaelis-Menten kinetics in the RAAD model reduced the $D_{z,O2}$ by 20%, from 10 to 8 times normal diffusion.[4] This leads us to believe that myoglobin facilitation fails to explain the enhanced diffusion suggested in Schubert's data.

4.3. Myoglobin and Axial Diffusion

The axial pO_2 profiles in Figs. 3 and 4 reflect features of elevated axial diffusion and axial diffusive coupling. Two of these features are the steep initial decline of pO_2 (Fig. 3) in the capillary, and the lack of a large pO_2 gradient between the capillary and tissue regions (Table 1). Both axial diffusion and diffusion coupling tend to reduce the inlet gradients and flatten the pO_2 profile.[6] At first it was thought that myoglobin facilitation might be enhanced in the presence of these mechanisms. But, the results provided by this simulation state otherwise. The coupling of axial diffusive transport in the capillary and tissue region appears to be of much greater importance in determining the pO_2 distribution than does myoglobin facilitation. This diffusive coupling reduces the capillary inlet pO_2 by 8%, in contrast to the 0.8% reduction provided by myoglobin facilitation.[6] These findings suggest that myoglobin facilitation is not a significant source of oxygen transport in the presence of axial diffusion.

4.3. Why Is Myoglobin Not Significant?

From Fig. 5, myoglobin remains almost completely saturated for about 85% of the capillary length. Only near the end of the capillary, where the tissue is lower in pO_2, oxymyoglobin begins to release its bound oxygen. This is expected since the 50% saturation pressure (P_{50}) for Mb is low, around 2.5 mmHg. This low P_{50} reduces the facilitative transport effects in the steady state, since much of the tissue is at a pO_2 near or above this pressure. Also, the low concentration of myoglobin, and low diffusibility of this species reduce its effectiveness as an oxygen transport facilitator. The finding that myoglobin facilitation is not significant in the steady state does not deny a storage or transient function for myoglobin.

5. CONCLUSION

The computer simulations show that myoglobin does facilitate oxygen diffusion in the presence of axial diffusion, but only to a small extent. The change in inlet capillary pO_2 was less than 1%. Facilitation is limited due to low tissue concentration of myoglobin, along with low myoglobin mobility in the tissue. These findings do not deny a storage function for myoglobin, but suggest that facilitation of oxygen transport is not myoglobin's main physiological function, at least in the steady state. It is conceivable that myocardial contractile activity could enhance D_{Mb}, thereby enhancing myoglobin's facilitative capacity. No experimental result of this effect has been reported.

At this writing the enhanced oxygen diffusion suggested by Schubert's experimental pO_2 measurements has not been explained. Stirring of tissue by the contractile elements during contraction remains a possible cause.[3] As the myosin filament "ratchets" along the actin filament during muscle contraction it is feasible that the hinging myosin molecules provide stirring effects. If this is true, the diffusion of many chemical species, including oxygen and myoglobin, should be enhanced by the "contractile-convection" provided during cross-bridge cycling. A measurement determining the transport of a diffusible species in living, working tissue is needed to further explore this theory.

PARAMETER LIST

z	=	axial position
z_o	=	normalizing length, capillary/Krogh cylinder length
$C_{O2,\,TIS}$	=	tissue oxygen concentration
$C_{O2,\,CAP}$	=	capillary oxygen concentration
C_o	=	normalizing concentration, usually $C_{Mb,TOT}$
$C_{Mb,TOT}$	=	total tissue concentration of myoglobin, 1.0×10^{-6} mol/cm^3
v_{CAP}	=	perfusate velocity in capillary
r_{CAP}	=	capillary radius
r_{TIS}	=	Krogh tissue cylinder radius
$D_{Z,\,TIS}$	=	tissue axial diffusion coefficient
$D_{Z,\,CAP}$	=	capillary axial diffusion coefficient
D_{MbO2}	=	MbO$_2$ tissue diffusion coefficient, 2.97×10^{-6} cm^2/s
k	=	O$_2$ metabolic rate in tissue
P	=	capillary wall mass transport coefficient (concentration driven)
k_1	=	oxygen-myoglobin on rate
k_2	=	oxygen-myoglobin off rate
Y	=	fraction of Mb saturated with oxygen

REFERENCES

1. Schubert, R.W., Fletcher, J.E. and Reneau, D.D., "An analytical model for axial diffusion in the Krogh cylinder," *Oxygen Transport to Tissue - VI*, New York:Plenum Press, pp. 433–442, 1985.
2. Schubert, R.W., Whalen, W.J. and Nair, P., "Myocardial pO$_2$ distribution in the autoregulation myocardium," *Am.J.Physiol.*, vol. 234, pp. H361-H370, 1978.
3. Schubert, R.W., and Fletcher, J.E., "Rethinking oxygen transport to tissue: model and experiment compared," *Comments on Theoretical Biology*, vol. 3, no. 1, pp. 23–42, 1993.
4. Napper, S.A. and R.W. Schubert, "Mathematical evidence for flow-induced changes in myocardial oxygen consumption," *Ann.Biomed. Eng.*, vol. 16, pp. 349–365, 1988.
5. Schubert, R.W., and Zhang, X., "The equivalent Krogh cylinder and axial oxygen transport," *Oxygen Transport to Tissue*, this volume, 1995.
6. Fletcher, J.E., and Schubert, R.W., "Axial diffusion and wall permeability effects in perfused capillary- tissue structures," *BioSystems*, vol. 20, pp. 153–174, 1987.
7. Zhang, X., "Theoretical oxygen distribution in tissue: effects of radial transport assumptions (Masters Thesis), Louisiana Tech University, Ruston, LA, 1992.
8. Baylor, S.M., and Pape, P.C., "Measurement of myoglobin diffusivity in the myoplasm of frog skeletal muscle fibres," *J.Phys.*, vol. 406, pp. 247–275, 1988.
9. Federspiel, W.J., "A model study of intracellular oxygen gradients in a myoglobin-containing skeletal muscle fiber," *Biophys.J.*, vol.49, pp. 857–868, 1986.
10. Jaquez, J.A., "The physiological role of myoglobin: more than a problem in reaction-diffusion kinetics," *Math.Biosci.*, vol. 68, pp. 57–97, 1984.
11. Covell, D.G., and Jacquez, J.A., "Does myoglobin contribute significantly to diffusion of oxygen in red skeletal muscle?," *Am.J.Physiol.*, vol. 252, pp. R341-R347, 1987.
12. Gonzalez-Fernandez, J.M., and Atta, S.E., "Facilitated transport of oxygen in the presence of membranes in the diffusion path," *Biophys.J.*, vol. 38, pp. 133–141, 1982.
13. Salathe, E.P., and Chaorong, C., "The role of myoglobin in retarding oxygen depletion in skeletal muscle," *Math. Biosci.*, vol. 116, pp. 1–20, 1993.
14. Fletcher, J.E., "Facilitated oxygen diffusion in muscle tissues," *Biophys.J.*, vol. 29, pp. 437–458, 1980.
15. Meng, H., Bentley, T.B., and Pittman, R.N., "Myoglobin content of hamster skeletal muscles," *J.Appl.Physiol.*, vol. 74, pp. 2194–2197, 1993.

16. Jurgens, K.D., Peters, T., and Gros, G., "Diffusivity of myoglobin in intact skeletal muscle cells," *Proc.NatlAcad.Sci. Physiology*, vol. 91, pp. 3829–3833, 1994.

17. Schuder, S., Wittenberg, J.B., Haseltine, B., and Wittenberg, B.A., "Spectrophotometric determination of myoglobin in cardiac and skeletal muscle: separation from hemoglobin by subunit-exchange chromatography," *Analytical Biochem.*, vol. 92, pp. 473–481, 1979.

18. Lentini, M., and Pereyra, V., "An adaptive finite difference solver for nonlinear two-point boundary problems with mild boundary layers," *SIAM J.Num.Anal.*, vol. 14, pp. 91–111, 1979.

21

MYOCARDIAL OXYGEN TENSION AND CAPILLARY DENSITY IN THE ISOLATED PERFUSED RAT HEART DURING PHARMACOLOGICAL INTERVENTION

Oleg Y. Grinberg,[1] Stalina A. Grinberg,[1] Bruce J. Friedman,[2] and Harold M. Swartz[1]

[1]Department of Radiology
[2]Section of Cardiology
Dartmouth-Hitchcock Medical Center
Hanover, New Hampshire 03755

ABSTRACT

Oxygen is essential for normal cardiac function and plays an important role in cardiac regulation. Electron paramagnetic resonance (EPR) oximetry appears to have some significant advantages for measuring oxygen tension (pO_2) in the beating heart. This study presents the serial measurement of myocardial pO_2 by EPR oximetry in the isolated crystalloid perfused heart during treatment with different cardioactive drugs: dobutamine, metoprolol, verapamil, vasopressin, and Nω-Nitro-L-Arginine Methyl Ester (L-NAME). Baseline myocardial pO_2 was 176 ± 14 mmHg (mean$\pm$S.E.). Myocardial capillary density in the intact contracting heart was calculated to be 2300 ± 100 mm^{-2}, using local myocardial pO_2 and a cylindrical model for oxygen diffusion in tissue. Each drug had characteristic effects on myocardial pO_2, myocardial oxygen consumption (MVO_2), and capillary density. Metoprolol and verapamil increased myocardial pO_2 by 51% and 18%, respectively, dobutamine decreased myocardial pO_2 by 84% while vasopressin and L-NAME had no significant effect on myocardial pO_2. Metoprolol and verapamil decreased MVO_2 by 9% and 56%, respectively, while dobutamine increased MVO_2 by 59%. A quantitative comparison of effects on the capillary bed based on changes in myocardial pO_2 and MVO_2 was made. Metoprolol and verapamil had opposite effects on the capillary bed. Verapamil decreased myocardial capillary density by 39%, while capillary density increased by 10% (n.s.) with metoprolol. Data following perfusion without drug is also presented. We conclude that: 1) The application of EPR oximetry with LiPc provides dynamic evaluation of local myocardial pO_2 in the contracting heart. 2) Using a cylindrical model of oxygen de-

Oxygen Transport to Tissue XVIII, edited by Nemoto and LaManna
Plenum Press, New York, 1997

livery and diffusion in tissue, these data may be used to describe the changes of capillary density during pharmacological interventions.

1. INTRODUCTION

Oxygen is essential for normal cardiac function and plays an important role in cardiac regulation[1,2]. The dynamic equilibrium between oxygen consumption (MVO_2) and oxygen delivery in myocardium is reflected by the myocardial oxygen tension (pO_2). This value is an important parameter that reflects the state of cardiac muscle and the capillary bed.

Many methods have been developed to measure pO_2 in tissue[3]. Electron paramagnetic resonance (EPR) oximetry appears to have some significant advantages for use in the beating heart[4,5]. Recently it was shown[6] that EPR oximetry used in conjunction with lithium phthalocyanine (LiPc) crystals as the O_2-sensitive probe, placed in the area of interest, provides accurate and dynamic evaluation of local myocardial pO_2 in the contracting isolated heart. Myocardial pO_2 increased as expected with increased delivery (concentration of oxygen or flow of perfusate) or decreased consumption. With increasing flow rate, myocardial pO_2 increased in a sigmoid fashion. When a critical flow or pressure was reached myocardial pO_2 increased more rapidly. Increased left ventricular end diastolic pressure decreased myocardial pO_2 due to local vascular compression. Myocardial pO_2 also was shown to increase significantly after recovery from repetitive ischemia, in conjunction with an increase in coronary vascular resistance. Increased myocardial pO_2 in normoperfused hearts may be due to decreased oxygen consumption after ischemia and/or increased local delivery, while in hypoperfused hearts the data were consistent with increased local oxygen delivery. Measurement of myocardial pO_2 and capillary density determined from a cylindrical model for oxygen diffusion may be used to study cardiac drug effects.

The effects of calcium channel blockers, nitric oxide, agonists and antagonists and vasopressin on arterioles and arteries have been well described[7,8]. It also is hypothesized that some drugs may have effects on the microcirculation and capillary bed[9–12]. These effects could have an important role in controlling myocardial function. Accurate measurement of the changes in local pO_2 and capillary density caused by different drugs may improve our understanding of the microcirculation and facilitate appropriate drug selection.

In the present report we investigated the affects on myocardial pO_2 of the commonly used beta-adrenergic agonist—dobutamine, a beta-adrenoreceptor antagonist—metoprolol, a calcium channel blocker—verapamil, a vasoconstrictor—vasopressin, and a nitric oxide inhibitor—Nω-Nitro-L-Arginine Methyl Ester (L-NAME) a relatively new agent that has attracted great interest. Myocardial pO_2 and the variations of oxygen consumption, perfusion pressure and left ventricular contractility were measured. Using these data we assessed the influence of these drugs on the capillary bed.

2. EXPERIMENTAL

2.1. Lithium Phthalocyanine as the O_2-Sensitive Probe and EPR Measurements

LiPc is a neutral π-radical crystalline substance that has a strong narrow EPR signal, whose line width is sensitive to oxygen[13] and therefore a convenient probe for EPR oximetry[14]. Four to ten small LiPc crystals (LETI, Grenoble, France) with total volume 0.5 x 0.2 x 0.2 mm^3, were loaded into a 26 gauge needle and implanted in the posterolateral wall of the left ventricle in the mid myocardium at a depth of 1 mm. For EPR measurements a L-band (1.18 GHz) spectrometer that utilizes a homemade microwave bridge specially designed for in vivo experiments was used. Movement of the heart, which can produce noise and adversely affect measurements, was diminished by placing the heart in a rigid plastic vessel in which the level of media was kept constant (Figure 1). All spectra were recorded, with careful regard to avoid power saturation and over modulation, on a PC computer (Gateway 2000) with scan time varying from 30 to 50 sec. The data were obtained by averaging 2 or 3 scans, depending on the noise level. The first derivative of the EPR absorption line was recorded and the line width measured as the distance between the peaks of these spectra. Myocardial pO$_2$ was calculated from a calibration curve made for this batch of LiPc[6].

2.2. Animal Preparation and Experimental Protocol

Male Wistar rats were given heparin (5 IU/gm) intraperitoneally 30–40 minutes before anesthesia with pentobarbital (40–60 mg/kg) intraperitoneally. The study conformed to the guidelines of the animal research laboratory of Dartmouth Medical School that is accredited by the American Association of Laboratory Animal Care. Following the onset of general anesthesia the rat heart was harvested in the usual fashion and perfused by the

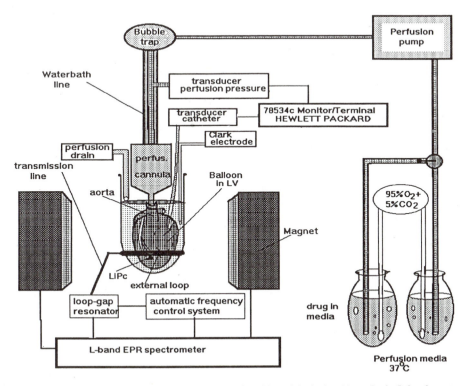

Figure 1. Diagram illustrating the perfusion apparatus and position of the isolated heart in the L-band spectrometers, showing pressure monitors and Clark electrode.

Langendorff technique. The rate of coronary flow was adjusted and kept constant with a variable speed peristaltic pump (Masterflex) for an initial aortic perfusion pressure (PP) around 70 mmHg. Pressure and heart rate (HR) were monitored with a disposable transducer (Transpac II Abbott, North Chicago, Illinois) and a hemodynamic monitor (Hewlett Packard 78534c). The perfused heart with implanted crystals was placed just above the external loop and maintained at a temperature of 37°C. Modified Krebs Henseleit solution (in mmol/l) 118 NaCl, 5.9 KCl, 3 $CaCl_2$, 1.2 $MgSO_4$, 0.5 NaEDTA, 25 Na-HCO_3 and 11 glucose, pH 7.4, in equilibrium with 5% CO_2 & 95% O_2 was used for perfusion.

Trans aortic leakage of perfusion media can affect the measured value for MVO_2[6], therefore, special care was taken when hanging the heart to minimize leakage through the vent in the left ventricle. After implantation of the LiPc crystals a latex balloon was inserted into the left ventricule and filled with a volume of distilled water sufficient to produce an end diastolic pressure of 8–12 mmHg. It was used to determine left ventricular isovolumetric parameters including systolic and diastolic pressure, developed pressure (DP) (difference between peak systolic and end diastolic pressure) and left ventricular contractility (HRxDP, product of heart rate and developed pressure). Clark electrodes were used to monitor pO_2 in the influent at various flow rates and the pO_2 of the effluent was measured throughout the experiment. MVO_2 was calculated from the product of flow rate and the difference between influent and effluent pO_2, assuming the concentration of oxygen in media and pure water was the same (210 μM in air, 760 mmHg, 37°C) and normalized to the wet weight of each heart. The Clark electrode was calibrated with a gas mixture 5% CO_2 & 95% O_2.

Measurements were made at three periods: *baseline* (before pharmacologic intervention); *with drug* (drug present in media) and *after drug* (following perfusion with drug free media). Separate animals were used for each set of measurements.

Twenty minutes were usually required for preparation of the heart and for initial equilibration. Measurements were then taken in triplicate five minutes apart. After the baseline measurements, Krebs Henseleit solution with a known concentration of a drug, also equilibrated with 5% CO_2 & 95% O_2 was infused. (Fig. 1). The measurements with drug were performed using standard concentrations: dobutamine hydrochloride (Eli Lilly & Co., Indianapolis)—1 μM, metoprolol tartrate (Schein Pharmaceutical, Inc.) —7 μM, verapamil HCL (American Regent Laboratories, Inc.)—0.2 μM, vasopressin 20Un/ml (American Regent Laboratories, Inc.)—20 μM and Nw-Nitro-L-Arginine Methyl Ester (Sigma)—30 μM. In a similar fashion to baseline measurements, fifteen minutes were allowed for stabilization with the drug, then three sets of measurements were made every five minutes. After measurements with drug, fifteen minutes were allowed for perfusion with drug free media (or media with 0.1 mM L-arginine (Sigma) for experiments using L-NAME) before repeating three sets of measurements five minutes apart. The mean value of these three measurements was used for analysis. Change was determined as the difference between this value and baseline measurement. Relative change was determined by dividing the change by the baseline value for each heart. The values for the last two periods are presented as changes from the baseline values and relative changes in each animal.

2.3. Calculation of Capillary Density

The measured myocardial pO_2 may be used to calculate relative myocardial capillary density[6]. The cylindrical steady state model for radial diffusion of oxygen from the capillary in striated muscle, which was developed seventy five years ago by Krogh[15,16] with Erlang, has been the basis for most attempts to calculate oxygen levels in tissue or to calculate capillary density if oxygen tension and MVO_2 are known. According to this model,

$$P_R = P_c - MVO_2(R^2\ln(R/r)^2 - (R^2 - r^2))/4D,$$

where P_R is the tissue pO_2 at distance R, R is the radius of the diffusion cylinder and 2R is the intercapillary distance (capillary density = $1/4R^2$), P_c is the capillary pO_2, r is the capillary radius (2.5 μm) and D is the tissue oxygen diffusion coefficient. D = 1.5×10^{-5} cm^2/sec, as reported for myocardial tissue[17].

As predicted by this equation, tissue pO_2 increases with increasing influent capillary pO_2 or decreasing MVO_2 or decreasing intercapillary distance (equivalent to increasing capillary density) or increasing capillary radius.

Kety[18] estimated $P_c = (pO_2IN + pO_2OUT)/2$ from systemic arterial (pO_2IN) and venous (pO_2OUT) oxygen tension in tissue. Using line width measurements for myocardial pO_2 which represents the mean value of P_R[6], the Krogh Erlang equation, the Kety estimation of P_c and assuming that capillary radius does not change significantly, the number of open capillaries was calculated.

2.4. Statistical Analysis

Summed results are expressed as mean ± standard error. A paired t-test is used to compare effects with the drug and effects following perfusion without drug versus baseline for line width, perfusion pressure, oxygen consumption and left ventricle contractility. Data are considered to be significantly different at p<.05.

3. RESULTS

The mean wet heart weight, initial flow, and perfusion pressure for all (34) hearts was 1.04±0.07g, 16±1 ml/min and 71.9±3 mmHg, respectively. Baseline myocardial pO_2 was 176±14 mmHg. Left ventricular contractility was 34500±1700 mmHg/min. Myocardial MVO_2 was 7.5±0.4 μmol/g/min. Table 1 presents the mean initial data for each group (segregated by drug) of animals, the number of animals in each group (shown in brackets), and changes of the measured parameters with drug intervention and after drug. The drugs had different effects on myocardial oxygen tension: it increased with metoprolol and verapamil, decreased with dobutamine, and did not change with L-NAME or vasopressin. The drugs also had different effects on perfusion pressure: it increased with vasopressin and L-NAME, decreased with dobutamine and was unchanged with metoprolol and verapamil. MVO_2 increased with dobutamine, and decreased with verapamil and metoprolol and was unchanged with vasopressin and L-NAME. Left ventricular contractility increased with dobutamine, decreased with verapamil or metoprolol, and was unchanged with vasopressin and L-NAME.Myocardial capillary density (n=34) in the contracting heart, calculated using local myocardial pO_2 and a cylindrical model for oxygen diffusion in tissue, was 2300±80 mm^{-2}. Calculated capillary density decreased significantly with verapamil and was not significantly changed with metoprolol, dobutamine, vasopressin, or L-NAME.

Table 1. Initial data and change of oxygen tension (pO_2, mmHg), perfusion pressure (PP, mmHg), oxygen consumption (MVO_2, μmol/min/g), left ventricle contractility (HRxDP, mmHg/min) and capillary density (CD, mm^{-2}) with drug (D) and after drug (d) treatment (mean±S.E) for groups of rat hearts (number is shown in brackets). Change was determined as the difference between the value and baseline measurement. The rate of coronary flow (Flow, ml/min) was kept constant

	Metoprolol (5)	Dobutamine (5)	Verapamil (6)	Vasopressin (7)	L-NAME (11)
Flow	16.9 ± 1	17.0 ± 1.4	17.5 ± 0.8	15.8 ± 1	14.5 ± 1
pO_2	145 ± 27	155 ± 11	168 ± 11	196 ± 17	192 ± 12
$D(pO_2)$	53 ± 15 *	−129 ± 15 *	30 ± 15 *	−11 ± 11	−30 ± 15
$d(pO_2)$	53 ± 23	53 ± 15 *	15 ± 8	23 ± 8 *	8 ± 15
PP	67.8 ± 1.9	75.0 ± 3.6	78.3 ± 4.1	72.0 ± 3.1	68.7 ± 2.5
D(PP)	0 ± 3	−19 ± 4 *	−2 ± 2	32 ± 6 *	26 ± 4 *
d(PP)	11 ± 4	17 ± 6 *	8 ± 4	19 ± 7 *	25 ± 5 *
MVO_2	9.2 ± 0.4	7.5 ± 0.4	7.6 ± 0.4	7.4 ± 0.4	6.7 ± 0.4
$D(MVO_2)$	−53 ± 19 *	250 ± 30 *	−320 ± 30 *	−25 ± 20	−6 ± 15
$d(MVO_2)$	−92 ± 4 *	−100 ± 20 *	−54 ± 20 *	−85 ± 30 *	−18 ± 15
HRxDP	36400 ± 2000	33800 ± 1500	33900 ± 900	31800 ± 1800	36100 ± 2200
D(HRxDP)	−3360 ± 880 *	19900 ± 3400 *	−19000 ± 1100 *	−1080 ± 1090	−1610 ± 970
d(HRxDP)	−5640 ± 980 *	−4530 ± 680 *	−5440 ± 540 *	−4530 ± 1190 *	−3640 ± 870 *
CD	2500 ± 140	2100 ± 120	2100 ± 90	2500 ± 160	2300 ± 150
D(CD)	240 ± 120	−180 ± 200	−840 ± 80 *	−160 ± 190	−120 ± 130
d(CD)	120 ± 180	340 ± 290	−110 ± 90	−90 ± 90	75 ± 180

*Data are significantly different by paired two tail t-test (p < .05)

Table 1 also summarizes changes of the measured parameters after drug. Myocardial oxygen tension increased after dobutamine and vasopressin. Perfusion pressure increased after dobutamine and did not return to baseline after vasopressin and L-NAME. MVO_2 decreased after dobutamine and vasopressin and did not return to baseline after verapamil and metoprolol. Calculated capillary density returned to baseline after verapamil.

Figure 2 demonstrates relative changes (%) of the measured parameters with pharmacological interventions. Myocardial oxygen tension increased 51% with metoprolol and 18% with verapamil and decreased 84% with dobutamine. Perfusion pressure increased 46% and 38% with vasopressin and L-NAME, respectively and decreased 25% with dobutamine. MVO_2 increased 34% with dobutamine and decreased 41% and 6% with verapamil and metoprolol, respectively. Left ventricular contractility increased 59% with dobutamine, decreased 56% and 9% with verapamil and metoprolol, respectively. Calculated capillary density changed significantly only with verapamil.

Figure 3 demonstrates relative changes (%) of the measured parameters after drug. Myocardial oxygen tension increased after dobutamine (34%) and vasopressin (11%). Perfusion pressure increased 24% after dobutamine, decreased but remained above baseline after vasopressin and L-NAME. MVO_2 decreased after dobutamine (13%) and vasopressin (10%), increased but remained above baseline after verapamil. Left ventricular contractility decreased after dobutamine (13%), vasopressin (14%) and L-NAME (10%); increased but remained below baseline for metoprolol and verapamil. Calculated capillary density returned to baseline after verapamil.

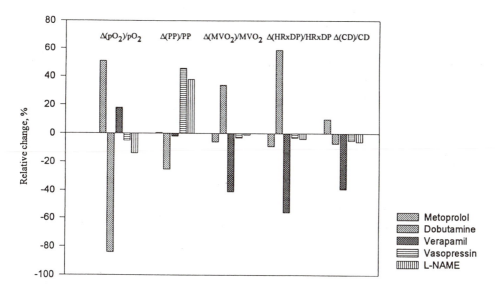

Figure 2. Relative change (%) of oxygen tension (pO_2) perfusion pressure (PP), oxygen consumption (MVO_2), left ventricle contractility (HR×DP), and capillary density (CD) with metoprolol, dobutamine, verapamil, vasopressin, and L-NAME.

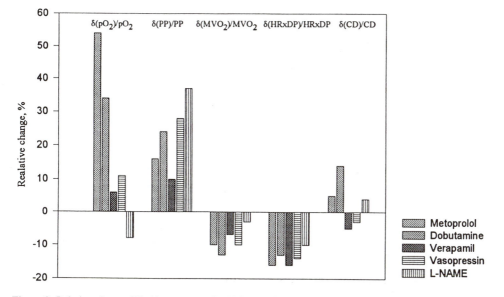

Figure 3. Relative change (%) of oxygen tension (pO_2), perfusion pressure (PP), oxygen consumption (MVO_2), left ventricle contractility (HR×DP) and capillary density (CD) following perfusion without drag.

4. DISCUSSION

4.1. Measurement of Myocardial pO_2 and MVO_2

Baseline myocardial pO_2 measured by EPR oximetry was 176 ± 14 mmHg which agrees with previous reports of myocardial oxygen tension in crystalloid perfused isolated hearts[6]. The mild variations in initial myocardial oxygen tension between animals (Table 1) may be explained in terms of crystal placement relative to the microvasculature and by the myocardial oxygen distribution of pO_2[6]. The mild variations in initial MVO_2 (Table 1) presumably reflects the difference in trans aortic leakage of perfusion media. Since coronary flow and influent oxygen concentration were kept constant during the experiments and the position of the crystal was fixed in each heart, the changes in myocardial pO_2 and MVO_2 were caused by the various drug treatments.

4.2. Pharmacological Effects

Our results demonstrate that effective drug concentrations were used as seen by the changes in MVO_2, contractility, and perfusion pressure (see Table 1). Each pharmacological intervention was accompanied by characteristic physiologic changes. Metoprolol and verapamil decreased left ventricular contractility and MVO_2. Dobutamine, which is an inotropic agent, increased left ventricular contractility and oxygen consumption. Vasopressin a vasoconstrictor and L-NAME which inhibits nitric oxide a vasodilator both increased perfusion pressure but had no significant effect on other parameters.

As expected local myocardial pO_2 changed with pharmacological manipulation of myocardial oxygen consumption and contractility. Myocardial pO_2 increased 7 mmHg with the beta blocker metoprolol and 4 mmHg with verapamil, a calcium channel blocker. Both these agents are known to decrease MVO_2[19,20] as confirmed by our results (Table 1). Dobutamine, an inotropic agent which increases MVO_2[21], resulted in a 17 mmHg decrease of myocardial pO_2.

Perfusion with drug free media also effected the measured parameters and may help explain actions of the drug. Although pO_2 decreased significantly with dobutamine and did not change significantly with vasopressin, after perfusion with drug free media pO_2 increased significantly in both cases. After dobutamine and vasopressin the decrease of MVO_2 presumably accounts for the increase of pO_2.

4.3. Relative Capillary Density

The 320 μmol/min/g decrease in MVO_2 observed with verapamil, had a smaller effect on myocardial pO_2 than the 53 μmol/min/g decrease of MVO_2 induced by metoprolol (Table 1). This discrepancy can be explained by changes in capillary density. Baseline myocardial capillary density (2300 ± 100 mm^{-2}) from these experiments agrees with previous reports of capillary density in rat hearts 2200 mm^{-2} [22], 2650 mm^{-2} [23] and 2300 ± 110 mm^{-2} [6]. Capillary density decreased 39% ($p<.05$) with verapamil while there was no significant change with dobutamine, L-NAME, metoprolol and vasopressin.

The slight increase in capillary density with metoprolol as compared to the significant decrease with verapamil may have important clinical implications and may explain some of the recognized benefits of beta blockers (such as metoprolol) in ischemic heart disease.

Drugs have discordant effects on the coronary vasculature [24], their effects on the capillary bed have been difficult to study. Vasopressin and L-NAME, which are known to affect larger vessels and arterioles[25–27], increased coronary resistance presumably by effects on arterioles. Determination of myocardial pO_2 by EPR oximetry shows that the capillary bed did not change significantly with these drugs. Thus, these data suggest that vasopressin and L-NAME affect the larger vessels but not the capillary bed.

4.4. Potential Limitations

Potential limitations of this study include use of the isolated perfused heart and a hemoglobin free perfusion media. Drug effects may be different in the intact animal. Perfusion with crystalloid media requires higher than usual perfusion pressure/flow and may result in early capillary recruitment. In these experiments the absence of drug effect on capillary density may be due to the use of high flow in crystalloid perfused hearts which are believed to operate at near maximal capillary density[28]. The changes of capillary density observed with verapamil, is a result of capillary closing.

To calculate relative capillary density, in addition to the usual limitations of the Krogh Erlang cylindrical model[18,29,30], assumptions must also be made regarding capillary radius and capillary pO_2.

5. CONCLUSION

The changes in the observed values of myocardial pO_2 in isolated contracting rat heart with drug treatment are consistent with the known pharmacological actions of the drugs.

The drugs had different effects on myocardial oxygen tension which increased 51% with metoprolol and 18% with verapamil and decreased 84% with dobutamine and did not change with L-NAME or vasopressin. The measured pO_2 values could not be inferred simply from measurements of single physiological parameters such as MVO_2 and therefore direct measurement of pO_2 is useful.

Myocardial pO_2 in the contracting heart may be used in conjunction with a cylindrical model of oxygen delivery and diffusion in tissue to describe changes of capillary density during pharmacological intervention. Two drugs that reduce MVO_2 had different effects on the capillary bed. Verapamil decreased myocardial capillary density by 39%, while capillary density increased 10% (n.s.) with metoprolol. Dobutamine, vasopressin and L-NAME did not change capillary density significantly.

We conclude that it is feasible and useful to make the accurate and dynamic measurement of local myocardial pO_2 in the isolated contracting heart and relative capillary density by EPR oximetry with LiPc.

ACKNOWLEDGMENTS

This work was supported by AHA, New Hampshire Affiliate Grant in Aid 9407770S and NIH grant GM 34250 and used the facilities of the EPR center at Dartmouth Medical School which was supported by NIH grant RR 01811.

REFERENCES

1. Relationship between carbohydrate and lipid metabolism and the energy balance of heart muscle. Neely JR, et al. *Ann Rev Physiol*, 1974;36:413–459.
2. Quantification of O_2 consumption and arterial pressure as independent determinants of coronary flow. Vergroesen I, et al. *Am J Physiol*, 1987;252:H5435 -5530.
3. Oxygen in mammalian tissue:methods of measurement and affinities of various reactions. Vanderkooi J M, et al. *Am J Physiol*, 1991;260:C1131-C1150.
4. Measurement of oxygen concentrations in the intact beating heart using EPR spectroscopy: A technique for measuring oxygen concentrations in situ. Zweier JL, et al. *J Bioener Biomem*, 1991;23(6):855–871.
5. The use of EPR for measurement of concentration of oxygen in vivo in tissues under physiologically pertinent conditions and concentrations. Swartz HM, et al. *Adv in Exp Med and Biol*, 1992;317:221–228.
6. Myocardial Oxygen Tension and Relative Capillary Density in Isolated Perfused Rat Hearts. Friedman BJ, et al. *J Molec Cell Cardiology*, 1995 in press.
7. EDRF coordinates the behavior of vascular resistance vessels. Griffith TM, et al. *Nature*, 1987;329: 442–445.
8. Mechanisms of disease. Franklin HE. *New England J Med*, 1982;307(26): 1618–1627.
9. Vasopressin, renin and norepinephrine level before and after failure due to idiopathic dilated cardiomyopathy. Rakusan GA, et al. *Am J Cardiol*, 1986;58: 300–303.
10. Effect of vasopressin on capillary recruitment and coronary blood flow in anesthetized rabbit. Funk W, et al. *Can J Physiol Pharmacol*, 1991;69:170–175.
11. Calcium Antagonist and Microperfusion. Tillmans H, et al. *Drugs*, 1991;42 (Suppl.1).
12. Changes in myocardial capillary diffusion capacity during infusion of vasoactive drugs. Whlander H, et al. *Acta Physiol Scand*, 1993;147:49–58.
13. Septet spin state in lithium phthalocyanine 1 radical compound. Turek P, et al. *Mol Crys Liq Cryst*, 1989;176:535–542.
14. Lithium phthalocyanine: A probe for EPR oximetry in viable biological systems. Liu KJ, et al. *Proc Natl Acad Sci USA*, 1993;90:5438–5442.
15. The number and distribution of capillaries in muscles with calculations of the oxygen pressure head necessary for supplying the tissue. Krogh A. *J Physiol (Lond)*, 1919;52:409–415.
16. The supply of oxygen to the tissues and the regulation of the capillary circulation. Krogh A. *J Physiol (Lond)*, 1919;52:457–474.
17. Die Sauerstoffdrucke im Herzmuskelgewebe. Thews G. *Pfluger Arch*, 1962; 276:166–181.
18. Determinants of tissue oxygen tension. Kety SS. *Fed Proc*, 1957;16:666–670.
19. LV oxygen consumption and pressure-volume area: role of norepinephrine and verapamil. Chung N, *Am J Physiol*, 1991;261(1 Pt 2):H77–82.
20. Effect of metoprolol on left ventricular function in rats with myocardial infarction. Cherng WJ, et al. *Am J Physiol*, 1994;266(2 Pt 2):H787–94.
21. Effect of intracoronary infusions of amrinone and dobutamine on segment shortening, blood flow and oxygen consumption in in situ canine hearts. Crystal GL, et al. *Anesthesia and analgesia*, 1994;76(6):1066–74.
22. Direct measurement of intercapillary distance in beating rat heart in situ under various conditions of O_2 supply. Martini J, et al. *Microvas Res*, 1969;1:244–256.
23. Microcirculation of the epimyocardial layer of the heart. I. A method for in vivo observation of the microcirculation of superficial ventricular myocardium of the heart and capillary flow pattern under normal and hypoxic conditions. Steinhausen M, et al. *Pflugers Arch*, 1978;378:9–14.
24. Differential response of large and small coronary arteries to nitroglycerine and angiotensin. Cohen MV, et al. *Circ. Res.* 1973;33:445–453
25. Hemodynamic effects of infused arginine vasopressin in congestive heart failure. Goldsmith SR, et al. *J Am Coll Cardiol*, 1986; 8:779–773.

26. Role of vasopressin in cardiovascular and blood pressure regulation. Abboud FM, et al. *Blood vessel*, 1990;27(2–5):106–15.

27. L-NAME, nitric oxide and jejunal motility, blood flow and oxygen uptake in dogs. Alemayehu A, et al. *British journal of pharmacology*, 1994:111(1):205–12.

28. Changes in myocardial capillary diffusion capacity during infusion of vasoactive drugs. Wahlander H, et al. *Acta Physiol Scand.* 1993;147:49–58

29. Oxygen supply to tissues: the Krogh model and its assumptions. Kreuzer F. *Experientia Basel*, 1982;38:1415–1426.

30. Analysis of oxygen delivery and uptake relationships in the Krogh tissue model. Schumacker PT, et al. *J Appl Physiol*, 1989;67:1234–1244.

22

INFLUENCE OF ISOKINETIC AND ERGOMETRIC EXERCISES ON OXYGEN PARTIAL PRESSURE MEASUREMENT IN THE HUMAN KNEE JOINT

O. Miltner, U. Schneider, J. Graf, and F. U. Niethard

Department of Orthopedic Surgery
University of Heidelberg

1. SUMMARY

We conducted the first in vivo investigation on the influence of joint movement on intraarticular oxygen partial pressure. The development of a special flexible micro-catheter allowed measurements of intraarticular oxygen partial pressure under both physiological and pathological conditions. The aim of this study was to evaluate the influence of different knee joint stresses on intraarticular oxygen partial pressure under physiological (healthy patients) and pathological (patients with osteoarthritis) conditions.

The results show that the different exercise patterns influence the intraarticular oxygen partial pressure. Patients with osteoarthritis showed a lower increase of intraarticular oxygen partial pressure compared with healthy patients. This phenomenon is directly correlated to the degree velocity of the isokinetic exercises. We found the same results under ergometric conditions. This method allows functional, intraarticular in vivo measurements under different exercise patterns. For the first time, we were able to measure the influence of joint movement on the intraarticular process of nutrition under physiological and pathological conditions. Also, to evaluate for the first time in vivo different concepts for osteoarthritis therapy.

2. INTRODUCTION

The human knee joint is similar to an organ with regard to its position, function and performance; moreover, it has a special nutritive condition (1,2). Nutrition of cartilage depends on the undisturbed diffusion between synovial membrane, synovia and cartilage (Fig. 1).

Oxygen Transport to Tissue XVIII, edited by Nemoto and LaManna
Plenum Press, New York, 1997

DIFFUSION

SYNOVIAL MEMBRANE ⟷ SYNOVIA ⟷ CARTILAGE

Figure 1. Cartilage nutrition.

Disturbance factors of the cartilage nutritions include:

1. Bad blood circulation / bulb of the vessel wall;
2. Fibrotic synovial membrane;
3. Change in quality and quantity of the synovia;
4. Immobilization;
5. Quality change of the matrix.

An arthritic knee joint has some, or all, of these disturbance factors. Therefore, a deficit of oxygen and substrate arise in the arthritic knee joint. Up to now, no in vivo investigation has been conducted to measure the influence of joint movement on intraarticular oxygen partial pressure. The development of a flexible micro-catheter (named Licox) allowed us to measure the intraarticular oxygen partial pressure under physiological and pathological conditions for the first time.

3. MATERIAL / METHOD

3.1. Material

The study population included 15 patients (8 females and 7 males) with typical clinical and radiological signs of osteoarthritis (Lequesne—Index > 15 points, Kellgren stage III–IV) (3,4), average age 69.8 years (range 56–79); and 10 healthy subjects (6 female and 4 males) with no clinical or radiological signs of osteoarthritis, average age 27.9 years (range 25–32 years), served as controls.

3.2. Method

The flexible Clark-type probe (named LICOX) was used for oxygen partial pressure measurement, and the microcatheter *thermocouple* for temperature measurement (Fig. 2).

The microcatheter po_2 sensor is a flexible Clark-type probe of small diameter (470 mm). Local tissue po_2 values are averaged over the 5 mm long sensitive area, i.e. the cylindrical outer surface of the probe situated near the catheter's tip. On-line temperature compensation is performed by the temperature probe. (pic. 1 in: GMS Mess systeme)

3.3. Measurement of pO_2

The osteoarthritic patients and the healthy subjects lay down for 30 min before the process begins. After repeat disinfection, local anesthesia with Carbostesin 0.5% and draping with sterile sheets, a trochar cannula (average 1.7 mm) was inserted into the recessus suprapatellaris. During this procedure the guidelines of the German Organization of Orthopedics and Traumatology were strictly followed. The flexible probe for oxygen partial pressure measurement and the microcatheter *thermocouple* for temperature measurement were inserted through the cannula into the knee (Fig. 2). Then the cannula was removed and the site of the puncture bandaged.

3.4. Isokinetic Exercise Program

The isokinetic exercise is an accommodating resistance exercise (5). An electrome-chanical device keeps the limb in motion at a constant, predetermined velocity.

The *Cybex 6000 weight lifting system* was used for the isokinetic exercise.

The intraarticular oxygen partial pressure was measured during slow dynamic tension (60°/sec) and rapid dynamic tension (180°/sec).

Test velocity: Repetitions:
60°/sec   5 X
180°/sec   20 X

The subjects were seated with the hips flexed around 90°, a position maintained by the back of the chair. The lever of the dynamometer was attached to the lower leg a few centimeters proximal to the ankle joint.

Afterwards, both groups participated for 5 min in an ergometric exercise program (with 90 rounds per min) on the *Fitron-Cybex Ergometer*.

3.5. Statistical Analysis

Means (x), and standard deviations (SD) were calculated using standard methods. The data of the two groups were compared using the t-test (5).

Differences were considered significant at a p-value < 0.05.

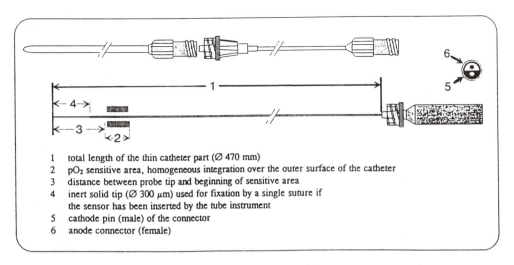

1   total length of the thin catheter part (Ø 470 mm)
2   pO₂ sensitive area, homogeneous integration over the outer surface of the catheter
3   distance between probe tip and beginning of sensitive area
4   inert solid tip (Ø 300 μm) used for fixation by a single suture if
    the sensor has been inserted by the tube instrument
5   cathode pin (male) of the connector
6   anode connector (female)

Figure 2. LICOX flexible Clark type oxygen probe with temperature compensation.

4. RESULTS

4.1. Resting Value

Figure 3 shows that the mean resting value of the oxygen partial pressure of the control group was 48.53 +/- 11.21 mmHg; the mean intraarticular temperature was 32.06 +/- 1.35 °C. The mean resting value of the osteoarthritis group was 29.98 +/- 3.90 mmHg; the mean intraarticular temperature was 35.71 +/- 1.04 °C. Mean values of both the oxygen partial pressure and temperature of the two groups were significantly different ($p < 0.001$).

4.2. Isokinetic Exercise

Figure 4 shows that after 5 repetitions with a test velocity of 60°/ sec the oxygen partial pressure of the control group increased by 36.35 +/- 31.45%, compared with the much smaller increase of 8.13 +/- 9.3% ($p < 0.05$) in the osteoarthritis group. One minute after the 5 repetitions the oxygen partial pressure of the patient group decreased below the initial value. After 7 minutes rest the oxygen partial pressure was reduced compare with the initial value, whereas the control group showed an improvement in oxygen partial pressure.

Figure 5 shows that after 20 repetitions with a test velocity of 180°/sec the oxygen partial pressure of the control group increased 25.28 $\pm$ 4.88%, whereas the increase in the patient group was only 13.02 +/- 7.93 ($p < 0.001$).

These results suggest that a test velocity of 60°/sec leads to the highest increase in oxygen partial pressure for the control group, whereas the osteoarthritis group shows the highest increase at a test velocity of 180°/sec.

4.3. Ergometric Exercise

Figure 6 shows that after 5 minute ergometric exercise the increase in oxygen partial pressure for the control group is 17.00 mmHg, and 1.7 mmHg for the osteoarthritis group.

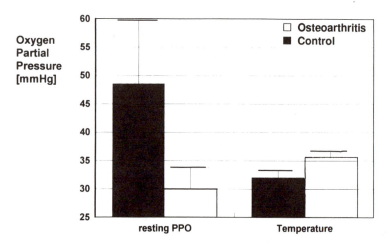

Figure 3. Resting values (mean ±SD) of intraarticular oxygen partial pressure and temperature of control and osteoarthritic groups.

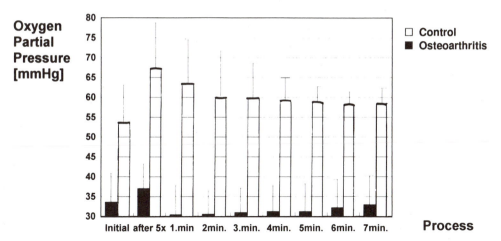

Figure 4. Effects of isokinetic exercise on intraarticular oxygen partial pressure (mean ± SD) after 5 repetitions at a velocity of 60°/sec. in osteoarthritic and control groups.

This is equivalent to an increase of 33.03 +/- 15.08% for the control group and an increase of 5.56 +/- 10.11% for the osteoarthritis group. The difference between these values was significant ($p < 0.001$).

5. DISCUSSION

The described method permits functional, intraarticular in vivo measurements under different exercise patterns. For the first time we were able to measure the influence of the joint movement on intraarticular oxygen partial pressure under physiological and pathological conditions.

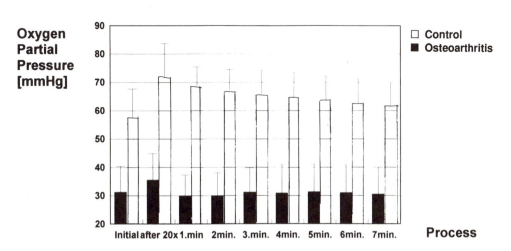

Figure 5. Effect of isokinetic oxygen (20 repetitions, 180°/sec. test velocity) on intraarticular oxygen partial pressure (mean ± SD) in osteoarthritic and control groups.

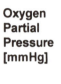

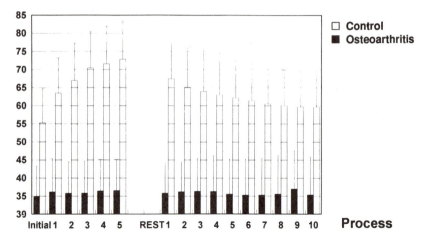

Figure 6. Effect of 5 min of ergometric exercise on intraarticular oxygen partial pressure (mean ± SD) in control and osteoarthritic groups.

The results obtained in osteoarthritis patients show that the resting value of the intraarticular oxygen partial pressure is significantly lower compared with healthy persons. We assume that the reduced blood flow and disturbed diffusion are the reasons for the lower resting value in arthritic knee joints.

It is known that pathological reduction of the intraarticular oxygen partial pressure leads to a reduction of the local cartilage oxygen partial pressure (6). Therefore, a reduction of the oxygen partial pressure has consequences for the articular cartilage, because of the special supply conditions of the knee joint (1,2,7).

Our results show that different exercise patterns influence the intraarticular oxygen partial pressure.

A test velocity of 60° sec (slow dynamic tension) leads to a decrease of the intraarticular oxygen partial pressure in the arthritic knee joint. A test velocity of 180° sec (fast dynamic tension), in contrast, leads to a very small decrease, and the ergometric exercise leads to a rise of oxygen partial pressure in an arthritic knee joint.

We conclude, that a velocity of 180° sec and ergometric exercise lead to an improvement of the intraarticular metabolic condition and support the regenerative process. A velocity of 60° sec on the other hand leads to a deterioration of the intraarticular oxygen partial pressure.

This method of intraarticular oxygen partial pressure measurement allows to determine the best exercise velocity in order to increase or decease the intraarticular oxygen partial pressure.

6. REFERENCES

1. Fassbender H-G. Pathogenetischen Aspekte der Arthrose und ihre therapeutische Aspekte. Z Rheumatologie 1991; 50: Suppl 1: 65–68.
2. Stevens CR, Blake DR, Merry P, Revell PA, Levick JR. A comparative study by morphometry of the microvasculature in normal and rheumatoid synovium. Arthritis Rheum 1991; 34 (12): 1508–1513.
3. Kellgren J, Lawrence J. Atlas of Standard Radiography: The epidemiology of chronic rheumatism. Vol 2, Oxford, Blackwell Scientific Publications, 1963.

4. Lequesne M. Clinical features, diagnostic criteria, functional assessment and radiological classification of osteoarthritis. Radiology 1982; 7: 2.
5. Moffroid M, Whipple R, Hofkosh J. A study of isokinetic exercise. J Physical Therapy 1968; 49(7): 735–747.
6. Köhler W, Schachtel G, Volesek P. Biometrie. Springer-Verlag Berlin, New York, Tokyo, 1984.
7. Brighton C, Lane JM, Koh JK. In vivo rabbit articular cartilage organ model, II 35 S Incorporation in various oxygen tensions. Arthritis Rheum 1974; 17: 245–252.
8. Geiler G. Pathologie des primär entzündlich und primär entzündlich degenerativ veränderten Gelenkes. Z gesamte inn Med 1987; 42 (15): 409–413.

THE EQUIVALENT KROGH CYLINDER AND AXIAL OXYGEN TRANSPORT

Roy W. Schubert and Xuejun Zhang

Biomedical Engineering
Louisiana Tech University
Ruston, Louisiana 71272

1. ABSTRACT

The Krogh-Erlang model has served as a basis of understanding of oxygen supply to resting and working muscle. Considerable discrepancy was found between pO_2 microsensor data and results from that model. A modification was made to the transport mechanisms implied by the Krogh-Erlang model by averaging the tissue radially, using a mass-transfer coefficient to maintain radial transport, and adding axial diffusion in the capillary and tissue. This radially-averaged, axially distributed (RAAD) modified Krogh model is used to evaluate the hypothesis that axial transport is important in Krogh-geometry capillary-tissue structures. Analytic solutions for the modified model were developed. RAAD model histograms bear a striking resemblance to experimental data, while results from the classic model do not. The former has an SSE (sum of squared error) of 10.2 with respect to experimental histograms, while the Krogh model has an SSE of 238.6. The effect of using a radial mass-transfer coefficient was evaluated by comparing the RAAD model with a fully distributed model. It had been shown that the modified Krogh model predicts tissue level data well when the length-to-tissue radius ratio is 50. It was expected that the predictions would be degraded for smaller ratios and then the Krogh model would suffice. By supplying a fixed volume of tissue at different radius/length ratios, it will be shown that the modified Krogh model is superior in all aspects to the Krogh model. The results are slightly different from those of the distributed model, but these differences are limited to the first 10% of the arteriolar region. It is concluded that the RAAD model is a better overall predictor of oxygen distribution and may be useful in furthering our understanding of oxygen transport to tissue in hemoglobinless perfusion situations. We suggest that this radially-averaged, axially-distributed model be used in place of the classic Krogh cylinder model for all biological situations.

Oxygen Transport to Tissue XVIII, edited by Nemoto and LaManna
Plenum Press, New York, 1997

2. INTRODUCTION

Models of oxygen(substrate) transport to tissue date back to the work of August Krogh[1] who found that capillaries were distributed somewhat uniformly in a cross-section of striated muscle. He proposed a repeated unit in which a central capillary supplies oxygen to a concentric tissue cylinder by radial diffusion, the Krogh cylinder geometry. Erlang provided a mathematical model based on Krogh's geometry. The adequacy of this model has been checked against an isolated, hemoglobinless-perfused, heart preparation[2] by comparing their pO_2 histograms (oxygen distributions). Krogh's model was unable to predict experimental results[3].

An alternative model[4] was derived by radially averaging the tissue oxygen concentration and substituting radial diffusive transport with an equivalent permeability coefficient (mass transfer coefficient) and adding axial diffusive transport. The model has been shown to be superior to the Krogh model in predicting experimental pO_2 distribution[4,5]. This radially-averaged, axially-distributed (RAAD) model (without capillary axial diffusion) was useful in an investigation into Gregg's phenomena[6], where Michaelis-Menten kinetics was added. Nevertheless, in some predictions, the RAAD model required the use of a high value of tissue axial diffusion coefficient (about 8 to 10 times higher than the value accepted in the literature). This led to questions about the appropriateness of the radially averaging used in the derivation of the RAAD model for heart tissue. Consequently, a fully distributed axially symmetric model (two-dimensional tissue, capillary axial diffusion) has been explored for parameters of physiologic interest and initial comparisons were made with experimental histograms[3,5]. It was found that the pO_2 histograms predicted by the fully distributed model and the RAAD model were identical (±0.3% max., ±0.05% ave.) for parameters describing heart tissue. Thus the applications and conclusions developed from the RAAD model, which were histogram-based, appeared to be valid for heart tissue. This seemed reasonable since the length-to-radius ratio was high, 50.

An extremely important benefit concerns extensions of the radially-averaged modeling efforts. Since extensive computational procedures were needed to obtain the results for the fully distributed model, it would be helpful to find out whether the fully distributed model and the analytic RAAD model can yield similar, or at least acceptable, results when the length/radius is smaller. Modifications to the RAAD model are considerably easier to carry out than those to the fully distributed model. An example comes from Napper and Schubert[6] who produced a nonlinear model by adding Michaelis-Menten kinetics to the RAAD model that required a mainframe computer for numerical solution, but allowed parameter optimization. It is easily recognized that use of the fully distributed model, with added Michaelis-Menten kinetics, would have been considerably labor intensive. When is it justified to proceed with the RAAD model? And, if one does, what kinds of "errors" could be introduced? The objective of this investigation is to compare and contrast the RAAD model (axial diffusion in tissue, with capillary axial diffusion), and the fully distributed model (radial and axial diffusion in tissue, with capillary axial diffusion) for a wide range of length/radius ratios. See Fletcher and Schubert[5] for an explanation of the need for capillary axial diffusion.

3. THE RAAD OF O_2 SUPPLY TO TISSUE

Shown in Figure 1 is a differential element used to derive the RAAD model. See Appendix I for definition of variables. Both capillary and tissue regions are radially averaged and h represents an equivalent permeability that replaces radial transport in the tissue region (see below).

The resultant model is an "equivalent" description because uniformly spaced capillaries of the same length with identical perfusate velocities and kinetics do not exist in any living tissue. Diffusion properties and O_2 consumption are not perfectly homogeneous. Yet in some sense, this model, and the organ it represents, can be thought of as "equivalent." In particular, the intention is to use the word "equivalent" to mean similarity of the distribution of O_2 in the metabolizing tissue region (as sampled randomly[2]).

3.1. Capillary Region

Axial transport is added to the basic model described in[4] because of its coupling to tissue axial diffusion[7]. The capillary equation then becomes

$$V_z \frac{dP(z)_c}{\partial z} - D_c \frac{d^2 P(z)_c}{\partial z^2} - \frac{2\sigma h}{R_c}(P(z)_t - P(z)_c) \qquad 0 \le z \le L, \ 0 \le r \le R_c \tag{1}$$

where V_z is the perfusate axial velocity, P_c is the partial pressure of oxygen (pO_2) in the capillary, D_c is the axial diffusion coefficient in the capillary, P_t is the tissue pO_2, σ is the partition coefficient (S_t/S_c), and S_c is the solubility of oxygen in the capillary. The radial mass transfer coefficient, h, represents a permeability equivalent of diffusion in the interstitium and tissue and is a function or R_t, R_c, and D_r. If one assigns a separate capillary wall permeability, ϑ (see reference 5), then h is replaced by $h_{eff} = h\vartheta/(h + \vartheta)$, since the resistance to transport is serial.

3.2. Tissue Region

Radial averaging the tissue over the region $R_c \le r \le R_t$ yields

$$S_t \ D_z \frac{d^2 P_t}{dz^2} + \frac{2 R_c \ S_t \ h \ (P_c - P_t)}{R_t^2 - R_c^2} = k \qquad 0 \le z \le L, \ R_c \le r \le R_t \tag{2}$$

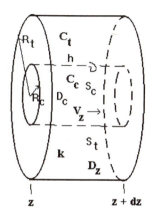

Figure 1. Capillary-tissue differential shell used to derive a radially-averaged, axially-distributed (RAAD) modification to Krogh's model.

where k is the substrate metabolism. This equation reflects that all the oxygen leaving the capillary enters the tissue at each z. Rearrangement of equation (1) into an expression for P_t and substitution of it and its second derivative into equation (2) produces a differential equation for $P_c(y)$.

3.3. Analytic Solution

After normalizing z, V_z, and r by L to y, V_y, and x, respectively, and solving, $P_c(y)$ is

$$P_c(y) = C_1 + \frac{L_4}{L_3} y + C_2 e^{r_1 y} + C_3 e^{r_2 y} + C_4 e^{r_3 y} \tag{3}$$

where r_i are roots of $D^3 + L_1 D^2 + L_2 D + L_3 = 0$, when

$$D = \frac{d()}{dy}, \quad L_1 = \frac{\beta}{\gamma}, \quad L_2 = \frac{1}{\gamma} = -\alpha, \quad L_3 = -\alpha L_1, \quad L_4 = \frac{L^2 k}{\gamma D_z S_t}$$

with

$$\alpha = \frac{2 x_c h L}{D_z (x_t^2 - x_c^2)}, \quad \beta = \frac{x_c V_y L}{2 \sigma h}, \quad \gamma = -\frac{x_c D_c}{2 \sigma h L}$$

Pt(y), the tissue pO2, can be found by substituting equation (3) and its derivatives into equation (1) after it has been normalized The result is:

$$P_t(y) = P_c(y) + \frac{L_4}{L_3} \beta + C_2 \delta_1 e^{r_1 y} + C_3 \delta_2 e^{r_2 y} + C_4 \delta_3 e^{r_3 y} \tag{4}$$

where $\delta_i = r_i (\beta + \gamma_i r_i)$.

The C_i are found by applying no flux boundaries and known capillary inlet P_{cA}:

$$\frac{dP_c}{dy}(1) = 0 \quad \frac{dP_t}{dy}(1) = 0 \quad \frac{dP_t}{dy}(0) = 0 \quad P_c(0) = P_{cA} \tag{5}$$

Using the inlet condition determines C_1 as

$$C_1 = P_{cA} - C_2 - C_3 - C_4 \tag{6}$$

The remaining constants need to be determined carefully because of extremely large terms and terms close to zero. An approximate solution was developed that used Gaussian elimination to identify terms close to zero and ratios of largeterms that tend to cancel. See Zhang8 for details. If r1 is the largest root and r2 is the smallest root, then:

$$C_2 = 0$$

$$C_3 = -\frac{1}{r_2\,(1+\delta_2)}\left(\frac{L_4}{L_3}+r_3\,(1+\delta_3)\,C_4\right)$$

$$C_4 = \frac{-L_4}{L_3\,r_3\,e^{r_3}\left(1-\dfrac{\delta_3}{\delta_1}\right)} \tag{7}$$

To make radial transport from the RAAD model and distributed model equivalent, the RAAD radial flux is assumed to be driven by a Krogh-based space-averaged pO2 when the capillary wall is freely permeable. ϑ is an additional finite capillary permeability. The result can be shown as:

$$h = \frac{-4\,S_t\,D_r\,(R_c^{\,2}-R_t^{\,2})^2}{R_c\,[\,3R_t^{\,4}-4\,(R_t^{\,2}-R_c^{\,2})+R_c^{\,4}+4\,R_t^{\,4}\,\ln(\frac{R_c}{R_t})\,]} \qquad h_{eff}=\frac{h\,\vartheta}{h+\vartheta} \tag{8}$$

3.4. Histograms

A histogram for the model is constructed by dividing the equivalent Krogh geometry into a mesh of curvilinear regions and computing the region average pO_2 and associated region's volume. Accumulation of these volumes into histograms by pO_2 range yields an estimate of the sample probability distribution[7,9]. Regions were chosen to be $1 um^3$ to reflect the volume sampled by the Whalen-Nair pO_2 microelectrode. While this approach allows model-to-data comparisons, it has the disadvantage that there is not a direct relationship between the predicted values and the corresponding measured values. In such cases, it is possible that more than one model may produce results that yield similar histograms; that is, the model may not be unique.

Table I. Parameters for modeling and associated nomenclature

Parameter	Value (units) or range	Description
L	0.01-0.05 (cm)	Capillary length in z
V_z	3.228 (cm/min)	Perfusate velocity in capillary
R_c	2.5×10^{-4} (cm)	Capillary radius
R_t	$1.049\text{-}22.92 \times 10^{-3}$ (cm)	Tissue radius
D_r	$9.9\text{-}99 \times 10^{-4}$ (cm^2/min)	Radial diffusion coefficient in tissue
D_z	$9.9\text{-}99 \times 10^{-4}$ (cm^2/min)	Axial diffusion coefficient in tissue
D_c	1.5×10^{-3} (cm^2/min)	Axial diffusion coefficient in capillary
S_t	1.31×10^{-9} (mol/g-mmhg)	Oxygen solubility in tissue
S_c	1.31×10^{-9} (mol/g-mmhg)	Oxygen solubility in capillary perfusate
k	3.2×10^{-9} (mol/g-min)	Tissue oxygen consumption

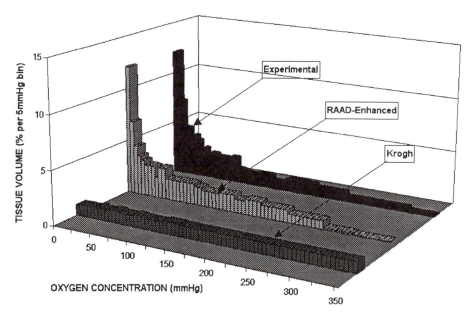

Figure 2. Theoretical histograms from the Krogh and RAAD model in comparison to experimental histograms from the beating cat heart.

4. RESULTS

Histograms (tissue pO_2 distributions) and tissue and capillary pO_2 profiles will be presented and compared for the RAAD model and the fully distributed model[5] for parameters representing the isolated heart, shown in Table I. Note that in Table I the radial oxygen diffusion coefficient D_r is equal to the axial oxygen diffusion coefficient D_z, and

Table II. Sum of the squared error

Comparison	Lum	$R_t$um	D	SSE
Krogh vs. Experimental	500	10.5	1&10	238.6
Distributed vs. Experimental	500	10.5	10	9.9
RAAD vs Experimental	500	10.5	10	10.2
Distributed vs RAAD-Heart	500	10.5	10	0.4
Distributed vs RAAD	250	14.6	10	2.6
Distributed vs RAAD	200	16.3	10	9.6
Distributed vs RAAD	100	22.9	10	60.9
Distributed vs RAAD	500	10.5	1	0.2
Distributed vs RAAD	200	16.3	1	0.2
Distributed vs RAAD	250	14.6	1	0.1
Distributed vs RAAD	100	22.9	1	4.1
Distributed vs RAAD-Skeletal Mus.	500	26.4	1	0.2
Distributed vs RAAD-Skeletal Mus.	500	26.4	10	9.2
Distributed vs RAAD-Brain	180	30	1	0.6
Distributed vs RAAD-Sciatic Nerve	1000	63	1	2.8

ranges from 1 (normal) to 10 (enhanced) times the nominal values in the literature. The interest in an enhanced diffusion coefficient in tissue reflects our interest in matching experimental data from isolated beating heart.

4.1. Histograms

Figure 2 displays the pO_2 distribution (histogram) from the Krogh model, from the RAAD model and from experimental data. The histograms are generated by sampling the tissue region at volume resolutions comparable with the region sampled by the Whalen-Nair pO_2 microelectrode[3]. The experimental data summarize approximately 1800 random microelectrode pO_2 samples from the free wall of the beating left ventricle. Measurements were taken with assurance that the electrode was not moving through the tissue[2]. Figure 3 is similar to Figure 2 but the histograms are generated at a much finer spatial resolution and compare predictions made by the RAAD and distributed model. In this figure the length-to-radius ratio (L/R_t) ranges from 4 to 50, while the volume of tissue, and all other parameters, remains fixed. Figure 4 contains histograms for the same L/R range, for normal diffusion. Table II quantified the goodness-of-fit between the histograms, measured as a squared difference between corresponding histogram bins, summed over all 22 histogram bins (SSE).

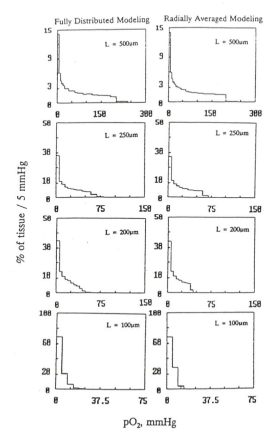

Figure 3. Theoretical histograms from the RAAD and fully distributed model for progressively shorter capillaries. Diffusion is enhanced (10X normal). Tissue volume is kept constant by enlarging the tissue radius as L decreases. Note that the histogram labeled "RAAD-Enhanced" in Figure 2 is generated from the same parameters as the top right hand panel of this figure.

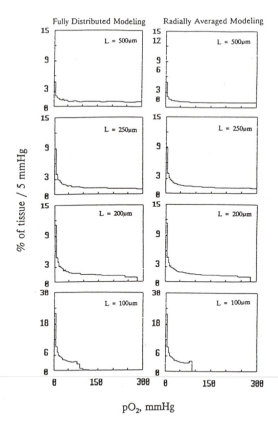

Figure 4. Theoretical histograms from the RAAD and fully distributed model for progressively shorter capillaries. Diffusion is normal. Tissue radius is 10.49, 14.62, 16.30 and 22.92 μm when L is 500, 250, 200, and 100 μm respectively.

4.2. Capillary and Tissue Axial Profiles

Axial pO_2 profiles are shown in Figure 5 for all the histograms shown in Figures 3 and 4 for various L/R. The capillary data are contained in the top half of the figure, while the tissue data comprise the lower half. The right-hand set of panels are generated by the distributed model, while the RAAD model was used to simulate the right-hand set of panels. Note that the first and third panel in the right-hand column, topmost dotted line, are associated with the histogram of Figure 2, "RAAD-Enhanced".

5. DISCUSSION

The Krogh geometry is the most common system used to model oxygen transport to tissue at the microcirculatory level. The same can probably be said for the Krogh mathematical model. However, axial diffusion in the capillary or tissue was not included in that model. From Figure 2 it can be seen that the predicted histogram is featureless. It has a constant value for the whole range of tissue pO_2. A priori, it was expected that the radial diffusion to increasingly larger volumes of tissue, as r increases(Figure 1) would produce a leftward shift in the histograms, but this only occurs if the capillary pO_2 is invariant in the axial direction, which is totally well mixed. This condition is unrealistic for a capillary length that is two hundred times the capillary radius. When the capillary is axially distrib-

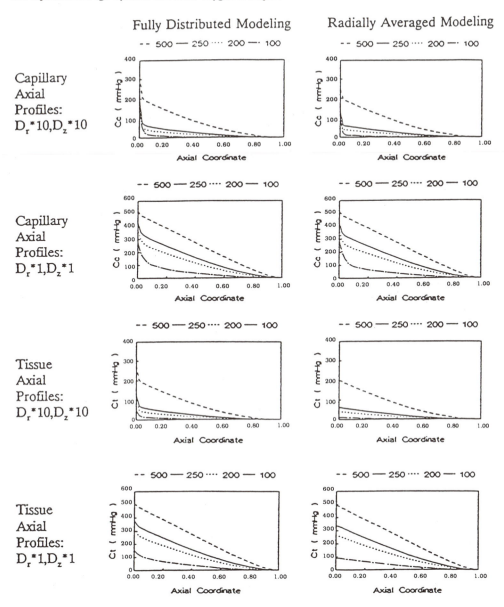

Figure 5. Axial pO$_2$ profiles from the distributed model (left column) and RAAD model (right column) as capillary length is decreased. Capillary profiles are featured in the top two rows, while the tissue profiles are pictured in the bottom two rows. Histograms associated with these profiles are provided in Figures 3 and 4.

uted, then the tissue becomes uniformly distributed in the absence of tissue axial diffusion. To be sure, there is distribution in the radial direction, but the radial domain is small compared to the axial domain (L/R$_t$). The sum of squared error (SSE) is very large between the Krogh model and experimental data, suggesting a significant mismatch between theory and experiment. It is concluded that the Krogh model is unable to predict experimental histograms. In contrast, the experimental histogram shows an increase in the percentage of tissue as pO$_2$ decreases. This leftward shift is a feature of all experimental histograms.

Therefore, axial diffusion in the tissue and in the capillary with a permeability barrier at the capillary wall (this paper) was considered.

The effect of the axial transport mechanisms on the histograms can also be seen in Figure 2 (see RAAD-Enhanced) and Table II. The parameters used are from Table I. Previous efforts[3,5] have found that these values produce histograms that bear a striking resemblance to experimental data. Histograms from the fully distributed and the RAAD simulation have an SSE of 9.9 and 10.2, respectively, with respect to the experimental data. Both the distributed and RAAD models are much better at simulating histograms than the Krogh model (SSE=238.6). The enhanced diffusion (high D_z) is troublesome, but may have a physiologic basis in the recycling of the heart's actin-myosin crossbridges[3]. Nonetheless, the fourth entry in Table II is evidence that the RAAD model and the distributed model produce similar results. This low SSE suggests that the far simpler RAAD model contains most of the useful transport in the hemoglobinless-perfused working heart. The SSEs for the normal diffusion (Table II, eighth entry) is less than 0.2 and less than 0.4 for the enhanced diffusion (Table II, fourth entry). Both of these SSEs are small in comparison to 238.6 for the Krogh model and less than either the experimental-distributed SSE (Table II, entry 2) or the experimental-RAAD SSE (Table II, entry 3). Thus, pO_2 histograms from the RAAD and the distributed models are practically the same for heart tissue parameters. We have observed that the differences in the histograms between the two models are within 0.3%. Thus it is concluded that the RAAD and fully distributed models produce very similar results and conclusions developed from the RAAD model are valid for the isolated perfused heart.

An important benefit concerns extensions of the modeling efforts as has been done by Napper and Schubert[6] and Gardner and Schubert[10]. In both papers, non-linear stiff differential equations were developed. This would have been considerably more complex had a fully distributed model been used. The work on sciatic nerve[11] showed that this type of non-linear model required a huge computer capacity (Cray computer). It is concluded that modifications to the radially average model are considerably easier to implement than modifications to the fully distributed model.

The larger question is: When is it justified to proceed with the RAAD model? Could the modification have been implemented by use of the RAAD concept or is a Cray solution justified? The preceding discussion makes a conclusion for isolated heart parameters clear: the RAAD model works well. But what would happen if other parameters were used in other ranges? This question has been answered by progressively shortening the capillary (increasing the tissue radius to keep the supplied tissue volume, and flow/tissue volume, constant) while keeping all other parameters fixed at the values shown in Table I. This documents the RAAD model under conditions where the radial diffusive transport is expected to play an increasingly bigger role. For enhanced diffusion in tissue, Figure 5 shows that the axial capillary and tissue profiles look similar in both models. Note that the top traces in four of the panels use the same parameters as the simulated histogram in Figure 2, "RAAD-Enhanced". A significant increase in SSE occurs when the capillary length drops from 250 µm to 200 µm (radial distance increases from 14.62 µm to 16.30 µm); SSE increases from 2.61 to 9.55. When the capillary length decreases to 100 µm (radial distance increases to 22.92 µm), the SSE reaches the highest level SSE = 60.9. For the normal diffusion, Figure 4 and Table II also show similar trends, but the SSE never exceeds 4.1. Thus, it seems that the RAAD model can have satisfactory performance when the capillary length is as small as 100 µm (radial distance is less than 22.92 µm) for normal diffusion. For enhanced diffusion, the SSE seems to become large at L=100 µm. We have observed that, with this parameter combination, the histogram difference is less than

1.44% for the low pO_2 region and the tissue profile differences approaches 66 mmHg, which occurs at the capillary inlet. These differences in prediction are expected because the potential for radial diffusion (O_2 gradient) is largest at the capillary entrance when the tissue is perfused with Krebs-Hensleit solution equilibrated with 95% O_2.

The last three entries in Table II are SSEs for other tissues and listed for comparative purposes. Listed only are L and R_t, but perfusate velocity and metabolism also reflect the listed organ. These SSEs are quite low and seem to indicate that the RAAD model would work well in all listed biological cases. Parameter values were taken from Klitzman, Popel and Duling[12] and Popel, Charny and Dvinsky for resting skeletal muscle[13], from Reneau and Knisely[14] for brain and Lagerlund and Low[11] for sciatic nerve. The working skeletal muscle parameters reflect our suspicion that the diffusion parameters may be enhanced by a factor of 10 by the contraction mechanism.

Space limits presentation of all the differences between the RAAD and distributed model. But note that the largest differences occur at the capillary inlet (Figure 5, y=0). Since radial averaging eliminates the steep gradients that the distributed model preserves, significant differences exist in the entrance region. Thus, caution is advised in the use of the RAAD model in estimating substrate levels in the entrance region. Nonetheless, the importance of axial transport is revealed by the RAAD model. We just caution that the effects are underestimated in the first 5–10% of the equivalent Krogh cylinder. However, the remaining 95% of the cylinder shows good agreement. Our unpublished observation is that for over 60% of the length ($0.4 \leq y \leq 1$) the RAAD-distributed differences are not academically interesting. The tissue pO_2 differences (for heart) are less than 0.015% in that range, but approach 2.7% for normal diffusion, and 13% for enhanced diffusion at y=0.

In conclusion, axial transport in the tissue and the capillary is significant. Histogram character is dependent on this transport phenomena. The results from the present project indicate that the RAAD model and the fully distributed model produce similar histograms and almost exactly the same capillary and radially averaged tissue pO_2, except at the arteriolar region. Since this is an analytic model, we recommend that the RAAD model be used to replace the classic Krogh-Erlang model for Krogh geometry situations. Since our observations and modeling are in a hemoglobinless perfused preparation, all preceding comments are restricted to that condition.

6. APPENDIX

Table III Parameter List.

Table III. Parameters for modeling and associated nomenclature

Parameter	Value (units) or range	Description
L	0.05 (cm)	Capillary length in z
V_z	3.2 (cm/min)	Perfusate velocity in capillary
R_c	2.5×10^{-4} (cm)	Capillary radius
R_t	1.049×10^{-3} (cm)	Tissue radius
D_r	9.9×10^{-3} (cm^2/min)	Radial diffusion coefficient in tissue
D_z	9.9×10^{-3} (cm^2/min)	Axial diffusion coefficient in tissue

(continued)

Table III. (*Continued*)

Parameter	Vakue (units) or range	Description
D_c	1.5×10^{-3} (cm^2/min)	Axial diffusion coefficient in capillary
S_t	1.31×10^{-9} (mol/g-mmhg)	Oxygen solubility in tissue
S_c	1.31×10^{-9} (mol/g-mmhg)	Oxygen solubility in capillary perfusate
k	3.2×10^{-9} (mol/g-min)	Tissue oxygen consumption
z	$0 \leq y \leq L$ (cm)	Axial coordinate
y	$0 \leq y \leq 1$	Normalized axial coordinate, z/L
r	$0 \leq r \leq R_c$ (cm)	Radial coordinate
x		Normalized radial coordinate, r/L
r_i		Roots of a polynomial
R	(cm)	Specific value of r
σ		Partition coefficient, S_t/S_c
h	(cm/min)	Equivalent permeability , replaces radial diffusion the tissue
ϑ	(cm/min)	Capillary permeability
h_{eff}	(cm/min)	Combined equivalent and capillary permeability
N	(mol-cm/g-min)	Radial flux from capillary to tissue
c,t	subscripts	Denotes capillary or tissue
$\alpha,\beta,\delta,\gamma,\varepsilon,\eta$		Parameters of the mathematical development
L_i		Coefficients of Differential Equation
D		Differential operator, d( )/dz

7. REFERENCES

1. Krogh, A. The number and distribution of capillaries in muscles with calculations of the oxygen pressure head necessary for supplying tissue. *J Physiol (London)* 1919;52:409–415.
2. Schubert, R.W., Whalen, W.J., Nair, P. Myocardial PO2 distribution: relationship to coronary autoregulation. *Am J Physiol* 1978;234(4):H361-H370.
3. Schubert, R.W., Fletcher, J.E. Rethinking oxygen transport to tissue: model and experiment compared. *Comments on Theoretical Biology* 1993;3:23–42.
4. Schubert, R.W., Fletcher, J.E., Reneau, D.D. An analytical model for axial diffusion in the Krogh cylinder. *Oxygen Transport to Tissue* 1984;433–442.
5. Fletcher, J.E., Schubert, R.W. Axial diffusion and wall permeability effects in perfused capillary-tissue structures. *BioSystems* 1987;20:153–174.
6. Napper, S.A., Schubert, R.W. Mathematical evidence for flow-induced changes in myocardial oxygen consumption. *Ann Biomed Eng* 1988;16:349–365.
7. Fletcher, J.E., Schubert, R.W. On the computation of substrate levels in perfused tissue. *Math Biosci* 1982;62:75–106.
8. Zhang, X. Theoretical Oxygen Distribution in Tissue: Effects of Radial Transport Assumptions (Masters Thesis). *Louisiana Tech University* 1992;Ruston, Louisiana.
9. Schubert, R.W. A Physiological and Mathematical Study of Oxygen Distribution in the Autoregulating Isolated Heart (Ph.D. Thesis). *Case Western Reserve University* 1976.
10. Gardner, J.D., Schubert, R.W. Evaluation of myoglobin function in the presence of axial diffusion. *Oxygen Transport to Tissue* 1995;this-volume.
11. Lagerlund, T.D., Low, P.A. Axial diffusion and Michaelis-Menten kinetics in oxygen delivery in rat peripheral nerve. *Am J Physiol* 1991;260:R430-R440.
12. Klitzman, B., Popel, A.S., Duling, B.R. Oxygen transport in resting and contracting cremaster muscles: Experimental and theoretical studies. *Microvascular Res* 1983;25:108–131.
13. Popel, A.S., Charny, C.K., Dvinsky, A.S. Effect of heterogeneous oxygen delivery on the oxygen distribution in skeletal muscle. *Math Biosci* 1986;81:91–113.
14. Reneau, D.D., Knisely, M.H. A mathematical simulation of oxygen transport in the human brain under conditions of countercurrent capillary blood flow. *Chemical Engineering Progress Symposium Series: Advances in Bioengineering* 1971;67:18–27.

24

INFLUENCE OF O_2-H_b KINETICS AND THE FÄHRAEUS EFFECT ON THE ARTERIOLAR ROLE IN GAS EXCHANGE

Guo-Fan Ye,[1] Donald G. Buerk,[2] Lei Ye[3] and Dov Jaron[1]

[1]Biomedical Engineering and Science Institute
Drexel University
Philadelphia, Pennsylvania 19104
[2]Department of Physiology
[3]School of Arts and Sciences
University of Pennsylvania
Philadelphia, Pennsylvania 19104

1. INTRODUCTION

The role of precapillary and postcapillary vessels in microcirculatory gas exchange have received considerable attention[1] ever since experimental findings indicated that significant amount of oxygen is exchanged between arterioles and the surrounding tissue[2–4]. Roth & Wade[5] simulated O_2-CO_2 coupled transport in the rat skeletal muscle microcirculation using a multicompartmental model. One of the noticeable results of their simulation was a dominant precapillary CO_2 flux leading to the conclusion that virtually all of the CO_2 exchange takes place in precapillary vessels during rest. They also concluded that, during exercise, 80% of CO_2 is exchanged before the capillary bed. Our simulation[6] for cat cerebral O_2-CO_2 transport predicted that the arteriolar contribution to total CO_2 flux was less than 20% and therefore suggested that capillaries were the prime site of CO_2 exchange in the microcirculation. Our later work[7], using a multicompartmental model for O_2-CO_2 coupled transport in the rat skeletal microcirculation under various rest/exercise conditions, suggested that a number of factors in model formulation or in simulation parameters may affect model prediction regarding the roles of arterioles and capillaries in microcirculatory gas exchange, particularly in CO_2 exchange. Simplifying assumption for compartmental concentration gradient, which was used by a number of earlier models, may significantly alter the result depending on the conditions. In addition, omission of radial blood diffusion resistance, which was also assumed by many investigators, may lead to an overestimation of arteriolar fluxes (F_a). Lower blood flow rate, higher arteriolar diffusion conductances, or higher CO_2/O_2 respiratory quotient may result in a higher contribution ratio of arterioles versus capillaries (F_a/F_c). These factors may contribute to the differences in predictions of F_a/F_c for different body organs or species of animals. In contrast with earlier models in the literature, our model usually predicts capillary dominance for O_2 and CO_2 exchange, and reveals the existence of negative venular flux contribution.

The effects of two other factors in model formulation, O_2-H_b kinetics and the Fähraeus effect, were not included in the above studies as well as in our earlier models. Most microcirculatory O_2 transport models have utilized the relationship between equilibrium O_2 saturation and partial pressure to express O_2 dissociation behavior. However, due to the existence of O_2 diffusion, the O_2-H_b reaction for blood in the microvessels is not in equilibrium even in the steady state. The O_2-H_b reaction kinetics limit the rate of O_2 offloading from hemoglobin and thus may affect the behavior of O_2 distribution[8]. Furthermore, Robin Fähraeus demonstrated that the apparent hematocrit (H_{app}) decreases from the larger microvessels to smaller microvessels[9] . This implies a corresponding decrease in the distribution of hemoglobin.

In our present study, we have included both O_2-H_b kinetics and the Fähraeus effect into our previous multicompartmental model for O_2-CO_2 coupled transport in the cat brain microcirculation[10][6]. This communication summarizes the investigation of the effects of O_2-H_b kinetics, the Fähraeus effect and their interaction on the arteriolar and capillary role in CO_2 and O_2 exchange under steady state.

2. METHODS

The detailed formulation of the model was described elsewhere[10][6]. Briefly, the cerebral microcirculation was simulated by 3 arteriole compartments (a1, a2, a3), 1 capillary compartment (cap), 3 venule compartments (v3, v2, v1), and 1 tissue compartment. The governing equations of the compartmental model for O_2 transport were developed by spatial averaging of the following distributed governing equations:

$$D_d \nabla^2 c_d - \mathbf{v} \nabla c_d - \beta R = 0 \quad \text{for the blood plasma}$$

(1)

where $R = k[H_b](S_{eq} - S)/(1 - S_{eq})$

$$D_{HbO_2} \nabla^2 c_{HbO_2} - \mathbf{v} \nabla c_{HbO_2} + R = 0 \quad \text{for } H_bO_2,$$

(2)

$$D_w \nabla^2 c_w + M_w = 0 \qquad \text{for the vessel wall, and}$$

(3)

$$D_T \nabla^2 c_T + M_T = 0 \qquad \text{for tissue}$$

(4)

where c is the concentration of O_2 at a given point, D is O_2 diffusivity, $\mathbf{v}$ is a vector representing blood velocity at the point, β is a constant, and M is O_2 metabolic rate per unit volume. The subscripts d, H_bO_2, w and T stand for the dissolved oxygen in plasma and in the hemoglobin solution inside erythrocytes, oxyhemoglobin, vessel wall and tissue, respectively. R is the rate of O_2-H_b transform kinetics. R is expressed in a form of single step re-action with a reaction constant k (44/sec). It varies with the actual O_2-H_b saturation (S), O_2-H_b saturation in equilibrium for the same Po_2 (Seq) and total hemoglobin concentration ($[H_b]$)[11][1]. Seq acts as a reference state for the reaction. Instead of the simple Hill expression for S_{eq} used in some previously published models[11][1], the modified Easton formula[12] was employed here. The modified Easton formula is valid for S_{eq} values from 0 to 95%. Hill's expression is, in contrast, valid only for the Seq range between 10% and 80%. This makes the Hill expression inappropriate for severe hypoxic cases or, conversely, for normal blood in large arterioles.

The Fähraeus effect was incorporated into the terms for diffusion and O_2-H_b kinetics in the governing equations. H_{app} was used to calculate the diffusive fluxes and the O_2-H_b kinetics rate. A gradual drop in the value of H_{app} from artery (A) to capillaries (60% reduction) and a gradual recovery from capillaries to vein (V) were assumed in the simulation. For the steady state study, it was assumed that the convective terms in the governing equations are not affected by the Fähraeus effect because of the continuity of hemoglobin flow.

Appropriate boundary conditions were incorporated to determine the lumped parameters for the compartmental governing equations, taking into consideration the effects of radial blood diffusion resistance, discrete nature of capillary blood, difference in metabolism between vessel wall and tissue, and dependence of tissue metabolic rate on tissue oxygen partial pressure. Corresponding equations and procedures were also set up for the parallel CO_2 transport. The Newton-Raphson method was adopted to solve the set of nonlinear algebraic governing equations. The model was used to predict the compartmental distribution of Po_2, Pco_2, S, pH and the difference between Seq and S (Seq-S). The distribution of O_2 and CO_2 fluxes along the arterioles, capillaries and venules were then obtained from the lumped form of the first term on the left side of Eq.1. Ratios of arteriolar and venular fluxes to capillary flux including and excluding O_2-H_b kinetics and the

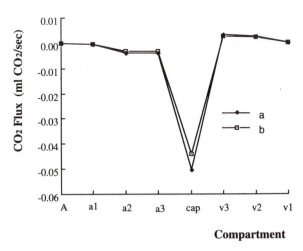

Figure 1. Compartmental CO_2 flux distribution predicted by the O_2-CO_2 coupled model under low cerebral blood flow (Q=0.5 Qnormal): **a**: excluding O_2-H_b kinetics and the Fähraeus effect; **b**: including O_2-H_b kinetics and the Fähraeus effect. In the figure, A represents the input artery, a1, a2 and a3 represent arteriole compartments, cap represents the capillary compartment, and v3, v2 and v1 represent venule compartments.

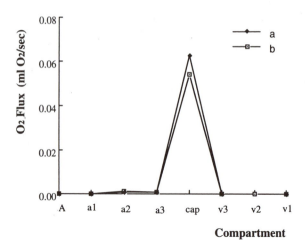

Figure 2. Compartmental O_2 flux distribution predicted by the O_2-CO_2 coupled model under low cerebral blood flow (Q=0.5 Q_{normal}): **a**: excluding O_2-H_b kinetics and the Fähraeus effect; **b**: including O_2-H_b kinetics and the Fähraeus effect.

Fähraeus effect were compared under three different values of cerebral blood flow rate (Q=2.0, 1.0 and 0.5 times Q_{normal}).

3. RESULTS

Figure 1 and Figure 2 compare the compartmental CO_2/O_2 flux distribution including and excluding O_2-H_b kinetics and the Fähraeus effect predicted by the O_2-CO_2 coupled model under low cerebral blood flow (Q=0.5 Q_{normal}). Table 1 summarizes the ratios of total arteriolar flux (F_a) to capillary flux (F_c) and the ratios of total venular flux (F_v) to capillary flux for four combinations that exclude or include O_2-H_b kinetics and the Fähraeus effect. Results are listed for both CO_2 and O_2 fluxes under low cerebral blood flow (Q=0.5 Q_{normal}) and high flow (Q=2 Q_{normal}). Results suggest that O_2-H_b kinetics reduce both arteriolar fluxes and capillary flux very slightly, and thus has no significant effect on the resulting F_a/F_c. The Fähraeus effect decreases CO_2 F_a by as much as 15% and F_c to a lesser extent, and thus reduces CO_2 F_a/F_c only minimally. In the case of O_2 exchange, the Fähraeus effect increased F_a/F_c slightly.

Table 1. Relative total arteriolar and venular CO_2/O_2 fluxes

	Q/Qnormal	CO_2				O_2			
		nk-nF	k-nF	nk-F	k-F	nk-nF	k-nF	nk-F	k-F
Fa/Fc	0.5	0.1585	0.1590	0.1546	0.1550	0.0288	0.0294	0.0361	0.0366
Fv/Fc	0.5	−0.1266	−0.1268	−0.1245	−0.1247	−0.0065	−0.0058	0.0024	0.0028
Fa/Fc	2.0	0.0327	0.0324	0.0323	0.0322	0.0225	0.0225	0.0297	0.0300
Fv/Fc	2.0	−0.0296	−0.0293	−0.0293	−0.0294	0.0016	0.0017	0.0092	0.0096

Note: Fa: total arteriolar flux; Fc: capillary flux; Fv: total venular flux; Q: cerebral blood flow rate;
nk-nF: excluding O2-Hb kinetics and the Fähraeus effect; k-nF: including the kinetics and excluding the Fähraeus effect; nk-F: excluding the kinetics and including the Fähraeus effect; k-F: including the kinetics and the Fähraeus effect

4. DISCUSSION

Our results suggest that the incorporation of O_2-H$_b$ kinetics and the Fähraeus effect into the model did not affect the capillary dominance in gas exchange predicted by our model. Furthermore, the relative arteriolar and venular contributions to CO_2 exchange were apparently greater than those to O_2 exchange under condition of low blood flow. "Negative" CO_2 venular flux and "negative" O_2 venular flux exist under some conditions. These observations are consistent with predictions of our previous investigations.

ACKNOWLEDGMENTS

This research was supported in part by the National Science Foundation under grant No. BES 9400329.

REFERENCES

1. Popel, A. S. Theory of oxygen transport to tissue. *Crit. Rev. Biomed. Eng.* **17**, 257–321, 1989.
2. Davies, P. W., and Bronk, D. W. Oxygen tension in mammalian brain. *Federation Proceedings* **16**, 689–692, 1957.
3. Duling, B. R., and Berne, R. M. Longitudinal gradients in periarteriolar oxygen tension: a possible mechanism for the participation of oxygen in local regulation of blood flow. *Circ. Res.* **27**, 669–678, 1970.
4. Pittman, R. N. Oxygen delivery and transport in the microcirculation. in *Microvascular Perfusion and Transport in Health and Disease* McDonagh, P. F., Eds. Karger, Basel, pp. 60–79, 1978.
5. Roth, A. C., and Wade, K. The effects of transport in the microcirculation: a two gas species model. *Microvasc. Res.* **32**, 64–83, 1986.
6. Ye, G.-F., and Jaron, D. Regional delivery of oxygen and carbon dioxide in the microcirculation. in *Proc.16th Annual International Conf. of the IEEE Engineering in Medicine & Biology Society,* Baltimore, pp. 1166–1167, 1994.
7. Ye, G.-F., Buerk, D. G., and Jaron, D. Arteriolar contribution to microcirculatory CO_2/O_2 exchange, *Microvasc. Res.* , in press.
8. Gutierrez, G. The rate of release and its effect on capillary O2 tension: a mathematical analysis. *Respir. Physiol.* **63**, 79–96, 1986.
9. Goldsmith, H. L., Cokelet, G. R., and Gaehtgens, P. Robin Fahraeus: evolution of his concepts in cardiovascular physiology. *Am. J. Physiol.* **257**, H1005-H1015, 1989.
10. Ye, G.-F., Moore, T. W., Buerk, D. G., and Jaron, D. A compartmental model for oxygen-carbon dioxide coupled transport in the microcirculation. *Ann. Biomed. Eng.* **22(5)**, 464–479, 1994.
11. Moll, W. The influence of hemoglobin diffusion on oxygen uptake and release by red cells. *Respir. Physiol.* **6**, 1–15, 1969.
12. Buerk, D. G., and Bridges, E. W. A simplified algorithm for computing the variation in oxyhemoglobin saturation with pH, Pco₂, T and DPG. *Chem. Eng. Comm.* **47**, 113–124, 1986.

25

CAN NMR DIFFUSION-WEIGHTED IMAGING PROVIDE QUANTITATIVE INFORMATION ON TUMOR INTERSTITAL pO$_2$?

J. F. Dunn,[1] S. Ding,[1] J. A. O'Hara,[3] K. J. Liu,[2] E. Rhodes,[3] F. Goda,[2] and H. M. Swartz[2]

[1]NMR and
[2]EPR Research Centers
Department of Diagnostic Radiology
[3]Department of Radiation Oncology
Dartmouth Hitchcock Medical Center
HB 7786, Hanover, 03755 New Hampshire

1. OXYGEN AND TUMOR THERAPY

Oxygenation (pO$_2$) is a major variable in many types of cancer treatment. This includes radiation therapy[1-6], photodynamic therapy[7-9] and certain chemotherapeutic agents[10-17]. The pO$_2$ level can affect the response of tumors to therapy, especially in the critical range below 10 mmHg, where increasing hypoxia results in increased resistance to radiotherapy[18]. If it were possible to measure pO$_2$ in tumors, then it might be possible to optimize the type and timing of treatment.

2. A CLINICAL GOAL: NON-INVASIVE METHODS OF MEASURING OXYGEN

The goal of being able to obtain direct measurements of pO$_2$ in tumors under clinical conditions has been difficult to achieve (for review see[19]). Microelectrodes have been used, but they are restricted to superficial tumors and they are difficult to use for long-term repetitive measurements due to the problems of continuously reinserting the electrode. It is difficult to find the same location, and inserting the electrode repeatedly may cause significant tissue damage.

Phosphorescence techniques are relatively non-invasive. They are based on the effectiveness of oxygen as quenching agent for emissions from selected infused lumipho-

Oxygen Transport to Tissue XVIII, edited by Nemoto and LaManna
Plenum Press, New York, 1997

res[20]. Currently, however, they cannot provide data under clinical conditions beyond a depth of 1 mm.

Electron paramagnetic resonance (EPR) provides another option. Recently we have demonstrated that EPR oximetry and paramagnetic oxygen sensitive probes can be used to measure pO_2 repeatedly in implantable murine tumors[21, 22]. While this procedure meets many of the requirements for clinical application, it currently can measure non-invasively only to a depth of 10 mm, and the oxygen sensitive paramagnetic particles (except for india ink) need to be evaluated for human use.

Another alternative involves nuclear magnetic resonance techniques, which offer the advantage of being non-invasive, widely available and capable of interrogating any region of the body. Measuring the relaxation times of fluorinated hydrocarbons (which are proportional to pO_2) show promise for time course studies as the technique combines spatial information with the capacity for multiple measurements, but at this time the sensitivity of the technique is much less than that of microelectrodes[23].

Instead of directly measuring oxygen, however, one can also adopt the strategy of measuring parameters which correlate with pO_2. ^{31}P-NMR studies have been used with some success for correlating oxygenation (or tumor hypoxic fraction) with tumor energy status[24–29]. The hypoxic fraction of murine tumor models increases as the tumors increase in size[30] and these changes are matched by a decline in PCr/Pi and PCr/(Pi + phosphomonoesters) in a murine fibrosarcoma FSa-II tumor on the foot of a rat[31]. Vaupel *et al.*[26] also found a significant correlation of tumor pO_2 and some indexes of ^{31}P metabolites with tumor size in the FSa-II. After increasing inspired pO_2 in rats with rhabdomyosarcomas, ^{31}P-spectroscopic measurements showed an increase in tumor energetics in conjunction with increased tumor pO_2, and decreased hypoxic fraction [29].

On the other hand, the changes in tumor energetics post-irradiation may not always track with expected changes in oxygenation[27, 32–34]. Such conflicting results have led some to conclude that the severity of oxygen depletion necessary to confer radiobiological hypoxia is insufficient to cause detectable changes in tumor metabolism as measured by ^{31}P-NMR[35].

Our goal is to combine the techniques of NMR with those of EPR oximetry in order to "calibrate" those NMR techniques which might correlate with pO_2 in tumors.

3. DIFFUSION IMAGING, A NEW POSSIBILITY

Recently, diffusion weighted nuclear magnetic resonance imaging (DWI), which measures an apparent diffusion constant (ADC), was shown to highlight changes in the brain in response to hypoxia or ischemia[36,37]. This phenomenon may correlate with impaired osmotic regulation as changes in ADC may reflect movement of water from the extra-cellular to the intra-cellular space where mobility is restricted[36,38,39]. Also, the intensities of DWIs increase at flow rates similar to those required for maintenance of ion gradients and high energy phosphates[37, 40].

We theorized that live cells in a chronically hypoxic environment such as a solid tumor also may have an impaired capacity for osmotic regulation. If this were the case, then hypoxic regions of specific tumors would differ from "normoxic" regions and so may be identifiable through diffusion imaging techniques. Such a relationship may hold in areas where necrosis has *not* occurred to the extent that cellularity declines and extracellular volume increases, but rather where living cells are subjected to a level of chronic hypoxia which induces cell swelling and a decline in extracellular volume (ECV). If necrosis did occur, then there would be an increase in ECV and an increase in ADC[41].

To answer the question of whether ADC correlates with pO$_2$, we correlated EPR oximetry measurements of oxygenation[21, 42–46] with MR measurements of the ADC in a RIF-1 murine fibrosarcoma[47].

4. MRI AND EPR MEASUREMENTS

4.1. The Technique of Correlating ADC and pO$_2$: ADC Measurements

The pulse sequence used for diffusion data acquisition was of the conventional "Stejskal-Tanner" spin-echo design[48, 49], using strong balanced gradients on both sides of the 180° RF pulse. The signal is attenuated by the diffusion of water molecules in the presence of the strong field gradients. This attenuation is an exponential function of the apparent diffusion coefficient ADC, $A=exp(-b*ADC)$, where the gradient factor b is a function of the amplitude and duration of the gradients[48, 49].

The ADC is not a simple measurement of the diffusion rate of water protons. It measures the distance that protons diffuse within a given time. If protons are restricted within a boundary, they will appear to diffuse more slowly than those which are not restricted. This is the basis for the distinction between a diffusion constant and an "apparent" diffusion constant or ADC, and in these experiments we can be certain only that we have measured an ADC.

4.2. Electron Paramagnetic Resonance Techniques

A crystalline EPR oximetry probe lithium phthalocyanine (LiPc), was implanted into the tumor. Details of the methods used for acquiring data on pO$_2$ in tissues *in vivo* using EPR oximetry and the LiPc probe have been previously described [21, 22, 42–47, 50]. Although EPR oximetry has been previously used for *in vivo* work[22], this is the first project to utilize the LiPc crystal as a probe in tumors.

A linear magnetic field gradient of 0.05mT/cm was applied along the direction of the largest separation of the two LiPc crystals. This was sufficient to separate the signals without causing distortion of the EPR line and permitted simultaneous measurements of tissue pO$_2$ at two sites[50].

The ADC map was calculated immediately after MR imaging and two regions in the tumor with differing ADC values were chosen by visually identifying regions which represented the extremes in ADC. The crystalline EPR oximetry probe LiPc, approximately 200 μm in diameter, was implanted as closely as possible to these sites using a 26 gauge needle. EPR oximetry was performed within 1.5 hours of measuring the ADC. Animals were anesthetized with an I.P. injection of ketamine/xylazine (90/9 mg/kg).

The LiPc did not cause a local inflammatory response over the time-course of the experiment as shown by H&E sections (Fig. 1).

5. CORRELATION OF ADC WITH pO$_2$ IN RADIATION INDUCED FIBROSARCOMAS

The radiation induced fibrosarcoma or RIF-1[51] was chosen as a model because it has a relatively homogeneous structure (in that there are no cysts or large areas of

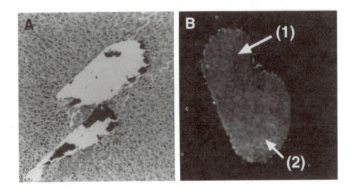

Figure 1. (A) An H&E section of a RIF-1 tumor containing LiPc. The holes in the section are caused by the knife catching on the LiPc as the crystal is difficult to cut. There is no evidence of lymphocyte infiltration or edema around the implant sites. (B) Pixel by pixel ADC map (from[47]) calculated from 5 diffusion weighted images with b values ranging from 0 to 2.249×10^9 s/m^2 (the diffusion gradient strength was varied up to 143 mT/m, δ = 12 ms, Δ = 15 ms). The image had a 3.0 cm FOV, a 2 mm slice thickness and a 128x128 matrix zero filled to 256x256. The tumor is 1020 mm^3. The arrows (1) and (2) correspond to the location of LiPc (EPR oximetry probe) as determined by the gradient echo image. The ADCs at positions 1 and 2 were 0.28 ± 0.04 and $0.59\pm0.07 \times 10^{-9}$ m/s^2 respectively (mean$\pm$S.D.) and the pO$_2$ values were 4 and 7 mmHg.

edema)(Figs. 1 and 2). It is important to have cell structure throughout the field of view as the ADC would be increased if cell content declined and if cells were replaced by fluid. Also, as solid morphology approximates many human tumors which often have very small changes in susceptibility across the tumor.

Figure 1A shows a calculated ADC map. The image shows small but significant changes in ADC across the tumor. Histological sections as well as the GE and spin-echo images showed that these tumors were relatively homogeneous with no areas of major

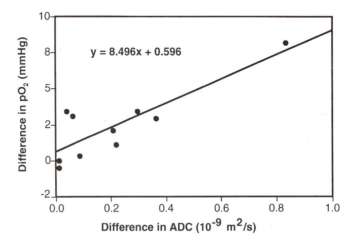

Figure 2. The relationship between tissue pO$_2$ and apparent diffusion constant (ADC), measured using MRI, in a RIF-1 tumor. The data show the difference between the high and low ADC value in each tumor vs. the difference between the pO$_2$ values taken at the respective points. The line is a least squared regression fit to all the data and the correlation coefficent = 0.8. In all tumors, the high ADC points corresponded to the regions of high pO$_2$.

lymphocyte infiltration or cysts. Figure 1B shows an H&E section of a tumor containing LiPc. The track of the implanting needle can be seen. The LiPc crystals are too hard for the knife to cut in paraffin sections and so holes in the block occur around the LiPc during sectioning. The slide shows that the LiPc was in close proximity to tumor cells and was not surrounded by clots, fluid or lymphocytes.

6. CONCLUSIONS

The results summarized here suggest that magnetic resonance techniques may provide non-invasive correlates of tissue oxygenation, either by direct measurement or by correlations with oxygen sensitive processes in cell metabolism and ion regulation. We propose that the ADC will correlate with oxygenation and hypothesize that the mechanism is based on the impairment of ion regulation during hypoxia.

Additional studies are underway to try to confirm and extend these findings. If the correlation of DWI with pO$_2$ is established, regardless of the mechanism, it could be of significant clinical value as the technique can be applied to any region of the body, and the technique can be implemented on most clinical MRI instruments.

ACKNOWLEDGMENTS

Supported in part by an American Cancer Society grant BE-186, an ACS Institutional grant IRG 157I from the Norris Cotton Cancer Center, NIH grant GM 34250 and used facilities of the Dartmouth EPR Center (supported by NIH grant RR01811).

REFERENCES

1. Churchill-Davidson, I. in *Hyperbaric oxygen and radiation therapy of cancer; proceedings* (ed. Vaeth, J.) 1–15 (S Karger, Basel, 1968).
2. Cater, D.B. *Tumori* 1964; 50:435–444.
3. Hockel, M., Schlenger, K., Knoop, C. and Vaupel, P. *Cancer Res.* 1991; 51:6098–6102.
4. Gatenby, R., Kessler, H., Rosenblum, J., Coia, L. and Broder, P. *Int J. Radiat. Oncol. Biol. Phys.* 1987; 14:831–838.
5. Hockel, M., Knoop, C., Schlenger, K., Vorndran, B., Baussmann, E., Mitze, M., Knapstein, P.G. and Vaupel, P. *Radiother. Oncol.* 1993; 26:45–50.
6. Okunieff, P., Hoeckel, M., Dunphy, E.P., Schlenger, K., Knoop, C. and Vaupel, P. *Int. J. Radiat. Oncol. Biol. Phys.* 1993; 26:631–636.
7. Chapman, J., Stobbe, C., Arnfield, M., Santus, R., Lee, J. and McPhee, M. *Radiat. Res.* 1991; 126:73–79.
8. Gibson, S.L. and Hilf, R. *Photochem. Photobiol.* 1985; 42: 367–373.
9. Henderson, B.W. and Fingar, V.H. *Photochem. Photobiol.* 1989; 49:299–304.
10. Teicher, B., lazo, J. and Sartorelli, A. *Cancer Res.* 1981; 41:73–81.
11. Suzuki, M., Hori, K., Abe, I., Saito, S. and Sato, H. *J. Natl. Cancer Inst.* 1981; 67:663–669.
12. Moulder, J.E. and Rockwell, S. *Cancer and metastasis reviews* 1987; 5:313–342.
13. Tremper, K., Friedman, A., Levine, E., Lapin, R. and Camarillo, D. *New Engl. J. Med.* 1982; 307:277–283.
14. Chaplin, D. and Horsman, M. *Int. J. Radiat. Oncol. Biol. Phys.* 1992; 22:459–462.
15. Vaeth, J.M. *Frontiers of Radiation Therapy and Oncology* 1968; 1:195.
16. Adams, G. *Cancer* 1980; 48:696–707.
17. Wilson, W.R., Zijl, P.v. and Denny, W.A. *Int. J. Radiat. Oncol. Biol. Phys.* 1992; 22:693–696.
18. Hall, E.J. *Radiobiology for the Radiologist* 1–534 (JB Lippincott, Philadelphia, 1988).
19. Stone, H.B., Brown, J.M., Phillips, T.L. and Sutherland, R.M. *Radiat. Res.* 1993; 136:422–434.
20. Wilson, D.F. and Cerniglia, G.J. *Adv. Exp. Med. Biol.* 1994; 345:539–47.

21. Bacic, G., Liu, K.J., O'Hara, J.A., Harris, R.D., Szybinski, K., Goda, F. and Swartz, H.M. *Magn. Reson. Med.* 1993; 30:568–572.
22. Goda, F., O'Hara, J.A., Rhodes, E.S., Liu, K.J., Dunn, J.F., Bacic, G. and Swartz, H.M. *Cancer Res* 1995; 55:2249–2252.
23. Dardzinski, B.J. and Sotak, C.H. *Magn. Reson. Med.* 1994; 32:88–97.
24. Rofstad, E.K., Howell, R.L., DeMuth, P., Ceckler, T.L. and Sutherland, R.M. *Int. J. Radiat. Biol.* 1988; 54:635–649.
25. Rofstad, E.K., DeMuth, P., Fenton, B.M. and Sutherland, R.M. *Cancer Res.* 1988; 48:5440–5446.
26. Vaupel, P., Okunieff, P., Kallinowski, F. and Neuringer, L.J. *Radiat. Res.* 1989; 120:477–93.
27. Tozer, G.M., Bhujwalla, Z.M., Griffiths, J.R. and Maxwell, R.J. *Int. J. Radiat. Oncol. Biol. Phys.* 1989; 16:155–164.
28. Dunn, J.F., Frostick, S., Adams, G.E., Stratford, I.J., Howells, N., Hogan, G. and Radda, G.K. *FEBS Letters* 1989; 249:343–347.
29. Sostman, H.D., Rockwell, S., Sylvia, A.L., Madwed, D., Cofer, G., Charles, H.C., Negro-Vilar, R. and Moore, D. *Magn. Reson. Med.* 1991; 20:253–267.
30. Gerweck, L.E., Urano, M., Koutcher, J., Fellenz, M.P. and Kahn, J. *Radiat. Res.* 1989; 117:448–58.
31. Okunieff, P.G., Koutcher, J.A., Gerweck, L., McFarland, E., Hitzig, B., Urano, M., Brady, T., Neuringer, L. and Suit, H.D. *Int. J. Radiat. Oncol. Biol. Phys.* 1986; 12:793–799.
32. Rofstad, E.K. *Int. J. Radiat. Biol.* 1990; 57:1–5.
33. Koutcher, J.A., Okunieff, P. and Neuringer, L. *Int. J. Radiat. Oncol. Biol. Phys.* 1987; 13:1851–1855.
34. Koutcher, J.A., Alfieri, A.A., Devitt, M.L., Rhee, J.G., Kornblith, A.B., Mahmood, U., Merchant, T.E. and Cowburn, D. *Cancer Res.* 1992; 52:4620–4627.
35. Adams, G.E., Bremner, J.C.M., Stratford, I.J. and Wood, P.J. *Brit J Radiology* 1992; Suppl 24. Radiation Science-of molecules, mice and men:137–141.
36. Moseley, M.E., Mintorovitch, J., Cohen, Y., Asgari, H.S., Derugin, N., Norman, D. and Kucharczyk, J. *Acta Neurochirurgica Suppl.* 1990; 51:207–209.
37. Busza, A.L., Allen, K.L., King, M.D., Bruggen, N.v., Williams, S.R. and Gadian, D.G. *Stroke* 1992; 23:1602–1612.
38. Busza, A.L., Allen, K.L., Williams, S.R. and Gadian, D.G. *Proc. Soc. Magn. Reson. Med.* 1993; p1497.
39. Beaulieu, C. and Allen, P.S. *Magn. Reson. Med.* 1994; 31:394–400.
40. Kohno, K., Hoehn-Berlage, M., Mies, G., Back, T. and Hossmann, K.A. *Magn. Reson. Imaging* 1995; 13:73–80.
41. Dardzinski, B.J., Helmer, K.G. and Sotak, C.H. *Proc. Soc. Magn. Reson.* 1994; p864.
42. Swartz, H.M., Boyer, S., Gast, P., Glockner, J.F., Hu, H., Liu, K.J., Moussavi, M., Norby, S.W., Vahidi, N., Walczak, T., Wu, M. and R.B.Clarkson. *Magn. Reson. Med.* 1991; 20:333–339.
43. Vahidi, N., Clarkson, R., Liu, K., Norby, S., Wu, M. and Swartz, H. *Magn. Reson. Med.* 1994; 31:139–146.
44. Glockner, J.F. and Swartz, H.M. in *Oxygen Transport to Tissue* (eds. Erdmann, W. & Bruley, D.F.) 229–245 (Plenum Publishing Corp, New York, 1992).
45. Liu, K., Gast, P., Moussavi, M., Norby, S., Vahidi, N., Wu, M. and Swartz, H. *Proc. Nat. Acad. Sci. USA* 1993; 90:5438–42.
46. Swartz, H.M., Liu, K.J., Goda, F. and Walczak, T. *Magn. Reson. Med.* 1994; 32:229–232.
47. Dunn, J.F., Ding, S., O'Hara, J.A., Liu, K.J., Rhodes, E., Weaver, J.B. and Swartz, H.M. *Magn. Reson. Med.* 1995; 34:515–519.
48. Chien, D., Buxton, R.B., Kwong, K.K., Brady, T.J. and Rosen, B.R. *J. Comp. Assist. Tomogr.* 1990; 14:514–520.
49. Stejskal, E.O. and Tanner, J.E. *J. Chem. Phys.* 1965; 42:288–292.
50. Smirnov, A.I., Norby, S., Clarkson, R.B., Walczak, T. and Swartz, H.M. *Magn. Reson. Med.* 1993; 30:213–220.
51. Twentyman, P.R., Brown, J.M., Gray, J.W., Franko, A.J., Scoles, M.A. and Kallman, R.F. *J. Natl. Canc. Inst.* 1980; 64:595–604.

26

EVALUATION OF THE CONCEPT OF "HYPOXIC FRACTION" AS A DESCRIPTOR OF TUMOR OXYGENATION STATUS[*]

S. M. Evans,[1] W. T. Jenkins,[2] M. Shapiro,[2] and C. J. Koch[2]

[1]School of Veterinary Medicine (Clinical Studies)
[2]School of Medicine (Radiation Oncology)
University of Pennsylvania
Philadelphia, Pennsylvania

ABSTRACT

The presence and significance of tumor hypoxia has been recognized since the 1950's. Hypoxic cells *in vitro* and in animal tumors *in vivo* are documented to be three times more resistant to radiation-induced killing compared to aerobic cells. There is now evidence that tumor hypoxia is treatment-limiting in many human cancers. One common way to describe the extent of hypoxia in individual and groups of tumors is the "hypoxic fraction." This measurement infers that cells are present in only two radiobiologically significant states: oxygenated and hypoxic. In this paper, we demonstrate the qualitative and quantitative presence of hypoxic tumor cells using the oxygen dependent metabolism of the 2-nitroimidazole, EF5. Two assumptions concerning the calculation and interpretation of the hypoxic fraction are considered. The first is the use of multiple animals to describe the radiation response at a given radiation dose. We hypothesize that the presence of inter-tumor variability in radiation response due to hypoxia could negatively influenced the characterization of the change in slope required to calculate the hypoxic fraction. The studies presented herein demonstrate heterogeneity of radioresponse due to hypoxic fraction within and between tumor lines. The 9L subcutaneous tumor studied in air-breathing rats demonstrates a 2 log variation in surviving fraction at 17 Gy. The Morris 7777 hepatoma, in contrast, showed little variability of radiation response. Our second question addresses the limitations of using the "hypoxic fraction" to describe the radiation response of a tumor. This calculated value infers that radiobiological hypoxia is a binary measurement: that a tumor contains two cell populations, aerobic cells with maximal radiosensitiv-

* Work supported by grants CA-56679 (SME, CJK) and CA-62331 (SME) from National Institutes of Health, and the Department of Radiation Oncology, University of Pennsylvania.

ity and hypoxic cells with maximal radioresistance. The classic work of Thomlinson and Gray, however, implies the presence of an oxygen gradient from tumors vessel through the tissues. In both the 9L and Q7 tumors, flow cytometric analysis of EF5 binding demonstrates a continuous range of cellular pO2 levels. These studies suggest that: 1) there is extensive intertumor variability of radiation response in certain tumor lines; 2) the variability in radiation response between individual tumors in a group may affect the ability to describe a particular tumor type's "hypoxic fraction" and 3) The oxygen status of tumor cells is a continuum. This realization affects the ability to apply a binary concept such as the "hypoxic fraction" effectively in radiobiology.

INTRODUCTION

Hypoxic cells are known to influence tumor growth, malignant potential, and treatment response in many experimental models. There is substantial evidence that the presence of hypoxic tumor cells influences treatment outcome in human cancers as well (1–3). In both experimental and clinical studies, commonly measured endpoints are the "hypoxic fraction" (4) and percentage of a tumor with pO_2 less than a certain value (usually pO_2 <5–10 mm Hg) (1, 5). Clinical trials in humans have been performed with the Eppendorf electrode and correlations between tumor response and the percentage of measurements under 5–10 mm Hg have been made (1). In experimental studies, the measurement of hypoxic fraction is classically based on the relative position of the radiation survival curves generated in tumor-bearing, air-breathing animals compared to tumors in hypoxic (euthanized) animals (4, 6). For tumors containing hypoxia studied in air-breathing animals, the radiation response curve is expected to be biphasic; the low dose portion of the curve describes the response of oxygenated cells and the high dose portion of the curve describes the response of the hypoxic cells. As with all experimental procedures, the analysis and interpretation of this data requires certain assumptions. Moulder and Rockwell (4) have reviewed many of the assumptions and limitations related to calculating the hypoxic fraction from paired survival curves. In the studies described herein, we investigate two additional questions concerning the measurement and interpretation of the hypoxic fraction. The first is the use of multiple animals to describe the radiation response at a given radiation dose. We have previously shown in the 9L subcutaneous tumor that, in air-breathing animals, there is extensive inter-tumor variation in radioresponse (7). This variability could be almost completely attributed to the presence of hypoxia and was not correlated to tumor size. We hypothesize that such inter-tumor variability in radiation response and hypoxic fraction could negatively influenced the ability to characterize the slope change required to calculate the hypoxic fraction. Our second question addressed the limitations of using the "hypoxic fraction" (or % of measurements less than a certain pO_2) to describe the radiation response of a tumor. The original work of Thomlinson and Gray (8) implied the presence of an oxygen gradient from the blood vessel into the tumor tissues. The gradient resulting from the diffusion and consumption of oxygen implies that there should be a continuum of radiation response in the tumor cells. Under these circumstances, the most hypoxic cells may not be the most treatment limiting (9).

Herein, we demonstrate the presence of a variation in inter- and intra-tumoral heterogeneity between cell lines and discuss the impact of these observations on the calculation and application of the hypoxic fraction. We also illustrate, *in vivo*, the continuum of oxygen diffusion and hypoxic cell binding using nitroimidazole binding techniques. Using

Hoescht 33342 binding to demonstrate blood flow, we show a negative correlation with cellular EF5 binding to hypoxic cells.

MATERIALS AND METHODS

Drug Synthesis

A pentafluorinated derivative of etanidazole was synthesized by Dr. M. Tracy and colleagues at Stanford Research International, Palo Alto, CA, and is referred to as EF5 in this manuscript.

Cell Preparation

Tumors were grown from cells derived from 9L rat glioma (10, 11) obtained from Dr. K.T. Wheeler (Bowman Gray School of Medicine, Winston Salem, NC). Morris hepatoma 7777 cells were obtained from American Tissue Culture Collection (ATCC). Tumor cell dissociation was based on a modification of previously described methods (12, 13).

Preparation of Monoclonal Antibodies

Monoclonal antibodies were made against radiochemically-produced adducts of EF5 and thiol-containing proteins as described previously (14). The antibodies used in the present study are a single clone, designated as ELK3–51. The monoclonal antibodies were conjugated with the green-excited, orange-emitting fluorescent dye, Cy3 (15). This dye is available in an amine reactive form from Biological Detection Systems (Pittsburgh, PA.).

EF5 Binding—Fluorescence Microscopy

The freezing, sectioning, fixing, blocking and staining of tissue sections with ELK3–51:Cy3 have been previously described (7). Briefly, tissues were rapidly removed from a live, anesthetized animal, placed in -50º isopentane for 30 seconds, rinsed rapidly in iced brine, then iced water, and placed onto dry ice pellets. Tissues were placed in a -80º freezer until sectioning. Fourteen micron frozen sections were cut onto poly-L-lysine coated slides, fixed in 4% paraformaldehyde for 1 hour, rinsed and blocked overnight. After removing the block, sections were stained for 4–6 hours in 75μM ELK3–51:Cy3 and rinsed twice in PBS containing 0.3% Tween 20. The final rinse was in PBS, and sections were stored in 1% paraformaldehyde until photographed and analyzed. All procedures and storage were at 0–4º.

EF5 Binding—Flow Cytometric Assay

The blocking and staining of cells with ELK3–51:Cy3 and preparation for flow cytometric analysis have been previously described and are similar to the above description for tissue sections (7). The Flow Cytometry Facility at the Cancer Center, University of Pennsylvania, has a FACstar Plus instrument (Becton Dickinson, Mountain View, CA) equipped with a water-cooled 200 mW Argon laser. Although the Cy3 dye is optimally excited at 565 nm, the highest available wavelength was 514 nm (Argon line). Reproducibility of this instrument was excellent on a week-to-week basis, based on the signal from tetramethyl rhodamine calibration beads. The voltage on the photomultiplier tube was adjusted to give a signal on these very bright beads of 5000 (approximately 450 volts). A minimum of 10,000 events (*ex vivo* cells from the tumor) were collected on each sample. Immunofluorescence data were displayed on a four decade log scale. Flow cytometric data analyses were performed using the Becton Dickinson software program Lysys II. Samples were gated on low angle (forward scatter) vs. 90° angle (side scatter) to select cell populations of interest. Cells for flow cytometric analysis were selected based upon the dot plot distributions of forward (reflecting cell size) and side (reflecting cell complexity) scatter. Cells with very low forward scatter and variable side scatter represented dead cells, cellular debris and red blood cells and were not included in the analysis. Data were analyzed using the remaining cells (R1, figure 4).

Tumor Tissue Samples

All animal studies were performed under the regulations provided by the University of Pennsylvania Institutional Animal Care and Use Committee (IACUC). 9L and Q7 tumors were grown as subcutaneous implants over the thigh musculature. Tumor bearing rats were given EF5 as an intravenous tail injection of 10 mM EF5 prepared in 0.9% saline. The mass of solution administered was 1% of the animal's mass and the resulting equivalent whole-body concentration was 100 µM. Recent pharmacologic studies in mice and cats show that this drug distributes evenly to all tissues ((16) and Northrop, unpublished data). Two hours and forty five minutes following EF5 administration, the animal was anesthetized with xylazine (1.3 mg/kg intraperitoneally) and ketamine (140 mg/kg intraperitoneally). At that time, 15 mg/kg Hoescht 33342 was given intravenously. Radiation was administered 15 minutes later (see below), the tumor rapidly removed and immediately cooled. The serum half-life of EF5 in rats is about 150 minutes, so rapid cooling is necessary to prevent depletion of oxygen and then binding of the residual drug in the excised tissue (17). The tumor was weighed and bisected. Half of the tumor was disaggregated (13) for plating efficiency and flow cytometric analyses and the other half quick-frozen for fluorescence and light microscopic analyses.

Plating Efficiency

Cells dissociated from tumors were counted using both a particle counter (Coulter®) and hemocytometer. For the clonogenic assay of 9L and Q7 tumors, suitable numbers of cells were plated into 100 mm plastic Petri dishes. Each dish contained 9 ml of Eagle's Minimal Essential medium made with 9% v/v bovine calf serum, 4% fetal calf serum and 1% antibiotics (GIBCO). For the 9L cell line, 50,000 feeder cells were also plated (feeder cells were prepared by irradiating aerobic 9L cells in tissue culture with 25 Gy). The number of cells plated was varied over a range in order to yield 100–200 colonies per plate. In this range, the number of colonies varies linearly with the number of cells seeded. Multiple replicates were plated at each of several dilutions. The plates were incubated for 10–15 days followed by fixation, staining and counting of colonies. Surviving cells produced colonies containing at least 50 cells. The plating efficiency of individual tumors was calculated based on hemocytometer counts of the numbers of tumor cells plated.

Irradiation Studies

Radiation was performed on an orthovoltage X-ray unit operated at 225 kV and 10 mA, 0.2 mm copper filter. The dose rate was 4.0 Gy/min. For all *in vivo* irradiations, thermoluminescent devices were placed on the tumor surface, and were exposed for one minute during the time the beam was on. Total exposures were then calculated for each tumor. Hypoxia was induced in tumors by allowing 10 minutes following euthanasia before irradiation. Hypoxic tumors were irradiated with doses of 0–30 Gy; cells dissociated from tumors and irradiated in suspension were given doses between 0 and 11 Gy.

Data Analysis

The hypoxia curve was generated from tumors irradiated in euthanized rats and the aerated curve was generated by irradiating cells from tumors with graded radiation doses. The survival model used was $S = S_o e^{-\alpha D - \beta D^2}$ and a quadratic fit was made to determine the best fit coefficients.

RESULTS

Figures 1 and 2 contrast the range of variability of radiation response in 2 tumor types. In the subcutaneous 9L glioma irradiated in air-breathing Fischer rats, a 2-log variation in response can be seen at 17 Gy. In contrast, Q7 tumors irradiated in air-breathing Buffalo rats demonstrate minimal inter-tumor variability, despite that these tumors were studied over 9 months time, were different passages and varied in size from 800 mg to 3.2 gm. In both the Q7 and 9L tumors irradiated in hypoxic, euthanized rats or tumor cells irradiated in suspension, there is little variability around the best fit curves ($R^2 = 0.89$ - 0.99). This is in contrast to the radiation response in air-breathing Fischer rats bearing 9L subcutaneous tumors. We have previously demonstrated that most of this variability in

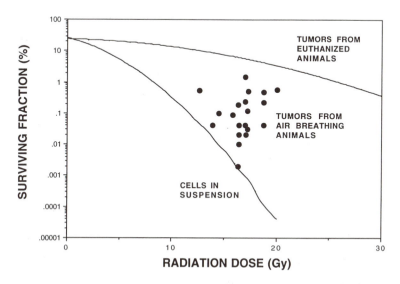

Figure 1. Survival curves from *in vivo-in vitro* plating efficiency experiments using 9L subcutaneous tumors. Data for cells dissociated from tumors and irradiated in suspension and for tumors irradiated under hypoxic conditions (euthanized rat) are solid lines which are the calculated best quadratic fit (R^2 for hypoxic tumors = 0.93 and for cells in suspension = 0.99). Individual data points obtained in air-breathing rats are shown (closed circles).

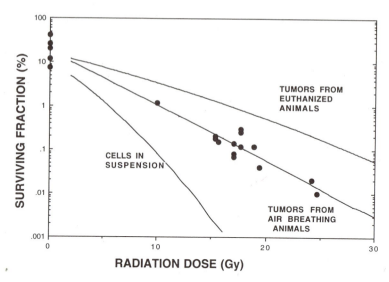

Figure 2. Survival curves from *in vivo-in vitro* plating efficiency experiments using subcutaneous Morris hepatoma 7777 tumors. Data for cells dissociated from tumors and irradiated in suspension and for tumors irradiated under hypoxic (euthanized) conditions are represented as solid lines which are the calculated best quadratic fit (R^2 for hypoxic tumors = 0.96 and for cells in suspension = 0.89). Individual data points obtained in air-breathing rats are shown (closed circles); for aerobic tumors the best fit line has a correlation coefficient of 0.96.

plating efficiency can be attributed to hypoxia using flow cytometric techniques (18). Conversely, in Q7 tumors, the percentage of moderately hypoxic cells as identified by flow cytometric analysis, is uniform among tumors (Evans, unpublished data).

Figure 3 illustrates fluorescent microscopic sections of EF5 binding compared with the identical sections following Hoescht dye administration. In this small 9L tumor (225 gr.), there is no necrosis present and there is bright binding in vascularized, oxygenated regions compared to absence of binding in avascular, hypoxic regions. These two images are negatives of each other, as would be expected; regions near blood flow are generally oxygenated and should not bind EF5. The flow cytometric analysis of cells dissociated from this tumor is illustrated in figure 4. Here, the continuum of cells from high binding (relative fluorescence up to 1,000) down to low binding cells (10–100 relative fluorescence) is shown.

DISCUSSION

The assessment of the hypoxic fraction in animal tumors is classically based on assay techniques which rely on comparisons of tumor *groups* irradiated under 'normal conditions' *vs.* those irradiated under conditions of complete artificial hypoxia (such as clamping the tumor vasculature or euthanizing the animal). Three endpoints for tumor cell survival/viability can be assessed: the relative survival of excised tumor cells (paired survival curves), the doses needed for tumor control (clamped TCD_{50} technique) or analysis of post- irradiation tumor growth (clamped growth delay technique). All three methods re-

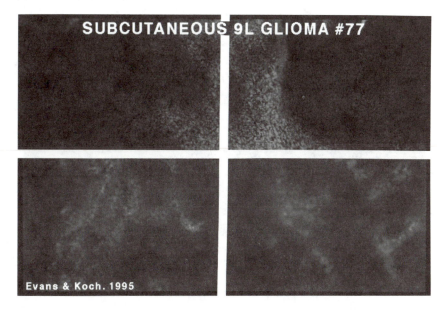

Figure 3. Fluorescent photomicrograph of 14 μm thick frozen section of a subcutaneous 9L glioma. Rat was intravenously injected with 100μM EF5 3 hours and 5μM Hoescht dye 15 minutes preceding tumor excision. Upper panels represent adjacent 1050 x 750 μm sections of tumor as viewed with green light and demonstrates EF5 binding to hypoxic tumor cells. Lower panels are the same as the upper sections but are viewed with blue light. This section demonstrates *in vivo* binding of cells adjacent to vessels patent during the 15 minutes following Hoescht injection and preceding euthanasia. Note the negative correlation between EF5 and Hoescht 33342 binding.

quire assumptions for both the methodology and calculation of the hypoxic fraction; these have been evaluated and discussed in detail by Moulder and Rockwell (4, 19). In this paper we have reassessed one of these assumptions: that the use of *groups* of animals for the calculation of the hypoxic fraction is appropriate in all tumor models. Secondly, we have evaluated the concept of the "hypoxic fraction" in terms of its relevance to the radiobiological endpoint of cell and tumor survival.

The paired survival curve assay compares the survival curves for tumor cells irradiated under normal aeration and acute hypoxia. Following irradiation under each of these environmental conditions, the tumors are removed from the host, dissociated into single cells and then assayed for viability; herein we used the *in vitro* colony forming assay to determine cell viability. Classically (and in contradistinction to the work presented herein), in order to obtain statistical significance, data from groups of 5 or more animals are pooled at each radiation dose. The assumptions made in using pooled data is that tumors grown from the same line, implanted into the same site, in similar hosts and studied at the same size will have a similar hypoxic fraction. Therefore, any variability around the best fit line will be due to causes other than hypoxia. This assumption was tested in detail in the BA1112 rhabdomyosarcoma grown in WAG/Rij rats (20); the variability around the best fit line for the radiation response of normally aerated and artificially hypoxic tumors was similar, but in each case there was a large standard deviation. The authors concluded that factors other than the fraction of hypoxic cells in individual tumors at the time of irradiation were responsible for the tumor response variation. Our data on the 9L subcutaneous tumor lead to a different conclusion. We find that there is minimal variability

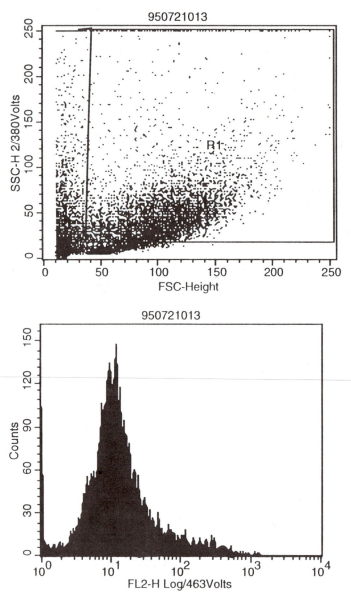

Figure 4. Dot plot distribution and flow cytometric analysis of cells dissociated from 9L subcutaneous tumor #77, 3 hours following 100 μM EF5 administration. Debris and red cells, characterized by a low forward scatter were gated out of the analysis (region 1). Analyses was performed based upon the remaining cells which are assumed to be a combination of tumor and host cells.

surrounding the best fit line describing hypoxic tumor response (R^2 = 0.99) and as much as a 2 log variation surrounding the response of tumors irradiated under aerated conditions. Analysis of the EF5 binding and flow cytometric data suggests that in this tumor line, hypoxia plays a major role in the variation of radiation response (7). Interestingly, the variation around the best fit line of both hypoxic and aerated Morris 7777 tumors is minimal and identical ($R^2 = 0.96$). "Classic" analysis of these data would lead to conclusions similar to those reported by Moulder in the BA1112 rhabdomyosarcoma (20).

The hypoxic fraction assigned to any tumor type is calculated from the extrapolation numbers of parallel lines fitted to the air and hypoxic curves for 'high' radiation doses. This presents another problem in calculating the hypoxic fraction using data from groups of animals where there is a large standard deviation around the data points: there is uncertainty in the exact position of the best fit line as well as an inherent difficulty in deciding where the linear portion of the curve begins. In the classic example of the paired survival curves from EMT6 mammary carcinoma (4, 6),the variability around portions of the fitted line was a factor of 8–10. These observations suggest the need to characterize the presence and extent of hypoxia in *individual* tumors rather than in tumor groups.

The second consideration is the biological relevance of the concept of the "hypoxic fraction". This calculated value infers that radiobiological hypoxia is a binary measurement: that a tumor contains two cell populations, aerobic cells with maximal radiosensitivity and hypoxic cells with maximal radioresistance. In fact, however, the original work of Thomlinson and Gray (8), and other more recent studies (21) suggest that a spectrum of radiosensitivity should exist in solid tumors. Recent work from this laboratory (7, 18), as well as the data presented herein (figures 4,5) document the existence and significance of a continuum of oxygen tensions in tumor cells. Our observation of the negative correlation between *in vivo* Hoescht 33342 and EF5 binding are a visual confirmation of Thomlinson and Gray's original hypothesis. Of interest is the consistent presence of an unlabelled zone when these two binding assays are superimposed. This can be predicted by the following observations and calculations: The average cell diameter is approximately 10 μm and oxygen is predicted to diffuse approximately 150–200 μm (15 cell layers). Hoescht is known to diffuse out of blood vessels, but only a short distance because it is avidly bound by the viable cells near the nourishing blood vessels (5–6 cell layers). Therefore, an unlabelled zone of 9–10 cell layers would be expected, and is demonstrated.

As noted above, three methods are classically used to calculate the hypoxic fraction of tumors: excision assays, clamped tumor control assays and growth delay assays. Because of their nature, excision assays are commonly performed at the lowest radiation doses (up to 30 Gy), compared to clamped tumor control assays (up to 80 Gy); growth delay assays are intermediate (up to 60 Gy). The implication of the presence of a continuum of hypoxic and aerobic cells is that the lower the radiation doses used in an assay, the greater the number of cells will be measured as resistant. Because of this, hypoxic fractions based upon excision assays should overestimate the number of hypoxic cells compared to the other methods of measurement.

Recently, the Eppendorf electrode has been used to characterize the presence of hypoxia in tumors. Several Eppendorf-based studies are now reported in humans showing that hypoxia is present and predictive for tumor response (1, 3, 22, 23). Despite the technical ability of this technique to describe the continuum of cellular oxygen, the most commonly cited endpoint is the percentage of measurements less than or equal to a certain value, essentially a hypoxic fraction measured using the electrode technique. In a number of experimental tumor lines (5, 24), it has been impossible to correlate this value to the classically measured hypoxic fraction. The commonly cited explanation for this is that the electrode may be measuring low pO2 values in areas that are not viable. Recent studies using the EF5 binding techniques have indeed shown the presence of hypoxic, metabolically active cells, but non-clonogenic cells in EMT6 spheroids (9). Other studies from our laboratories have shown that the percentage of moderately, not severely hypoxic cells in animal tumors determine radiation response (18). However, the work presented herein suggest another potential explanation. It may be that, in certain tumor types, the value, or the concept of the "hypoxic fraction" is unreliable. Now that sophisticated methods to measure individual tumor hypoxia and identify hypoxic subpopulations are available, it may be time to more closely evaluate the time honored endpoint of "hypoxic fraction".

REFERENCES

1. Hockel, M., Knoop, C., Schlenger, K., Vordran, B., Baussmann, E., Mitze, M., Knapstein, P. G., and Vaupel, P. Intratumor pO2 predicts survival in advanced cancer of the uterine cervix. Radiotherapy and Oncology, *26*:45–50, 1993.
2. Gatenby, R. A., Kessler, H. B., Rosenblum, J. S., Coia, L. R., Moldofsky, P. J., Hartz, W. H., and Broder, G. J. Oxygen distribution in squamous cell carcinoma metastases and its relationship to outcome of therapy. Int. J. Radiat. Oncol. Biol. Phys., *14*:831–838, 1988.
3. Kallinowski, F., and Buhr, H. J. Can the oxygenation status of rectal carcinomas be improved by hyperoxia? pp. 291–296, 1995. *In:* Tumor Oxygenation. *Eds.* Vaupel, Kelleher, Gunderoth. Gustav Fischer Verlag, Stuttgart, 1995.
4. Moulder, J. E., and Rockwell, S. C. Hypoxic fractions of solid tumors: experimental techniques, methods of analysis and a survey of existing data. Int. J. Radiat. Oncol. Biol. Phys., *10*:695–712, 1984.
5. Horsman, M. R., Khalil, A. A., Nordsmark, M., Siemann, D. W., Hill S. A.,Lynch, E. M., Chaplin, D. J., Stern, S., Thamas, C. D., Guichard, M., Grau, C., and Overgaard, J. The use of oxygen electrodes to predict radiobiological hypoxia in tumors. pp. 49–58, *In:* Tumor Oxygenation. *Eds.* Vaupel, Kelleher, Gunderoth. Gustav Fischer Verlag, Stuttgart, 1995.
6. Rockwell, S., Moulder, J. E., and Douglas, F. M. Tumor-to-tumor variability in the hypoxic fractions of experimental rodent tumors. Radiotherapy and Oncology, *2*:57–64, 1984.
7. Evans, S. M., Joiner, B. J., Jenkins, W. T., Laughlin, K. M., Lord, E. M., and Koch, C. J. Identification of hypoxia in cells and tissues of epigastric 9L rat tumours using EF5. Br. J. Cancer, *72*: 875–882, 1995.
8. Thomlinson, R. H., and Gray, L. H. The histological structure of some human lung cancers and the possible implications for radiotherapy. Br. J. Cancer, *9*:539–579, 1955.
9. Woods, M. R., Lord, E. M., and Koch, C. J. Prediction of hypoxic radioresistance by monoclonal antibody reactive with 2-nitroimidazole adducts. Int. J. Radiat. Oncol. Biol. Phys., *34*: 93–101, 1996.
10. Leith, J. T., Schilling, W. A., and Wheeler, K. T. Cellular radiosensitivity of a rat brain tumor. Cancer, *35*:1545–1550, 1975.
11. Wallen, C. A., Michaelson, S. M., and Wheeler, K. T. Evidence for an unconventional radiosensitivity of rat 9L subcutaneous tumors. Radiat. Res., *85*:529–541, 1980.
12. Howell, R. L., and Koch, C. J. The disaggregation, separation and identification of cells from irradiated and unirradiated EMT6 mouse tumors. Int. J. Radiat. Oncol. Biol. Phys., *6*:311–318, 1980.
13. Evans, S. M., and Koch, C. J. Characterization of the 9L glioma as a tissue isolated epigastric implant. Radiat. Oncol. Invest., *2*:134–143, 1994.
14. Lord, E. M., Harwell, L., and Koch, C. J. Detection of hypoxic cells by monoclonal antibody recognizing 2-nitroimidazole adducts. Cancer Res., *53*:5271–5276, 1993.
15. Southwick, P. L., Ernst, L. A., Tauriello, E. W., Parker, S. R., Mujumdar, R. B., Mujumbdar, S. R., Clever, H. A., and Waggoner, A. S. Cyanine dye labeling reagents - carboxymethylindocyanine succinimidyl esters. Cytometry, *11*:418–430, 1990.
16. Laughlin, K. M., Evans, S. M., Lord, E. M., and Koch, C. J. Biodistribution of EF5 [2-(2-nitro-iH-imidazole-1yl)-N-(2,2,3,3,3-pentafluoropropyl)acetamide] in BALB/c mice bearing EMT6tumors; implications for oxygen measurements in normal and tumor tissues. Journal of Pharmacology and Experimental Therapeutics, *277*: 1049–1057, 1996.
17. Koch, C. J., Giandomenico, A. R., and Lee Iyengar, C. W. Bioreductive metabolism of AF-2 [2(2-furyl)-3-(5-nitro-2-furyl)acrylamide] combined with 2-nitroimidazole radiosensitizing agents. Biochem. Pharmacol., *46*:1029–1036, 1993.
18. Evans S.M., Jenkins W.T., Joiner B., Lord E.M. and Koch C.J. 2-nitroimidazole (EF5) binding predicts radiation resistance in individual 9L subcutaneous tumors Cancer Res., *56*: 405–411, 1996.
19. Moulder, J. E., and Rockwell, S. Tumor hypoxia: its impact on cancer therapy. Cancer and Metastasis Rev., *5*:313–341, 1987.
20. Moulder, J. E., and Martin, D. F. Hypoxic fraction determinations in the BA1112 rat sarcoma: variations within and among assay techniques. Rad. Res., *99*, 1984.

21. Tannock, I. F. Oxygen diffusion and the distribution of radiosensitivity in tumours. Br. J. Radiol., *45*:515–524, 1972.

22. Lartigau, E., Lusinchi, A., Randrianarivelo, H., Weeger, P., Wibault, P., Luboinski, B., Eschwege, F., and Guichard, M. Oxygen tension distribution before and during accelerated radiotherapy and carbogen breathing: preliminary results. pp. 305–312 *In:* Tumor Oxygenation. *Eds.* Vaupel, Kelleher, Gunderoth. Gustav Fischer Verlag, Stuttgart, 1995.

23. Lawrence, V., Ward, R., and Bleenen, N. Tumor pO2 distribution in patients treated with the combination of nicotinamide and carbogen breathing. *In:* Tumor Oxygenation. *Eds.* Vaupel, Kelleher, Gunderoth. Gustav Fischer Verlag, Stuttgart, 1995.

24. Biade, S., Yeh, K. A., Milito, S. J., Brown, D. Q., Lanciano, R. M., and Chapman, J. D. Electrode measurements of oxygen tensions in rat prostate carcinomas and comparisons with other assays. pp. 83–94. *In:* Tumor Oxygenation. *Eds.* Vaupel, Kelleher, Gunderoth. Gustav Fischer Verlag, Stuttgart, 1995.

27

OPTICAL IMAGING OF BREAST TUMOR BY MEANS OF CONTINUOUS WAVES

S. Nioka,[1] Y. Yung,[1] M. Shnall,[2] S. Zhao,[1] S. Orel,[2] C. Xie,[1] B. Chance,[1] and L. Solin[3]

[1]Department of Biochemistry/Biophysics
[2]Department of Radiology
[3]Department of Oncology
 University of Pennsylvania
 Philadelphia, Pennsylvania 19104

INTRODUCTION

Early detection of breast cancer is one of the keys to decrease the mortality of this epidemic disease. Since the time that the NIH recommended X-ray mammography for an annual screening for women over 50 years of age (1), the mortality has indeed dramatically reduced (2). However, there are some concerns about the use of X-ray mammography; we consider the X-ray to be an unsatisfactory technique for this screening purpose. X-ray mammography is insensitive to one-fourth of cancer cases and itself is carcinogenic. It does not penetrate dense breasts, and is generally not applied to women under 40 years of age.

We have tested three optical technologies: TRS (time resolved spectroscopy), CWS (continuous wave spectroscopy), and PMS (phase modulated spectroscopy) (3). We have reported breast imaging with TRS previously (4). While CWS has been used for diaphanography, it has been shown repeatedly to lack specificity and imaging capabilities. Here we employ a tumor-occupying contrast agent and an image reconstruction algorithm to overcome the existing problems. This CWS imaging study is a series of our efforts to try to find a best screening method for early breast tumors. We use small tungsten bulbs (less than 1 watt) and silicon diode detectors to transilluminate and to detect through a breast, from all angles, in a coronal section of the breast. The light intensities from the detectors can be analyzed to reconstruct images using a back-projection algorithm. An optical contrast agent clearly enhances a location of a lesion and is a key element of the success of the current technique (5).

Oxygen Transport to Tissue XVIII, edited by Nemoto and LaManna
Plenum Press, New York, 1997

METHOD

Eight or 16 combinations of light sources (tungsten bulbs) and light detectors (silicon photodiodes) are located on a two-dimension circle line at an equal distance from each other (22.5° or 11° angle apart, Figure 1A, 1B). In the circle, we placed a breast model subject using 0.5% intralipid and ink (about the same scattering and absorption coefficients as those in the breast tissue), or a human breast with the probes touching the tissue lightly. We turn on one of the light sources with less than 1 watt at a time and acquire the light intensities received by the 8 or 16 detectors located on the circle line. The data acquisition for an image takes 4–8 seconds with 8x8 or 16x16 data points. A contrast agent; Indocyanine Green (ICG, 0.25–0.5 mg/kg) is injected in the model system or in the human intravenously, while data are being acquired continuously every few seconds over 10–15 min as the ICG absorption signal appears and disappears. Data are processed as OD changes due to ICG from the iv injection at the beginning. Some data points are averaged in several time windows and, as a result, several images are reconstructed using a back-projection algorithm.

Ten subjects were volunteers with found breast tumors; some had undergone lumpectomy and radiation therapy for cancer. We report here the examples of lumpectomized breasts or tumors of a relatively large size (1 cm or more).

RESULTS

The Model Studies

Figure 2A shows two tumor-like objects made of 1 cm diameter tubes in a 8 cm diameter container, filled with 0.5% intralipid solution (approx. μ_a and μ_s' of 0.03 and 6 cm^{-1}, re-

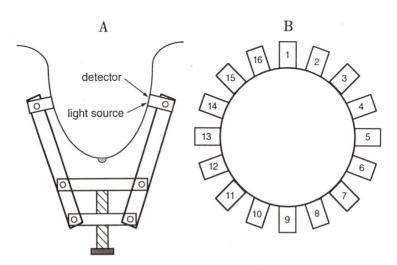

Figure 1. Scheme A describes the cut section of the 16 light source-detector device, holding a human breast inside. The diameter can be fitted easily with set screws. The 16 light source-detector combinations in each arm are located at equal distance (11° angle apart), but when the device fits a breast, only the diameter changes.

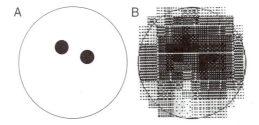

Figure 2. A model study of optical imaging with the 8x8 device. Intralipid 0.5% and ink resembles the optical characteristics of the human breasts. Two 1 cm objects are located 1 cm apart. When 8x8 images are made, the two objects are depicted in the reconstructed image by a back-projection algorithm.

spectively). A contrast agent (ICG) is circulated in the tubes (each has 1 mm diameter, bundled to yield 1 cm total diameter), which has approximately some nanomolar concentration of ICG. This concentration is assumed to be similar to that obtained in human breasts injected intravenously with 0.25 to 0.5 mg/Kg of ICG. Eight source-detector is used and 144 pixels are made out of the 8x8 light intensity information. The resolution is 7 mm. Thus, this CWS image appears to detect two 1 cm objects which are 1 cm apart in a model system (Figure 2B).

Human Breast Imaging

Case 1: A Cancer Breast. This patient is a 64 year-old woman, who has a tumor about 1.5 cm in diameter and located 2.5 cm deep in the skin. The source and detector are located at 90° when the ICG accumulation is most sensitively detected (Figure 3). This figure depicts the ICG accumulation in the lesion in the early periods, as well as the later period after the contrast agent injection, compared with that on the same place in the other normal breast. The result is consistent with animal studies with transplanted rat tumor models. According to our animal studies, the increased circulation has been recognized very early, even when the tumor is still too small to be visible (less than a few mm).

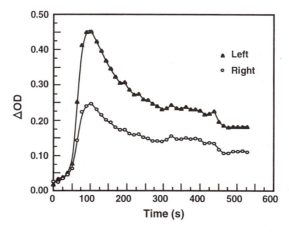

Figure 3. Continuous wave spectra of ICG time course. The breast with cancer shows much higher absorption than in the normal breast.

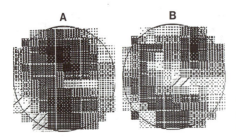

Figure 4. optical image of a lumpectomized breast as a poorly circulating area with ICG injection. A: 1 min after the ICG injection. B: 2 min after the injection.

Case 2: A Lumpectomized Breast. This patient had a lumpectomy 14 days prior to the optical imaging. There is a seroma formation with some fluid retention in the artificial cyst at 3 o'clock. At the beginning after the ICG injection, the ICG began to appear mainly in the central area, and the lesion is seen as a cold spot at 3 o'clock (Figure 4A). A few minutes later, ICG redistributed towards the outside, but there is still a low ICG concentration in the lesion, suggesting a poor circulation in the seroma (Figure 4B).

Case 3: A Fibrous Cyst. The patient (56-years-old) has a long history of a palpable tumor. The lump swells with menstral cycle, and sometimes lactates. MRI shows a colony of small fibrous cysts, whose ducts are hypertrophic and connected to the nipple (Figure 5). When ICG is injected, optical image depicts the lesion area (Figure 6B), and contrast of the lesion is high during the following minutes (2–4 minutes) (Figure 6C–6E) in the 16x16 image. It reveals that a functional tumor like this also has increased circulation and is associated with a high accumulation of ICG. The contrast agent enabled the depiction of the tumor in this case.

DISCUSSION

We demonstrate that the diffusive Continuous Wave NIR has a potential for imaging human breast lesions. The key to its success is to produce higher contrast by the use of contrast agents. Furthermore, the back-projection algorithm can provide better resolution

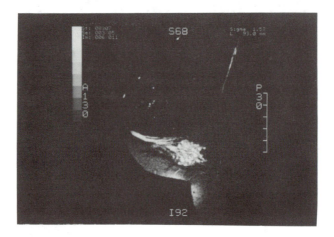

Figure 5. MRI of a cystic fibrosis disease. Gadolinium accumulation is seen in the swelling ducts of the cyst.

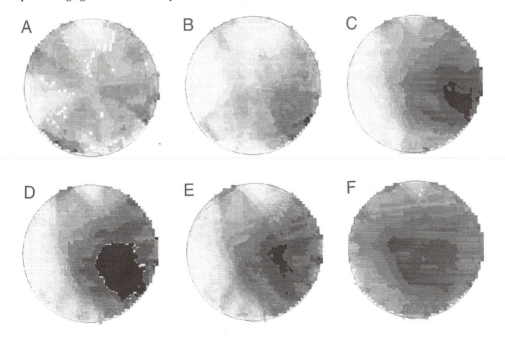

Figure 6. Optical images of the cystic fibrosis with ICG injection at B. A: pre-injection. B–F: correspond to images at one-minute intervals after the ICG injection (1–5 min).

than the current diaphanography. However, shown here is an example of the benign tumor, which clearly indicates greater blood flow and blood volume in the hyperactive benign tumor. The question here is, does the blood flow–blood volume image really diagnose malignant tumor? We can only answer this question by experiencing more cancer cases as well as benign tumors and comparing the two.

The next step is to search for the specificity of a malignant tumor. We now know that to image the high circulation and blood volume does not necessarily identify the malignancy because it shows a hyperactive metabolism or the heterogeneity of the tissue metabolism. The other function of high circulation high blood volume image has to be considered. For example, unusually high permeability constant or diffusion coefficient of ICG into the lesion may identify malignancy. The contrast method we used may help identify malignancy by observing time-distribution relationship of the contrast agent.

Many previous investigations have indicated that oxygen concentration in the tumor is much lower than in the normal tissues (6). Benign tumors do not have such low oxygen concentrations (6). The oxygen image should be considered as a potential diagnostic image for cancer. Oxygen image can be easily obtained by adding the information of multiple wavelength data.

ACKNOWLEDGMENT

This research is supported by DOD grant USAMRDC DAMD17-93-C-3071.

REFERENCES

1. Shapiro, S., Venet,L et al. Ten to fourteen year effect of screening on breast cancer mortality. J. Natl. Cancer Inst. 69:349–355, 1982.
2. National Institute of Health Consensus Development Conference Statement: Treatment of Early Breast Cancer. (June 18–21, 1990) Bethesda, MD.
3. Cardio Green (CG), SterileIndocyanine Green USP. Becton Dickenson and Company, 1990.
4. O'Leary, MA, DA. Boas, B. Chance, AG. Yodh. Simultaneous scattering and absorption images of heterogeneous media using diffusive waves within the Rytov approximation. SPIE 2389:320–327, 1995.
5. Nioka,S. M. Shnall, M. Miwa, S. Orel, M. Haida, S. Zhao and B. Chance. Photon imaging of human breast cancer. Adv. Exp. Med. Biol. 16:171–179, 1994
6. Vaupel, P. DK. Kelleher, M. Gunderoth(eds) Tumor oxygenation. Stuttgart, New York Fisher, 1995

28

POTENTIAL FOR EPR OXIMETRY TO GUIDE TREATMENT PLANNING FOR TUMORS

Julia A. O'Hara,[1] Fuminori Goda,[2] Jeffrey F. Dunn,[2] and Harold M. Swartz[2]

[1]Department of Medicine (Radiation Oncology)
[2]Department of Diagnostic Radiology
Dartmouth Medical School
Norris Cotton Cancer Center, Hanover, New Hampshire 03755

1. INTRODUCTION AND THEORETICAL CONSIDERATIONS

A major contributing factor in the failure of solid tumors to be locally controlled by radiation therapy (RT) is the relative radiation resistance of hypoxic cells of tumors compared to well-oxygenated cells. Recently clinical studies have established the presence of hypoxic regions in human tumors (1, 2). Further studies confirmed that relatively high tissue pO_2 in human tumors correlated with positive outcomes of radiation therapy and that poor outcomes were associated with tumors with low pO_2 (3–6). As a result of available studies, the conclusion has been drawn that the effective level of oxygenation in individuals could not be predicted based on tumor type, histology, staging, or even size, but had to be measured (7). With the development of methods to measure the pO_2 in tumors (8), it now seems feasible to determine if this parameter, which can be of crucial importance in radiation therapy, can be used to improve treatment by permitting individualized optimization of therapy on the basis of the pO_2 in the tumor.

Measurements of pO_2 by electron paramagnetic resonance (EPR Oximetry) are particularly promising for using pO_2 measurements to guide therapy because of the capability of this technique to make repeated measurements of pO_2 noninvasively and with adequate accuracy (< 1 torr) and sensitivity for the radiobiologically crucial levels (~ 5 torr or less) (9, 10). In this paper we summarize the rationale for such an approach and the initial results that are available to test the hypothesis that EPR oximetry can provide data that will be of practical use to guide tumor therapy.

Oxygen plays a critical role in the metabolism of tumors and normal tissues and is a key determinant of sensitivity of tissues to ionizing radiation (11). Reoxygenation after radiation was described in 1968 by Van Putten and Kallman (12) and has subsequently been found in virtually all animal tumors. Most of the evidence for reoxygenation has been made by measuring the hypoxic cell fraction by radiobiological methods using the paired survival curve method (13). Recent studies have shown that while in many animal tumors the radiobiological hypoxic fraction correlates with pO_2 (14), different assays may give different hypoxic fractions in the same type of tumor (13, 15) and consequently the subject remains controversial. Lack of adequate techniques to monitor pO_2 repeatedly in individual tumors may be the reason for failure to resolve these issues and to determine how reoxygenation can best be used to improve radiation therapy.

The level of oxygen may also affect chemotherapy. Well-oxygenated tissue is likely to be more accessible to drugs than poorly oxygenated tissues, if oxygenation is proportional to perfusion (16). Chemotherapeutic drugs may have differential toxicities for hypoxic versus oxic cells (17); this potential difference has been used in strategies which exploit the presence of hypoxic regions in tumors by using drugs selectively toxic to hypoxic cells or drugs that are activated to toxic products under hypoxic conditions (18, 19). Chemotherapeutic drugs may also have vasoactive effects that could modify tumor oxygenation, drug metabolism, cytotoxicity, drug access, radiation sensitivity, and length of time of exposure to the drug (20). Recently, information about pO_2 after chemotherapy has identified several classes of drugs that produce reoxygenation measured radiobiologically (21–23). Using microelectrodes it has been shown that chemotherapy can affect tumor pO_2 (21, 24), although in some cases the difference in tumor pO_2 has been explained by differences in tumor volumes (25).

The role of oxygen in chemotherapy plus radiation is even more complex, because of the different ways that chemotherapy (one or more drugs) can affect tissues, especially when combined with radiation. An understanding of the effects of combined therapy is desirable because, while most of the primary non-surgical treatment of tumors is still done by fractionated radiation therapy, combinations of radiation with chemotherapy have been used increasingly over the last three decades (26). Empirical methods most often have been used in developing the sequence, timing, and dosages of effective combinations, which has resulted in the evolution of clinical protocols that may not be optimal for the specific cancer under treatment, especially if the treatments affect the pO_2 in the tumor and/or adjacent tissues (27). The principles of how chemotherapeutic drugs can improve treatment by radiation have been outlined by Steel and Peckham (28) and recently summarized (26) The general types of interactions that occur in tumors include: 1) *spatial cooperation*, that is each agent is effective against a target that is missed by the other. This mechanism can operate when radiation and drug targets are in different parts of the body, as in local treatment of a tumor with radiation and adjuvant chemotherapy used to attack micro-metastases at distant sites in the body. In addition, a drug that has access to a tumor may produce additional kill above that by radiation. 2) *Addition of anti-tumor effects*, which assumes that the use of two or more agents will kill more cells than could be killed by one alone, and 3) *enhancement of tumor response*, the anti-tumor effect is greater than the effects expected with the agents used separately (29). Exploitable mechanisms for *enhancement of tumor response* include reoxygenation following drug treatment and before irradiation and improved drug access following irradiation (28).

A premise of the current study and discussion is that reoxygenation plays a critical role in the response of tumors to radiation and chemotherapy. Our work and that of others has shown that the timing of reoxygenation is dependent on tumor type, the type of chemotherapy, radiation dose, and the schedule by which they are combined. The number and complexity of these factors makes it very difficult to predict the timing of reoxygenation and, therefore, the pO_2 in tumors needs to be measured directly. If reoxygenation occurs under conditions of clinical delivery of radiation and chemotherapeutic agents, then knowledge of the timing and degree of reoxygenation could contribute to rational design of protocols for effective combination treatment. Identification of tumors that are hypoxic or fail to reoxygenate could aid in customizing treatment so that appropriate therapies could be designed. EPR oximetry appears to have the characteristics needed for such measurements, since it can measure pO_2 sequentially and with the temporal resolution required to show transient alterations in pO_2.

EPR oximetry involves the placement of an oxygen-sensitive probe into the tumor that then reports the pO_2 in the region of the tumor in equilibrium with the probe (30, 31). The volume of measurement is the tissue in contact with the slurry of the insoluble carbonaceous material. Using EPR oximetry, pO_2 can be monitored from the same position in a tumor repeatedly in the same animal over the whole course of treatment, without need for anesthesia. The ability to monitor pO_2 non-invasively and repeatedly at the same point in a tumor has direct applicability for measuring reoxygenation in animal tumors and with further technological developments, in human tumors.

In this study we monitored intratumoral pO_2 using EPR oximetry and investigated the effect of changes in pO_2 caused by single doses of radiation or cyclophosphamide on the subsequent administration of radiation. Cyclophosphamide (CY) was chosen as the cytotoxic agent for this study since the combination of CY with radiation has shown schedule dependent effectiveness in several tumor systems (32–34) possibly related to reoxygenation. Studies in support of this demonstrate vascular effects of CY that might affect its efficacy (21, 35, 36). Bleomycin, cisplatin, mitomycin C, and taxol also have been shown to produce drug-induced oxygenation changes (21, 23).

2. MATERIALS AND METHODS

All animal procedures were approved by the Institutional Animal Care and Use Committee of Dartmouth Medical School.

2.1. Animal Tumor Models

These studies were carried out using the radiation induced fibrosarcoma (RIF-1) and mouse mammary adenocarcinoma (MTG-B). All tumors were grown on 6-week-old female C3H/HeJ mice (Jackson Laboratories, Bar Harbor, ME) and mice were randomly assigned to treatment protocols at the time of implantation. RIF-1 was grown according to the protocols of Twentyman et al. (37) as previously described (10). The cells were supplied by Dr. Janna Wehrle, Johns Hopkins University. An intradermal injection (50 μl) of the tumor cell suspension i.d. (2.0 x 10^5 cells) in the right flank, resulted in tumors of approximately 7 to 8 mm in diameter 12 days post transplantation.

The MTG-B tumor is a murine adenocarcinoma maintained by serial passage in five to seven week-old female C3H/HeJ mice (Jackson Lab, Bar Harbor, ME). This tumor was initially obtained from a spontaneous C3H mouse mammary tumor originating in the glandular epithelium, and first characterized by Clifton et al. (38). It has been used extensively in our laboratory for the study of the effects of radiation and chemotherapy (39, 40). For transplantation, tumors were removed aseptically from mice and minced in minimum essential media (MEM) without serum (GIBCO, Grand Island NY). The minced tumor particles were pressed through a nylon 70 μM cytosieve [Fisher] and centrifuged at 60 x g for 5 minutes. The pellet of tumor cells was resuspended in fresh MEM. A subcutaneous injection of 0.05 ml (10^6 cells) tumor cell suspension in the right flank typically grows to a flattened sphere of approximately 7 to 8 mm within 7 to 10 days.

2.2. Drug Administration

Cyclophosphamide (SIGMA, St Louis, MO) was dissolved immediately before use in 0.9% sterile saline and injected i.p. (0.2 ml/25 g mouse).

2.3. Radiation

Tumors were irradiated using a Maxitron-300 orthovoltage machine (General Electric, Milwaukee, WI) with a 1.5 cm cone portal (positioned in direct contact with the skin overlying the tumor) using a 3 mm Al filter at 140 kVp and 20 mA. The dose-rate at the skin was 4.72 Gy/min. Half the dose was delivered, then the tumor was inverted to deliver the second half. The control group was sham irradiated. Mice were restrained during the time of irradiation (about 5 minutes, including set up) but were not anesthetized.

2.4. Tumor Regrowth Delay Analysis

Tumor diameters in three orthogonal directions (d_1, d_2, d_3) were measured daily using calipers. Tumor volumes were calculated using the formula: $V_t = \frac{1}{6}(d_1 {}_* d_2 {}_* d_3)$. The response of the individual tumors to radiation was quantified by computing the growth delay to reach the doubling volume (GD_{DV}) for individual mice in each treatment group using the method of Jones *et al.* (39).

2.5. *In Vivo* EPR Oximetry

EPR spectra of India ink in tumors were obtained using a 1.2 GHz ("L-band") EPR spectrometer which we constructed. Typical settings for the spectrometer were: magnetic field, 425 Gauss; modulation frequency, 27 kHz; modulation amplitude, 0.2 Gauss; incident microwave power, 15 mW. The mice were restrained in a plastic holder with a hole through which the tumors were exposed. The detecting EPR coil was positioned over the tumor and five spectra were recorded per animal (30 seconds per spectrum, total measurement time was less than 10 min including positioning of the animal and spectrometer adjustment). Spectral line widths of India ink were measured and the pO_2 values calculated from a calibration curve of linewidth at various pO_2.

The calibration curve of pO_2 *vs.* line width of India ink was determined using a Bruker, ER 220D-SRC EPR spectrometer (9.6 GHz, X-band) and a commercial oxygen analyzer (Sensor Medics. Co., Model OM-11, Anaheim CA). The calibration procedure was the same as described previously, including verification of its validity for 1.2 GHz studies (31, 41). Control and experimental animals were restrained in the same manner and for similar time periods.

2.6. Statistics

For tumor growth delay experiments, the calculated tumor doubling and tripling volume growth delays were used as end points in analysis of variance (42) to determine the effect of treatment. A subset of 5 mice per group was measured for pO_2 each day up to 10 days post treatment. A repeated measures analysis was used to test differences of pO_2 measurements relative to baseline values between treatment groups at each of three time periods (24 hr, 72 hr and 7 day). All statistical tests were performed at the 0.05 level of significance and were two-sided. We assessed the relationship between volume and pO_2 using longitudinal methods (43). Figures given for tumor size or pO_2 are Mean ± SEM.

3. RESULTS AND DISCUSSION

3.1. Radiation-Induced pO_2 Changes in MTG-B and RIF-1 Tumors

Using direct measurements of tumor partial pressure of oxygen (pO_2) in two different murine tumors, we have shown that tumor pO_2 changes after radiation in a tumor-specific biphasic pattern (9, 10). The two tumors studied were a relatively hypoxic, heterogeneous metastatic tumor, the mouse mammary adenocarcinoma, MTG-B (9, 10) and the radiation-induced fibrosarcoma, RIF-1 (10). Note that the baseline pO_2 in RIF-1 tumors is higher than that of MTG-B (10). After single doses of radiation the pO_2 drops and this is followed by an increase in pO_2 to pretreatment or higher values. The pattern is the same in both types of tumors studied but the timing of minimal and maximal pO_2 differ. In one tumor, the RIF-1, the pO_2 changes occur at times of hypoxic cell fraction changes (10, 44). This pattern was exploited by timing a second dose of radiation (10Gy) to correspond with the highest pO_2 after a priming dose of 10 Gy. The time course of pO_2 changes in the two tumors is shown in Figure 1.

As can be seen in both tumor systems the pO_2 dropped after irradiation, followed by a recovery to at least the pretreatment pO_2. The timing of maximum hypoxia was different however: 6 hr for MTG-B and 24 hr for RIF-1. The timing of maximum pO_2 was 48 hr for MTG-B and 72 hr for RIF-1. Similar effects on pO_2 were seen in tumors when the radiation dose was 10 Gy (10). The pO_2 in normal tissue (contralateral leg muscle) was higher than in the tumor and varied but had no definite trend. Thus these results present a tumor-specific radiation-induced time course of pO_2 changes that is dependent on the type of tumor and was not found in unirradiated normal or tumor tissue. The pO_2 in unirradiated tumors showed a downward course as the tumor volume increased, but the rate and magni-

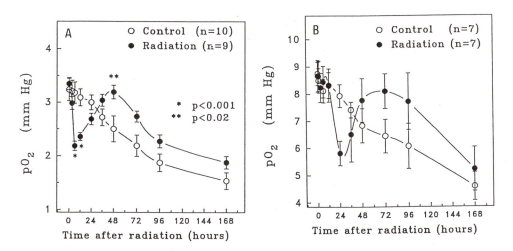

Figure 1. Time Course of Average pO_2 Changes in Irradiated Tumors (20 Gy). A. MTG-B, B. RIF-1. Values are Mean ± SEM. Adapted from Reference (10).

tude of these changes varied in individual tumors. For the remaining experiments described, we have used the RIF-1 tumor.

3.2. Effect of Interval on Split Dose Radiation in RIF-1

We then investigated whether two radiation (10 Gy) fractions would be more effective if the second dose was delivered at the time of highest pO_2 than at the time of minimum pO_2. RIF-1 tumors were divided into four treatment groups on the 11th day post transplantation (Taken as Day O) when the average volume was 106 ± 10 mm^3. Treatment Groups were: Group 1 (Control) = Sham Irradiated, Group 2 (Single) received 20 Gy on Day O, Group 3 (Hypoxic) received 10 Gy on Day O and another 10 Gy one day later, Group 4 (Oxic) received 10 Gy on Day O and another 10 Gy three days later. The calculated growth delay to double the treatment volume was used as the end point in analysis of variance (45) to assess the effect of treatment. The doubling volume growth delay for Group 3 (Oxic treatment) was significantly different from Group 4 (Hypoxic group) ($F[1,33] = 4.23$, $p = 0.05$). A significant difference was found between the four groups for G_{DV} ($F[3,33] = 5.86$, $p = 0.003$). Mean times to double the volume at the time of treatment are shown in Table 1.

These results are consistent with the hypothesis that the directly measured pO_2 in the tumor can be used to predict the response to a subsequent dose of radiation. As indicated by the growth of the tumors, they were more radioresistant 1 day after an initial dose of radiation than 2 days later, when reoxygenation has occurred as measured by pO_2. Further work is required to determine whether similar effects will be found at lower doses of radiation and if measurements of pO_2 will be similarly predictive of biological responses of other tumors such as the MTG-B tumors.

It should also be noted that the localized pO_2 measurements obtained with EPR oximetry did predict the response of the tumor, indicating that such measurements can be representative of the whole tumor.

3.3. Effect of Cyclophosphamide on Tumor pO_2

Cyclophosphamide treatment of RIF-1 tumors causes dramatic pO_2 changes in RIF-1 tumors, as shown in Figure 2 Panel A. The average pretreatment volume was 220 mm^3. Pretreatment pO_2 was 8.9 ± 1.0 torr which was followed by a drop to 3.3 ± 0.4 torr. This initial drop of 6 torr was followed by a recovery within three hours and a return to pretreatment pO_2 by 24 hours post cyclophosphamide treatment (46). The difference in pO_2 at the 1 hr time point between treated animals and untreated controls was highly significant

Table 1. Effect of 20 Gy on time to double the treatment volume of RIF-1 tumors

		Doubling time (days)	
Treatment group	n	Mean	SEM
1. Sham control	10	3.74	0.86
2. Single	7	8.67	1.15
3. Oxic (3 day interval)	8	9.17	1.46
4. Hypoxic (1 day interval)	9	6.09	0.77

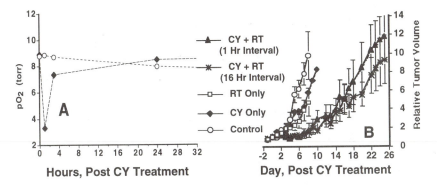

Figure 2. Panel A: pO_2 changes after CY treatment of RIF-1 tumors. Panel B: Tumor volume changes after CY alone or plus irradiation at 1 hour or 16 hours post CY. The cyclophosphamide dose was 50 mg/kg. The radiation dose was 10 Gy.

(p < .002). Our results on the time of pO_2 changes in RIF-1 tumors after cyclophosphamide agree with a previous report by Dorie and Kallman (21) on the time of maximum hypoxia (1 hr) and they also observed that this was followed by reoxygenation, as measured by radiobiological methods.

Figure 2B shows the tumor volume changes in the same mice for each treatment group (n=3). There was no significant difference in volume between controls and CY treated tumors one day post CY. Therefore these changes in pO_2 (0–3 days post CY) occurred in the absence of significant changes in the tumor volume, indicating that the effect was not due to the loss of cells.

3.4. Effect of Radiation and Cyclophosphamide on Tumor Volume

In this study the time course shown in Figure 2A was exploited by timing a single dose of radiation to coincide with the time of lowest pO_2 (at 1 hr) or after pO_2 had recovered (at 16 hr) post CY. Tumor volume was monitored, and the results are shown in Figure 2 Panel B. While there appeared to be a trend for the radiation delivered after pO_2 had recovered to be more effective than at the time of maximum hypoxia, this difference was not significant.

In split dose radiation treatments with ionizing radiation, the second radiation dose was more effective when delivered at the time of minimum versus maximum hypoxia. However, when chemotherapy perturbed the pO_2, there was no difference in the amount of tumor growth delay caused by a radiation dose at this time of maximum hypoxia versus the effect observed when the radiation was delivered a time when the pO_2 had returned to the pretreatment value (reoxygenation). We have no clear explanation for this at the present time. It may simply reflect the relatively small numbers of animals used in these studies. Although the hypoxia experienced after the chemotherapy was of very short duration (about 1 hr) as opposed to longer duration after radiation, the duration of hypoxia per se seems unlikely to alter the radiobiological sensitivity of the cells, because at the molecular level at least, the effects of oxygen occur on the basis of the very rapid reactions whose rate is proportional to the concentration of molecular oxygen. It has been argued that chronic hypoxia is more significant for radioresistance than acute hypoxia (47) and the changes after cyclophosphamide certainly do appear to represent 'acute' hypoxia; if this does occur it must be due to some biological changes because, as noted, the fundamental radiation chemistry should not be affected. It seems more likely that the lower pO_2 did lead to a decreased response to ionizing radiation, but that this was offset by other effects of the chemotherapy, such as a shift of the cells to a more resistant phase of the cell cycle and/or that the repair systems for the cells were affected differently at the two time intervals that were tested. Another factor may be the difference in the type and/or amount of active metabolites of cyclophosphamide at the different time periods, making the combination more effective at 1 hr than predicted by pO_2.

4. CONCLUSIONS

Consistent with the basic hypothesis, the results with split doses of radiation indicate the potential value of EPR oximetry to predict the optimal timing for split dose radiotherapy. Additional studies need to be done, however, to determine if similar effects will be observed with fractionation schemes more similar to those used in clinical medicine. The results of the preliminary study with CY do not support the hypothesis, but in view of their limited nature and the possibilities of other offsetting effects by this drug, it is clear that additional studies are also needed for these experiments. The work of Begg *et al.* and others reported that alternating cyclophosphamide and radiation with longer intervals than used here might be more effective than short intervals (36, 48, 49) and it should be useful to measure the pO_2 levels in tumors at those time points, as well as expand the data on measurements at short intervals after chemotherapy.

The experiments summarized here indicate that EPR oximetry can measure both pO_2 and tumor response with the frequency and duration needed to follow the effects of treatment in individual tumors after single and combined therapy. It seems possible that further studies using this methodology will resolve whether reoxygenation contributes to improved tumor response after different modalities and whether measuring pO_2 can lead to more effective cancer therapies.

ACKNOWLEDGMENTS

This work was supported by ACS Grant BE-186, the Core Grant of the Norris Cotton Cancer Center CA23108, NIH Grant GM51630 and used the facilities of the IERC at Dartmouth supported by NIH grant RR-0811.

REFERENCES

1. R. A. Gatenby, L. R. Coia, M. P. Richter, H. Katz, P. J. Moldofsky, P. Engstrom, D. Q. Brown, R. Brookland and G. J. Broder, Oxygen tension in human tumors: In vivo mapping using CT-guided probes. *Radiology.* **156,** 211–214 (1985).
2. M. Hockel, K. Schlenger, C. Knoop and P. Vaupel, Oxygenation of carcinomas of the uterine cervix: evaluation by computerized O_2 tension measurements. *Cancer Research.* **51,** 6098–6102 (1991).
3. P. Okunieff, M. Hoeckel, E. P. Dunphy, K. Schlenger, C. Knoop and P. Vaupel, Oxygen tension distributions are sufficient to explain the local response of human breast tumors treated with radiation alone. *Int J Radiat Oncol Biol Phys.* **26,** (4), 631–6 (1993).
4. M. Hockel, C. Knoop, K. Schlenger, B. Vorndran, E. Baussmann, M. Mitze, P. G. Knapstein and P. Vaupel, Intratumoral pO_2 predicts survival in advanced cancer of the uterine cervix. *Radiother Oncol.* **26,** (1), 45–50 (1993).

5. E. Lartigau, A. M. Le Ridant, P. Lambin, P. Weeger, L. Martin, R. Sigal, A. Lusinchi, B. Luboinski, F. Eschwege and M. Guichard, Oxygenation of head and neck tumors. *Cancer.* **71**, (7), 2319–25 (1993).

6. R. A. Gatenby, H. B. Kessler, J. S. Rosenblum, L. R. Coia and P. J. Broder, Oxygen distribution in squamous cell carcinoma metastases and its relationship to outcome of radiation therapy. *Int J Radiat Oncol Biol Phys.* **14**, 831–838 (1987).

7. P. W. Vaupel, Oxygenation of solid tumors. In *Drug Resistance in Oncology* (B. A. Teicher, Ed.), pp. 53–86. Marcel Dekker, New York, 1993.

8. H. B. Stone, J. M. Brown, T. L. Phillips and R. M. Sutherland, Oxygen in human tumors: correlations between methods of measurement and response to therapy. Summary of a workshop held November 19–20, 1992, at the National Cancer Institute, Bethesda, Maryland. *Radiat Res.* **136**, (3), 422–34 (1993).

9. J. A. O'Hara, F. Goda, K. J. Liu, G. A. Bacic, P. J. Hoopes and H. M. Swartz, Oxygenation in a murine tumor following radiation: an in vivo electron paramagnetic resonance oximetry study. *Radiat Res.* **144**, (2), 222–229 (1995).

10. F. Goda, J. A. O'Hara, E. S. Rhodes, K. J. Liu, J. F. Dunn, G. Bacic and H. M. Swartz, Changes of oxygen tension in experimental tumors after a single dose of X-ray irradiation. *Cancer Res.* **55**, (1 Jun), 2249–2252 (1995).

11. E. J. Hall, Radiobiology for the Radiologist. In Ed.), pp. 143. JB Lippincott, Philadelphia, 1988.

12. L. M. Van Putten and R. F. Kallman, Oxygenation status of a transplantable tumor during fractionated radiation therapy. *JNCI.* **140**, (3), 441–451 (1968).

13. J. E. Moulder and S. Rockwell, Hypoxic fractions of solid tumors: experimental techniques, methods of analysis and a survey of existing data. *Int J Radiat Oncol Biol Phys.* **10**, 695–712 (1984).

14. M. R. Horsman, A. A. Khalil, D. W. Siemann, C. Grau, S. A. Hill, E. M. Lynch, D. J. Chaplin and J. Overgaard, Relationship between radiobiological hypoxia in tumors and electrode measurements of tumor oxygenation. *Int J Radiat Oncol Biol Phys.* **29**, (3), 439–42 (1994).

15. K. Sasai and J. M. Brown, Discrepancies between measured changes of radiobiological hypoxic fraction and oxygen tension monitoring using two assay systems. *Int J Radiat Oncol Biol Phys.* **30**, (2), 355–61 (1994).

16. R. K. Jain, Physiological resistance to the treatment of solid tumors. In *Drug Resistance in Oncology* (B. A. Teicher, Ed.), pp. 87–105. Marcel Dekker, New York, 1993.

17. J. E. Moulder and S. Rockwell, Tumor hypoxia: its impact on cancer therapy. *Cancer and metastasis reviews.* **5**, 313–342 (1987).

18. I. J. Stratford, Bioreductive drugs in cancer therapy. *Br J Radiol.* **Suppl**, (24), 128–13 (1992).

19. J. M. Brown and M. J. Lemmon, Tumor hypoxia can be exploited to preferentially sensitize tumors to fractionated irradiation [see comments]. *Int J Radiat Oncol Biol Phys.* **20**, (3), 457–61 (1991).

20. R. E. Durand and N. E. LePard, Modulation of tumor hypoxia by conventional chemotherapeutic agents. *Int J Radiat Oncol Biol Phys.* **29**, (3), 481–486 (1994).

21. M. J. Dorie and R. F. Kallman, Reoxygenation in the RIF-1 tumor after chemotherapy. *Int J Radiat Oncol Biol Phys.* **24**, (2), 295–9 (1992).

22. E. Jahde, S. Roszinski, T. Volk, K. H. Glusenkamp, G. Wiedemann and M. F. Rajewsky, Metabolic response of AH13r rat tumours to cyclophosphamide as monitored by pO_2 and pH semi-microelectrodes. *Eur J Cancer.* **1**, 116–22 (1992).

23. L. Milas, N. Hunter, K. A. Mason, C. Milross and L. J. Peters, Tumor reoxygenation as a mechanism of taxol-induced enhancement of tumor radioresponse. *Acta Oncol.* **34**, (3), 409–12 (1995).

24. B. A. Teicher, N. P. Dupuis, T. Kusumoto, M. Liu, F. Liu, K. Menon, G. N. Schwartz and I. E Frei, Decreased tumor oxygenation after cyclophosphamide, reoxygenation and therapeutic enhancement with a perflubron emulsion/carbogen breathing. *Int J Oncol.* **3**, 197–203 (1993).

25. M. Busse and P. W. Vaupel, The role of tumor volume in 'reoxygenation' upon cyclophosphamide treatment. *Acta Oncologica.* **34**, (3), 405–408 (1995).

26. T. L. Phillips, Terminology for chemoradiation effects. In *Chemoradiation: An Integrated Approach to Cancer Treatment* (M. J. John, Ed.), pp. 11–17. Lea & Febiger, Philadelphia, 1993.

27. W. B. Looney and H. A. Hopkins, Rationale for different chemotherapeutic and radiation therapy strategies in cancer management. *Cancer.* **67**, (6), 1471–83 (1991).

28. G. G. Steel and M. J. Peckham, Exploitable mechanisms in combined radiotherapy-chemotherapy: The concept of additivity. *Int J Radiat Oncol Biol Phys.* **5**, 85 (1979).

29. G. G. Steel, The combination of radiotherapy and chemotherapy. In *The Biological Basis of Radiotherapy* (G. G. Steel, G. E. Adams, and M. J. Peckham, Ed.), pp. 239–248. Elsevier, Amsterdam, 1983.

30. H. M. Swartz, G. Bacic, B. Friedman, F. Goda, O. Grinberg, P. J. Hoopes, J. Jiang, K. J. Liu, T. Nakashima, J. A. O'Hara and T. Walczak, Measurements of pO_2 in vivo, including human subjects, by electron param-

agnetic resonance. In *Oxygen Transport to Tissue* (e. a. M.C. Hogan, Ed.), pp. 119–128. Plenum Press, New York, 1994.

31. H. M. Swartz, K. J. Liu, F. Goda and T. Walczak, India ink: A potential clinically applicable EPR oximetry probe. *Magn Reson Med.* **31,** (2), 229–232 (1994).

32. W. B. Looney, H. A. Hopkins and M. Tubiana, Experimental and clinical studies alternating chemotherapy and radiotherapy. *Cancer Metastasis Rev.* **8,** (1), 53–79 (1989).

33. B. A. Teicher, S. A. Holden, S. M. Jones, J. P. Eder and T. S. Herman, Influence of scheduling on two-drug combinations of alkylating agents in vivo. *Cancer Chemother Pharmacol.* **25,** (3), 161–6 (1989).

34. R. F. Kallman, D. Rapacchietta and M. S. Zaghloul, Schedule-dependent therapeutic gain from the combination of fractionated irradiation plus c-DDP and 5-FU or plus c-DDP and cyclophosphamide in C3H/ Km mouse model systems. *Int J Radiat Oncol Biol Phys.* **20,** (2), 227–32 (1991).

35. P. G. Braunschweiger, Effect of cyclophosphamide on the pathophysiology of RIF-1 solid tumors. *Cancer Res.* **48,** 4206–4210 (1988).

36. A. C. Begg, K. K. Fu, D. C. Shrieve and T. L. Phillips, Combination therapy of a solid murine tumor with cyclophosphamide and radiation: The effects of time, dose and assay method. *Int J Radiat Oncol Biol Phys.* **5,** 1433–1439 (1979).

37. P. Twentyman, Timing of Assays: an important consideration in the determination of clonogenic cell survival both in vitro and in vivo. *Int J Radiat Oncol Biol Phys.* **5,** 1213–1220 (1979).

38. K. H. Clifton, R. C. Briggs and H. B. Stone, Quantitative radiosensitivity studies of solid carcinomas *in vivo*: methodology and effect of anoxia. *J Natl Canc Inst.* **36,** 965–974 (1966).

39. E. Jones, B. Lyons, E. Douple, A. Filimonov and B. Dain, Response of a brachytherapy model using ^{125}I in a murine tumor system. *Rad Res.* **118,** 112–130 (1989).

40. E. B. Douple, J. A. O'Hara and E. L. Jones, Paraplatin enhancement of radiation therapy in a murine tumor (MTG-B). In *Anticancer Drug Research* (K. Lapis S. Eckhardt, Ed.), pp. 71–80. Akademiai Kiado, Budapest, 1987.

41. F. Goda, K. J. Liu, T. Walczak, J. A. O'Hara and H. M. Swartz, In vivo oximetry using EPR and India ink. *Magn Reson Med.* **33,** (2), 237–245 (1995).

42. D. Hand and C. C. Taylor, *Multivariate Analysis of Variance and Repeated Measures,* ed. Chapman and Hall, New York, 1987.

43. S. L. Zeger and K. Y. Liang, Longitudinal data analysis for discrete and continuous outcomes. *Biometrics.* **42,** 121–130 (1986).

44. M. J. Dorie and R. F. Kallman, Reoxygenation of the RIF-1 tumor after fractionated radiotherapy. *Int J Radiat Oncol Biol Phys.* **12,** 1853–1859 (1986).

45. J. Neter, W. Wasserman and M. H. Kutner, *Applied Linear Statistical Models,* 2nd ed. RD Irwin Inc, Homewood, IL, 1985.

46. J. A. O'Hara, F. Goda and H. M. Swartz, The pO_2 changes in RIF-1 tumors after combined therapy with cyclophosphamide and radiation. *Br J Canc.* **Submitted,** (1995).

47. M. R. Horsman, C. Grau and J. Overgaard, Reoxygenation in a C3H mouse mammary carcinoma. The importance of chronic rather than acute hypoxia. *Acta Oncol.* **34,** (3), 325–8 (1995).

48. W. B. Looney and H. A. Hopkins, Experimental and clinical rationale for alternating chemotherapy and radiotherapy in human cancer management. In *Chemoradiation: An Integrated Approach to Cancer Management* (M. J. John, Ed.), pp. 27–51. Lea & Febiger, Philadelphia, 1993.

49. P. R. Twentyman, R. F. Kallman and J. M. Brown, The effect of time between x-irradiation and chemotherapy on the growth of three solid mouse tumors. II. Cyclophosphamide. *Int J Radiat Oncol Biol Phys.* **5,** 1425–1427 (1979).

29

VASCULARIZATION, BLOOD FLOW, OXYGENATION, TISSUE pH, AND BIOENERGETIC STATUS OF HUMAN BREAST CANCER[*]

Peter Vaupel

Institute of Physiology and Pathophysiology
University of Mainz
D-55099 Mainz, Germany

INTRODUCTION

Many solid tumors are relatively resistant to conventional irradiation, chemotherapy and other non-surgical treatment modalities. A variety of factors are involved in the lack of responsiveness of these neoplasms, including (a) an intrinsic, genetically determined resistance and (b) physiological properties primarily created by inadequate and non-uniform vascular networks. Physiological factors which are usually closely linked encompass microcirculatory parameters (including transvascular and interstitial transport), tissue oxygen and nutrient supply, tumor pH and bioenergetic status. Despite the important role of physiological properties for tumor growth and metastasis, for early tumor response to treatment, for tumor detection, and probably for prediction of long-term outcome, reliable data on human solid tumors are scarce although the number of clinical investigations dealing with this subject is rapidly increasing.

Breast cancer is a leading cause of cancer-related deaths of women, yet there is a striking paucity of information concerning the above mentioned parameters. In this presentation, relevant clinical findings available so far on blood supply and flow-related physiological properties of human breast cancers will be reviewed and emphasis will be given to the relevance of these factors in clinical oncology.

VASCULARIZATION AND BLOOD FLOW OF BREAST CANCERS

Most, if not all solid tumors begin as avascular aggregates of malignant cells. "Microscopic tumors" exchange nutrients and metabolic waste products with their surround-

---

[*] This paper is dedicated to Professor Dr. Dr. Gerhard Thews on the occasion of his 70th birthday.

ings by simple diffusion. Therefore, the growth of an avascular three-dimensional aggregate of tumor cells is self-limiting. The establishment of progressive expansion of malignant tumors is possible only if supply and drainage are initiated via blood flow through exchange vessels of the tumor microcirculatory bed. When considering the origin of blood vessels in a growing tumor, one must take into account the existence of two different types of vessels:

- pre-existing normal host vessels incorporated into the tumor, and
- newly formed tumor vessels arising from neovascularization stimulated by release of (one or more) angiogenesis factors. These vessels are in general void of smooth muscle cells and are not innervated.

Newly formed microvessels in most solid tumors do not conform to the normal morphology of the host tissue vasculature. Microvessels in solid tumors exhibit a series of severe structural and functional abnormalities. They are often dilated, tortuous, elongated and saccular. There is significant arterio-venous shunt perfusion accompanied by an anarchic vascular organization. Excessive branching is a common finding often coinciding with blind vascular endings. Incomplete or even missing endothelial lining and interrupted basement membranes result in an increased vascular permeability with RBC extravasation, significant interstitial fluid flow and a rise in viscous resistance to flow mainly due to hemoconcentration. Aberrant vascular morphology and a decrease of vessel density are responsible for an increase in geometric resistance to flow which, together with an enlargement of diffusion distances due to the expansion of the extravascular space can lead to perfusion with hypoxemic and nutrient deprived blood. Substantial spatial heterogeneity in the distribution of tumor vessels and significant temporal heterogeneity in the microcirculation within a tumor may result in a considerably anisotropic distribution of tumor tissue oxygenation, nutrient supply, drainage of catabolites, tissue pH and bioenergetic status, factors which are usually closely linked and which define the so-called metabolic microenvironment. Variations in these relevant parameters between tumors (even of the same grade and stage) are often more pronounced than differences occurring between different locations or microareas within a tumor (for a review see [1]).

Morphological appearance of the tumor vascular bed does not necessarily allow direct judgements concerning functional aspects of the tumor microcirculation or of the nutritive blood flow. In experimental tumor systems, only 20–85% of the tumor vessels are perfused at a given time. This fraction is dependent on the tumor cell line investigated [2].

Little is known about the clinical importance and the prognostic value of tumor angiogenesis in human tumors. The vessel density evaluated exclusively in the most vascularized areas of the tumor has been shown to be an independent prognostic factor in human breast cancer [3,4]. Meanwhile, other studies have confirmed the relationship between increased intratumoral microvessel density and the risk of metastasis and/or decreased patient survival with breast carcinoma [e.g., 5–10]. In contrast, several groups have shown that greater vascular density was associated with longer patient survival (e.g. [11]) or that assessment of vascularity is not an independent prognostic factor in lymph node negative, invasive breast cancer [12]. There are relevant data available indicating that the markers used and the method chosen to determine vascular density may significantly influence the results obtained (e.g. [13]). Thus, it is not absolutely clear whether microvessel counts in histological sections of tumor samples might be of use in predicting the outcome of breast cancer patients and additional studies are needed to provide a clear and more detailed picture of the prognostic significance of tumor vascularization [14].

Only few studies on blood flow through breast carcinomas have been reported so far [15–18]. Some of them are anectodal reports rather than systematic investigations, and therefore, definite conclusions cannot be drawn. Considering the presently available data, the following (preliminary) conclusions can be drawn when flow data derived from different reports are pooled:

a. Blood flow (and thus O_2 supply) can vary considerably ranging from flow values found in the normal postmenopausal breast to those measured in the lactating breast (0.08–0.8 ml·g⁻¹·min⁻¹; see Fig. 1). Breast cancers, thus can have flow rates similar to those measured in breast tissue with a high metabolic rate, or can exhibit flow rates comparable to that of tissues with a low metabolic turnover (postmenopausal breast tissue [19]).

b. The average perfusion rate of breast carcinomas does not deviate substantially from that of other solid malignancies.

c. Flow data from multiple sites of measurement show marked heterogeneity within individual breast cancers. However, tumor-to-tumor variability seems to be more pronounced than intra-tumor heterogeneity.

d. There is no association between tumor size and blood flow. No apparent correlation can be drawn between flow and prognosis [18].

e. Blood flow values are found to be similar for metastatic lesions and breast primaries [18].

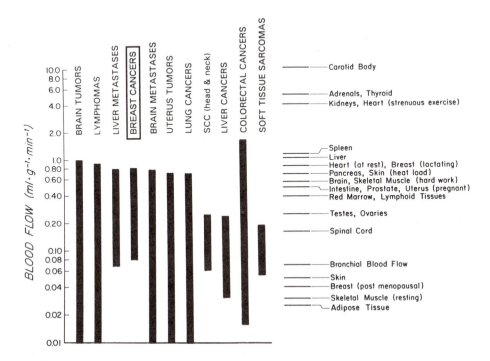

Figure 1. Variability of blood flow in human malignancies (black bars) and mean flow values of normal tissues and organs (pooled data, for a review see [1]). SCC = Squamous cell carcinoma.

FLUID PRESSURE AND CONVECTIVE CURRENTS IN THE INTERSTITIAL SPACE

The growing tumor produces new, often abnormally leaky microvessels but is unable to form its own functioning lymphatic system. As a result of this and due to a large hydraulic conductivity, in breast cancers—like in many other solid tumors—there is a significant bulk flow of free fluid in the interstitial space. Whereas in the normal tissue convective currents in the interstitial compartment are estimated to be about 0.5–1% of plasma flow, in xenografted humen breast cancers interstitial water flux can reach 15% of the respective plasma flow ([1], see Fig. 2).

After seeping copiously out of the highly permeable tumor microvessels, fluid accumulates in the tumor matrix and a high interstitial pressure builds up in solid tumors [20]. Whereas in normal breast tissue the interstitial fluid pressure is slightly subatmospheric or just above atmospheric values, an interstitial hypertension with mean values of 15 mmHg and higher develops in breast cancers [20]. These increased interstitial fluid pressures, which drop precipitously in the outermost rim of the tumor, can wash out therapeutic agents, especially larger molecules, from the tumor into the surrounding tissue, i.e., fluid is squeezed out from the high- to the low-pressure regions at the tumor/normal tissue interface.

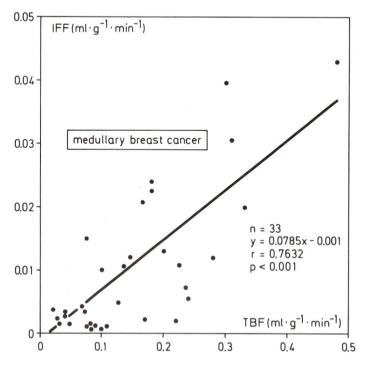

Figure 2. Interstitial fluid flow (IFF) as a function of blood flow (TBF) in xenografted human breast cancer (adapted from [1]).

OXYGEN CONSUMPTION RATE AND TISSUE OXYGENATION IN BREAST CANCERS

Oxygen consumption rates of breast cancers are in the range of $3–10$ $\mu l \cdot g^{-1} \cdot min^{-1}$, whereas in the normal postmenopausal breast the respective values range from $3–6$ $\mu l \cdot g^{-1} \cdot min^{-1}$ [19]. There is ample evidence to suggest that oxygen extraction is not impaired in breast cancer cells and that the cellular respiratory function is not deficient (10–35% in breast cancer vs. 50–75% in postmenopausal breast). When considering tumoral oxygen extraction data derived from $^{15}O_2$-PET studies using the O_2 steady state technique, an underestimation of the mean values has to be considered on the basis of computer simulation studies mimicking tissue heterogeneity [21]. PET studies published to date may thus not be accurate enough for the assessment of oxygen extraction in breast cancer and other malignancies.

Extensive studies on the tissue oxygenation of primary breast cancers have been performed by several groups [22–28]. As a result of a compromised and anisotropic microcirculation, many breast cancers reveal hypoxic tissue areas which are heterogeneously distributed within the tumor mass. Mean and median O_2 tensions (pO_2) obtained from different pathological stages and histological grades are, on average, distinctly lower than in the normal tissue [22,27]. Oxygen tensions measured in the normal breast revealed a mean (and median) pO_2 of 65 mmHg, whereas in cancers of the breast of stages pT1–4, the median pO_2 was 28 mmHg (Fig. 3). Thus far, one third of the breast cancers investigated exhibited pO_2 values between 0 and 2.5 mmHg, i.e., tissue areas with less than half maximum radiosensitivity. In contrast, in the normal breast pO_2 values ≤ 12.5 mmHg could not be detected [22]. In all systematic studies on breast cancers, bimodal pO_2 distribution curves have been obtained [22,23,27], either indicating the co-existence of normoxic and hypoxic tumor areas or a relevant contribution of pO_2 readings in the stromal compartment of breast cancers.

When pooled data for stages pT1 & 2, and pT3 & 4 breast cancers are compared, there is no evidence of statistically significant differences between the two groups (median pO_2 in pT1 & 2 tumors: 26 mmHg; pT3 & 4 tumors: 30 mmHg, Fig. 3). This implies that the oxygenation in breast cancers and the occurrence of hypoxia and/or anoxia does not correlate with the clinical stage [22,25,27,29]. Similarly, there was no association between tumor size and blood flow [18,30]. The proportion of pO_2 values between 0 and 2.5 mmHg was $\approx 6\%$ in pT1 & 2, and $\approx 7\%$ in pT3 & 4 tumors. In addition, there is substantial evidence that the oxygenation patterns do not correlate with the histological grade [22,25,27], the menopausal status, the tumor histology (ductal vs. lobular), the extent of necrosis of fibrosis, and with a series of other clinically relevant parameters (e.g., hormone receptor status, hemoglobin level, smoking habits [22,25]).

When comparing pO_2 data of breast cancers from different institutions, there is good agreement in the oxygenation status observed. The tumor data are nearly identical whereas the pO_2 data for the normal breast exhibit some differences [22,27]. Most probably, the lower pO_2 values in the study by Runkel et al. [27] are due to a higher number of postmenopausal breasts being included (94% vs. 67% in the study by Vaupel et al. [22]).

As was the case with the primary tumors, the oxygenation of metastatic lesions is generally anisotropic and compromised as compared to normal tissues at the site of metastatic growth. The median pO_2 values of the secondary tumors are distinctly lower than those recorded in the tumor surroundings. This holds true for a series of metastatic lesions [28]. Metastatic lesions of breast cancers exhibited a poorer oxygenation status than the

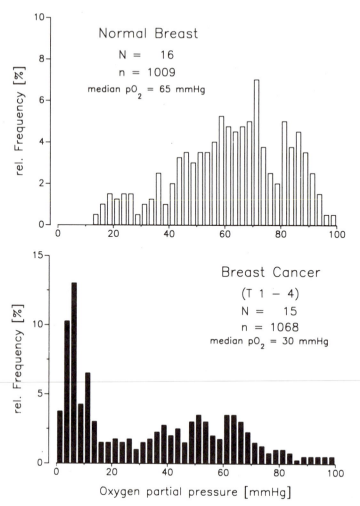

Figure 3. pO$_2$ histograms for normal breast (upper panel) and for breast cancers (lower panel, clinical stages T1–4). N = number of breast cancers investigated, n = number of pO$_2$ measurements (adapted from [22]).

primaries [29]. Whether this pattern is a characteristic of this tumor entity or a general biological phenomenon has to be elucidated in ongoing studies. Local recurrencies of breast cancers also seem to have a higher hypoxic fraction than the primary tumors [29].

Summarizing the information on the oxygenation status of breast cancers available so far (for reviews see [19,23,24,26,31]), several investigations have clearly shown that

    a. tumor oxygenation, as a rule, is anisotropic and compromised as compared to normal tissues,

    b. on average, the median pO$_2$ values in primary, metastasic and recurrent tumors are lower than in the normal tissue at the site of growth,

    c. many solid tumors (~30–35%) contain hypoxic tissue areas (pO$_2$ ≤ 2.5 mmHg),

    d. tumor-to-tumor variability in oxygenation is significantly greater than intratumor variability,

    e. tumor oxygenation is unpredictable considering staging and grading, and

f. tumor oxygenation is independent of other known oncologic parameters.

TUMOR pH

Warburg´s classic work in the 1920s showed that cancer cells intensively split glucose to lactic acid even in the presence of oxygen. Because of this excessive lactic acid production it was assumed for many decades that tumors are acidic. However, the unfolding story of tumor pH and its consequences have recently become clearer, due to techniques which are able to preferentially measure intra- or extracellular pH in malignancies. Under many conditions it has now been confirmed that the intracellular pH in tumor cells is neutral to alkaline as long as tumors are not oxygen- and energy-deprived [32]. Tumor cells have efficient mechanisms for exporting protons into the extracellular space, which represents the acidic compartment in tumors. For this reason, a pH gradient exists across the cell membrane in tumors ($pH_i > pH_e$). Interestingly this gradient is the reverse of normal tissues where pH_i is lower than pH_e (see Fig. 4, for reviews see [19,33,34]).

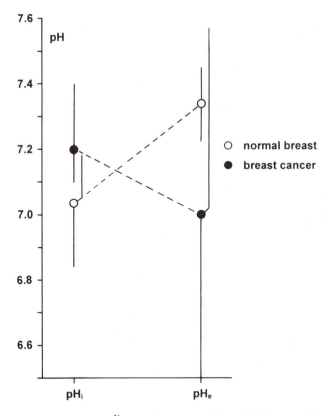

Figure 4. Intracellular (pH_i measured with ^{31}P-NMR) and extracellular pH (pH_e assessed by pH-sensitive electrodes) values in normal breast (open circles) and in breast cancers of patients (filled circles). Values shown are means and the range of pH data measured [19,34].

BIOENERGETIC STATUS OF BREAST CANCERS

Human breast cancer cells have an average ATP content of 8.4 ± 1.1 fmole/cell in cell culture (S. Singer, personal communication), which is similar to the ATP content of human colon cancer cells (7.6 ± 0.6 fmole/cell, [35]), but distinctly higher than the cellular ATP concentration reported for fibroblasts fed daily with growth medium (≈ 3 fmole/cell, [36]).

In vivo ^{31}P-NMR spectroscopy has been employed in monitoring the energy metabolism of human tumors since 1983 [37]. From the studies available, information is provided that may be beneficial in the clinical treatment of cancer. Furthermore, there are indications that serial monitoring of tumor response can assist in optimizing the timing of treatments [38].

In Fig. 5, ^{31}P-NMR spectra from normal breast tissue are compared with tumor spectra (spectra are redrawn from original recordings [39,40]). According to these exemplary spectra, in many human malignancies high concentrations of phosphomonoesters (PME, precursors of membrane lipids), phosphodiesters (PDE, metabolites) and inorganic phosphate (P_i) and low phosphocreatine (PCr) levels are often characteristically found [21].

In order to describe the bioenergetic status of normal tissues and malignancies relevant metabolite ratios have been compiled in Figs. 6 and 7. PCr/P_i ratios for various human malignancies and normal tissues are depicted in Fig. 6. The data show that PCr/P_i in

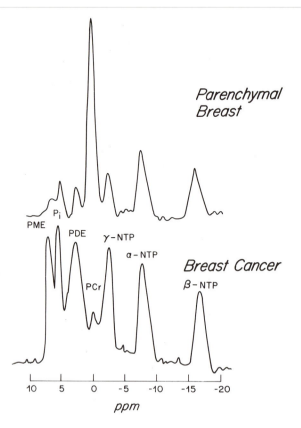

Figure 5. Typical ^{31}P-NMR spectra of parenchymal breast and a human breast cancer (adapted from [1]).

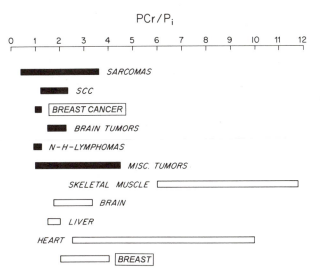

Figure 6. PCr/P$_i$ ratios calculated for human malignancies (black bars) and for normal tissues (white bars). All ratios represent pooled data. SCC = Squamous cell carcinoma, N-H-Lymphomas = Non-Hodgkin-lymphomas.

normal brain and in brain tumors is similar (for a review see [1]), whereas this ratio is significantly higher in parenchymal breast vs. breast cancer (p < 0.001).

ß-NTP/P$_i$ ratios for human tumors and normal tissues are presented in Fig. 7. Here, no clear differences are seen between normal breast and breast cancer. Significant differences are only obtained for sarcomas vs. skeletal muscle.

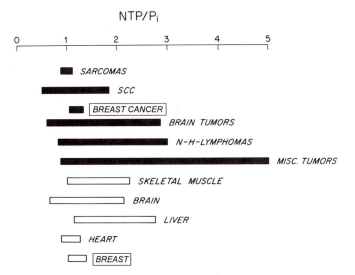

Figure 7. Pooled NTP/P$_i$ ratios for human tumors (black bars) and for normal tissues (white bars). For further explanation see legend to Fig. 6.

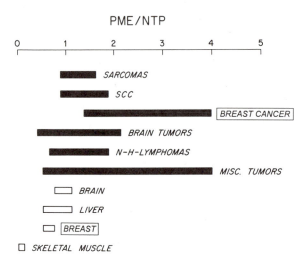

PME/NTP

Figure 8. Pooled PME/NTP ratios for various human tumors (black bars) and for normal tissues (white bars). For further explanation see legend to Fig. 6.

Due to relatively high concentrations of mobile phosphomonoesters, the PME/NTP (Fig. 8) and PME/P$_i$ ratios (Fig. 9) are consistently higher in breast cancers compared to normal breast and in sarcomas relative to skeletal muscle.

CONCLUSIONS

According to currently available information on blood flow and flow-related parameters of the so-called metabolic microenvironment (e.g., oxygenation, tissue pH and bioenergetic status), significant variations in these relevant parameters are likely to occur between different locations within breast cancers and between tumors of the same grade and clinical stage. Therefore, evaluation of these parameters which are usually closely linked in individual tumors before therapy may enable pretherapeutic selection of tumors for modified treatment approaches to improve local control and patient survival.

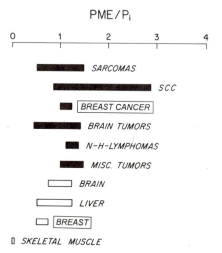

PME/P$_i$

Figure 9. Pooled PME/P$_i$ ratios for human malignancies (black bars) and for normal tissues (white bars). For further explanation see legend to Fig. 6.

REFERENCES

1. P. Vaupel. Blood flow, oxygenation, tissue pH distribution and bioenergetic status of tumors. Ernst Schering Research Foundation, Lecture 23, Berlin (1994).
2. H.J.J.A. Bernsen, P.F.J.W. Rijken, T. Oostendorp & A.J. van der Kogel. Vascularity and perfusion of human gliomas xenografted in the athymic nude mouse. Brit. J. Cancer 71, 721–726 (1995)
3. N. Weidner, J. Folkman, F. Pozza, P. Bevilacqua, E.N. Allred, D.H. Moore, S. Meli & G. Gasparini. Tumor angiogenesis: A new significant and independent prognostic indicator in early-stage breast carcinoma. J. Natl. Cancer Inst. 84, 1875–1887 (1992).
4. N. Weidner, J.P. Semple, W.R. Welch & J. Folkman. Tumor angiogenesis and metastasis—correlation in invasive breast carcinoma. New Engl. J. Med. 324, 1–8 (1991).
5. E.R. Horak, R. Leek, N. Klenk, S. Lejeune, K. Smith, N. Stuart, M. Greenall, K. Stepniewska & A.L. Harris. Angiogenesis, assessed by platelet/endothelial cell adhesion molecule antibodies, as indicator of node metastasès and survival in breast cancer. Lancet 340, 1120–1124 (1992).
6. S. Bosari, A.K.C. Lee, R.A. DeLellis, G. Heatley, B. Wiley & M.L. Silverman. Microvessel quantitation and prognosis in invasive breast carcinoma. Hum. Pathol. 23, 755–761 (1992).
7. M. Toi, J. Kashitani & T. Tominaga. Tumor angiogenesis is an independent prognostic indicator in primary breast carcinoma. Int. J. Cancer 55, 371–374 (1993).
8. A. Obermair, K. Czerwenka, C. Kurz, P. Buxbaum, M. Schemper & P. Sevelda. Influence of tumoral microvessel density on the recurrence-free survival in human breast cancer: Primary results. Onkologie 17, 44–49 (1994).
9. A. Obermair, K. Czerwenka, C. Kurz, A. Kaider & P. Sevelda. Tumorale Gefäßdichte bei Mammatumoren und ihr Einfluß auf das rezidivfreie Überleben. Chirurg 65, 611–615 (1994).
10. Y. Ogawa, Y.-S. Chung, B. Nakata, S. Takatsuka, K. Maeda, T. Sawada, Y. Kato, K. Yoshikawa, M. Sakurai & M. Sowa. Microvessel quantitation in invasive breast cancer by staining for factor VIII-related antigen. Brit. J. Cancer 71, 1297–1301 (1995).
11. E. Protopapa, G.S. Delides & L. Révész. Vascular density and the response of breast carcinomas to mastectomy and adjuvant chemotherapy. Eur. J. Cancer 29A, 1391–1393 (1993).
12. M.E.H.M. van Hoef, W.F. Knox, S.S. Dhesi, A. Howell & A.M. Schor. Assessment of tumour vascularity as a prognostic factor in lymph node negative invasive breast cancer. Eur. J. Cancer 29A, 1141–1145 (1993).
13. J.M. Wang, S. Kumar, D. Pye, N. Haboubi & L. Al-Nakib. Breast carcinoma: Comparative study of tumor vasculature using two endothelial cell markers. J. Natl. Cancer Inst. 86, 386–388 (1994)
14. B. Endrich & P. Vaupel. Tumorale Gefäßdichte bei Mammatumoren und ihr Einfluß auf das rezidivfreie Überleben. Chirurg 66, 76–77 (1995).
15. R.P. Beaney. Positron emission tomography in the study of human tumors. Semin. Nucl. Med. 14, 324–341 (1984).
16. R.P. Beaney, A.A. Lammertsma, T. Jones, C.G. McKenzie & K.E. Halnan. Positron emission tomography for in-vivo measurements of regional blood flow, oxygen utilisation, and blood volume in patients with breast carcinoma. Lancet 1, 131–134 (1984).
17. R. Johnson. A thermodynamic method for investigation of radiation induced changes in the microcirculation of human tumors. Int. J. Radiat. Oncol. Biol. Phys. 1, 659–670 (1976).
18. C.B.J.H. Wilson, A.A. Lammertsma, C.G. McKenzie, K. Sikora & T. Jones. Measurements of blood flow and exchanging water space in breast tumors using positron emission tomography: A rapid and noninvasive dynamic method. Cancer Res. 52, 1592–1597 (1992).
19. P. Vaupel, F. Kallinowski & P. Okunieff. Blood flow, oxygen and nutrient supply, and metabolic microenvironment of human tumors: a review. Cancer Res. 49, 6449–6465 (1989).
20. R.K. Jain. Barriers to drug delivery in solid tumors. Sci. American 271, 58–65 (1994).
21. P. Vaupel. Blood flow and metabolic microenvironment of brain tumors. J. Neuro-Oncol. 22, 261–267 (1994).
22. P. Vaupel, K. Schlenger, C. Knoop & M. Höckel. Oxygenation of human tumors: Evaluation of tissue oxygen distribution in breast cancers by computerized pO_2 tension measurements. Cancer Res. 51, 3316–3322 (1991).
23. P. Vaupel. Oxygenation of human tumors. Strahlenther. Onkol. 166, 377–386 (1990).
24. P. Vaupel, K. Schlenger & M. Höckel . Blood flow and tissue oxygenation of human tumors: an update. Adv. Exp. Med. Biol. 317, 139–151 (1992).
25. S.J. Falk, R. Ward & N.M. Bleehen. The influence of carbogen breathing on tumour tissue oxygenation in man evaluated by computerised pO_2 histography. Br. J. Cancer 66, 919–924 (1992).

26. P.W. Vaupel. Oxygenation of solid tumors. In: Drug Resistance in Oncology. Ed. Teicher, B.A. Marcel Dekker, New York, pp. 53–85 (1993).

27. S. Runkel, A. Wischnik, J. Teubner, E. Kaven, J. Gaa & F. Melchert. Oxygenation of mammary tumors as evaluated by ultrasound-guided computerized-pO_2-histography. Adv. Exp. Med. Biol. *345*, 451–458 (1994).

28. P.W. Vaupel, D.K. Kelleher & M. Günderoth (eds.).Tumor Oxygenation, Stuttgart, Jena, New York: Fischer (1995).

29. J. Füller, H.J. Feldmann, M. Molls & H. Sack. Untersuchungen zum Sauerstoffpartialdruck im Tumorgewebe unter Radio- und Thermoradiotherapie. Strahlenther. Onkol. *170*, 453–460 (1994).

30. E.M. Grischke, M. Kaufmann, M. Eberlein-Gonska, T. Mattfeldt, Ch. Sohn & G. Bastert. Angiogenesis as a diagnostic factor in primary breast cancer: Microvessel quantitation by stereological methods and correlation with color Doppler sonography. Onkologie *17*, 35–42 (1994).

31. P. Vaupel. Oxygen transport in tumors: Characteristics and clinical implications. Adv. Exp. Med. Biol. in press (1995)

32. P. Vaupel, C. Schaefer & P. Okunieff. Intracellular acidosis in murine fibrosarcomas coincides with ATP depletion, hypoxia, and high levels of lactate and total P_i. NMR Biomed. *7*, 128–136 (1994).

33. J.R. Griffiths. Are cancer cells acidic? Br. J. Cancer *64*, 425–427 (1991).

34. P. Vaupel. Physiological properties of malignant tumours. NMR Biomed. *5*, 220–225 (1992).

35. H.S. Garewal, F.R. Ahmann, R.B. Schifman & A. Celniker. ATP assay: Ability to distinguish cytostatic from cytocidal anticancer drug effects. J. Natl. Cancer Inst. *77*, 1039–1045 (1986).

36. S.K. Calderwood, E.A. Bump, M.A. Stevenson, I. van Kersen & G.M. Hahn. Investigation of adenylate energy charge, phosphorylation potential, and ATP concentration in cells stressed with starvation and heat. J. Cell. Physiol. *124*, 261–268 (1985).

37. J.R. Griffiths, E. Cady, R.H.T. Edwards, V.R. McCready, D.R. Wilkie & E. Wiltshaw. ^{31}P-NMR studies of a human tumour in situ. Lancet *1*, 1435–1436 (1983).

38. T.C. Ng, S. Vijayakumar, A.W. Majors, F.J. Thomas, T.F. Meaney & N.J. Baldwin. Response of a non-Hodgkin lymphoma to ^{60}Co therapy monitored by ^{31}P MRS in situ. Int J. Radiat. Oncol. Biol. Phys. *13*, 1545–1551 (1987).

39. W. Negendak, M. Crowley, N. Keller, M. Nussdorfer & J.L. Evelhoch. In vivo ^{31}P MRS of normal human breasts: Age dependence and comparison with breast cancers. Proc. 7th Ann. Meeting Soc. Magn. Res. Med., San Francisco, CA, Vol. *1*, 336 (1988).

40. R.D. Oberhaensli, D. Hilton-Jones, P.J. Bore, L.J. Hands, R.P. Rampling & G.K. Radda. Biochemical investigation of human tumours in vivo with phosphorus-31 magnetic resonance spectroscopy. Lancet *1*, 8–11 (1986).

30

OXYGEN TENSIONS IN RODENT TUMORS AFTER IRRADIATION WITH NEUTRONS

L. Weissfloch,[1] T. Auberger,[1] R. Senekowitsch-Schmidtke,[2] F. M. Wagner,[3] K. Tempel,[4] and M. Molls[1]

[1]Clinic and Policlinic for Radiotherapy and Radiation Oncology
[2]Clinic and Policlinic for Nuclear Medicine
 Klinikum rechts der Isar
 Technische Universitaet Munich
[3]Reactor Station Garching
 Technische Universitaet Munich
[4]Institute for Pharmacology, Toxicology, and Pharmacy
 Veterinary Faculty, LMU Munich
 Germany

1. ABSTRACT

We started investigations on intratumoral oxygen tension after irradiations with reactor fission neutrons using the *Eppendorf-pO$_2$ Histograph*[R]. Isotransplanted AT17-mammary carcinomas on C3H-mice and osteosarcomas OTS-64 on balb C-mice received 2 or 6 Gy neutrons single dose. Before and at certain points of time after treatment the pO$_2$ values were evaluated.

Some tumors with initially low median pO$_2$ values showed a short-lasting increase between 2 and 24 h after irradiation. In those tumors with relatively high pretherapeutic pO$_2$ values the pO$_2$ decreased to the range of hypoxia. A third group of tumors showed no marked changes after irradiation. No tumor stopped growth during the observation period.

2. INTRODUCTION

In conventional radiotherapy low oxygen tension correlates with low radiosensivity. This oxygen effect is less pronounced in neutron therapy (4, 6, 16). A novel technique of intratumoral oxygen tension measurement with polarographic needle probes opens a new field to validate the reactions after irradiation (1, 9, 18, 19). We started to investigate pO$_2$ distributions in murine tumors before and after irradiation with neutrons.

Oxygen Transport to Tissue XVIII, edited by Nemoto and LaManna
Plenum Press, New York, 1997

3. MATERIALS AND METHODS

Animals and Tumors

The studies were performed on two different mouse tumors.

Into the right abdominal wall of female C3H-mice, the AT17-mammary carcinoma was isotransplanted. This tumor is known as a slow-growing adenocarcinoma with very rare necrosis up to large sizes (12).

The osteosarcoma OTS-64 was isotransplanted into the right hind foot of balb C-mice.

Anesthesia and Temperature

For tumor transplantation and pO_2 measurement the mice were anesthetized by intraperitoneal injection of 0.1 mg/g Ketamine [Ketanest[R], Parke-Davis] and 0.016 mg/g Xylazine [Rompun[R], Bayer], solved in 0.9 % NaCl (3).

The temperature was measured by a rectal, thermosensitive catheter probe and maintained at 36°C, using an infrared lamp.

pO_2 Measurement

The tissue oxygenation was determined with the *Eppendorf pO_2 Histograph*[R] (Eppendorf-Netheler-Hinz, Hamburg, Germany) using polarographic needle electrodes of 0.3 mm diameter. Via a trocar the needle probe was placed into the tumor periphery. The probe was automatically moved through the tumor in steps of 0.7 mm and the local pO_2 was measured at each step. Before irradiation and at 2, 12 and 24 h as well as 1, 2 and 3 weeks after irradiation the pO_2 values were evaluated in this way.

Technical data of this equipment have been described elsewhere (1, 5, 9, 18).

Neutron Irradiation

The irradiation with fission neutrons was performed with the RENT II beam (75% neutrons, 25% photons, maximum of energy 2 MeV) at the research reactor of the Technische Universitaet Munich in Garching. Eight AT17-tumors received 2 Gy single dose, 7 AT17-tumors 6 Gy single dose and 4 OTS-64-osteosarcomas 6 Gy single dose.

4. RESULTS

AT17-mammary carcinomas irradiated with 2 Gy showed in 4 of 8 cases an increase of median pO_2 at 2 h after irradiation (Fig.1). In 2 well-oxygenated tumors with median oxygen tensions of 25 and 16 mmHg the pO_2 values decreased within 2 h to 4 and 9 mmHg, followed by an increase to 14 and 13 mmHg at 12 h. One AT17-mammary carcinoma revealed a steady increase of the median pO_2 up to 24 h. After the time point of 24 h all oxygen tensions decreased up to day 14. Afterwards, a slight increase of pO_2 values could be observed within the third week. One tumor did not respond in any described way, but the median pO_2 declined from the beginning. In 2 carcinomas with very low oxygen values during the whole period, tumor necrosis developed within 2 weeks after irradiation.

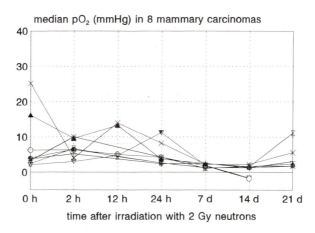

Figure 1. Median pO$_2$ in 8 mammary carcinomas after irradiation with 2 Gy neutrons single dose.

All tumor volumes, also of tumors with necrosis, enlarged constantly, ranging from 520 to 780 mm^3 before treatment and from 890 to 3.140 mm^3 at the end of observation.

All mammary carcinomas irradiated with 6 Gy showed a decrease of the median pO$_2$ within 2 h after irradiation (Fig.2). Increases could be observed in 2 tumors at 12 h and 24 h. Two tumors presented with an extreme variation of values. In one AT17-tumor the median pO$_2$ was 12 mmHg before irradiation, declined to 8 mmHg at 2 h, increased to 15 and 27 mmHg at 12 and 24 h respectively and declined again afterwards. Another tumor started at 2 mmHg before and 3 mmHg at 2 h after irradiation, increased to 26 mmHg at 12 h, decreased again to 4 mmHg at 24 h and developed a necrosis within 2 weeks after irradiation. In three tumors a continuous pO$_2$ decrease could be observed up to days 7 and 14. Later on, a slight increase was observed. The AT17-tumor with the highest pO$_2$ value before treatment responded most significantly. The pO$_2$ started at 33 mmHg, went down to 9, 2 and 1 mmHg at 2, 12 and 24 h respectively. On day 7 it was near 0 mmHg and increased again to 3 and 6 mmHg on days 14 and 21 respectively. During this period the tu-

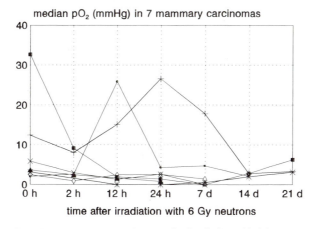

Figure 2. Median pO$_2$ in 7 mammary carcinomas after irradiation with 6 Gy neutrons single dose.

mor volume decreased from 520 to 330 mm³ on day 7 and enlarged again to 520 and 900 mm³ on days 14 and 21 respectively. Tumors with a pre-treatment-volume of 1.180 mm³ grew up to 3.000 mm³ without interruption, while those of 520 mm³ enlarged within the third week to 680 and 810 mm³.

All of the 4 osteosarcomas showed a decrease of the median pO_2 within 2 h after 6 Gy irradiation (Fig.3). In three cases the pO_2 values increased remarkably at 12 h, which was followed by a continous decrease up to day 14 and a slight increase on day 21 in two tumors. This was accompanied by a steady increase of the volumes of 2 tumors from 630 mm³ both on day 0 up to 2.350 and 3.140 mm³ respectively on day 21. The third tumor-pO_2 started to increase on day 7, associated with a rapid growth up to 4.900 mm³ of volume. The best-oxygenated osteosarcoma was one of the largest tumors (2.090 mm³) at the start of the investigation. After irradiation the median pO_2 decreased rapidly within 2 h from 29 mmHg to 19 mmHg and continued to be low on day 7. This tumor showed neither a pO_2 increase nor growth.

5. DISCUSSION

Changes in tumor oxygenation could be observed after irradiation with neutrons. Some of the tumors with initially low median pO_2 values showed a short-lasting increase within 2 and 24 h after treatment. In those tumors with relatively high median pO_2 values before irradiation the pO_2 decreased and finally came down to the range of hypoxia (about 5 mmHg) and a third group of tumors showed no marked changes after irradiation.

The interpretation of these results has to be with caution. The increase of oxygen tension after neutron irradiation occurred earlier than described in the literature of photon treatment (11, 16, 17). The reason for this is unclear. It might be a hyperaemia-like state after an increase in tumor blood supply, which would be an interesting observation with regard to clinical radiooncology. The increase of blood flow and oxygen supply might influence the bioavailability of drugs in a positive way. In consideration of BNCT, this is of special interest. However, whether this fast increase is based on irradiation processes or influenced by anesthetic side effects must be studied furtheron. Observations of Howes (7)

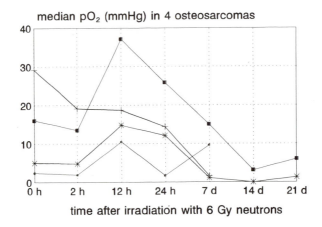

Figure 3. Median pO_2 in 4 osteosarcomas after irradiation with 6 Gy neutrons single dose.

and Rockwell et al. (15) in mammary carcinomas indicate, that the extent and rapidity of reoxygenation in different tumors is extremly variable and impossible to predict.

In our first investigations a correlation of oxygen tension with tumor size was observed in mammary carcinomas, but not in osteosarcomas. Generally, the pO_2 values of osteosarcomas revealed a better oxygenation status than mammary carcinomas of comparable volumes. Different results have been published on the correlation of tumor oxygenation with tumor size. Kallinowski et al. (10) described a distinct worsening of the tissue oxygenation at larger tumor volumes in pO_2 histograms measured in FSa II mouse fibrosarcoma and in MCa IV mouse mammary adenocarcinoma. Vaupel et al. (19) also reported a decrease of pO_2 in murine fibrosarcomas as tumor size enlarged. However, in contrast, the oxygenation of xenografted human gliomas remained uncharged up to large volumes. In several human tumors, like breast and cervix cancer, the oxygenation status did not correlate with tumor size (2, 5, 13, 14, 18). Finally, Kallinowski et al. (8, 10) pointed out, that tumors of the same cell line and growth stage can exhibit pronounced variations in their tissue oxygenation. They described remarkable differences in median pO_2 in tumors growing in the thigh and in the dorsal hind leg.

We have found that no tumor stopped growth during the observation period. Therefore, at present we do not know whether the increased tumor volume at the end of the observation period was due to an increase of the tumor cell number or/and growth of connective tissue or/and tumor necrosis.

6. ACKNOWLEDGMENT

The financal support by the Bayerisches Staatministerium fuer Landesentwicklung und Umweltfragen, Munich, is gratefully acknowledged.

REFERENCES

1. Fleckenstein W, Weiss C, Heinrich R, Schomerus H, Kersting T (1984): A new method for the bed-side recording of tissue pO_2 histograms. *Verh. Dtsch. Ges. Inn.Med.* 90, 439–443
2. Füller J, Feldmann HJ, Molls M, Sack H (1994): Untersuchungen zum Sauerstoffpartialdruck im Tumorgewebe unter Radio- und Thermoradio-therapie. *Strahlenther.Onkol.* 170, 453–460
3. Gabrisch K, Zwart P (1987): *Krankheiten der Heimtiere.* Schluetersche Verlagsanstalt, Hannover
4. Gatenby R, Kessler HB, Rosenblum JS, Coia LR, Moldofsky PJ, Harz WH, Broder GJ (1988): Oxygen distribution in squamous cell carcinoma metastases and its relationship to outcome of radiation therapy. *Int.J.Radiat. Oncol.Biol.Phys.* 14, 831–838
5. Hoeckel M, Schlenger K, Knoop C, Vaupel P (1991): Oxygenation of carcinomas of the uterine cervix: evaluation by computerized O_2-tension measurements. *Cancer Res.* 51, 6098–6102
6. Horsman MR, Khalil AA, Nordsmark M, Grau C, Overgaard J (1993): Relationship between radiobiological hypoxia and direct estimates of tumor oxygenation in a mouse tumour model. *Radiother.Oncol.* 28, 69–71
7. Howes SE. (1969): An estimation of changes in the proportion and absolute numbers of hypoxic cells after irradiation of transplanted C3H mouse mammary tumors. *Br.J.Radiol.* 42, 441–447
8. Kallinowski F, Schlenger KH, Runkel S, Kloes M, Stohrer M, Okunieff P, Vaupel P (1989): Blood flow metabolism, cellular microenvironment and growth rate of human tumor xenografts. *Cancer Res.* 49, 3759–3764
9. Kallinowski F, Zander R, Hoeckel M, Vaupel P (1990): Tumor tissue oxygenation as evaluated by computerized pO_2 histography. *Int.J.Radiat. Oncol.Biol.Phys.* 19, 953–961
10. Kallinowski F, Wilkerson, Moore R, Strauss W, Vaupel P (1991): Vascularity, perfusion rate and local tissue oxygenation of tumors derived from ras-transformed fibroblasts. *Int.J.Cancer* 48, 121–127

11. Kallman RF, Bleehen NM (1968): Post-irridiation cyclic radiosensivity changes in tumors and normal tissues. *In: Proc. of the Symposium on Dose Rate in Mammalian Radiolbiology.* Eds. Brown DG, Cragle RG, Nooman JR. Oak Ridge, pp. 20.1–20.23

12. Kummermehr J (1985): Measurement of tumour clonogenes in situ. *In: Cell Clones: Manual of Mammalian Cell Techniques.* Eds. Potten CS, Hendry JH. Churchill Livingstone, Edinburgh, pp. 215–222

13. Lartigau E, Vitu L, Haie.Meder C, Cosset MF, Delapierre M, Gebaulet A, Eschwege F, Guichard M (1992): Direct oxygen tension measurement in carcinoma of the uterine cervix: preliminary results. *In: Clinical Oxygen Pressure Measurements III.* Ed. Ehrly AM, Blackwell Wissenschaft, Berlin, pp. 117–120

14. Okunieff P, Hoeckel M, Dunphy EP, Schlenger K, Knoop C, Vaupel P (1993): Oxygen tension distributions are sufficient to explain the local response of human breast tumors treated with radiation alone. *Int.J.Radiat. Oncol.Biol.Phys.* 26, 631–636

15. Rockwell S, Moulder JE (1985): Biological factors of importance in split-course radiotherapy. *In: Optimization of Cancer Radiotherapy.* Eds. Paliwal BR, Herbert DE, Orton CG. American Institue of Physics, New York, pp. 171–182

16. Thomlinson RH (1968): Changes of oxygenation in tumors in relation to irradiation. *Front.Radiat.Ther.Oncol.* 3, 109–121

17. van Putten LM, Kallmann RF (1968): Oxygenation status of a transplantable tumor during fractionated radiotherapy. *J.Natl.Cancer Inst.* 40, 441–451.

18. Vaupel P, Schlenger K, Knoop C, Hoeckel M (1991): Oxygenation of human tumors: evaluation of tissue oxygen distribution in breast cancer by computerized O_2 tension measurement. *Cancer Res.* 52, 3316–3322

19. Vaupel P (1993): Oxygenation in solid tumors. *In: Drug Resistance in Oncology.* Ed. Teicher BA. Marcel Dekker, New York, pp. 53–85

31

PERIPHERAL PERFUSION AND TISSUE OXYGENATION IMPROVEMENT INDUCED BY ANTIHYPERTENSIVE MEDICATION COMBINED WITH LIPOIDOPROTEINOSIS TREATMENT

G. Cicco,[1] P. Vicenti,[1] A. Pirrelli,[1] and A J. van der Kleij[2]

[1]Department of Internal Medicine and Oncology
Hypertension Center, University of Bari
Italy
[2]Academic Medical Center/University of Amsterdam
Department of Surgery, Amsterdam
The Netherlands

INTRODUCTION

The presence of microcirculatory disorders (i.e. increase in blood viscosity) as well as increased aggregation rate of erythrocytes has been described (1,2) in non-treated hypertensive patients. The increased aggregation rate has been linked to microvasculopathy and hyperfibrinogenemia frequently present in treated hypertensive patients with metabolic disturbances (such as diabetes, lipoidoproteinosis) (3,4,5). Lipoidoproteinosis, haemorheological and clotting disorders are often the underlying base for serious pathology (ictus, myocardial infarction, etc.) complicating hypertension (6). It is noted that hypertension itself not only represents an independent atherogenic risk factor, but also low "shear stress" within the vessel wall and in addition the level of systolic-diastolic oscillation favours the formation of atherosclerotic patches. All these events are notably increased in the presence of other risk factors for cardiovascular pathology such as smoking, diabetes, blood hyperviscosity and lipoidoproteinosis (7). Furthermore, microcirculatory disorders in hypertensive patients are often associated with a reduction in peripheral oxygen delivery (8). Reduction of blood pressure values and metabolic disturbances in hypertensive patients may improve peripheral perfusion and cellular oxygen delivery.

Oxygen Transport to Tissue XVIII, edited by Nemoto and LaManna
Plenum Press, New York, 1997

Table 1. Low Calorie Diet (1200): Bromatogical composition

Protide	76 g
Glycide	117 g
Lipids	55 g
Cholesterol	180 mg
Saturated fatty acids	12.7 g
Unsaturated fatty acids	19.4 g

AIM OF THE STUDY

The aim of this study was to evaluate in mild hypertensive patients the effect of anti-hypertensive medication combined with lipoidoproteinosis treatment and adjusted diet on peripheral perfusion and peripheral oxygenation .

MATERIALS AND METHODS

After 90 days treatment with Fosinopril (20 mg OD), Pravastatine (20 mg OD) and a low caloric diet (1200 Kcal) (Table 1), 22 patients were evaluated (Table 2). These patients (12 male and 10 female, age 55 ± 4 years) were characterized by mild hypertension 1st Stage (WHO), peripheral arterial occlusive disease (POAD) II° type A (Leriche-Fontaine classification) (Table 3) and lipoidoproteinosis. At the beginning of every 2nd week and at the end of the study period the systolic blood pressure (SBP), diastolic blood pressure (DBP), mean arterial blood pressure [MAP = DBP + 1/3(SBP-DBP)], heart rate (in supine and standing position) and lipid pattern were measured. The ankle/ brachial pressure index was used to assess peripheral perfusion. Three transcutanoeus oximeters were contemporarily applied to evaluate peripheral oxygen delivery (Figure 1). At both calfs a Clark PO_2 sensor (Cutan PO_2 Monitor 820 Kontron Instrum.) was used to measured the transcutaneous PO_2 value and a Combi sensor (Microgas 7640 MK-2-Kontron Instrum.) (Figure 2A, B) was used in the subclavian area to measure the transcutaneous PO_2 ($TcPO_2$) value as well as the PCO_2 ($TcPCO_2$) value. The computerized Microgas 7640 MK2 instruments consists of a calibrator, and a combi sensor simultaneously measuring $TcPO_2$ and $TcPCO_2$. The Combi sensor is based on a Clark type sensor for the oxygen (O_2) and a Severinghaus sensor for carbon dioxide (CO_2). The oxygen is measured with a Amperometer via a reduction in the microcathode which is negatively polarized with a refer-

Table 2. Patients characteristics, 12 male and 10 female

Age range 51 - 59 years	No family history of diabetes
Non-smokers	Family history of lipoidoproteinosis
Family history of hypertension	Non-diabetic
Moderate obesity-body lean index	M: 25 ± 1.6 F: 26 ± 3.9
Systolic Blood Pressure	167 ± 7 mmHg
Diastolic Blood Pressure	99 ± 4 mmHg
Mean Blood Pressure	121 ± 3 mmHg
Heart Rate	82 ±7 beats/min.

Table 3. Leriche-Fontaine Peripheral Arterial Disease Classification

Stage I:	Patients with the presence of varied undefined symptoms, paraesthesias, heaviness in legs, and uncertain objectivity.
Stage II:	"Claudicatio intermittens" -IIa pain free time in legs whilst walking more than 100 m -IIb: pain free time in legs whilst walking less than 100 m
Stage III:	Patients with spontaneous or nocturnal leg pain reduced by sitting or movement.
Stage IV:	Presence of trophic lesions.

ence electrode and the measured current is proportional to the PO_2. The PCO_2 is measured using a Potentiometer by determining the pH of an electrode. The variations in pH are directly correlated to the logarithm of the PCO_2 variations. The pH is taken by measuring the potential present between a glass electrode (for the pH) and a silver/ silverchloride reference electrode. The silver/silverchloride reference electrode is used for both sensors. To maintain arterialization of the skin the sensor is kept at a constant temperature of 44°C. The Cutan PO_2 monitor 820 Kontron Instrum. uses a Clark sensor for PO_2 only. Transcutaneous measurements were registered before and after a 3' step test and after 10' rest (Figure 3). All measurements were performed during standard environmental conditions.

RESULTS

After 3 months treatment with Fosinopril, Pravastatine and a Low Calorie Diet a relative improvement in tissue perfusion and oxygen delivery was observed during baseline conditions (Table 4) and after exercise (Table 5). The haemodynamic parameters and

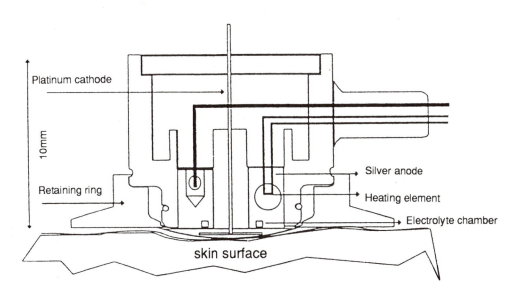

Figure 1. Diagram of the transcutanoeus oxygen electrode (Cutan PO_2 monitor, 820 Kontron Instruments).

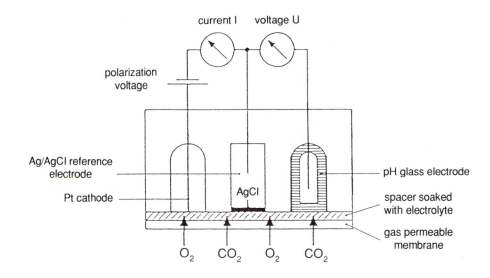

Figure 2. Diagrammatic illustration of the comb; sensor (Microgas 764, MK-2 Konton Instruments) for simultaneous transcutaneous PO_2 and PCO_2 measurements.

Table 4. Peripheral perfusion and oxygenation parameters registed every 2 weeks during 3 months of treatment; all values are expressed in mean±SD

WEEKS	0*	2*	4*	6	8	10	12*	Δ%
TcPO₂ (Infraclav. BSL)	69±4	70±2	72±2	73±3	74±3	76±4	77±4	+12
TcPO₂ (Foot BSL)	45±4	47±3	49±2	51±4	51±3	53±6	53±5	+19
TcPO₂ (Infraclav.Aft.Ex.)	74±3	74±4	76±3	76±5	77±3	79±4	80±5	+10
TcPO₂ (Right calf Aft. Ex.)	59±4	53±3	55±2	56±3	57±3	60±4	62±5	+18
TcPO₂ (Left calf Aft. Ex.)	53±5	54±2	54±3	55±2	58±4	58±5	59±5	+12
RPI	0.65±0.07	0.67±0.04	0.68±0.02	0.68±0.04	0.69±0.03	0.69±0.02	*** 0.69±0.04	+6
Ankle/Brachial Press. Index	0.68±0.1	0.69±0.01	0.71±0.2	0.73±0.1	0.74±0.2	0.76±0.1	** 0.76±0.2	+12

*p < 0.01   **p < 0.02   ***p < 0.05

Steptest

It is necessary to make the patient step up and down thirty times per minute during three minutes. Step height male 50 cm., female 40 cm.; children & patients < 160cm. 30 cm.

Figure 3. Steptest paradigm.

Table 5. Haemodynamic parameters registered every 2 weeks during 3 months of treatment; all values are expressed in mean±SD

WEEKS	0*	2	4*	6	8	10	12*	Δ%
SBP (Supine)	167±7	165±6	160±5	154±4	150±3	150±4	147±7	-12
DBP	99±2	98±3	95±4	95±4	94±4	90±4	89±3	-10
MAP	121±4	120±3	117±4	115±3	113±3	110±4	108±4	-11
HR	82±7	82±4	84±3	80±4	82±5	83±3	84±6 **	+3
SBP (Standing)	152±8	158±6	153±5	150±6	147±4	145±6	141±7	-11
DBP	94±4	92±3	92±4	90±2	99±3	85±4	84±4	-11
MAP	116±3	114±4	112±3	110±5	108±4	105±3	103±4	-12
HR	88±7	87±4	88±5	86±4	88±3	87±4	89±7 **	+10

* $p < 0.01$ ** < NS

Table 6. Lipid patterns registered every 2 weeks during 3 months of treatment; all values are expressed in mean±SD

WEEKS	0	2	4*	6	8	10	12*	Δ%
TOT. CHOL.	286±18	259±15	238±14	236±19	226±20	220±12	214±14	-25
TRIGLICERIDES	198±7	195±6	190±5	188±6	183±5	180±6	179±7	-10
HDL-CHOL.	34±3	34±2	35±3	35±4	36±2	36±3	37±2	+9
LDL-CHOL-	211±16	186±12	165±12	163±14	153±12	144±10	143±12	-32
TOT-CHOL./HDL	8.3±0.7	7.6±0.5	6.8±0.5	6.7±0.8	6.2±0.8	6.1±0.6	5.7±0.4	-31
LDL/HDL	6.1±0.6	5.4±0.5	4.7±0.4	4.6±0.4	4.2±0.5	4±0.4	3.7±0.3	-39

* $p < 0.01$

the lipid pattern (cholesterolemia, trigliceridemia, HDL-chol. LDL-chol., total chol./HDL chol. ratio, LDL/HDL chol. ratio) also revealed a significant improvement.

CONCLUSION

Mild hypertensive patients with PAOD stage II^a and lipoidoproteneinosis may benefit from treatment with Fosinopril, Pravastatine, and a low calorie diet as was shown by the improvement in the peripheral perfusion and peripheral oxygenation before and after exercise test.

REFERENCES

1. Harris I., Loughlin G., The viscosity of blood in high blood pressure. *Am. J.Med. 1980,* 23:451–464.
2. Lorient-Roudat M.F., Roudat R., Freyburger G.L. Hemorheological abnormalities in essential hypertension. *Clin. Hemorheol.* 1987, 7:537.
3. Petraliot A., Malatino L.S., Fione C.F. Erythrocyte aggregation in different stages of arterial hypertension. *Tromb. Haemost.* 1985, 54:555.
4. Tsinahdzvbishvili B., Beritashvili N., Mcheolishvili G., Erythrocyte aggregability in essential hypertension. *Abstract book, Proc. 1. ICCH/8 ECCH Vienna* 1993, 13 - 3:401.
5. Cicco G., Dolce E., Mancini M., Pirrelli A., Atherosclerosis and hemorheology in hypertension; Organ damage. *Medit. J. Surg. Med.* 1994, 3: 131 - 138.
6. McGill M.C., Adria S.Stella J., Corbonell L.M. General lindings of international atherosclerosis. *Project Lab. Inv.* 1968, 18: 498.
7. Kannel W.B., Wolf P.A., McGee D.L. Systolic blood pressure arterial, rigidity and risk of stroke. The Framingham study. *J. Am. Med.* 1981, 245: 1225.
8. Cesarone M.R., Laurora G., Belcardo G.U., Microcirculation in systemic hypertension. *Angiology.* 1992, 43 (11): 899 - 903.

32

PO$_2$-DEPENDENT GLOMERULAR ULTRAFILTRATION OF MIDDLE-WEIGHT PROTEIN IS MODIFIED BY PROTECTIVE AMINO ACIDS

Gernot Gronow,[1] Miklós Mályusz,[1] and Norbert Klause[2]

[1]Department of Physiology
[2]Clinic of Nephrology
University of Kiel
24098 Kiel, Germany

1. INTRODUCTION

In vivo, hypoxia may reduce tubular transport activity in the kidney, leading to an increased diuresis and the urinary excretion of filtered protein (Maack, 1992). Whether hypoxic proteinuria originates exclusively from a reduced tubular reabsorption or, at least in part, from an altered glomerular permeability for plasma proteins remains unclear. Investigations on glomerular permeability at low oxygen tension are complicated *in vivo* by an increased sympathetic neuronal activity, accompanied by renal arterial vasoconstriction and a reduction of renal blood flow as well as of glomerular filtration rate (Bursaux et al., 1976). An isolated kidney preparation offers the advantage of a maintained perfusion flow rate even at extreme low oxygen tension (Gronow & Kossmann, 1985; Gronow et al., 1986; Mályusz & Gronow, 1987). An additional advantage of this preparation appears to be the observation that at extreme low oxygen tension lack of metabolic energy prevents tubular reabsorption of filtered protein (Park & Maack, 1984). Thus, under experimental conditions of extreme hypoxia, GFR-corrected alterations in urinary excretion of perfusate protein may represent changes in glomerular permeability.

According to our own observations (Gronow et al., 1986; Mályusz & Gronow, 1987; Gronow & Klause, 1989), amino acids in an isolated kidney preparation stimulated hypoxic glomerular filtration and reduced as well urinary protein loss. These opposite effects of amino acids are not fully understood. Usually the renal glomerulotubular feed-back mechanism, i.e. preglomerular afferent vasoconstriction (Schnermann et al., 1992) would have reduced at high rates of hypoxic Na(Cl) excretion glomerular filtration as well as protein excretion, A suppression of protein excretion at high rates of hypoxic glomerular filtration may than indicate an amino acid-induced permeability changes in the glomerular membrane itself.

Oxygen Transport to Tissue XVIII, edited by Nemoto and LaManna
Plenum Press, New York, 1997

To test this hypothesis we measured renal function at extreme low oxygen tension (PO_2 << 1 mm Hg) in an isolated rat kidney preparation with and without amino acids in the perfusate. In a first series of experiments, hypoxic renal function was tested with an improved mixture of glycine, proline and aspartate in the perfusate (Mályusz & Gronow, 1987). In a second experimental design, glycine served as the sole amino acid in the perfusate. Tested renal parameters were perfusion flow rate (PFR), glomerular filtration rate (GFR), fractional glomerular filtration of fluid (FF), glomerular siewing of α-amylase (AML) and of albumin, and the excretion of the brush border enzyme γ-glutamyltransferase (γGT). Our data provide evidence for a stabilizing effect of glycine on glomerular siewing of middle-weight protein at low oxygen tension.

2. MATERIAL AND METHODS

Preparation, cannulation, and perfusion of the rat kidney has been described elsewhere (Gronow and Cohen,1984; Gronow and Kossmann, 1985). Briefly, the isolated right kidney of starved, male Sprague-Dawley rats (mean body weight 384 ±38 g) was recirculating perfused with Krebs-Ringer-bicarbonate medium (250 ml, pH 7.35, 38°C, 10 mM lactate) at a mean "arterial" pressure of 100 ±4 mmHg.•6 g•dl^{-1} bovine albumin, analytical grade (Serva, Heidelberg, FRG) served as colloid in the perfusate. Additionally, a marker of glomerular permeability for middle-weight protein, 32.7 ±0.23 Units·ml^{-1} of homologous pancreatic α-amylase (AML) was added to the perfusate. AML was prepared from rat pancreatic tissue by affinity chromatography according to the method of Burril et al. (1981) and was described in detail elsewhere (Mályusz et al., 1990). The tested amino acid mixture consisted of glycine, L-proline, and L-aspartic acid, each 2 mM. In perfusions performed with either L-proline, glycine or L-aspartate, single amino acids were added at a concentration of 5 mM to the perfusate. An "arterial" oxygen tension << 1 mm Hg was introduced by gassing the perfusate with 95% N_2 : 5% CO_2. Perfusate oxygenation was controlled polarographically by means of Clark-Type electrodes.

Perfusion flow rate (PFR) and glomerular filtration rate (GFR) were measured according to earlier reports (Gronow & Cohen, 1984; Gronow & Kossmann, 1985; Gronow et al., 1987). Glomerular filtration fraction (FF) was calculated as GFR·100·PFR^{-1}. Perfusate and urine activities of enzymes were estimated by standard enzyme assays, brush border γ-glutamyltransferase (γGT) according to Monotest 235075 (Boehringer Mannheim, FRG), α-amylase according to Monoamyltest (Biomed, Munic, FRG). Fractional filtration of AML was calculated as urinary excretion rate·100·perfusate activity^{-1} ·GFR^{-1}. Excretion of γGt was calculated as urinary excretion rate•GFR^{-1}. Protein measurements were performed according to the method of Lowry et al. (1951). Fractional excretion of protein was calculated as mg excreted protein•!00•GFR^{-1} •60 mg^{-1} . A P-value of 0.05 or less in statistical comparisons (Student's T-test) was assumed to indicate a significant difference.

3. RESULTS AND DISCUSSION

3.1. Effects of Amino Acid Mixture on Hypoxic Renal Function

In a first series of experiments isolated rat kidneys were 30 min recirculating perfused at an arterial PO_2 << 1 mm Hg. The effect of a mixture of 3 amino acids (3AA) on hypoxic kidney function was compared with the effect of its single components glycine (Gly), L-proline (Pro), and L-aspartate (Asp):

Without amino acids in the perfusate (Tab. 1), perfusion flow rate (PFR) remained at extreme low arterial oxygen tension nearly unchanged. Glomerular filtration rate (GFR) decreased significantly from 0.90 ±0.06 to 0.32 ±0.04 ml•g^{-1}•min^{-1}. In consequence, filtration fraction (FF) fell to about one third of its initial value. Fractional excretion of protein and α-amylase (AML) rose significantly despite the observed reduction in GFR, protein excretion from 0.6% to 2.7%, AML-excretion from 8.1% to 26%. Severity of hypoxic damage was indicated by an about sevenfold increase in urinary losses of γ-glutamyltransferase (γGT). Addition of the 3AA-mixture to the perfusate stimulated hypoxic PFR by about 10%, and GFR by about 116%. Glomerular siewing of protein fell markedly in the presence of 3AA: protein by 63%, AML by 53.8%. The losses of γGt were markedly suppressed in the presence of 3AA, γGT activity fell from 2.17 ±0.34 to 0.21 ±0.04 mU•g^{-1}•min^{-1}.

With one of 3 amino acid tested, the observed effects were similar to those described above when glycine (Gly) was present in the perfusate (Tab. 1). Hypoxic renal function in presence of L-proline (Pro) or L-aspartate (Asp) was not significant different from values obtained with no added amino acids in the perfusate ("no AA" in Tab. 1). The protective effect of glycine on hypoxic cellular enzyme losses has already been described by other authors (Weinberg et al., 1987) and our own laboratory (Gronow et al., 1994). In the isolated perfused rat kidney, glycine and/or L-alanine also reduced hypoxic cellular damage in the thick ascending limb of Henle (Silva et al., 1991) and suppressed hypoxic protein and enzyme leakage (Gronow & Klause, 1989). Thus, it appeared reasonable to assume that in the present experiments most if not all of the observed beneficial effects of the 3AA-mixture were mediated by glycine. To verify this hypothesis in a final series of ex-

Table 1. Effect of amino acids on renal function in an isolated rat kidney preparation perfused 30 min at extreme low oxygen tension (PO$_2$ < 1 mm Hg)

	Oxygenated control	Extreme hypoxia				
		no AA	3AA	Pro	Asp	Gly
PFR	32.5	33.3	36.4	34.2	32.4	36.6
±SD	±2.3	±2.5	±1.8	±2.2	±2.6	±1.4
GFR	0.90*	0.32	0.69*	0.35	0.31	0.69*
±SD	±0.06	±0.05	±0.04	±0.05	±0.04	±0.05
FF	2.77*	0.96	1.90*	1.02	0.96	1.89*
±SD	±0.21	±0.13	±0.22	±0.13	±0.09	±0.24
Prot	0.60*	2.70	1.01*	2.30	2.70	0.95*
±SD	±0.10	±0.40	±0.13	±0.38	±0.47	±0.12
AML	8.10*	26.2	12.0*	23.1	25.2	11.3*
±SD	±0.56	±4.70	±2.10	±3.70	±3.90	±2.60
gGT	0.34*	2.17	0.23*	2.05	2.22	0.18*
±SD	±0.06	±0.34	±0.04	±0.42	±0.47	±0.04

* significant difference at p 0.05 with respect to hypoxic control (no AA)
No AA = no amino acids added; 3AA = amino acid mixture with glycine (Gly), L-proline (Pro), and L-aspartate (Asp) added, 2 mM each. Single amino acids were added at 5 mM. PFR = perfusion flow rate; GFR = glomerular filtration rate; FF = filtration fraction; Prot = fractional protein exretion; AML = fractional α-amylase excretion; γGT = exretion of γ-glutamyltransferase. For further information see text (x ±SD, n = 6)

periments isolated rat kidneys were perfused with glycine as the sole amino acid added to the perfusate.

3.2. Glycine Effects on Renal Hemodynamics

According to our own observations (Mályusz & Gronow, 1987; Gronow & Klause, 1989) and reports of other investigators (Sayed et al., 1990) the addition of amino acids to the perfusate induced a small increase in perfusion flow rate (Fig.1, upper panel, triangles). Without glycine in the perfusate (solid circles) and a maintained PFR, glomerular filtration rate (GFR, middle panel) fell dramatically due to the activation of the tubulo-glomerular feed-back mechanism (Schnermann et al., 1992), This hypoxic decrease in GFR was prevented by about 50% in the presence of glycine. The fractional amount of filtered fluid, i.e. the glomerular filration fraction (FF, lower panel in Fig. 1) rose in the presence of glycine from 0.99 ±0.12% to 1.97 ±0.1%. These observations are in accordance with experiments of Sayed et al. (1990) who observed in the oxygen-limited perfused kidney a support of FF by glycine. Thus, glomerular filtration in extreme hypoxia was supported by glycine via a direct effect on glomerular membrane permeability and/or by a reduction of tubular cell swellng.

3.3. Effect of Glycine on Protein Excretion and Filtration

To test our hypothesis that glycine might have affected glomerular permeability we added a glomerular marker for middle-weight protein, α-amylase (AML), to the perfusate. Under control conditions (see Tab. 1), a small fraction of AML (molecular weight 54 kda) passed the glomerular filter (siewing coefficient = 0.118). Albumin (MW 69 kda), in contrast, is nearly reflected at the glomerular barrier (siewing coefficient << 0.01). Under our experimental conditions, i.e. at extreme low oxygen tension (PO_2 << 1 mm Hg), inhibition of metabolic energy generation reduced renal tubular reabsorption of filtered protein to values near zero (Park & Maack, 1984). Thus, in the albumin-perfused rat kidney, excreted protein was assumed to represent nearly all filtered protein. Indeed, the recovery of urinary AML-activity equalled the decline of AML-activity in the perfusate, and analysis of excreted protein revealed an albumin fraction of 98.6 ±3.2%.

In the time course of extreme hypoxia, protein excretion rose without glycine in the perfusate by about 62% from 0.32 ±0.02 mg•g^{-1}•min^{-1} at the beginning to 0.52 ±0.11 mg•g^{-1}•min^{-1} after 40 min. Addition of glycine to the perfusate suppressed protein losses significantly to about one third of control values. The observed simultaneous hypoxic reduction in GFR (Fig. 1, middle panel) and the concomitant fall in filtered load did not reduce the protective glycine effect: In contrast, after correction for GFR-variation, the suppression of fractional excretion of protein by glycine was even more pronounced: protein excretion rose in controls (Fig. 2, upper panel, solid circles) by 2.15% from 0.59 ±0.04% to 2.7 ±0.19%. With glycine in the perfusate (triangles), protein excretion fell by only 0.2% from 0.20 ±0.04% to 0.42 ±0.14%. A similar stabilizing effect of glycine on albumin filtration excretion has been described by Sayed et al., (1990)

Excretion of the brush border enzyme, γ-glutamyltransferase (γGT), increased without glycine in the perfusate about sevenfold in extreme hypoxia, γGT-activity rose from 0.31 ±0.01 mU•g^{-1}•min^{-1} at the beginning to 2.17 ±0.03 mU•g^{-1}•min^{-1} after 40 min. Addition of glycine to the perfusate dramatically reduced brush border losses, as indicated by a significant lower γGT-liberation, γGT-activity fell by about 89% from 0.15 ±0.01 mU•g^{-1}•min^{-1} at the beginning to 0.23 ±0.03 mU•g^{-1}•min^{-1} after 40 min. Reduction

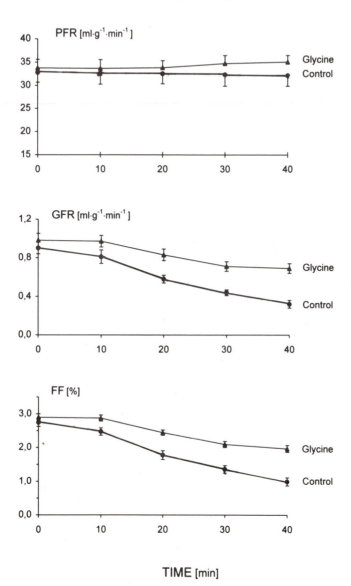

Figure 1. Time courses of perfusion flow rate (PFR), glomerular filtration rate (GFR), and of fractional glomerular filtration (FF) at extreme low oxygen tension (PO$_2$ $\ll$ 1 mm Hg) in the isolated, recirculating perfused rat kidney. Perfusions were performed with (solid triangles) or without glycine (solid circles) in the perfusate (x ±SD, n=6)

of γGT-excretion may have also been influenced by the concomitant variations in diuresis. To compensate for this we calculated γGT-excretion over GFR in the time course of hypoxic perfusion. GFR-corrected γGT-losses (Fig. 2, middle panel) rose without glycine in the perfusate (solid circles) by more than two orders of magnitude from 0.34 ±0.08

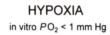

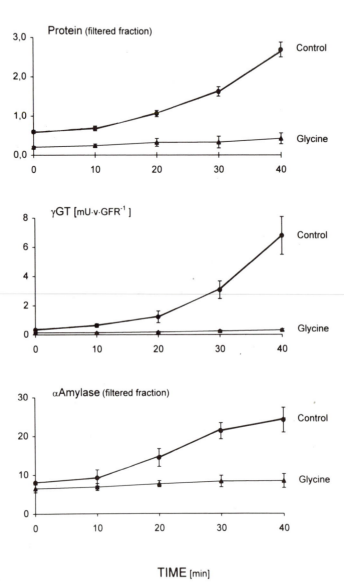

Figure 2. Time courses of fractional excretion (% of filtered load) of perfusate protein (albumin), of α-amylase (AML), and of GFR-corrected excretion of γ-glutamyltransferase (γGT) at extreme low oxygen tension (PO$_2$ << 1 mm Hg) in the isolated, recirculating perfused rat kidney. Perfusions were performed with (solid triangles) or without glycine (solid circles) in the perfusate (x ±SD, n=6)

mU•g^{-1} •min^{-1} to 6.78 ±1.3 mU•g^{-1}•min^{-1}. Addition of glycine to the perfusate (solid triangles) suppressed γGT-losses to the range of aerobic control values (Tab. 1), γGT-activity rose from 0.15 ±0.08 mU•g^{-1}•min^{-1} to 0.33 ±0.07 mU•g^{-1}•min^{-1}.

Protective effects of glycine on hypoxic enzyme losses are well known in the literature (Weinberg et al., 1987). The observed reduction of cellular enzyme losses in the presence of glycine significantly correlated with the support of tubular cell volume regulation in extreme hypoxia (Gronow et al., 1994). Thus, it appeared reasonable to assume that in our present experiments hypoxic cell swelling was also suppressed by glycine. Reduced tissue swelling would have then in turn facilitated glomerular filtration by a reduced intratubular pressure (Gronow and Cohen, 1984). Accordingly, with glycine in the perfusate, a significantly smaller loss of γGT (Fig. 2) was accompanied by an increase in glomerular filtration rate (Fig. 1).

Without glycine in the perfusate, absolute α-amylase (AML) excretion rose in extreme hypoxia by about 48% from 2.38 ±0.48 mU•g^{-1}•min^{-1} to 3.51 ±0.68 mU•g^{-1}•min^{-1}. Glycine reduced AML-excretion about half from 2.11 ±0.30 mU•g^{-1}•min^{-1} at the beginning to 1.87 ±0.36 mU•g^{-1}•min^{-1} at the end. GFR-corrected fractional AML-filtration rose in parallel (solid circles in Fig. 2, lower panel), AML.siewing increased about threefold from 8.01 ±0.32% to 24.2 ±3.2%. Addition of glycine to the perfusate (triangles) lowered AML-excretion markedly by about 200%, fractional AML-filtration only rose from 6.52 ±1.0% to 8.46 ±1.8%.

4. CONCLUSIONS

Our results support the hypothesis that beneficial effects of amino acid mixtures on hypoxic kidney function reported earlier from our labarotory (Mályusz & Gronow, 1987) were mediated, at least in part, by glycine (Tab. 1). This neutral, non-essential amino acid probably improved hypoxic renal glomerular filtration not by vasodilation or changes in the perfusion flow rate, as indicated in the present experiments by a significant gain in glomerular filtration fraction (FF, Fig. 1). This increase in FF may have been mediated by a reduction of intratubular pressure in consequence of less hypoxic cell swelling (Gronow and Cohen, 1984), indicated by a significant decrease in brush border γGT-losses in the presence of glycine (Fig. 2).

Glomerular siewing of middle-weight protein increased significantly at extreme low oxygen tension, the smaller molecule α-amylase (AML, MW 54 kda) to a greater extent (24.2%) than albumin (MW 69 kda) with a siewing coefficient of 2.7%. Addition of glycine to the perfusate reduced protein filtration in the hypoxic kidney, albumin filtration fell to 0.4%, and AML.filtration to 8.5%. This reduction of hypoxic protein filtration at an increased rate of fluid filtration may be explained by two different sites of glycine action: a) as discussed above, by a facilitation of glomerular fluid filtration via a reduction of intratubular backpressure, and b) by a preservation of the the filtering slit membrane of glomerular podocytes via the membrane-stabilizing effect of glycine.

5. REFERENCES

Burril, P. H., P. M. Brannon, N. Kretchmer (1981): A single-step purification of rat pancreatic and salivary amylase by affinity chromatography. Anal. Biochem. 17, 402–405

Bursaux, E., C. Poyart, B. Bohn (1976): Renal hemodynamics and renal O_2-uptake during hypoxia in the anaesthetized rabbit. Pflugers Arch 365, 213–220

Gronow, G., J. J. Cohen (1984): Substrate support for renal functions during hypoxia in the perfused rat kidney. Am. J. Physiol. 247, F618-F631

Gronow, G., Th. Kelting, Ch. Skrezek, J.v.d. Plas, J. C. Bakker (1987): Oxygen transport to renal tissue: Effect of oxygen carriers. Adv. Exp. Med. Biol. 215, 117–128

Gronow, G., N. Klause (1989): Support of posthypoxic renal respiratory function by specific amino acids. Funktionsanalyse biologischer Systeme 19, 225–231

Gronow, G., N. Klause, M. Mályusz (1994): Restriction of hypoxic membrane defect by glycine improves mitochondrial and cellular function in reoxygenated renal tubules. Adv. Exp. Med. Biol. 361, 585–589

Gronow, G., and H. Kossmann (1985): Perfusate oxygenation and renal function in the isolated rat kidney. Adv. Exp. Biol. Med. 191, 675–682,

Gronow, G., Ch. Skrezek, H. Kossmann (1986): Correlation between mitochondrial respiratory dysfunction and Na^+-reabsorption in the reoxygenated rat kidney. Adv. Exp. Med. Biol. 200, 515–522

Lowry, O.H., N. J. Rosebrough, A. L. Farr, R. J. Randall (1951): Protein measurement with the Folin phenol reagent. J. Biol. Chem. 193, 265–275

Maack, T.: Renal handling of proteins and polypeptides. In: Handbook of physiology. Renal physiology (Ed. E. E. Windhager), 2039–2080. Oxford University Press, New York 1992

Mályusz, M., G. Gronow (1987): Contrasting effects of amino acid mixtures on hypoxic dysfunction in the rat kidney. In: Molecular nephrology (Eds. Z. Kovacevic, W. G. Guder), 353–359

Mályusz, M., P. Wrigge, D. Kaliebe, J. Das (1990): Differences in the renal handling of pancreatic and salivary amylase in the rat. Enzyme 43, 129–136

Park, C. H., T. Maack (1984): Albumin absorption and catabolism by isolated perfused proximal convoluted tubules of the rabbit. J. Clin. Invest. 73, 767–777

Sayed, A. A. E., J. Haylor, A. M. E. Nahas (1990): Differential effects of amino acids on the isolated perfused rat kidney. Clinical Science 79, 381–386

Schnermann, J., D. A. Haberle, J. M. Davis, K. Thurau: Tubuloglomerular feed-back control of renal vascular resistance. In: Handbook of physiology. Renal physiology (Ed. E. E. Windhager), 1675–1705. Oxford University Press, New York 1992

Silva, P., S. Rosen, K. Spokes, F. H. Epstein (1991): Effect of glycine on medullary thick ascending limb injury in perfused kidneys. Kidney Int. 39, 653–658

Weinberg, J. M., J. A. Davis, M. Abarzua, T. Rajan (1987): Cytoprotective effects of glycine and glutathione against hypoxic injury ito renal tubules. J. Clin. Invest. 80, 1446–1454

33

FIXED ACID UPTAKE BY VISCERAL ORGANS DURING EARLY ENDOTOXEMIA

John A. Kellum, Rinaldo Bellomo, David J. Kramer, and Michael R. Pinsky

Department of Anesthesiology/CCM
University of Pittsburgh Medical Center
Pittsburgh, Pennsylvania

INTRODUCTION

Metabolic acidosis commonly occurs in patients with the sepsis syndrome (1). Acidosis correlates with increased mortality even in the absence of increased lactate levels and is a more reliable predictor of outcome (2). Although many studies have focused on the pathophysiology, clinical significance, and treatment of lactic acidosis (3–9), relatively few have investigated other sources of metabolic acidosis in sepsis. This is surprising because lactate ion accounts for less than 50% of the "unmeasured" anions present in patients with sepsis and metabolic acidosis (10). We have previously demonstrated that during normal physiologic conditions the liver takes up some of these other anions. However, following administration of endotoxin the liver switches to release of unexplained anions (11). This might account for the appearance of unexplained anions in the circulation of patients with sepsis (10) and liver disease (12) and may result in systemic acidosis if these anions accumulate in excess of strong cations. However, a non-anion gap metabolic acidosis occurs within several minutes of the administration of endotoxin to healthy animals (13). In addition, patients with sepsis frequently exhibit an acidosis which has a significant non-anion gap component (14). This acidosis cannot be explained by the release of anions by the liver. Accordingly, we reanalyzed the data from our original study (11) and included analysis of net acid flux in order to determine the sites of fixed acid production and clearance in acute endotoxemia.

METHODS

Surgical Preparation

The study was approved by the Animal Care and Use Committee of the University of Pittsburgh. Ten male mongrel dogs were anesthetized with pentobarbital sodium (30 mg/kg iv) following an overnight fast. The trachea was intubated and each dog was ventilated (Siemens-Servo 900B, Solna, Sweden) at a tidal volume of 12 ml/kg. End-tidal CO_2 was continually monitored (Hewlett-Packard, Palo Alto, CA). Arterial blood gases were periodically sampled, and ventilation was adjusted to maintain an arterial pH between 7.35 and 7.45. A 7-Fr balloon-tipped pulmonary artery thermodilution catheter with a 15-cm proximal port (American Edwards model 93A-095, Irvine, CA) was advanced into the pulmonary artery via the left external jugular vein. A 7-Fr polyethylene catheter was advanced from the right external jugular vein into the left hepatic vein to a distance of approximately 3 cm beyond the inferior vena cava under fluoroscopic guidance. For measurement of arterial pressure, a 5-Fr catheter with multiple side holes was inserted into the high abdominal aorta via the right femoral artery. A 7-Fr polyvinylchloride catheter was also inserted into the right femoral vein for the administration of a continuous infusion of pentobarbital at 2–4 $mg \cdot kg^{-1} \cdot h^{-1}$.

A splenectomy was performed after maximal splenic contraction to 0.5 ml of topical epinephrine (1:10,000). The splenic vein was cannulated with a 5-Fr polyethylene catheter that was passed into the portal vein to the level of the porta hepatis. The portal vein and common hepatic artery distal to the origin of the gastroduodenal artery were isolated, and ultrasonic flow probes (Transonic Systems, Ithaca, NY) were placed around each vessel.

The left renal artery was isolated, and an ultrasonic flow probe was placed around it. A 5-Fr polyethylene catheter was advanced through the left external jugular vein into the left renal vein at the level of the renal pelvis. The infrahepatic vena cava was isolated, and a hydraulic vascular occluder was placed around it for the purpose of a parallel study.

The abdomen was loosely closed with interrupted sutures. All the animals were fluid resuscitated with 0.9% saline as necessary to maintain the right atrial pressure between 2 and 5 mm Hg. The animals were then allowed to stabilize. Stability was defined as constant heart rate, arterial pressure, end-tidal CO_2, and organ flow signals for at least 30 min.

Experimental Protocol

Each animal served as its own control. Before receiving endotoxin blood was collected from all the catheters in heparinized syringes for the determination of blood gases, oxygen content, hematocrit, and levels of phosphate, and albumin. Blood flows to organs were measured on a strip-chart recorder (Gould Inc., Cleveland, OH). After obtaining these control measurements, *E. coli* endotoxin (L-2880 lipopolysaccharide, Sigma, St. Louis, MO) (1 mg/kg) was infused over 5 min via the right atrial port and the hemodynamic response of the animal was monitored without resuscitation. This was done to avoid any confounding effect of resuscitation fluid on ion concentrations and system acid-base balance. Thirty to 45 min after the administration of endotoxin, once the dog was again in a hemodynamic steady state, measurements were repeated as during the control condition.

Measurements and Calculations

Blood O_2 saturation, O_2 content, and hemoglobin concentration were measured using a cooximeter calibrated for dog blood (Instrumentation Laboratories model 282, Lexington, MA). Blood gases and pH were analyzed using a blood gas analyzer (Radiometer ABL-30, Copenhagen, Denmark). Organ flow data were obtained from ultrasonic flowmeters calibrated *ex vivo* using a standard perfusion circuit as recommended by the manufacturer (Transonic Systems, Ithaca, NY). Sodium, chloride, potassium, calcium, magnesium, phosphate and albumin were analyzed using an Ektachem 700 analyzer (Kodak, Rochester, NY) and standard reagents.

For the analysis, fixed acid was determined using two methods. First, the standard base excess was calculated according to the Siggaard-Andersen equations (15). Next, the effective strong ion difference (SIDe) was calculated from the pCO_2, phosphate, and albumin levels according to the methods described by Figge and coworkers (16). Fixed acid uptake for the gut and kidney was determined by subtracting the arterial concentration from the venous concentration and then multiplying by flow. For the kidney, total flow was estimated as the sum of left renal artery flow plus (left renal artery flow x the ratio of right to left kidney wet weight). For the liver, metabolic acid uptake was determined as follows: ([hepatic vein] x hepatic vein flow) - ([arterial] x hepatic artery flow) - ([portal vein] x portal vein flow).

Statistical Analysis

Statistical comparisons were carried out using the Wilcoxon rank sum test and correlations were tested for using Spearman's rank correlation test. Error values given in the text are standard deviations. A $P < 0.05$ was considered statistically significant.

RESULTS

Following the administration of endotoxin, the mean arterial pressure decreased from 113.6 ±19.2 to 57.0 ±14.2 mmHg ($P < 0.01$), the cardiac output decreased from 2.1 ±0.4 to 1.5 ±0.4 L/min ($P < 0.05$), and the systemic oxygen consumption was unchanged (131.2 vs 125.2 ml/min). During the control period the arterial pH was 7.34 ± 0.04. During the endotoxemic condition the arterial pH decreased to 7.22 ± 0.05 ($P < 0.001$). This was purely a metabolic acidosis, as the arterial pCO_2 was unchanged (33.2 ± 3.2 vs 33.7 ± 5.2 mm Hg). Measurements of fixed acid from the viscera failed to demonstrate the site of acid production. Lactate, though increased during endotoxemia (mean difference: 0.69 ± 0.28 mmol/l) could explain only 16% of the total acid load.

Both methods of fixed acid measurement (base excess vs effective strong ion difference) produced similar results (r = 0.98). The direction of the effect and the statistical significance were identical regardless of the method used.

During the control period, the kidney removed fixed acid from the circulation (6.03 ± 4.97 mEq/h). The gut and liver were neutral for fixed acid. During early endotoxemia, however, only the gut had increased fixed acid uptake (36.60 ± 6.60 mEq/h, $P < 0.05$) (Table 1).

Arterio-venous desaturation across the gut increased from 25% during the control to 38% during endotoxemia conditions, but this increase did not correlate with the fixed acid gradient across the gut ($r^2 = 0.03$). The mean gradient of base excess across the gut changed from -0.55 mEq/l during control to 2.47 mEq/l during endotoxemic conditions (mean difference: 3.01 ± 1.48 mEq/l).

DISCUSSION

The etiology of metabolic acidosis in sepsis is largely unknown. Lactic acidosis appears to account for only part of the acid load, while a large portion remains unexplained.

Table 1. Mean lactate and fixed acid flux across each organ

	Control	Endotoxemia	*P*-value
Liver			
lactate	1.8 ± 2.4	1.8 ± 3.6	0.82
fixed acid	-14.4 ± 63.0	-4.2 ± 14.4	0.10
Gut			
lactate	-1.8 ± 2.4	-3.0 ± 3.0	0.94
fixed acid	-1.2 ± 43.8	-36.6 ± 21.0	0.04*
Kidney			
lactate	-0.6 ± 0.6	-1.8 ± 2.4	0.50
fixed acid	-6.0 ± 15.6	-13.2 ± 16.8	0.27

All fluxes shown in mEq/hr. Fixed acid was determined by the effective strong ion difference. All values are means ± standard deviation.
*Significant at $P < 0.05$.

The results of this study suggest that the role played by the visceral organs in early endotoxemia is more complex than previously recognized. Neither the gut nor the liver showed a net release of fixed acid during early endotoxemia. Thus, despite baseline uptake and later release of anions as reported previously (11), the liver did not show net fixed acid uptake or release. This can be explained by the movement of other ions balancing the effect on the SID (either exchange of other anions or the concomitant release or uptake of cations). In contrast, the gut actually takes up fixed acid (in addition to unexplained anions) in the early endotoxic condition.

It is unclear what the relationship this finding has with the development of splanchnic acidosis, as measured by the decrease in calculated intestinal pH (pHi). This presumed intracellular acidosis has recently been demonstrated to occur as a result of systemic acidosis, even in the absence of tissue ischemia or hypoxia (17). Furthermore, abnormal intestinal permeability has been shown to occur in relation to low pHi (17) and, although controversial, this altered permeability has been proposed as an important mechanism of multi-systems organ failure (18). Further study is needed to delineate the importance of fixed acid uptake by the gut as a mechanism for decreased intestinal pHi and altered permeability.

Decreases in fixed acid across any vascular bed are consistent with known physiologic mechanisms. Blood bicarbonate levels increase as blood passes from the arterial to the venous circulation due to the Haldane effect (19). This "effect" occurs by two mechanisms. First, carbamino carriage is greater in reduced than in oxygenated hemoglobin. Second, reduced hemoglobin exhibits greater buffering capacity than oxyhemoglobin (19). Thus, fully desaturated blood is more basic than saturated blood when CO_2 is held constant. It would be possible, then, to attribute fixed acid uptake across a vascular bed to the Haldane effect. However, in order to explain an increase in fixed acid uptake with endotoxin, there would need to be a major change in A/V desaturation. Although A/V desaturation across the gut increased from 25% during control to 38% during endotoxemia, this increase did not correlate with the fixed acid gradient across the gut. Furthermore, this amount of desaturation would be expected to increase the base excess by only about 0.375 mEq/l (20). The measured mean increase in base excess was 8 times that (3.01 mEq/l). Therefore, only a small fraction of the total fixed acid uptake by the gut can be attributed to the Haldane effect.

Another mechanism which can produce increased bicarbonate concentrations in venous blood relative to arterial blood is hemoconcentration. In certain situations, such as ischemia, fluid shifts may effect the concentration of bicarbonate. Changes in free water did not appear to play a role in this study. During endotoxemia, the serum Na^+ concentrations did not change from the artery to the portal vein (148.2 ±3.5 mEq/l vs 147.6 ±2.4 mEq/l). However, serum bicarbonate levels increased across the gut from 13.6 ±1.8 mEq/l to 15.7 ±1.6 mEq/l ($P < 0.05$). The results of this study do not reveal the site of fixed acid production. An increase in fixed acid as well as chloride levels in arterial blood during endotoxemia as compared to control values suggests that chloride movement into the intravascular space may be an important mechanism. The mean chloride levels in arterial blood were greater during early endotoxemia (124.7 ±2.1 vs 128.4 ±2.9 mEql/l, $P < 0.05$). This finding could be a result of Donnan equilibrium in the setting of increased protein transudation from the vascular space (21).

REFERENCES

1. Young, L.S. In GL Mandell, RG Douglas, Jr, JE Bennett (eds): *Principles and Practice of Infectious Diseases* New York: Churchill Livingstone; 1990: 611–632.
2. Stacpoole P.W., E.C. Wright, T.G. Baumgartner, et al. Natural history and course of acquired lactic acidosis in adults. *Am. J. Med.* 97: 47–54, 1994.
3. Cowan B.N., H.J. Burns, P. Boyle, et al. The relative prognostic value of lactate and haemodynamic measurements in early shock. *Anaesthesia* 39: 750–755, 1984.
4. Curtis S.E., and S.M. Cain. Regional and systemic oxygen delivery/uptake relations and lactate flux in hyperdynamic endotoxin-treated dogs. *Am. Rev. Respir. Dis* 145: 348–354. 1992.
5. Fowler A.A., R.F. Hamman, G.O. Zerbe, et al. Adult respiratory distress syndrome - Prognosis after onset. *Am. Rev. Respir. Dis.* 132: 472–478, 1985.
6. Mizock B.A., and J.L. Falk. Lactic acidosis in critical illness. *Crit. Care Med.* 20: 80–93, 1992.
7. Peretz D.I., H.M. Scott, J. Duff, et al. The significance of lactic acidemia in the shock syndrome. *Ann. NY Acad. Sci.* 119: 1133–1141, 1965.
8. Stacpoole P.W., E.M. Harman, S.H. Curry, T.J. Baumgartner, and R.I. Misbin. Treatment of lactic acidosis with dichloroacetate. *N. Engl. J. Med.* 309: 390–396, 1983.
9. Vincent J.L., P. DufaCrit. Care Medye, J. Berre, et al. Serial lactate determinations during circulatory shock. *Crit. Care Med.* 11: 449–451, 1983.
10. Mecher C., E.C. Rackow, M.E. Astiz, and M.H. Weil. Unaccounted for anion in metabolic acidosis during severe sepsis in humans. *Crit. Care Med.* 19: 705–711, 1991.
11. Kellum J.A., R. Bellomo, D.J. Kramer, and M.R. Pinksy. Hepatic anion flux during acute endotoxemia. *J. Appl. Physiol.* 78:2212–2217, 1995.
12. Kellum J.A., D.J. Kramer, and M.R. Pinsky. Unexplained positive anion gap metabolic acidosis in end stage liver disease. *Crit. Care Med.* 22: A209, 1994.
13. Kellum J.A., R. Bellomo, D.J. Kramer, and M.R. Pinsky. Etiology of metabolic acidosis during saline resuscitation in endotoxemia. *Am. J. Res. Crit. Care Med.* 151 (4): A318, 1995.
14. Gilfix, B.M., M. Bique, and S. Magder. A physical chemical approach to the analysis of acid-base balance in the clinical setting. *J. Crit. Care* 8(4): 187–197, 1993.
15. Siggaard-Andersen O. *The Acid-Base Status of Blood.* 4th ed. Copenhagen: Munksgaard; 1974; 97.
16. Figge J., T. Mydosh, and V. Fencl. Serum proteins and acid-base equilibria: a follow-up. *J. Lab. Clin. Med.* 120: 713–9, 1992.
17. Salzman A.L., H. Wang, P.S. Wollert, et al. Endotoxin-induced ileal mucosal hyperpermeability in pigs: role of tissue acidosis. *Am. J. Physiol.* 266: G633–46, 1994.
18. Fiddian-Green R. Hypotension, splanchnic hypoxia and arterial acidosis in ICU patients. *Circulatory Shock* 21:326, 1987.
19. Ferguson J.K.W., and F.J.W. Roughton. The direct chemical estimation of carbamino compounds of CO_2 with haemoglobin. *J. Physiol.* 83: 68–77, 1934.
20. Nunn J.F. *Nunn's Applied Respiratory Physiology.* 4th ed. Oxford: Butterworth-Heinemann, Oxford 1993: 219–227.
21. Ganong W.F. *Review of Medical Physiology.* 15th ed. Norwalk CT: Lanage; 1991:6.

34

RELEASE OF LACTATE BY THE LUNG IN ACUTE LUNG INJURY

John A. Kellum, David J. Kramer, Sunil Mankad, Rinaldo Bellomo,
Kang Lee, and Michael R. Pinsky

Department of Anesthesiology and Critical Care Medicine
University of Pittsburgh Medical Center
Pittsburgh, Pennsylvania

INTRODUCTION

The pathogenesis of hyperlactatemia during SIRS is poorly understood. Yet lactate is often used clinically as a marker of anaerobic metabolism and is thus assumed to represent inadequate tissue perfusion.[1-5] This belief is supported by the high mortality seen in patients with hyperlactatemia,[1-2] and by the disordered oxygen transport exhibited by patients with sepsis.[6] Many clinicians routinely use therapies to improve global oxygen transport on the assumption that such treatment will reverse tissue dysoxia and ameliorate hyperlactatemia.[7-8]

The belief that anaerobic glycolysis is primarily responsible for hyperlactatemia persists in the clinical literature despite increasing evidence to the contrary. Direct measurements of cellular hypoxia using ^{31}P-NMR techniques in animal models of sepsis appear to show ample intracellular oxygen.[9] In human studies, tissue pO_2 increases with worsening sepsis, further challenging the notion that cellular hypoxia is the major pathophysiologic abnormality in sepsis.[10] In clinical studies of patients with sepsis, increasing oxygen delivery is often not associated with a decrease in the serum lactate concentration[7] and may even result in an increase. Moreover, serum lactate levels correlate poorly with systemic oxygen delivery in patients with trauma or sepsis.[11]

Although the lung is not usually considered as a source of blood lactate even in patients with acute lung injury (ALI), over the past 25 years there have been reports of a positive lactate gradient across the lung in various disease states[6,13-16] while no such gradient exists in normal subjects.[16-17] We have previously described an increase in lactate concentration across the lung in the dog during early endotoxemia.[12] Accordingly, we sought to determine if the lung is a source of lactate release in humans with hyperlacticemia and to determine the relationship between lung lactate release and lung injury.

METHODS

After approval from our institution's Biomedical Investigational Review Board, 22 subjects were evaluated. ICU patients were eligible for the study if they had pulmonary arterial and peripheral arterial catheters in place and had at least one simultaneous arterial and mixed venous blood sample drawn. In most cases this was done as part of a hemodynamic profile. In addition, subjects were required to have a chest radiograph on the same day as the blood samples.

Simultaneous arterial and mixed venous blood samples were obtained and analyzed for serum lactate concentrations. These measurements were timed to coincide with arterial blood gases, mixed venous oxygen saturation and cardiac output determinations using thermodilution. For subjects with serum lactate levels > 2.0 mmol/l, a second arterial lactate measurement was made to determine the direction the lactate level over time.

Laboratory records for these 22 subjects were reviewed (including arterial blood gases, ventilator setting and total respiratory compliance) and the chest radiographs were examined by investigators who were blinded to the results of the lactate determinations. Using these data, a Murray Lung Injury Score[18] (LIS) was calculated and recorded for each subject.

For the primary analysis, subjects were divided into two groups. in Group I (ALI), subjects had ali as defined by LIS scores ≥ 2.0 and also hyperlactatemia, (Serum Lactate Concentrations > 2.0 mmol/L). There were nine subjects in this group. Group II (control) consisted of 12 subjects who had no acute lung injury (LIS scores ≤ 1.5), with or without increased lactate concentrations. One additional subject was excluded from the primary analysis because his LIS was 2.3 but he was not hyperlactatemic (arterial lactate 1.6 mmol/l).

Measurements and Calculations

Blood gases and pH were analyzed using a blood gas analyzer (Radiometer ABL-30, Copenhagen, Denmark). Cardiac output was measured using the thermodilution technique and averaging measurements from five bolus injections of 5 ml of room temperature saline administered at random intervals in the respiratory cycle as calculated using a cardiac output computer (American Edwards 9520 A). Hemoglobin and hematocrit were measured, and serum blood lactate was measured by the enzymatic method (YSI 2300 stat plus, Yellow Springs, OH).

The transpulmonary lactate gradient was determined as the mixed venous [lactate] - arterial [lactate]. Lactate flux is defined as the lactate gradient x flow (cardiac output). In order to avoid the confounding effects of changes in hemoconcentration on serum lactate levels, we further adjusted the calculation by using the hemoglobin (Hb) concentration to standardize the lactate content in each blood sample. This was done as follows:

$$\text{Adjusted Lactate Gradient} = (\text{arterial [lactate]} - \text{venous [lactate]}) - \left(\frac{(\text{arterial [Hb]} - \text{venous [Hb]}) \times \text{arterial [lactate]}}{\text{arterial [Hb]}} \right)$$

Statistical comparisons were carried out using Wilcoxon's rank sum test and correlations were tested for using Spearman's correlation test. A p < 0.05 was considered statistically significant. All data were expressed as standard deviation.

RESULTS

For each subject with ALI and hyperlacticemia (group I), an arterial-venous lactate gradient existed demonstrating release of lactate by the lung (Table 1). This gradient persisted after correction for changes in hemoconcentration across the lung. Arterial lactate levels were found to be increasing over time in 8 of 9 subjects in this group and stable in one subject. The mean transpulmonary lactate flux differed in each group (231.3 vs 5.0 mmol/hr; p = 0.001). The lactate flux and the arterial-venous lactate difference correlated with LIS both for the entire group and for the subgroup with hyperlacticemia (r = .69, p < 0.01). Pulmonary lactate flux was not related to arterial lactate levels (r = .25). The one patient with ALI (LIS 2.3) but with a normal lactate level (1.6 mmol/l) also had a small transpulmonary lactate gradient (0.1 mmol/l).

DISCUSSION

The results of this study suggest that the lung is an important source of lactate during acute lung injury in man. These data also suggest that lung lactate release is related to the extent of lung injury. In the 9 subjects with ALI, the transpulmonary contribution to circulating lactate was approximately 200 mmol/hr. This value is well in excess of what would
be required to produce a significant increase in blood lactate, assuming a volume of distribution of 20–30 L in these patients.[19]

Our finding of a positive transpulmonary lactate flux is consistent with reports by others[6,13–15] and with our own animal study using an endotoxemia model.[12] However, these data are inconsistent with the traditional view that hyperlacticemia of critical illness is caused by an inadequate tissue perfusion and anaerobic glycolysis.[2–3]

The etiology of lung lactate release in ALI is unclear. It is unlikely that the lung parenchyma was hypoxic as these patients were closely monitored and only one patient exhibited an arterial PO_2 of < 60 mm Hg. However, it is possible that some areas of the lung were collapsed and potentially hypoxic. Alternatively, the lungs have the largest and most

Table 1. Dynamics of lung lactate efflux in patients with acute lung injury (Group 1) compared to control subjects (Group 2)

	Group 1	Group 2	p-value
n	9	12	
Arterial lactate (mmol/l)	9.6 ± 7.5	3.4 ± 3.9	0.006
Cardiac Output (l/min)	10.4 ± 4.1	5.9 ± 1.9	0.014
Lung Injury Score	3.0 ± 0.5	0.8 ± 0.6	<0.001
Lactate gradient (mmol/l)	0.4 ± 0.2	0.05 ± 0.1	0.001
Lactate flux (mmol/hr)	273 ± 241	21 ± 54	0.001
Adj lact flux (mmol/hr)	231 ± 211	5.0 ± 37	0.001
LIS vs adj. lact flux r = 0.65	—		<0.01

dense vascular bed in the human body. Injury to the endothelial cells in this vasculature may result in lactate release from either aerobic or anaerobic metabolism or from the inhibition of pyruvate dehydrogenase. This latter mechanism is known to be exist *in vitro*[20–21] and would be expected to lead to pyruvate and lactate accumulation in the cell, deranged oxidative phosphorylation, and the release of lactate into the circulation. Furthermore, neutrophils are sequestered in the pulmonary circulation in ALI and they may also serve as a source of lactate release.

However, nonspecific lung injury itself does not appear to produce any significant lung lactate release. Lee et al. were unable to show lung lactate release using unilateral hydrochloric acid instillation in the dog.[22] This may have occurred because of the heterogenous injury, small amount of lung involved, and the resultant decrease in perfusion to the injured segments.

In conclusion, our study demonstrates that the pathogenesis of hyperlacticemia in critically ill patients with ALI is complex and challenge the simplistic view that a single mechanism (tissue hypoxia) is responsible for the hyperlacticemia seen in some patients with acute lung injury.

REFERENCES

1. Vitek V, Cowley RA (1971) Blood lactate in the prognosis of various forms of shock. Ann Surg 173:308–313.
2. Weil MH, Afifi AA. Experimental and clinical studies on lactate and pyruvate as indicators of the severity of acute circulatory failure (shock). Circulation 1970; 41:989–1001.
3. Vincent JL, Dufaye P, Berre J, Leeman M, Degaute JP, Kahn RJ. Serial lactate determinations during circulatory shock. Crit Care Med 1983;11:449–51.
4. Madias NE. Lactic acidosis. Kidney Int 1986; 28:752–74.
5. Mizock BA, Falk JL. Lactic acidosis in critical illness. Crit Care Med 1992; 20:80–93.
6. Sayeed MM. Pulmonary cellular dysfunction in endotoxin shock: metabolic and transport derangements. Circ Shock 1982; 9:335–55.
7. Vincent JL, Dufaye P, Berre J, Leeman M, Degaute JP, Kahn RJ. Serial lactate determinations during circulatory shock. Crit Care Med 1983; 11:449–51.
8. Fiddian-Green RG, Haglund U, Gutierrez G, Shoemaker WC. Goals for the resuscitation of shock. Crit Care Med 1993; 21:S25-S31.
9. Hotchkiss RS, Rust RS, Dence CS, et al. Evaluation of the role of cellular hypoxia in sepsis by hypoxic marker [18F] fluoromisonidazole. Am J Physiol 1991; 261: R965-R972.
10. Boekstegers P, Weidenhofer S, Kapsner T, Werdan K. Skeletal muscle partial pressure of oxygen in patients with sepsis. Crit Care Med 1994; 22: 640–650.
11. Ronco JJ, Fenwick JC, Tweeddale MG, Wiggs BR, Phang PT, Cooper DJ, Cunningham KF, Russell JA, Walley KR. Identification of the critical oxygen delivery for anaerobic metabolism in critically ill septic and nonseptic humans. JAMA 1993; 270:1724–30.
12. Bellomo R, Ondulick B, Kellum, JA, Pinsky MR. Visceral lactate fluxes during early endotoxemia in the dog. Am J Respir Crit Care Med 1994; 149: A413 (abstract).
13. Strauss B, Caldwell PRB, Fritss Jr. HW. Observations on a model of proliferative lung disease. I. Transpulmonary arteriovenous differences of lactate, pyuvate and glucose. J Clin Invest 1970; 49:1305–10.
14. Bowles SA, Schlichtig R, Kramer DJ, Klions HA. Arteriovenous pH and partial pressure of CO2 detect critical oxygen delivery during progressive hemorrhage in dogs. J Crit Care 1992; 7:95–105.
15. Gutierrez G, Clark C, Nelson C, Tiu A, Brown S. The lung as a source of lactate in sepsis and ARDS. Chest 1993; 104:S12 (abstract).
16. Mitchel AM, Cournaud A. The fate of circulating lactic acid in the human lung. J Clin Invest 1955; 34:471–6.
17. Harris P, Bailey T, Bateman M, et al. Lactate, pyruvate, glucose and free fatty acid in mixed venous and arterial blood. J Appl Physiol 1963; 18:933–6.
18. Murray JF, Matthay MA, Luce JM, Flick MR. An expanded definition of the adult respiratory distress syndrome. Am Rev Respir Dis 1988; 138:720–3.

19. Woods HF, Connor H. The role of liver dysfunction in the genesis of lactic acidosis. In: Woods HF, Connor H , eds. Lactate in acute conditions. Basel: Karger, 1979; 102–14.

20. Kilpatrick-Smith L, Erecinska M. Cellular effects of endotoxin in vitro. I. Effect of endotoxin on mitochondrial substrate metabolism and intracellular calcium. Circ Shock 1983; 11:85–99.

21. Kilpatrick-Smith L, Dears J, Erecinska M, Silver IA. Cellular effects of endotoxin in vitro II. Reversibility of endotoxic damage. Circ Shock 1983; 11:101–11.

22. Lee KH, Rico P, Ondulick BW, Pinsky MR. Hydrochloric acid-induced lung injury is not associated with a positive lung lacate flux. Am J Respir Crit Care Med 1995;151:A761.

35

ENDOTHELIAL AND SYMPATHETIC REGULATION OF VASCULAR TONE IN CANINE SKELETAL MUSCLE

C. E. King-VanVlack,[1,2] S. E. Curtis,[3,4] J. D. Mewburn,[2] S. M. Cain,[4] and
C. K. Chapler[2]

[1]School of Rehabilitation Therapy
[2]Department of Physiology
Queen's University
Kingston, ON, Canada, K7L 3N6
[3]Departments of Pediatrics
[4]Physiology and Biophysics
University of Alabama at Birmingham, 35294

INTRODUCTION

In vitro studies have shown that production of the vasoconstrictor endothelin-1 (ET) is inhibited by NO in porcine aorta (Boulanger & Lüscher, 1990) while in vivo studies have shown that the increase in total peripheral resistance following nitric oxide synthase (NOS) inhibition in anesthetized rats is blunted by blockade of endothelin receptors (Nafrialdi et al., 1994; Richard et al., 1995). In order to assess the role of endothelin in the regulation of resting vascular tone in skeletal muscle, it was first necessary to establish that we could effectively inhibit the vasoconstrictor actions of endothelin in our experimental preparation. Endothelin-1 binds to both ET_A receptors on vascular smooth muscle producing vasoconstriction (Barnes, 1994) and to ET_B receptors on endothelial cells to induce transient vasodilation through stimulation of NO production (Fujitani et al., 1993; Sakurai et al., 1992). The contribution of ET_B receptors in the vasoconstrictor response to ET is minimal, but some studies have demonstrated that the ET_A receptor antagonists BQ-123 and FR139317 were unable to fully prevent or reverse the vasoconstrictor effect of endothelin in (Bird & Waldron, 1993; McMurdo et al., 1993). Because the dilatory action of ET is transient, we elected to focus on the vasoconstrictor action of ET.

The purpose of these experiments was to determine the threshold concentration of exogenous endothelin that was required to elicit a significant elevation in muscle vascular resistance and to establish the concentration of the selective ET_A receptor antagonist, cyclo-(D-Trp-D-Asp-Pro-D-Val-Leu-) (BQ-123), that was required to overcome the constrictor action of endothelin. A second goal of this study was to demonstrate that the

Oxygen Transport to Tissue XVIII, edited by Nemoto and LaManna
Plenum Press, New York, 1997

inhibitory action of BQ-123 on endothelin-induced vasoconstriction was not associated with blockade of other receptors which mediate vascular smooth muscle constriction; namely α-adrenergic receptors.

METHODS

Mongrel dogs (n=5) were anesthetized with sodium pentobarbital (32 mg·kg^{-1} i.v.) with an additional 65 mg (i.v.) given hourly. The animals were intubated, ventilated to maintain arterial PCO_2 between 30–35 mmHg and paralyzed with succinylcholine chloride (30 mg·kg^{-1} i.m., 0.1 mg·min^{-1} i.v.). A catheter was placed in the brachial artery for withdrawal of arterial blood samples. The left gastrocnemius muscle was cleared of overlying tissue and the arterial and venous flows were isolated to the respective popliteal vessels. The animals were heparinized (1000 Units·kg^{-1} i.v.) and a catheter containing an electromagnetic flow probe was inserted into the popliteal vein for measurement of venous outflow; a second channel in the outflow path allowed for in situ zero flow calibration without occluding venous outflow from the muscle. Venous outflow was returned to the animal via a reservoir attached to a catheter in the right femoral vein. Arterial flow to the muscle was directed via a two-channel catheter from the right femoral artery to the left popliteal artery. One channel allowed for autoperfusion of the muscle while the second channel had an in-line pump by which blood flow to the muscle could be kept constant. Muscle perfusion pressure (MPP) was measured just prior to the insertion of the catheter.

Once surgical preparations were complete, a 30 minute period was allowed for stabilization of cardiovascular and metabolic parameters. Under constant flow conditions, the MPP responses of the left gastrocnemius muscle were recorded and arterial and muscle venous blood samples were taken during a control period. Endothelin was perfused in incremental concentrations of 0.1 and 0.5 µg·kg^{-1}·min^{-1}, i.a. and the above measurements were repeated after 20 min of perfusion with each concentration of ET (Figure 1). Once a substantial elevation in MPP was obtained (usually at the 0.5 µg·kg^{-1}·min^{-1}), BQ-123 (2x10^{-8} mol·kg^{-1}·min^{-1}, i.a.) was added to the perfusate to block ET_A receptors; measurements were obtained 45 min later. Norepinephrine (NE; 1.0 µg·min^{-1}) was then added to

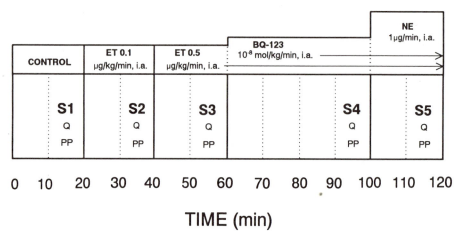

Figure 1. Schematic representation of the protocol.

the perfusate to stimulate α_1-adrenergic receptors (Kubes et al., 1992) and measurements were obtained when the peak vasoconstrictor response to NE occurred.

All blood samples were analyzed for PO_2, PCO_2, and pH using a Radiometer BMS-MKII blood gas analyzer and these data were corrected later to the temperature of the dog at the time of sampling. In addition, all blood samples were analyzed for O_2 concentration using an Instrumentation Laboratories Co-oximeter (model IL-482). The resulting values were corrected for O_2 in solution using the factor 0.003 ml $O_2 \cdot dl^{-1} \cdot mmHg\ PO_2^{-1}$. Muscle vascular resistance was calculated as MPP divided by muscle blood flow. Muscle oxygen uptake (VO_2) was calculated as muscle blood flow multiplied by the arteriovenous oxygen concentration difference. Oxygen extraction ratio was calculated as the arteriovenous difference divided by the arterial oxygen concentration. All measured and calculated variables were reported per gram of wet muscle weight.

All values are reported as means ± standard error (SE). Differences within each group were determined using a single repeated measures analysis of variance (ANOVA) and post hoc Duncan's Multiple Means test. Significance was accepted at $p<0.05$.

RESULTS

The values for muscle blood flow, perfusion pressure and resistance are shown in Figure 2. Despite attempts to maintain muscle blood flow constant throughout the experiment, the value for muscle blood flow during the final stage of the experiment (ET+BQ-123+NE) was less ($p<0.05$) than that observed during control. The lower concentration of ET (0.1 $\mu g \cdot kg^{-1} \cdot min^{-1}$) had no effect on muscle vascular resistance or MPP but infusion of 0.5 $\mu g \cdot kg^{-1} \cdot min^{-1}$ caused a significant increase in both MPP and muscle vascular resistance. Inhibition of ET_A receptors by infusion of BQ-123 caused MPP and muscle vascular resistance to return to control values. MPP and muscle vascular resistance increased ($p<0.05$) above control levels after addition of NE to the perfusate. The values for oxygen uptake and O_2 extraction ratio following ET, ET+BQ-123 or ET+BQ-123+NE were not different from values obtained during control (Figure 3).

DISCUSSION

Our findings indicate that the threshold concentration of endothelin required to produce significant vasoconstriction in canine skeletal muscle vasculature was 0.5 $\mu g \cdot kg^{-1} \cdot min^{-1}$ and that this vasoconstriction was reversed by ET_A receptor blockade using BQ-123. Further, the reversal of ET-induced vasoconstriction by BQ-123 was not due to additional antagonism of α-adrenergic receptors.

We examined the changes in vascular tone of the gastrocnemius muscle circulation following ET infusion. The lower concentration of ET used in this study (0.1 $\mu g \cdot kg^{-1} \cdot min^{-1}$) resulted in no significant change in muscle perfusion pressure, however, the higher concentration of ET (0.5 $\mu g \cdot kg^{-1} \cdot min^{-1}$) caused muscle perfusion pressure to increase from 131±16 to 191±22 mmHg ($p<0.05$). In anesthetized rats, iliac blood flow did not change appreciably until ET infusions of 3.0 $\mu g \cdot kg^{-1}$ but significant reductions in mesenteric and renal blood flow occurred at ET concentrations of 1.0 $\mu g \cdot kg^{-1}$ (Clozel & Clozel, 1989). Lerman et al. (1992) found significant elevations in total peripheral resistance and renal vascular resistance but not coronary or pulmonary vascular resistance when 2.5 $ng \cdot kg^{-1} \cdot min^{-1}$ was infused into anesthetized dogs. A 30% decrease in renal blood flow was ob-

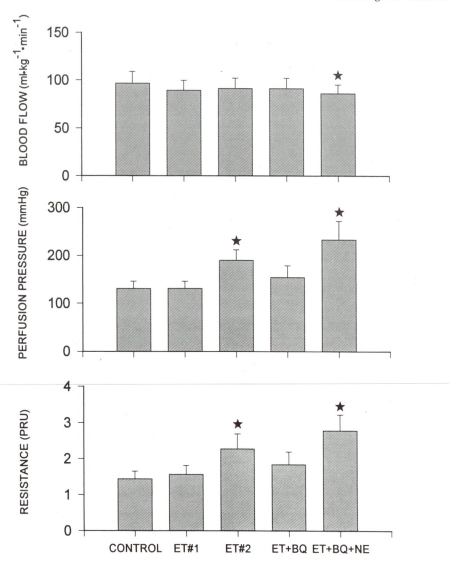

Figure 2. The mean values ± SE for blood flow, muscle perfusion pressure and muscle vascular resistance during control, following 0.1 µg·kg⁻¹·min⁻¹ ET (ET#1), and following 0.5 µg·kg⁻¹·min⁻¹ ET (ET#2) with subsequent inhibition of ET_A receptors (ET+BQ-123) and then addition of norepinephrine (ET+BQ- 123+NE). (★) represent significant difference from control value at $p<0.05$.

served in anesthetized rabbits following ET infusions of 20 pmol·kg⁻¹·min⁻¹ (Rogerson et al., 1993). Our results and those of others indicate that regional vascular differences in endothelin-induced vasoconstriction exist which may be related to the type and/or density of endothelin receptors in different vascular beds.

Other in vivo experiments in anesthetized dogs have reported whole body pressor responses following administration of ET that were similar to the increases observed in our muscle preparation. Mean arterial pressure increased 15 and 25 mmHg in conscious and anesthetized dogs respectively that received 300 ηmol·kg⁻¹ of ET intravenously (Given et al., 1989). Conscious dogs that received 1 µmol·kg⁻¹ of ET, had an average increase in

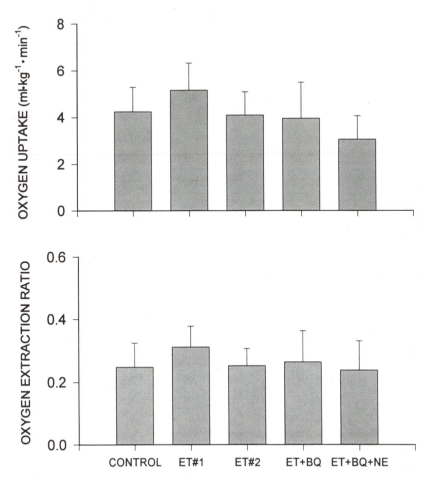

Figure 3. The mean values ± SE for skeletal muscle oxygen uptake and oxygen extraction ratio during control, following 0.1 μg·kg⁻¹·min⁻¹ ET (ET#1), and following 0.5 μg·kg⁻¹·min⁻¹ ET (ET#2) with subsequent inhibition of ET$_A$ receptors (ET+BQ-123) and then addition of norepinephrine (ET+BQ- 123+NE). (★) represents significant difference from control value at p<0.05.

mean arterial pressure of 45 mmHg but some animals also experienced emesis at this concentration of ET (Given et al., 1989). Mean arterial pressure increased 10 and 30 mmHg after infusion of 10 and 20 pmol·kg⁻¹·min⁻¹ of ET respectively in anesthetized dogs; these concentrations corresponded to plasma ET levels of 69 and 317 pmol·L⁻¹ respectively (Donicker et al., 1991). Lerman et al. (1992) also infused ET into anesthetized dogs at a rate of 2.5 μg·kg⁻¹·min⁻¹ with a resultant increase in plasma ET from normal resting values of 10 ρg·ml⁻¹ to those of 23 ρg·ml⁻¹. A significant increase in total peripheral resistance was observed, but no change in mean arterial pressure occurred because of a significant fall in cardiac output (Lerman et al., 1992). In other animal models, ET at concentrations of a) 10⁻¹¹mol·kg⁻¹·min⁻¹ caused a 35 mmHg increase in mean arterial pressure in anesthetized rats (Warner et al., 1994), b) 1.0 μg·kg⁻¹ increased mean arterial pressure in anesthetized monkeys (Clozel & CLozel, 1989), and c) 20–40 x 10⁻¹²mol·kg⁻¹·min⁻¹ increased mean arterial pressure 7 and 60 mmHg respectively in anesthetized rabbits (Rogerson et al., 1993).

We chose to use a selective ET_A receptor antagonist, because it appears that the predominant systemic effect of ET is that of vasoconstriction via ET_A receptors on vascular smooth muscle (Barnes, 1994; Fujitani et al., 1993; Sakurai et al., 1993). Our findings that $2x10^{-8}mol\cdot kg^{-1}\cdot min^{-1}$ BQ-123 significantly reversed the pressor effect of ET in canine skeletal muscle vasculature are in agreement with those of Warner et al., (1994) who found that infusion of BQ-123 at a concentration of $10^{-8}mol\cdot kg^{-1}\cdot min^{-1}$ significantly reversed the whole body pressor effect of ET in anesthetized rats.

Our data indicated that the pressor effect of ET could be reversed with ET_A receptor blockade without interference of α-adrenergic induced vascular smooth muscle contraction. The increase in muscle perfusion pressure and resistance that were observed following norepinephrine infusion were similar to those previously reported from our laboratory in the dog hindlimb (Kubes et al., 1992). Also in agreement with our findings are the in vivo findings for anesthetized rabbits in which adrenergic-induced vasoconstriction by phenylephrine was not affected by the ET_{A+B} receptor antagonist bosentan (Richard et al., 1995) and the in vitro findings in which BQ-123 had no effect on the contractile responses to norepinephrine in rat coronary arteries (Ihara et al., 1992).

The findings of this study provide the groundwork for future investigations of the nature of endothelial and sympathetic interaction in the regulation of canine skeletal muscle vascular tone. In our hands, we know the approximate concentration of endothelin required to elicit vasoconstrictor response in this vascular system and the effective dose of antagonist to reverse this effect without interference with sympathetic receptors. This pharmacological substantiation will now be used in experiments to determine the contribution of endothelin to the pressor response following nitric oxide synthase inhibition and sympathetic activation in canine skeletal muscle vasculature.

ACKNOWLEDGMENTS

These studies were supported by the Medical Research Council of Canada.

REFERENCES

Barnes, P.J. Endothelins and pulmonary disease. J. Appl. Physiol. 77:1051–1059, 1994.

Bird, J.E. and T.L. Waldron. Incomplete inhibition of endothelin-1 pressor effects by an endothelin ET_A receptor anatagonist. Eur. J. Pharmacol. 240:295–298, 1993.

Boulanger, C. and T.F. Lüscher. Release of endothelin from the porcine aorta: inhibition by endothelium-derived nitric oxide. J. Clin. Invest. 85:587–590, 1990.

Clozel, M. and J.-P. Clozel. Effects of endothelin on regional blood flows in squirrel monkeys. J. Pharmacol. Expt. Ther. 250:1125–1131, 1989.

Donicker, J.E., C. Hanet, A. Berbinschi, L. Galanti, A. Robert, H. VanMechelen, H. Pouleur and J-M. Ketelslegers. Cardiovascular and endocrine effects of endothelin-1 at pathophysiological and pharmacological plasma concentrations in conscious dogs. Circ. 84:2476–2484, 1991.

Fujitani, Y., H. Ueda, T. Okada, Y. Urade and H. Karaki. A selective agonist of endothelin Type B receptor, IRL 1620, stimulates cyclic GMP increase via nitric oxide formation in rat aorta. J. Pharmacol. Expt. Ther. 267:683–689, 1993.

Given, M.B., R.F. Lowe, H. Lippton, A.L. Hyman, G.E. Sander and T.D. Giles. Hemodynamic actions of endothelin in conscious and anesthetized dogs. Peptides 10:41–44, 1989.

Ihara, M., K. Noguchi, T. Saeki, T. Fukuroda, S. Tsuchida, S. Kimura, T. Fukami, K. Ishikawa, M. Nishikibe and M. Yano. Biological profiles of highly potent novel endothelin antagonists selective for the ET_A receptor. Life Sci. 50:247–255, 1992.

Kubes, P., M. Melinyshyn, K. Nesbitt, S.M. Cain and C.K. Chapler. Participation of α_2-adrenergic receptors in neural vascular tone of canine skeletal muscle. Am. J. Physiol. 262:H1705-H1710, 1992.

Lerman, K., E.K. Sandok, F.L. Hildebrand and J.C. Burnett. Inhibition of endothelium-derived relaxing factor enhances endothelin-mediated vasoconstriction. Circ. 85:1894–1898, 1992.

McMurdo, L., R. Corder, C. Thiemermann and J.R. Vane. Incomplete inhibition of the pressor effect of endothelin-1 and related peptides in the anaesthetized rat with BQ-123 provides evidence for more than one vasoconstrictor substance. Br. J. Pharmacol. 108:557–561, 1993.

Nafrialdi, N., B. Jover and A. Mimran. Endogenous vasoactive systems and the pressor effect of acute N^ω-nitro-L-arginine methyl ester administration. J. Cardiovasc. Pharmacol. 23:765–771, 1994.

Richard, V., M. Hogie, M. Clozel, B. Löffler and C. Thuillez. In vivo evidence of an endothelin-induced vasopressor tone after inhibition of nitric oxide synthesis in rats. Circ. 91:771–775, 1995.

Rogerson, M.E., H.S. Cairns, L.D. Fairbanks, J. Westwick and G.H. Neild. Endothelin-1 in the rabbit: interactions with cyclo-oxygenase and NO-synthase products. Br. J. Pharmacol. 108:838–843, 1993.

Sakurai, T., M. Yanagisawa and T. Masaki. Molecular characterization of endothelin receptors. Trends Pharmacol. Sci. 13:103–108, 1992.

Warner, T.D., G.H. Allcock and J.R. Vane. Reversal of established responses to endothelin-1 in vivo and in vitro by the endothelin receptor antagonist, BQ-123 and PD-145065. Br. J. Pharmacol. 112:207–213, 1994.

36

COLLOIDAL GOLD PARTICLES AS A MARKER OF PLASMA PERFUSION AND ENDOCYTOSIS IN KIDNEY, LIVER, AND SPLEEN

Martin F. König, Ewald R. Weibel, and Sanjay Batra

Institute of Anatomy
University of Berne, 3000 Berne 9
Switzerland

INTRODUCTION

Studies of *in vivo* microvascular perfusion are commonly performed by injection of plasma tracers such as labeled fluorescent dyes.[3,13–15] This method is suitable only at the light microscopic level and identifies only those capillaries which contain plasma tracer at sufficiently high concentrations.[7]

Only electronmicroscopy (EM) allows to identify all anatomically present capillaries, whereas for light microscpy (LM) a marker specific for the capillary wall such as alkaline phosphatase,[1,2] silver methenamine,[11] toluidine blue,[12] fibronectin or laminin needs to be used.

While the high resolution of EM is well suited for identification of appropriate plasma tracers, LM sections present a larger number of capillaries on the same section, which is convenient for studies of regional perfusion pattern. Therefore an ideal tracer would be detectable at both LM and EM levels. We recently developed a new plasma tracer, which is detectable by both electron and light microscopy,[6] in form of colloidal gold particles. Electron micrographs allow unambiguous capillary identification as well as detection of even minute amounts of tracer. In addition, colloidal gold particles were observed in endothelial endosomes, thus providing us with a marker of endocytosis.[7]

The aim of the present study was therefore to examine both *in vivo* capillary perfusion of several organs and endocytosis of colloidal gold particles in rabbits following 2 and 15 minutes circulation time.

Oxygen Transport to Tissue XVIII, edited by Nemoto and LaManna
Plenum Press, New York, 1997

MATERIAL AND METHODS

Preparation of RSA-Gold Complexes

The preparation of colloidal gold particles has been previously described.[6] Briefly, a volume of 3 liters of 8 nm diameter gold particles (corresponding to about $4 \cdot 10^{16}$ particles)[5] were prepared, labeled to rabbit serum albumin (RSA) and concentrated by centrifugation to 4–5 ml. After dialysing against Ringer solution (pH 7.4), the gold concentrate has been Millipore filtered.

Experimental Protocol

Six rabbits with a mean body weight of 3.9 kg (0.18 SE) were premedicated (atropine 50 mg, heparin 2500 ui, ketamine-hydrochloride 50 mg) and anaesthetized with pentobarbital injected into the ear vein. A thin catheter was advanced to the right atrium via the femoral vein. The chest was opened and the lung was ventilated by means of a small animal respirator (tidal volume 15 ml, frequency 40/min, end expiratory pressure 2 cm H_2O). A snare, consisting of a strong silk thread passed through a rigid tube to an external clamp system, was placed inside the pericardium around the base of the heart.

RSA-gold concentrate was infused over 15 seconds through the femoral catheter into the right atrium. Two minutes or fifteen minutes post-injection the circulation was arrested by rapidly closing the snare around the heart. Small pieces of the midportion of kidney, liver and spleen were subsequently immersion fixed in half concentrated Karnovsky fixative before further processing for EM and LM.

Histological Procedure

Standard electron microscopic techniques were followed to dehydrate and embed the tissue in Epon resin.[4,9] Sections were cut at 60 nm and mounted on uncoated 200 mesh grids. In order to improve the visibility of the gold particles, the sections were only lightly stained with lead citrate and uranyl acetate (each 5 minutes at 20°C).

For light microscopy routine paraffin embedding was performed. To visualize the gold label, particles were enlarged using silver enhancement applying silver acetate.[6] When this procedure was performed on control organs that did not contain gold particles, no specific silver staining resulted.

RESULTS

Kidney

Capillaries of cortex and medulla of the kidney showed homogeneously dispersed gold particles in plasma (Fig. 1). Examination of the glomeruli showed some gold particles in endothelial vesicles. Gold particles were observed in the glomerular basement membrane and appeared to have passed through the endothelial fenestrae. Further passage towards the urinary space seemed to be stopped by the basement mebrane, as no gold particles were detected in the urinary space. In medulla gold particles left blood plasma by endothelial fenestrae and were observed in the endothelial basement membrane, as well as in the entire connective tissue space. However, gold particles were not observed in the tu-

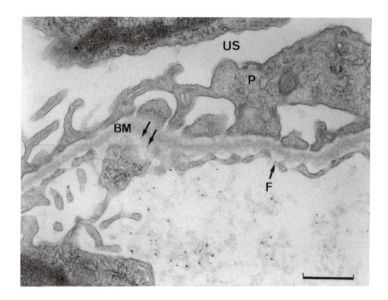

Figure 1. Kidney glomeruli show gold particles lying in basement membrane (BM, arrows) after having passed through endothelium (EN) fenestrae (F). Usually gold particles do not pass the podocyte (P) to the urinary space (US). Blood flow stop 2 minutes after injection. Scale marker 0.5 μm.

bular epithelium nor in the tubular urinary space, i.e. plasma clearance of gold particles was not accomplished by the kidney.

Photomicrographs of silver enhanced paraffin sections confirmed the distribution of gold particles as seen in EM. Silver enhanced glomerular capillaries were well demarcated as black convoluted vessels, allowing for a clear distinction between capillaries and urinary space.

Liver

Plasma contained a remarkable amount of gold particles in capillaries, and in the Dissé space (Fig. 2), from where they were seen to spread in the spaces between hepatocytes. No tracer was detected in billiary capillaries or in large billiary ducts as they are separated from plasma by tight junctions. Interlobular connective tissue also contained gold particles that passed through the fenestrated endothelium of capillaries related to the branches A. and V. interlobularis. Since lymphatic endothelium is fenestrated in this region, it is not surprising that lymphatic vessels also contained gold particles. Light microscopy showed black stained plasma in all blood vessels including liver sinusoids (Fig. 3). In addition, a variable degree of staining was noted in the interlobular connective tissue as well as in lymphatic vessels. EM revealed, that two minutes after particle infusion, all sinusoids contained colloidal gold particles.

Gold particles were found in endosomes of various cell types. Both, Kupffer cells and endothelial cells showed a marked amount of gold particles in their endosomes, often at a higher concentration than in plasma (Fig. 2). Also hepatocytes contained endocytosed gold particles which were mainly located in regions juxtaposed hepatocytes. Hepatocytes of zone 1 contained more gold particles than hepatocytes of zone 3. This effect was also demonstrated on lightmicroscopic sections where a gradient of labeled hepatocytes, de-

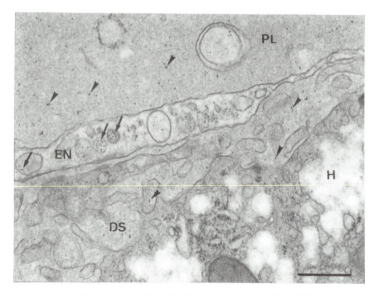

Figure 2. Endocytosis of particles by endothelial cell (EN, arrows) in liver sinusoid 2 minutes after colloidal gold injection. Dispersed gold particles (arrow heads) are found in plasma (PL) as well as in the Dissé space (DS) between hepatocyte (H) and endothelial cell (EN). Scale marker 0.5 μm.

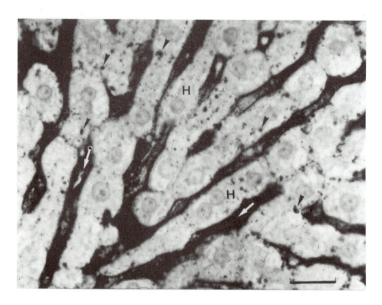

Figure 3. Liver after silver enhancement: Sinusoids (arrows) appear black between hepatocytes (H). Some hepatocytes show gold labeled endovesicles (arrowheads). Blood flow stop 2 minutes after injection. Scale marker 15 μm.

creasing from zone 1 to zone 3 was observed (Fig. 3). This reflects rates of endocytosis by hepatocytes.

Spleen

As in the case of liver, the spleen is a part of the reticuloendothelial system and therefore both plasma labeling and endocytosis is expected. Accordingly, we observed macrophages containing gold particles surrounded by labeled plasma (Fig. 4). In LM sections, the red and white pulpa were clearly distinguished due to the preferential black plasma labelling in the sinusoids of the red pulpa. In the white pulpa, the eccentric central artery was easily pointed out because of the black stained plasma.

DISCUSSION

In the present study we described RSA labeled colloidal gold particles as new in vivo plasma marker visible on both EM and LM sections of kidney, liver and spleen. The high number of colloidal gold nanospheres concentrated to 4–5 ml enabled us to detect plasma perfusion in all three organs. Even at the level of individual capillaries, plasma labelling was clearly observed in the face of dilution and clearance phenomena. Based on the direct observation of colloidal gold particles on electron micrographs, no uncertainties regarding tracer or capillary identification occurred as may be the case if only light micrographs are considered.[6]

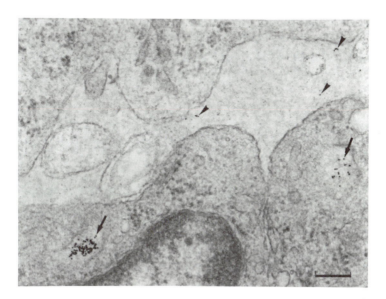

Figure 4. Spleen macrophages contain colloidal gold particles in endovesicles at high concentrations (arrows). They are surrounded by labeled blood plasma (arrowheads). Scale marker 0.2 μm.

Plasma Perfusion

Given the high resolution of EM, the presence of even a few gold particles is sufficient for indication of plasma perfusion on individual capillaries.[6,8] Gold particles may be detected even if capillaries were collapsed or filled with blood cells as gold particles were routinely distributed in remaining plasma. The time of circulation (2 and 15 minutes) did not ostensibly influence our observations on gold particle distribution in plasma. Despite the differences in organ structure and function, it was remarkable that capillary perfusion patterns were similar amongst various vascular beds.

Endocytosis

Gold particles were shown to be a useful tool for the description of endocytosis in various cells and organs. Gold particles were found in endothelial endosomes, particularly in liver and kidney. Organ specific macrophages also contained gold particles. These observations were noticed already after two minutes circulation time. After fifteen minutes circulation, only the magnitude of endocytosis was greater.

To date, studies on endocytosis using protein labeled colloidal gold particles have been performed by *in situ* perfusion of PBS containing gold.[10] In the present study, colloidal gold particles were directly injected into the blood stream of animals with intact circulatory systems. Accordingly, our observations regarding endocytosis are more representative of physiological conditions than *in situ* methods.

CONCLUSION

In the present study we demonstrated *in vivo* microvascular perfusion and endocytosis in kidney, liver and spleen by using small colloidal gold particles complexed to albumin as a new tracer for electron and light microscopic examination. From our electron microscopic observations we conclude that this tracer is excellent for quantitative studies of *in vivo* capillary perfusion. Colloidal gold particles are also useful for precise *in vivo* endocytosis studies at the EM level, and for semi-quantitative studies on plasma perfusion pattern at the LM level.

ACKNOWLEDGMENTS

The authors would like to thank Mrs. J. de los Reyes, Mr. M. Linder and Mr. K. Babl for their technical assistance.

REFERENCES

1. S. Batra, K. Rakusan, and S.E. Campbell, Geometry of capillary networks in hypertrophied rat heart, *Microvasc. Res.* 41:29–40 (1991).
2. J.M. Dawson, K.R. Tyler, and O. Hudlicka, A comparison of the microcirculation in rat fast glycolytic and slow oxidative muscles at rest and during contractions, *Microvasc. Res.* 33:167–182 (1987).
3. D. Hargreaves, S. Egginton, and O. Hudlicka, Changes in capillary perfusion induced by different patterns of activity in rat skeletal muscle, *Microvasc. Res.* 40:14–28 (1990).

4. H. Hoppeler, O. Mathieu, E.R. Weibel, R. Krauer, S.L. Lindstedt, and C.R. Taylor, Design of the mammalian respiratory system. VIII. Capillaries in skeletal muscles, *Respir. Physiol.* 44:129–150 (1981).
5. T. Kehle and V. Herzog, Interactions between protein-gold complexes and cell surfaces: a method for precise quantitation, *Eur. J. Cell Biol.* 45:80–87 (1987).
6. M.F. König, J.M. Lucocq, and E.R. Weibel, Demonstration of pulmonary vascular perfusion by electron and light microscopy, *J. Appl. Physiol.* 75:1–7 (1993).
7. M.F. König, E.R. Weibel, and S. Batra, Colloidal gold as an in vivo plasma marker in skeletal muscle and heart demonstrated by electron and light microscopy, *Am. J. Physiol.* submitted:(1995).
8. M.F. König, E.R. Weibel, and S. Batra, Comparison of in vivo microvascular perfusion pattern between skeletal muscle and heart. *Oxygen Transport to Tissue* in press:(1995).
9. L. Mermod, H. Hoppeler, S.R. Kayar, R. Straub, and E.R. Weibel, Variability of fiber size, capillary density and capillary length related to horse muscle fixation procedures, *Acta Anat.* 133:89–95 (1988).
10. D. Predescu and G.E. Palade, Plasmalemmal vesicles represent the large pore system of continuous microvascular endothelium, *Am. J. Physiol.* 265:H725-H733 (1993).
11. R.J. Tomanek and M.R. Aydelotte, Late onset renal hypertension in old rats alters left ventricular structure and function, *Am. J. Physiol.* 262:H531-H538 (1992).
12. R.J. Tomanek, M.R. Aydelotte, and C.A. Butters, Late-onset renal hypertension in old rats alters myocardial microvessels, *Am. J. Physiol.* 259:H1681-H1687 (1990).
13. F. Vetterlein, B. Demmerle, A. Bardosi, U. Göbel, and G. Schmidt, Determination of capillary perfusion pattern in rat brain by timed plasma labeling, *Am. J. Physiol.* 258:H80-H84 (1990).
14. H.R. Weiss, Measurement of cerebral capillary perfusion with a fluorescent label, *Microvasc. Res.* 36:172–180 (1988).
15. H.R. Weiss, E. Buchweitz, T.J. Murtha, and M. Auletta, Quantitative regional determination of morphometric indices of the total and perfused network in the rat brain, *Circ. Res.* 51:494–503 (1982).

37

MATHEMATICAL MODELLING OF LOCAL REGULATION OF BLOOD FLOW BY VENO-ARTERIAL DIFFUSION OF VASOACTIVE METABOLITES

A. V. Kopyltsov and K. Groebe

Institut für Physiologie und Pathophysiologie
Johannes Gutenberg-Universität Mainz
Duesbergweg 6, D-55099 Mainz, Germany

INTRODUCTION

It is widely accepted that vasoactive substances which are consumed or produced by tissue metabolism play a role in the adjustment of local perfusion rate to the metabolic needs of the tissue. In order to evoke a response of the vascular system, these substances — in the following for simplicity denoted by "vasodilators" even though oxygen, for example, is a vasoconstrictor — need to get into close contact with the small arterioles which represent the most powerful effectors in perfusion control. On the other hand, tissue sites in which supply with nutrients is most critical ("lethal corners") and in which a vasodilator signal may be generated earliest, are located hundreds of μm away from the arteriolar supply. In an attempt to explain how this gap in the signal chain may be bridged, it has been suggested that vasodilators released by the tissue cells are taken up by the blood stream and transported with the blood to the venules and from there by diffusion to the accompanying arterioles which are reactive to changes in vasodilator concentration [9, 16].

In order to study the potential role of this mechanism, a mathematical model describing the motion of blood through a symmetrically branching vascular network in oxidative skeletal muscle and the transport of oxygen and metabolic products in the tissue, in the vasculature, and between paired arterial and venous microvessels has been developed. This model considers oxygen transport from red blood cells to tissue, oxygen consumption and vasoactive metabolite formation in tissue, vasodilator transport from tissue to venules, its diffusion from venules to arterioles (v-a diffusion), and its influence on arteriolar diameters. Wherever available, the model is based on realistic dimensions and geometry of vessel segments, viscosity of blood and plasma, diffusion coefficients, etc. The total pressure drop across the vascular network is assumed to be constant. Blood flow in vessels is described by Poiseuille's law. Since detailed information on production rate and dose-effect curves of the various vasoactive metabolites is not known, it is assumed in the model that there is only one vasoactive metabolic product, the influence of which on arteriolar smooth muscle is equivalent to the accumulated influence of all metabolic products. The transport of oxygen and metabolic products in tissue are described by Laplace-type differential equations. The radius of arterioles is taken to be dependent on metabolic product concentrations in the arterioles. Altogether, this description of microvascular transport and substance exchange results in a system of algebraic and differential equations which can be solved numerically using the finite difference method.

The distribution of red blood cells and the velocities with which they move through arterioles, capillaries, and venules, both determining the conditions of transfer of respiratory gases and metabolic products in tissue microregions, depend upon the forces influencing blood flow, structure of vessel network, size of vessels, viscosity of plasma and blood [1, 4, 15]. In order to study the influence of a combination of all these factors upon blood flow or tissue metabolism, mathematical models are widely used [5, 6, 7, 8, 11, 12, 13, 14, 15, 17, 18]. Most of them describe either blood flow in vessels [1, 4, 12, 13, 14, 17] or transport of respiratory gases in erythrocytes, plasma, capillary endothelium, interstitial space, and tissue [5, 6, 7, 8, 11, 15, 18]. For a more realistic approximation of *in vivo* conditions, the development of a model simulating blood flow in vascular networks, transport of respiratory gases and metabolites in tissue, and the effects of metabolic products on the sizes of arterioles and thus on blood flow seems to be desirable. In the present paper, such a model is developed and used to analyze the relations between the most important parameters determining blood flow (which are the structure of the vascular network, the sizes of vessels, and viscosity of blood) and oxygen consumption by tissue.

MATHEMATICAL MODEL

The mathematical model includes three branching orders of a symmetric microvascular network which are arterioles A2, A3, and A4, venules V2, V3, and V4, and capillaries C (branching order 5) connecting arterioles A4 and venules V4 (Fig. 1). The blood successively moves through arterioles (A2, A3, A4), capillaries (C) and venules (V4, V3, V2). The total number of arterioles, venules, and capillaries in branching orders 2 to 5 is denoted by n_2 to n_5, respectively. The blood flow is driven by the pressure drop between the ends of the network and is described by Poiseuille's law in arterioles and venules. In capillaries, a generalization of Poiseuille's law is used which takes account of the pressure drop across individual red blood cells. According to [17], this pressure drop $\Delta\mathscr{P}$ is given by:

$$\Delta\mathscr{P} = \dot{Q}/G,$$

where $\dot{Q}$ is the bulk flow of plasma and red blood cells through the vessel, and G is a conductance which has the following form:

$$G = \left[\frac{128 \cdot \mu_B \cdot L}{\pi \cdot d^4}\right]^{-1} \quad \text{for arterioles and venules,}$$

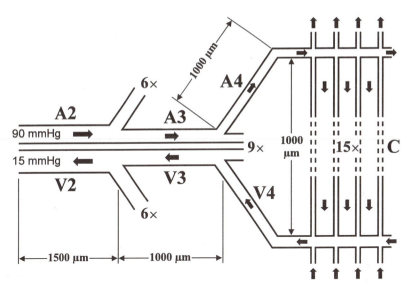

Figure 1. General form of the model of the vascular network. A2, A3, A4 are the arterioles, V2, V3, V4 are the venules, and C are the capillaries connecting fourth order arterioles and venules. The arrows indicate the directions of blood flow. Assumed pressures at the arterial and venous ends of the network are 90 mmHg and 15 mmHg, respectively. The multiplicities 6×, 9×, and 15× specify the ratios of number of vessels in each generation to number of feeding arterioles or draining venules, respectively. Thus the numbers n_i of vessels in each branching order are $n_2=1$, $n_3=6$, $n_4=54$, $n_5=810$.

$$G = \left[\frac{128 \cdot \mu_B \cdot L}{\pi \cdot d^4} + \frac{16 \cdot \mu_P}{\pi \cdot d^3} \cdot \sum_j \Delta \mathscr{P}_j \right]^{-1} \quad \text{for capillaries,}$$

where μ_B and μ_P are the viscosities of blood and plasma, respectively, L and d are vessel length and diameter, and $\Delta \mathscr{P}_j$ is the non-dimensional additional pressure drop for the j-th red blood cell.

Time dependent oxygen transport from capillary blood through a carrier-free region to myoglobin-containing muscle tissue is described by the well known system of partial differential equations [5, 8]:

$$\left. \begin{aligned} \frac{\partial P}{\partial t} + \vec{v} \cdot \nabla P &= D_{O_2 E} \cdot \nabla^2 P + \frac{\rho(P, \mathscr{S})}{\alpha_E} \\ \frac{\partial \mathscr{S}}{\partial t} + \vec{v} \cdot \nabla \mathscr{S} &= D_{Hb} \cdot \nabla^2 \mathscr{S} - \frac{\rho(P, \mathscr{S})}{[Hb]_T} \end{aligned} \right\} \text{ in the red blood cell,}$$

$$\frac{\partial P}{\partial t} + \vec{v} \cdot \nabla P = D_{O_2 CFR} \cdot \nabla^2 P \quad \text{in the carrier-free region}$$

$$\left. \begin{aligned} \frac{\partial P}{\partial t} &= D_{O_2 M} \cdot \nabla^2 P + \frac{\sigma(P,S)}{\alpha_M} - \frac{\dot{V}_{O_2}}{\alpha_M} \\ \frac{\partial S}{\partial t} &= D_{Mb} \cdot \nabla^2 S - \frac{\sigma(P,S)}{[Mb]_T} \end{aligned} \right\} \text{ in the muscle fiber,}$$

where the following conventions apply:

∇	gradient operator,
P	oxygen partial pressure,
$\mathscr{S}$	hemoglobin oxygen saturation,
S	myoglobin oxygen saturation,
$\vec{v}$	local velocity vector of fluid movement,
$D_{O_2 E}, D_{O_2 CFR}, D_{O_2 M}$	diffusion coefficients of oxygen in the erythrocyte, in the carrier-free region (consisting of a plasma sleeve, the capillary endothelium, and the interstitial space), and in the muscle fiber, respectively,
D_{Hb}, D_{Mb}	diffusion coefficients of hemoglobin and myoglobin,
α_E, α_M	Bunsen's solubility coefficient for oxygen inside the erythrocyte and the muscle fiber,
$[Hb]_T$	total hemoglobin concentration in the erythrocyte,
$[Mb]_T$	total myoglobin concentration in the muscle fiber,
$\rho(P,\mathscr{S})$	net exchange rate between free and hemoglobin-bound oxygen at P_{O_2} P and Hb-O_2 saturation $\mathscr{S}$
$\sigma(P,S)$	net exchange rate between free and myoglobin-bound oxygen at P_{O_2} P and Mb-O_2 saturation S,
$\dot{V}_{O_2}$	oxygen consumption rate by muscle tissue.

Formation and transport of metabolic products in tissue are described by a similar system of partial differential equations:

$$\frac{\partial C}{\partial t} = D_{Mp M} \cdot \nabla^2 C + \beta \cdot \dot{V}_{O_2}^n + \gamma \cdot \frac{\varepsilon}{P+\varepsilon} \text{ in the muscle fiber,}$$

$$\frac{\partial C}{\partial t} = D_{Mp IE} \cdot \nabla^2 C \text{ in interstitium and capillary endothelium,}$$

$$\frac{\partial C}{\partial t} + \vec{v} \cdot \nabla C = D_{Mp B} \cdot \nabla^2 C \text{ in capillary blood,}$$

where additionally:

C	concentration of metabolic product,

$D_{MpM}, D_{MpIE}, D_{MpB}$ diffusion coefficients of metabolic product in muscle fiber, interstitial space and capillary endothelium, and capillary blood, respectively,

$\beta, \gamma, \varepsilon, n$ coefficients describing the dependence of metabolic product formation on $\dot{V}_{O_2}$ and P_{O_2} (cf. Fig. 2a).

According to [11], the flux F of the metabolic product from the venules to the arterioles per unit length of vessel is described by the equation:

$$F = -2 \cdot \pi \cdot K \cdot (C_v - C_a) \cdot \ln(\sigma)^{-1},$$

where C_v and C_a are the concentrations of the metabolic product in the venules and arterioles, respectively, K is the tissue metabolic product diffusivity, and $-\ln(\sigma)^{-1}$ is a dimensionless shape factor specified by

$$\sigma = \frac{R_v}{2R_a} \cdot \left(c \cdot d - 1 - \sqrt{(c^2 - 1) \cdot (d^2 - 1)} \right),$$

with

$$c = 1 + \frac{\delta}{R_v} \quad \text{and} \quad d = 1 + \frac{\delta + 2R_a}{R_v},$$

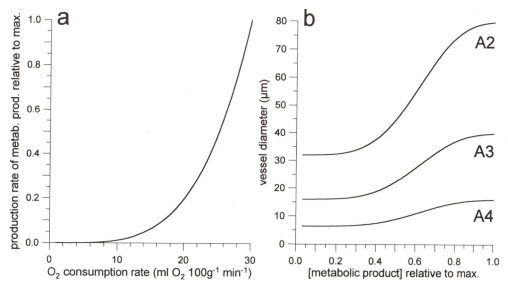

Figure 2. Metabolite-related input data to the model. *(a)* Changes in metabolite production rate at high P_{O_2}'s as a function of $\dot{V}_{O_2}$, normalized to metabolite production rate at 30 ml O2/100g/min. *(b)* Dose-response curves of arterioles A2 to A4 as functions of normalized metabolite concentration.

where R_a and R_v are the radii of arteriole and venule, respectively, and δ is the distance between them.

The metabolic product diffuses from venules to arterioles and affects arteriolar smooth muscle which relaxes. The pertinent increase in arteriolar radius R_a is described in the model by (cf. Fig. 2b)

$$R_a = R_{max} - (R_{max} - R_{min}) \cdot e^{-a \cdot C_a},$$

with

R_{max}, R_{min}	maximal and minimal radius of the arteriole, respectively,
C_a	concentration of metabolic product in arteriole,
a	"sensitivity" of arteriolar response to vasodilator.

Input data to the model for vascular dimensions and geometry, blood and plasma viscosity, diffusivities, etc. were selected to match the situation in cat tenuissimus muscle with adenosine as a vasodilator (cf. [2, 3, 19]). As experimental data for vasoactive metabolite production rates as functions of $\dot{V}_{O_2}$ and P_{O_2} and for arteriolar response curves to luminal vasodilator concentrations are not available, the corresponding parameters were chosen to mimic realistic interrelations between $\dot{V}_{O_2}$ and blood flow rate (cf. [8]). Altogether, the above relations form a system of equations which can be solved numerically. The calculations were performed on a VAX/VMS cluster at the University of Mainz.

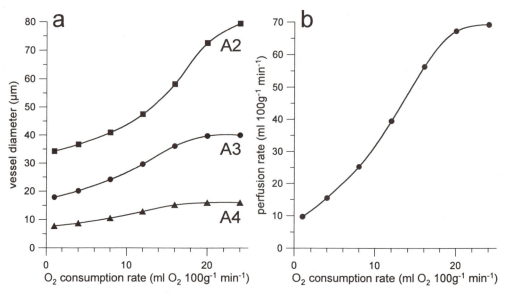

Figure 3. Calculated responses of the vascular network to changes in O_2 consumption rate. (a) Mean diameters in arteriolar generations A2 to A4 as functions of $\dot{V}_{O_2}$. (b) Calculated steady state perfusion rate as a function of $\dot{V}_{O_2}$.

RESULTS AND DISCUSSION

As expected, the calculated arteriolar radii increase with increasing oxygen consumption by tissue (Fig. 3a). In smaller arterioles, maximum diameter is attained at smaller values of oxygen consumption rate. For example, the arterioles in generation A4 become maximally dilated at $\dot{V}_{O_2} \approx 18$ ml/100g/min, A3 arterioles at $\dot{V}_{O_2} \approx 20$ ml/100g/min, and A2 arterioles at $\dot{V}_{O_2} \approx 24$ ml/100g/min. This is because in the vascular tree, the vasoactive metabolic product is partly shunted from venules to arterioles, and therefore its concentration increases more gradually with $\dot{V}_{O_2}$ in larger vessels. Corresponding to vascular dilation, calculated blood flow rate rises from 10 to 69 ml/100g/min (Fig. 3b).

Perfusion control in oxidative muscle primarily needs to satisfy the muscle cells' need for oxygen. In a very rough approximation, this implies that for doubling $\dot{V}_{O_2}$, twice the perfusion rate is necessary. This may be achieved by halving resistance to flow or — with regard to individual arterioles — by increasing their diameter by a factor of $\sqrt[4]{2}$. More precisely, at low to moderate performance, muscle enhances its O_2 extraction, so an underproportional growth of perfusion rate is sufficient. On the other hand, at highest levels of performance, extraction falls — at least in electrically stimulated muscles [10] —, so blood flow must rise overproportionately. As a consequence, there is no simple relation between $\dot{V}_{O_2}$ and perfusion rate. Moreover, at constant $\dot{V}_{O_2}$, perfusion rate varies inversely with arterial blood O_2 concentration, requiring that vasodilator production rate depends not only on $\dot{V}_{O_2}$ but also on some indicator of tissue energetic status, e.g., tissue P_{O_2}. As a further complication, flow conductance changes in proportion to the fourth root of vessel diameter, the dependence of which on vasodilator concentration exhibits some kind of saturation characteristics (see, e.g., [9]). In order to achieve an at least halfway realistic description of perfusion control, we had to find a suitable combination of a "vasodilator production function" and a dose-response curve for arteriolar diameter dependence on vasodilator concentration which came close to meeting the above requirements. By trial and error, we came up with a fourth power dependence on $\dot{V}_{O_2}$ and an inverse dependence on tissue P_{O_2} for vasodilator production rate, and with an asymptotic exponential growth of vessel diameter with vasodilator concentration (see section MATHEMATICAL MODEL). With these relations, blood flow increases 1.64-fold for an increase of $\dot{V}_{O_2}$ from 4 to 8 ml/100g/min and 2.23-fold for an increase in $\dot{V}_{O_2}$ from 8 to 16 ml/100g/min. Corresponding estimates from experimental data are 1.64- and 2.55-fold [8].

The above results were obtained by numerically solving the system of equations described in section MATHEMATICAL MODEL. Alternatively, one can start the calculations with a set of parameters pertinent to steady state conditions at some (low) performance, introduce a step increase in O_2 consumption rate, and iterate the system until a new steady state at the higher $\dot{V}_{O_2}$ is reached. The time courses resulting from this procedure may then be compared to experimentally observed response times in the microvasculature which are about 2 to 4 min [16]. Most surprisingly, calculated time courses are extremely slow, the slower, the higher the new performance level. Typically, it takes at least 20 to 30 min real time until vessel diameters and blood flows remain stable. According to the basic assumptions underlying the model, steady state vasodilator concentrations in the tissue and consequently also in draining blood represent an equilibrium between production and removal. While changes in vasodilator production rate caused by an increase in $\dot{V}_{O_2}$ and arteriolar response to luminal vasodilator concentrations are assumed to take place instantaneously, the consecutive changes in vasodilator removal and in tissue vasodilator concentration must occur much more slowly: Enhanced metabolite production will give rise to increases of concentration in tissue and outflow path, of v-a diffusional flux, and of arteriolar concentration, which, in turn, raises metabolite concentration in the tissue. Hence, in addition to being produced at a higher rate, the vasoactive metabolite is shunted between venules and arterioles and thus washed back into the tissue. Due to their small surface area (relative to the supplied tissue volume) and their unfavourable geometry, v-a pairs are highly inefficient in diffusional substance exchange, and therefore this washin process may be expected to proceed very slowly. This is what is actually observed in the computations at vasodilator production rates which are suitable to reproduce realistic steady state flows. Clearly, higher metabolite production rates would speed up vasodilator accumulation and arteriolar response. In this case, however, metabolites would still continue to accumulate in the tissue after vasodilation has reached its maximum. Consequently, following cessation of (long lasting) muscular work, it would take even longer for vasodilator concentration to fall below the level at which arterioles start to constrict. Even though this phenomenon has been found consistently for all parameter settings tested, additional investigations are needed in order to systematically assess the effects of varying parameter values, of different step changes in $\dot{V}_{O_2}$, of heterogeneous diffusivities or distribution coefficients of the metabolite, of changes in production functions and dose-response curves, of combined variations in arterial O_2 concentration and $\dot{V}_{O_2}$, etc. However, even based on the limited amount of data presently available, these observations strongly challenge the suitability of v-a diffusion of vasoactive metabolites for controlling arteriolar flow path resistance.

In conclusion, the model gives a reasonable approximation of the steady state dependencies of functional parameters of the vascular bed (diameters of arterioles, blood flow rates) on oxygen consumption by tissue. The reasons for the discrepancies between calculated and experimental time courses of vascular responses to changes in $\dot{V}_{O_2}$ remain to be clarified in more detail. Moreover, in future studies it is intended to take account of further metabolic products which influence blood flow through vascular networks in order to allow for a more adequate description of the processes taking place during local adjustment of perfusion to tissue metabolic needs.

ACKNOWLEDGMENT

This work was supported by the Deutsche Forschungsgemeinschaft (Grant 436 RUS 17/197/93 S).

REFERENCES

1. C.G. Caro, T.Y. Pedley, R.C. Schroter, W.A. Seed, The mechanics of the circulation, Oxford, Pergamon Press, 1978.
2. E. Eriksson, M. Myrhage, Microvascular dimensions and blood flow in skeletal muscle, *Acta Physiol.Scand.* 86:211–222 (1972)
3. K. Fronek, B.W. Zweifach, Microvascular pressure distribution in skeletal muscle and the effect of vasodilation, *Am.J.Physiol.* 228:791–796 (1975)
4. Y.-C. Fung, Biodynamics (Circulation), Springer-Verlag, New York, 1984.
5. K. Groebe, Effects of red cell spacing and red cell movement upon oxygen release under conditions of maximally working skeletal muscle, *Adv.Exp.Med.Biol.* 248:175–185 (1989).
6. K. Groebe, A versatile model of steady state O_2 supply to tissue: Application to skeletal muscle, *Biophys.J.* 57:485–498 (1990).

7. K.Groebe, O_2 transport in skeletal muscle: Development of concepts and current state, *Adv.Exp.Med.Biol.* 345:15–22 (1994).

8. K.Groebe, An easy-to-use model for oxygen supply to red muscle, *Biophys.J.* 68:1246–1269 (1995).

9. R.L. Hester, Venular-arteriolar diffusion of adenosine in hamster cremaster microcirculation, *Am.J.Physiol.* 258:H1918–H1924 (1990).

10. C.R. Honig, T.E.J. Gayeski, W. Federspiel, A. Clark, P. Clark, Muscle O_2 gradients from hemoglobin to cytochrome: new concepts, new complexities, *Adv.Exp.Med.Biol.* 169:23–38 (1984)

11. C.R. Honig, T.E.J. Gayeski, A. Clark, P.A.A. Clark, Arteriovenous oxygen diffusion shunt is negligible in resting and working gracilis muscles, *Am.J.Physiol.* 261:H2031–H2043 (1991).

12. Yu.Ya. Kislyakov, A.V. Kopyltsov, Erythrocyte in the capillary – the mathematical model, **in**: Biomechanical transport processes, F.Mosora *et al.* (eds.), pp. 217–222, Plenum Press, New York, 1990.

13. Yu.Ya. Kislyakov, A.V. Kopyltsov, Mathematical model of the movement of a non-symmetric erythrocyte along a capillary, *Biophysics* 3:484–489 (1990).

14. A.V. Kopyltsov, Effect of the viscosity of the plasma on the resistance to motion of erythrocytes along the capillaries, *Biophysics* 6:1131–1136 (1989).

15. A.S. Popel, Theory of oxygen transport to tissue, *Critical Rev.Biomed.Eng.* 17:257–321 (1989).

16. Y. Saito, A. Eraslan, R.L. Hester, Importance of venular flow in control of arteriolar diameter in hamster cremaster muscle, *Am.J.Physiol.* 265:H1294–H1300 (1993).

17. G.W. Schmid-Schoenbein, R. Skalak, S. Usami, S. Chien, Cell distribution in capillary networks, *Microvasc.Res.* 19:18–44 (1980).

18. G. Thews, Oxygen supply to the dynamically working skeletal muskle, **in**: Funktionsanalyse biologischer Systeme, Bd.16, M. Meyer, N. Heisler (eds.), pp. 63–75, Akademie der Wissenschaften und der Literatur, G.Fischer, Stuttgart, 1986.

19. B.J. Zweifach, H.H. Lipowsky, Pressure-flow relations in blood and lymph microcirculation, **in**: Handbook of Physiology, Sect. 2: The Cardiovascular System, Vol. IV: Microcirculation, E.M. Renkin, C.C. Michel, (eds.), pp. 251–307, American Physiological Society, Bethesda, 1984

38

REGIONAL CEREBRAL BLOOD FLOW AFTER SUBARACHNOID HEMORRHAGE (SAH) IN THE RAT

Edwin M. Nemoto, W. Andrew Kofke, Howard Yonas, Donald Williams, Marie Rose, Gutti Rao, and Elena Simplaceanau

Departments of Anesthesiology/CCM, Neurological Surgery, and Pathology
University of Pittsburgh School of Medicine, NMR Center
Carnegie Mellon University

INTRODUCTION

Current models of subarachnoid hemorrhage (SAH) in the rat involve either the direct injection of blood into the subarachnoid space[1,2] or arterial rupture after craniotomy.[3,4] Neither model simulates the phenomenon occurring in patients; the first, because it lacks an arterial rupture, and the second because of the need to open the cranium and thereby eliminating the acute and precipitous rise in ICP and a component of the ischemic insult that occurs after a SAH. Recently, a model involving the intravascular rupture of the middle cerebral artery (MCA) by a suture passed via the common carotid artery into the internal carotid artery to puncture the MCA has been described[5,6] which appears ideal because it duplicates the phenomenon in patients with respect to an arterial rupture, no craniotomy thereby allowing the rise in intracranial pressure to occur after rupture as it does in patients. Although changes in rCBF both qualitative and quantitative have been described for up to 2 hr after rupture, the changes occurring days after the hemorrhage to determine whether a delayed ischemic event occurs has not been determined. The objective of this study was to evaluate the changes in regional cerebral blood flow (rCBF) beyond days 1 and 3 postinsult.

METHODS

Male Wistar rats weighing 300 - 400g with free access to food and water up to the time of the studies are anesthetized with 4% halothane in 70% N_2O/ 30%O_2, their tracheas intubated with 14G catheters and mechanically ventilated with 1–2% halothane N_2O/O_2 70/30. Bicillin 60,000 units will be given IM. Gentamicin 4 mg is given IM. Atropine, 1 mg is given both prior to surgery and immediately post surgery IM (for a total of 2 mg). All surgical procedures were performed under aseptic conditions.

The right common carotid arteries were exposed and dissected to the juncture of the internal and external carotids, and to expose the pterygopalatine arteries.[5,6] In sham operated animals, at this point, the common carotid arteries are ligated and the wounds are sutured closed. In SAH animals, monofilament lines, 8lb test, were inserted in the common carotid arteries, through the internal carotid arteries, continuing past the pterygopalatine arteries, through the carotid canal, a total of 2.0 cm from the internal/external carotid bifurcation. (Monofilament is premarked in 0.5cm intervals). The monofilament punctures the internal carotid at the base of the brain. Monofilament is then removed and the common carotids are ligated. The wounds are closed and halothane/N_2O anesthesia is discontinued with continued ventilation on 100% O_2 until extubation. Animals requiring more than 2 h for extubation are excluded from the study. The animals are placed under close observation for up to 4 h after recovery and later housed overnight and watched for any respiratory difficulties.

Animals are transported to MRI facility at Carnegie Mellon University. There, the rats are anesthetized with 4% isoflurane in 50%N_2O/50%O_2, their tracheas are intubated with 14G catheters and mechanically ventilated with 1 to 1.5% isoflurane 70%N_2O/30%O_2. Femoral artery and vein cannulas were inserted for monitoring arterial blood pressure and infusion of replacement fluids and drug infusion. The rats were paralyzed with pancuronium bromide, 0.6 mg, IV, inspired isoflurane decreased to 0.4%.and atropine 1 mg was administered IM, and 3.0 mls 0.9% sodium chloride and 3.0 mls 5% dextrose in 0.9% sodium chloride was infused IV.

The rats were then secured in position in the carriage for the MRI and the ventilator adjusted to achieve a $PaCO_2$ between 35 and 40 mmHg, and PaO_2 greater than 100 mm Hg. with a positive end expiratory pressure of 5 cm H_2O.

Throughout the time in the magnet, arterial pressure is continuously monitored with intermittent arterial blood gas values obtained before the first MRI scan. Additional pavulon was provided as needed to insure paralysis of animal during scans.

Measurements of regional cerebral blood flow (rCBF) were made as previously described.[7] Briefly, proton MRI was done on a Biospec 4.7 T NMR spectrometer with a 40-cm magnet bore equipped with a 15 cm diameter gradient insert (Bruker Instruments, Billerica, MA). A Bruker 7-cm diameter volume coil was used. Image parameters were as follows: recovery time(TR)=2 s, echo time (TE) = 30 ms, field of view (FOV) =5 cm, slice thickness (SLTH)=2mm, and matrix size =64 X 64. To obtain a perfusion image, four pairs of images were obtained for each flow measurement. In addition, T2-weighted scans for tissue water assessment were made. Thereafter, the rats were removed from the MRI back to the surgical laboratory where isoflurane anesthesia was continued on 0.4%. 3.0 cc saline and the rats were rehydrated with 3.0 mls 5% dextrose in 0.9% saline over 2 minutes. The femoral artery and vein catheters were removed and the wounds sutured closed. The rats were finally treated with atropine, 1 mg, IM, and neostigmine 0.1 mg, IM, and Gentamicin, 4 mg IM. Isoflurane and nitrous oxide anesthesia were discontinued and the rats exposed to 100% O_2 until extubation and kept on 100% O_2 for 30 min post extubation, and the rats were returned to their cages after recovery.

On days 2, 3 or 8 post SAH or sham, the procedures were identical to those described for day 1. However, after the last study, the rats' brains were perfusion fixed with buffered formalin via the left cardiac ventricle, and the brain removed and the hemorrhage noted and labeled. Histopathological analysis of the brains were done by Dr. G. Rao , neuropathologist.

Regional cerebral blood flows were measured in 10 different brain regions on both right and left hemispheres (Fig. 1). All rCBF values were corrected to a $PaCO_2$ of 40

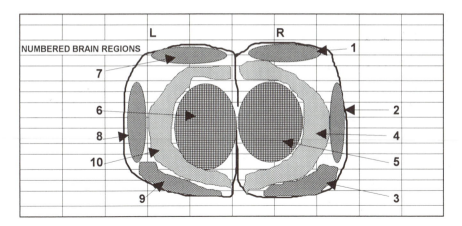

Figure 1. Diagrammatic illustration of the 10 brain regions analyzed for regional cerebral blood flow (rCBF). Numbered regions indicated as follows: 1,7= Rt and Lt Parietal Cortex; 2,8 =lateral temporal cortex; 3,9 =medial temporal cortex; 4,10 =Rt and Lt hippocampus; 5,6 =Rt and Lt basal ganglia.

mmHg using a value of 3% correction/mmHg difference in $PaCO_2$. Two way analysis of variance with posthoc testing of significance by the Student-Neuman Keuls test were done with a maximum P value ≤ 0.05 for statistical significance.

RESULTS

Physiological variables were controlled within normal limits (Table 1). Mean arterial PCO_2 ranged between 36 and 44 mmHg and PaO_2 well above 100 mmHg. Mean arterial pressure (MAP) ranged between 100 and 125 mmHg throughout in all groups.

Table 1. Physiological variables for up to 8 days after suture-induced subarachnoid hemorrhage in rats

Group		MAP (mmHg)	pH	pCO₂ (mmHg)	pO₂ (mmHg)	BE (mEq/L)
DAY 1						
SHAM(N=5)	X	126	7.35	44	118	-1.6
	SD	13	0.07	9	41	2.3
SAH(N=8)	X	130	7.41	38	177	-0.6
	SD	12	0.04	3	32	3.3
DAY 3						
SHAM(N=9)	X	128	7.38	39	177	-1.7
	SD	18	0.06	5	37	2.6
SAH (N=12)	X	121	7.40	36	201	-2.1
	SD	21	0.04	2	42	2.5
DAY 8						
SHAM(N=7)	X	133	7.38	39	157	-0.8
	SD	19	0.04	3	43	2.5
SAH(N=7)	X	134	7.42	37	188	0.1
	SD	14	0.03	2	19	1.1

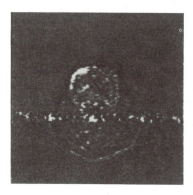

Figure 2. MRI rCBF image showing marked hyperemia in the right parietal cortex one day after SAH of the right middle cerebral artery. On the image, right is left and left is right.

Significant (P <0.001) hyperemia was observed in almost all brain regions examined at 1 day after SAH (Figs. 2 and 3). The hyperemia observed on day one post injury was followed by a relative hypoperfusion compared in the SAH compared to the SHAM treated rats (Fig. 4). By day 8 post SAH (Fig. 5), the hyperemia and at day 1 and hypoperfusion by day 3 had nearly completely disappeared and rCBF values between the two groups were essentially the same. The hyperemia observed on day one postSAH especially in the right parietal and right lateral temporal cortex was especially significant in brain regions that suffered infarction upon histopathological analysis at 3 or 8 days post SAH (Fig. 6). This pattern of cerebral infarction and ischemic neuronal necrosis was definitely limited to the distribution of the middle cerebral artery. Despite some rats showing severe cerebral infarction in some regions of the brain, the results were variable in that some rats did not show any hemorrhage.

DISCUSSION

The results show that suture induced middle cerebral artery rupture produces in some instances, severe ischemic infarction that is highly localized. Measurements of rCBF

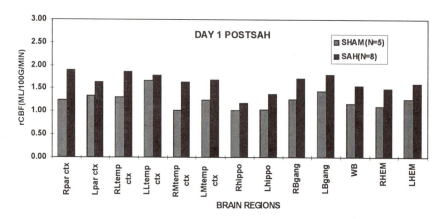

Figure 3. Regional cerebral blood flow (rCBF) in rats one day after suture-induced subarachnoid hemorrhage of the right middle cerebral artery. rCBF measurements were made during anesthesia with 0.4% isoflurane/70% N_2O/30% O_2 and mechanical ventilation. rCBF values of SAH rats were significantly higher (P<0.001) in all brain regions compared to SHAM operated rats.

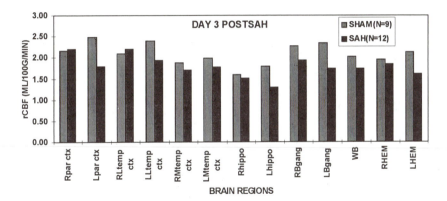

Figure 4. Regional cerebral blood flow (rCBF) values in rats 3 days after suture-induced subarachnoid hemorrhage (SAH) of the right middle cerebral artery. See legend Fig. 1 for other details of anesthesia. *= P<0.05 compared to corresponding value in the SAH group. **=P<0.01 compared to corresponding value in the SAH group.

also reveal a marked hyperemia as early as one day after hemorrhage which progressively subsides over 3 and 8 days postinjury. The results of this study are unique in that it is the first model of SAH in the rat capable of producing ischemia of sufficient severity so as to cause ischemic infarction. This has not been previously demonstrated in any rat model of SAH.

Despite the evidence of cerebral ischemic infarction and some indication that rCBF values in SAH rats at 3 days after injury were lower than in SHAM rats, there was no indication of ischemia sufficiently severe to cause the degree of infarction observed. The reason may be attributable to the fact that the ischemic insult may be occurring before one day post injury. Indeed, in rats subjected to the same method of SAH induction, but apparently of much greater severity in that the rats for the most part did not survive the insult although there were different grades of severity that were observed, rCBF values were minimal with the first 1-3 hours post injury. Bedersen et al, using laser doppler flowmetry

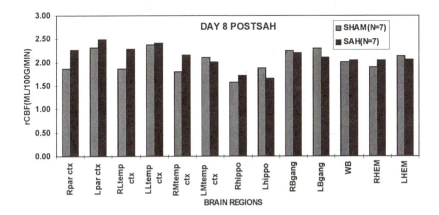

Figure 5. Regional cerebral blood flow (rCBF) values in rats 8 days after suture-induced subarachnoid hemorrhage (SAH) of the right middle cerebral artery. See legend Fig. 1 for other details of anesthesia. *= P<0.05 compared to corresponding value in the SAH group.

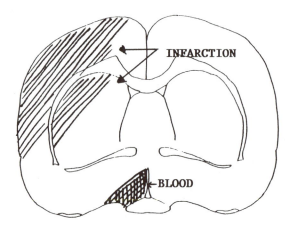

Figure 6. Diagrammatic illustration of the pattern of ischemic infarction observed in a rat 8 days after SAH. On the image, right is left and left is right.

showed that the minimum blood flow was achieved within the first 5 min after SAH and was restored to 50% of normal values within 25 min postSAH. Thus, it is very likely that the ischemic insult accounting for the histopathological damage sustained is attributable to ischemia occurring within the first few minutes after hemorrhage. There is a general appreciation that the ischemic insult in the rat after SAH occurs in the rat on a time scale that is highly accelerated compared to that occurring in patients, namely with cerebral hypoperfusion occurring much earlier than seen in patients. Our results suggest as did the studies by Bedersen et al[5] and Veelken et al[6] that indeed, postinsult cerebral hypoperfusion at least in this model occurs within the first 24 h and probably within the first 3-4 hours after the hemorrhage.

REFERENCES

1. Delgado TJ, Arbab MAR, Diemer NH, Svendgaard N-A. Subarachnoid hemorrhage in the rat: Cerebral blood flow and glucose metabolism during the late phase of cerebral vasospasm. J Cereb Blood Flow & Metab 1986;6:590–599.
2. Zuccarello M, Anderson DK. Protective effect of a 21-aminosteroid on the blood brain barrier following subarachnoid hemorrhage in rats. Stroke 1989;20:367–371.
3. Barry KJ, Gogjian MA, Stein BM. Small animal model for investigation of subarachnoid hemorrhage and cerebral vasospasm. Stroke 1979;10:538–541.
4. Kader A, Krauss WE, Onesti ST, Elliott JP, Solomon RA. Chronic cerebral blood flow changes following experimental subarachnoid hemorrhage in rats. Stroke 1990;21:577–581.
5. Bedersen JB, Germano IM, Guarino L. Cortical blood flow and cerebral perfusion pressure in a new non-craniotomy model of subarachnoid hemorrhage in the rat. Stroke 1995;26:1086–1092.
6. Veelken JA, Laing RJC, Jakubowski J. The Sheffield model of subarachnoid hemorrhage in rats. Stroke 1995;26:1279–1284.

39

EFFECT OF HYPOXIC HYPOXIA ON TRANSMURAL GUT AND SUBCUTANEOUS TISSUE OXYGEN TENSION

Mark D. Suski, David Zabel, Vitaly Levin, Heinz Scheuenstuhl, and Thomas K. Hunt

Department of Surgery
University of California, San Francisco
San Francisco, California 94143

1. INTRODUCTION

Multiple System Organ Failure develops in 15% of surgical intensive care unit patients despite being adequately resuscitated by conventional criteria. Of these, greater than 50% will eventually die[1]. Some current theories implicate the persistence of inadequate gut oxygenation as the principle inciting event[2,3]. It is proposed that gut hypoxia compromises both mucosal barrier integrity and transmural oxidative bacterial killing. The net effect is an increased rate of bacterial translocation, which if unchecked can rapidly progress to sepsis and death. The early detection of gut hypoxia offers an opportunity to intervene and possibly prevent this scenario.

Prior work in our laboratory has demonstrated the presence of a large transmural gut oxygen gradient. Under physiologic conditions, mucosal oxygen tension (PMO_2) is dramatically lower than its serosal counterpart (PSO_2)[4]. Because mucosal cells appear to function at the edge of viability in relation to oxygen tension, it is intuitively attractive that protective mechanisms may exist. However, mucosal PO_2 is already so low that it is difficult to imagine further protection from pathologic insult. Splanchnic blood flow is under both local and systemic autoregulatory control[5]. Perfusion to the splanchnic tissue bed is decreased during low flow states. The resultant mucosal damage has been well documented and is presumably due to ischemic hypoxia [6,7]. Little however is known about the effect of arterial hypoxia alone.

2. HYPOTHESIS

In the present study, transmural gut and subcutaneous oxygen tensions were evaluated during acute decreases in inspired oxygen concentrations and during normoxic resus-

Oxygen Transport to Tissue XVIII, edited by Nemoto and LaManna
Plenum Press, New York, 1997

citation. We proposed two hypotheses. First, the mucosal oxygen tension is not maintained during hypoxic insult. Second, the subcutaneous tissue oxygen tension ($PSQO_2$), which provides a direct, continuous and quantitative assessment of oxygen availability, correlates with the transmural gut oxygen gradient.

3. MATERIALS AND METHODS

All experiments were performed under protocols approved by the Committee on Animal Research at the University of California, San Francisco. Seven adult male Sprague-Dawley rats (350–375gms) underwent anesthesia (IM injection of 2.5 mg/kg of acepromazine maleate and 40 mg/kg of ketamine hydrochloride) prior to celiotomy. Anesthesia was maintained by periodic injection at half the initial dose. Euthermia was maintained with a heating blanket.

Oxygen measurements were obtained by using fluorescent oxygen sensors (TOPS™ Oxygen Optode, InnerSpace Medical, Irvine CA) placed within a silastic tonometer. These probes function by the principle of "Fluorescence Quenching". Light of a known wavelength is transmitted to the sensor where it excites the fluorescent dye on the tip to emit light of a second wavelength. This light in turn is quenched or diminished in direct proportion to the amount of oxygen present. Since the intensity of the emited light is inversely proportional to the oxygen concentration encountered, the partial pressure of oxygen can be determined. No oxygen is consumed in this process and the calibration is temperature corrected and linear over the range from 0–154 mm Hg. The silicone tonometers are freely permeable to oxygen, and therefore the recorded measurements reflect the mean oxygen tension of the surrounding tissue. The tonometers were placed in the subcutaneous tissue of the abdomen and on the serosal and mucosal antimesenteric surfaces of the colon approximately 2 cm distal to the cecum. The oxygen sensors were then inserted into the tonometers and the entire assembly flushed with hypoxic saline to eliminate air bubbles which delay equilibration. The sensors were allowed to equilibrate for 20 minutes at room air before measurements were begun.

The fraction of inspired oxygen (FiO2) was varied from a baseline of .21 to .15 and .09 before being returned to a baseline room air value. Measurements were obtained for 30 minutes during initial normoxic and subsequent hypoxic conditions and for 2 hours during normoxic recovery.

The respiratory gas mixture was delivered at 4 L/min via a modified face mask to ensure an adequate minute ventilation. Maintenance intravenous fluid was administered via a femoral venous cannula at 2.5 ml/kg/hr. Statistical significance was determined using a paired Student's t-test. All results are presented as mean ± standard deviation.

4. RESULTS

Our results confirm the presence of a steep transmural gut PO_2 gradient between mucosa and serosa under normoxic conditions. This gradient is maintained during hypoxic challenge as well as following normoxic resucitation. More importantly, mucosal PO_2 after falling during hypoxia does not return to baseline during normoxic recovery, in contrast to subcutaneous tissue and serosal PO_2. In addition, the subcutaneous tissue PO_2 approximates the serosal PO_2 at each FiO2 tested. Linear regression analysis reveals a strong correlation between decreases in the subcutaneous oxygen tension and a decreasing

Table 1. Mean subcutaneous (PSQO2), serosal (PSO2), and mucosal (PMO2) oxygen tensions for each FiO2. (± Standard Deviation mm Hg)

FiO_2	$PSQO_2$	PSO_2	PMO_2
0.21	62±6	67±4	11±1
0.15	30±4*	29±8*	08±2*
0.09	14±6*	14±6*	06±2*
0.21	64±8	65±8	09±1*

(*p<0.05 compared to initial room air value)

transmural gut gradient (PSO_2 - PMO_2) as depicted by a R^2 value of .95 and a p value of .001.

5. DISCUSSION

Our primary finding is that although acute respiratory hypoxia significantly reduced oxygen tension in all tissues measured, normoxic resuscitation did not fully restore mucosal PO_2 to baseline values. Though the difference is small, it is both statistically and biologically significant. A commonly held view of Multiple System Organ Failure is that it is initiated by an increased rate of bacterial translocation. This "Gut Hypothesis" states that either bacterial overgrowth, impaired host defense systems or the disruption of mucosal barrier integrity is required for clinically relevant bacterial translocation to occur [8]. Arterial hypoxia potentiates the translocation of bacteria across the bowel wall in experimental models[9]. The transmural gut oxygen tensions encountered in our study fall within a hypoxic range that can result in mucosal disruption and impaired oxidatative bacterial killing in neutrophils. The continuous monitoring of subcutaneous tissue PO_2 has been a long-standing interest of our laboratory. Past clinical studies have determined that the $PSQO_2$ accuratey predicts the risk of wound infection (unpublished data), is the most sensitive measure of volume status[10], and corresponds to decreases in bowel perfusion in response to hemorrhage[11]. This study now correlates a decreasing $PSQO_2$ with a decreasing transmural gut oxygen gradient. Subcutaneous PO_2 monitoring may allow more optimal management of critically ill patients by maintaining transmural gut oxygenation.

6. CONCLUSION

Acute respiratory hypoxia significantly reduces oxygen tension in the subcutaneous tissue of the abdomen and the serosal and mucosal surfaces of the colon. The mucosal PO_2, already near a critical level in normoxic conditions, falls with hypoxia to an extremely low level and more importantly appears not to recover from hypoxic insult. Though the differences are numerically small, they are proportionally great, and irreversible loss of mucosal barrier function and impaired oxidative bacterial killing may result. Subcutaneous tissue oxygen measurements may represent a useful clinical method for identifying gut hypoxia.

7. ACKNOWLEDGMENTS

This study was supported by NIH GM 27345.

8. REFERENCES

1. Haglund, U., Fiddian-Green, R. Assessment of adequate tissue oxygenation in shock and critical illness: Oxygen transport in sepsis, Bermuda, April 1 + 2, 1989. Intensive Care Med. 1989:15 (7):475–477.
2. Antonsson, J., Fiddian-Green, R. The role of the gut in shock and multiple system organ failure. European Journal of Surgery. 1991:157:3–12.
3. Deitch, E. Multiple organ failure - pathophysiology and potential future therapy. Annals of Surgery. 1992:16:117–134.
4. Zabel, D., Hopf, H., Hunt, T. Transmural gut oxygen gradients in shocked rats resuscitated with heparan. Archives of Surgery. 1995:130:59–63.
5. Granger, D., Richardson, P., Kvietys, P., Mortillaro, N. Intestinal blood flow. Gastroenterology. 1980:78:837–863.
6. Deitch, E., Morrison, J., Berg, R., Specian, R. Effect of hemorrhagic shock on bacterial translocation, intestinal morphology, and intestinal permeability in conventional and antibiotic-decontaminated rats. Critical Care Medicine. 1990:18:529–536.
7. Haglund, U., Abe, T., Bradie, I., Lundgren, O. The intestinal mucosal lesions in shock: studies of the pathogenesis. Eur. Surg. Res. 1976:8:448–460.
8. Deitch, E. Bacterial translocation of the gut flora. Journal of Trauma. 1990:30:s184-s189.
9. Lelli, J., Drongowoski, R., Coran, A., Abrams, G. Hypoxia-induced bacterial translocation in the puppy. Journal of Pediatric Surgery. 1992:27:974–982.
10. Jonsson, K., Jensen, J., Goodson, W., West, J Hunt, T. Assessment of perfusion in postoperative patients using tissue oxygen measurements. British Journal of Surgery:1987:74:263–267.
11. Gosain, A., Rabkin, J., Reymond, J., Jensen, J., Hunt, T., Upton, R. Tissue oxygen tension and other indicators of blood loss or organ perfusion during graded hemorrhage. Surgery:1991:109: 523–532.

40

EFFECTS OF HEMODILUTION AND OXYGEN BREATHING ON GUT OXYGENATION IN ANESTHETIZED DOGS

T. A. Walker,[1] S. E. Curtis,[1] P. E. Keipert,[3] W. E. Bradley,[2] and S. M. Cain[2]

[1]Departments of Pediatrics
[2]Physiology and Biophysics
University of Alabama at Birmingham
Birmingham, Alabama 35294–0005
[3]Alliance Pharmaceutical Corp.
San Diego, California 92121

INTRODUCTION

A heightened interest in perioperative strategies designed to reduce or avoid allogeneic blood transfusion has occurred as the list of potential transfusion-related complications has grown (Spahn, 1994). One such strategy, acute normovolemic hemodilution, involves the preoperative exchange of the patient's blood with colloid or crystalloid to a predetermined hematocrit. As a result, blood lost during surgery contains less red blood cells and the patient may be transfused with his own normal hematocrit blood as needed towards the completion of the procedure (Messmer, 1986). Because hemodilution reduces arterial oxygen content, cardiac output must increase in order to maintain systemic oxygen delivery. This is facilitated by a decrease in blood viscosity with resultant lowering of vascular resistance and left ventricular afterload (Cain, 1994). Also, flow need not increase in direct proportion to the decrease in systemic hematocrit for microvascular oxygen delivery to be maintained. This is because at the capillary level, hematocrit is normally only half that of systemic hematocrit and it remains nearly constant until systemic hematocrit falls to levels below 20% (Intaglietta, 1989). Therefore, tissue oxygenation is unlikely to be affected by moderate degrees of hemodilution, a concept which has been supported by direct measurements of tissue Po_2 in various organs (Messmer, 1973). Still, the limits of hemodilution remain ill-defined. Recent data suggest that hemodilution to a hemoglobin of ≈3 g/dl may be "clinically acceptable in young, healthy patients" (Fontana, 1995). Yet such conclusions are based on global measures of oxygen transport alone. Some of the animal data do suggest that tissue oxygenation is impaired during severe hemodilution. For example, Noldge et al. (1991) examined the effects of hemodilution (hemoglobin 4 g/dl) on splanchnic oxygenation in pigs and found that hepatic and small intestine serosal surface

Po$_2$ were significantly decreased. Because the gut mucosal layer appears to be especially vulnerable to hypoxia in other shock states (Vallet, 1994), we speculated that mucosal oxygenation may be even more affected by severe hemodilution than other tissues.

METHODS

Seven mongrel dogs were anesthetized with pentobarbital sodium (30 mg/kg iv initially), then supplemented as needed if a periodic toe pinch caused a change in arterial pressure or heart rate. The animals were volume ventilated through a cuffed endotracheal tube with room air to maintain Pco$_2$ between 30 and 35 Torr. Paralysis was achieved with succinylcholine (30 mg,im), followed by continuous infusion (0.1 mg/min iv). Catheters were placed in the carotid and pulmonary arteries for continuous measurement of blood pressure and for blood sampling. Through a midline laparotomy, the spleen was ligated and venous outflow from a segment of ileum was isolated as previously described by Vallet et al. (1994). Intestinal autoperfusion and innervation were maintained and all animals were anticoagulated with heparin. In an adjacent gut segment, mucosal and serosal surface Po$_2$ were measured with multiwire Po$_2$ electrodes (L. Eschweiler & Co, Kiel, Germany) and a saline-filled tonometer was inserted into the gut lumen to determine intramucosal pH (Vallet, 1994). Gut blood flow was measured with a Transonic^{tm} flow probe and oxygen uptake was calculated from flow and simultaneous measures of arterial and venous oxygen contents. Whole body oxygen uptake and cardiac output were determined from analysis of expired gases and arterial and mixed venous O$_2$ content differences. Gut lactate flux was calculated as the product of the arteriovenous difference and blood flow.

After an initial set of measurements, each animal was isovolemically hemodiluted with 5% albumin to a target hemoglobin of ≈8 g/dl. Following repeat measurements, the fraction of inspired O$_2$ was changed to 1.0 and progressive hemodilution was begun with 5% albumin at 0.75 ml/kg/min. Because the animals were anticoagulated and had undergone extensive surgery, they had ongoing blood loss which was compensated by volume infusion to maintain euvolemia. This allowed progressive hemodilution to a final hemoglobin of ≈3 g/dl over a one hour and 45 minute period. Blood volume was periodically assessed by Evans blue dye dilution. Hemodynamic and oxygen transport data were collected every 15 minutes and tissue Po$_2$ measurements with gut mucosal pH every 30 minutes.

RESULTS

Data for cardiac output and whole body oxygen delivery and oxygen uptake are shown in Figure 1. Cardiac output increased more than two-fold with hemodilution to a hemoglobin of 3 g/dl. Although oxygen delivery fell initially, it remained stable during the remainder of the protocol due to the increase in cardiac output and oxygen uptake never differed from baseline. Similar to the whole body, gut blood flow also more than doubled with progressive hemodilution (Figure 2). Initially, increased flow to the gut was unable to fully compensate for the reduction in oxygen content and oxygen delivery fell. Thereafter, oxygen delivery stabilized and always remained above reported critical levels (Nelson, 1987). Oxygen uptake followed a pattern similar to delivery.

Mean values for gut mucosal and serosal tissue Po$_2$ are depicted in Figure 3. Mucosal Po$_2$ decreased with hemodilution to 8 g/dl, was restored with hyperoxia, then fell

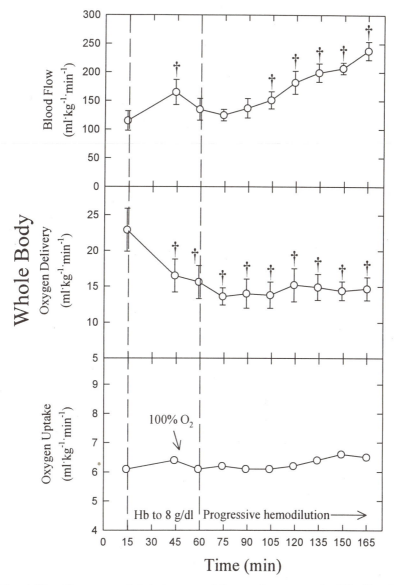

Figure 1. Mean ± SE cardiac output, whole body oxygen delivery and oxygen uptake. †Significantly different from baseline (p<.05).

significantly (p<.05) with progressive hemodilution to values 50% of baseline. Although there was some variability, serosal Po_2 did not change significantly over time. Coincident with reductions in mucosal Po_2 was an increase in gut lactate production (Figure 4, top). The initial increase in gut lactate was associated with the fall in oxygen delivery; however, the increase observed during progressive hemodilution occurred without any change in gut oxygen delivery or uptake. Compared to baseline (3.1 ± 1.4 mM/L), whole body arterial lactate was significantly increased during the first hour after the initial hemodilution (4.0 ± 1.5 mM/L), but returned to values not different from baseline (3.6 ± 1.1 mM/L) for

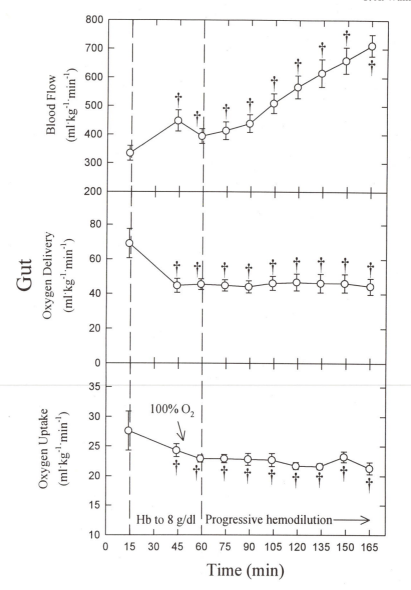

Figure 2. Mean ± SE gut blood flow, oxygen delivery, and oxygen uptake. †Significantly different from baseline (p<.05).

the remainder of the study. As illustrated in Figure 4 (bottom), mucosal pH remained unchanged despite evidence of impaired mucosal oxygenation.

DISCUSSION

The principle finding in this model of severe hemodilution was that the gut mucosa demonstrated greater sensitivity to anemic hypoxia than did gut serosa. This was suggested by significantly decreased surface tissue Po$_2$ measurements in the mucosa but not

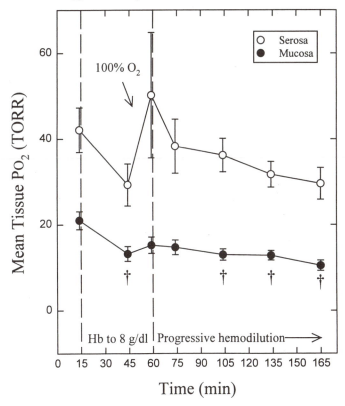

Figure 3. Mean ± SE gut mucosal and serosal tissue Po_2. †Significantly different from baseline (p<.05).

in the serosa. The fact that gut lactate output increased as mucosal Po_2 fell provides supportive evidence that the mucosa became significantly hypoxic with progressive hemodilution. These responses occurred without any measurable changes in gut oxygen uptake and in whole body arterial lactate and oxygen uptake. Although mucosal oxygen uptake per unit of weight may be greater than that of muscularis and the remainder of the gut wall, its proportion of total gut weight is smaller. It is reasonable, therefore, that a decrease in mucosal oxygen uptake alone may not have been detected by the global measurement. Methodology to determine regional oxygen uptake within the gut wall is not yet available.

Previous animal studies have demonstrated impaired gut oxygenation with hemodilution (Kiel, 1989; Noldge, 1991). Using a canine isolated jejunum prep, Kiel et al. (1989) found that hemodilution to a hematocrit of 20% caused a decrease in gut oxygen delivery despite an increase in blood flow and that, in addition, oxygen extraction was impaired. They and others (Fink, 1991) have suggested that the anatomic arrangement of villous arterioles may predispose the mucosa to hypoxia. Because these arterioles branch at right angles to the villi, a process termed plasma skimming (Jodal and Lundgren, 1970) may occur and, as a result, blood with a lower hematocrit is delivered to the mucosal villi. Indeed, if similar mechanisms were operative in our more severe hemodilution model, oxygen delivery may have been even further compromised and would explain the observed reductions in mucosal Po_2.

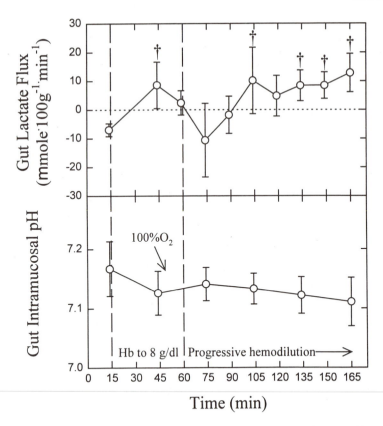

Figure 4. Mean ± SE gut lactate flux (top) and gut intramucosal pH (bottom). †Significantly different from baseline (p<.05).

Another finding of this study was that the observed mucosal dysoxia was not detected by intramucosal pH monitoring. Although mucosal pH was trending downward, the changes were not statistically significant. One explanation for this may be that the degree of dysoxia may have been insufficient to alter mucosal pH. However, as mucosal oxygenation decreased, the gut began to produce lactate and it is conceivable that with continued monitoring a pH change may have been detected.

In summary, the limits of hemodilution will ultimately be determined by tissue and cellular responses to anemic hypoxia. We have shown in dogs that the gut mucosa may experience impaired oxygenation during severe hemodilution without similar impairment evident at the serosal surface or from measures of systemic oxygen uptake. This may have direct clinical relevance particularly in view of the proposed role that the gut mucosa may play in the pathophysiology of sepsis and the multiple organ dysfunction syndrome.

ACKNOWLEDGMENTS

Supported by funds from Alliance Pharmaceutical Corp.

REFERENCES

Cain, S.M., 1994, Oxygen delivery and intentional hemodilution. *Adv. Exp. Biol. Med.* 361:271–278.

Fink, M.P., 1991, Gastrointestinal mucosal injury in experimental models of shock, trauma, and sepsis. *Crit. Care Med.* 19:627–641.

Fontana, J.L., Welborn, L., Mongan, P.D., Sturm, P., Martin, G., and Bunger, R., 1995, Oxygen consumption and cardiovascular function in children during profound intraoperative normovolemic hemodilution. *Anesth. Analg.* 80:219–225.

Intaglietta, M., 1989, Microcirculatory effects of hemodilution: background and analysis. In: Tuma, R.F., White, J.V., and Messmer, K. (eds.) *The Role of Hemodilution in Optimal Patient Care.* W. Zuckschwerdt Verlag Munchen, pp 21–40.

Jodal, M., and Lundgren, O., 1970, Plasma skimming in the intestinal tract. *Acta Physiol. Scand.* 80:50–60.

Kiel, J.W., Riedel, G.L., and Shepherd, A.P., 1989, Effects of hemodilution on gastric and intestinal oxygenation. *Am. J. Physiol.* 25:H171-H178.

Messmer, K., Kreimeier, U., and Intaglietta, M., 1986, Present state of intentional hemodilution. *Eur. Surg. Res.* 18:254–263.

Messmer, K., Sunder-Plassmann, L., Jesch, F., Gornandt, L., Sinagowitz, E., and Kessler, M., 1973, Oxygen supply to the tissues during limited normovolemic hemodilution. *Res. Exp. Med.* 159:152–166.

Nelson, D.P., King, C.E., Dodd, S.L., Schumacker, P.T., and Cain, S.M., 1987, Systemic and intestinal limits of oxygen extraction in the dog. *J. Appl. Physiol.* 63:387–394.

Noldge, G.F., Priebe, H.J., Bohle, W., Buttler, K.J., and Geiger, K., 1991, Effects of acute normovolemic hemodilution on splanchnic oxygenation and on hepatic histology and metabolism in anesthetized pigs. *Anesthesiology* 74:908–918.

Spahn, D.R., Leone, B.J., Reves, J.G., and Pasch, T., 1994, Cardiovascular and coronary physiology of acute isovolemic hemodilution: A review of nonoxygen-carrying and oxygen-carrying solutions. *Anesth. Analg.* 78:1000–1021.

Vallet, B., Lund, N., Curtis, S.E., Kelly, D., and Cain, S.M., 1994, Gut and muscle tissue PO_2 in endotoxemic dogs during shock and resuscitation. *J. Appl. Physiol.* 76:793–800.

41

EQUAL OXYGEN DELIVERY MAY NOT RESULT IN EQUAL OXYGEN CONSUMPTION

Guo-Fan Ye,[1] Frans F. Jöbsis-VanderVliet,[2] Paul D. Jöbsis,[2]
Stephen E. Dubin,[1] Wenyao Shi,[1] and Dov Jaron[1]

[1]Biomedical Engineering and Science Institute
Drexel University
Philadelphia, Pennsylvania 19104
[2]Department of Cell Biology
Duke University Medical Center
Durham, North Carolina 27710

1. INTRODUCTION

This communication presents our recent modeling and experimental study on the relationship between oxygen consumption rate and delivery rate. Oxygen consumption rate ($\dot{V}o_2$) by an organ is regarded to represent its tissue O_2 metabolic rate. Under steady state, $\dot{V}o_2$ is usually determined from the product of blood flow rate and the arteriovenous O_2 concentration difference across the organ. Oxygen delivery rate ($\dot{D}o_2$) is defined as the product of arterial O_2 concentration and blood flow rate. Numerous investigations of the relationship between $\dot{D}o_2$ and $\dot{V}o_2$ have been reported. Many of these studies were related to the biphasic supply-dependent O_2 consumption concept for tissue hypoxia determination[1][2]. The biphasic concept states that, for a given energy demand by the tissue, a plot of $\dot{V}o_2$ versus $\dot{D}o_2$ displays two distinct regions (or phases). In one region, $\dot{V}o_2$ remains constant regardless of changes in $\dot{D}o_2$. When $\dot{D}o_2$ declines below a threshold value (the "critical $\dot{D}o_2$"), $\dot{V}o_2$ becomes an approximately linear function of $\dot{D}o_2$.

This concept led to two conclusions[2]. First, that O_2 consumption rate is dependent only on O_2 delivery rate, i.e., the value of the critical $\dot{D}o_2$ is the same under stagnant hypoxia due to falling blood flow, hypoxic hypoxia due to falling arterial O_2-Hb saturation (So_2), or anemic hypoxia due to falling Hb concentration. Second, that augmenting O_2 delivery rate through elevation of blood flow rate, increased arterial So_2, or increased systemic hematocrit is, in principle, equally beneficial to ameliorating tissue hypoxia.

A number of microcirculatory mechanisms, such as O_2-Hb dissociation, O_2 convection, diffusion and metabolism, and the Bohr and Haldane effects, are involved in tissue oxygen transport. There are, however, few mathematical models that study the $\dot{D}o_2$-$\dot{V}o_2$ relationship in an organ by simulating oxygen transport in the microcirculation. We carried out a computer simulation and preliminary animal experiment to investigate the effects of microcirculatory input variables on cerebral $\dot{D}o_2$-$\dot{V}o_2$ relationship under steady state. The results were compared with the conclusions of the biphasic concept.

2. METHODS

2.1. Model Simulation

Our multicompartmental steady-state model for O_2-CO_2 coupled transport in the cat brain microcirculation[3][4] was employed to investigate the relationship between oxygen delivery rate and oxygen consumption rate. The model contains 3 arteriole compartments, 1 capillary compartment, 3 venule compartments and 1 tissue compartment (Fig.1). Gases diffuse between every vessel compartment and the metabolic tissue compartment. The governing equations and the relevant lumped parameters of the model were developed through space-averaging the corresponding distributed model[5][3] and include O_2-Hb dissociation, O_2 convection and diffusion, and the Bohr and Haldane effects. Different from earlier multicompartmental models, the effects of radial blood diffusion resistance, discrete nature of capillary blood, difference in metabolism between vessel wall and tissue, and dependence of tissue metabolic rate on tissue oxygen partial pressure were taken into consideration. These features have significant effects on the model predictions[6].

The simulation was first performed for two cases under normal cerebral oxygen delivery rate. For each case, the same oxygen delivery rate was employed by using different combinations of blood flow rate and arterial O_2 concentration. The two combinations were normal blood flow rate (0.68 ml/sec) with normal arterial O_2 concentration (corresponding to a Po_2A value of 98.5 mmHg under Pco_2A value of 40 mmHg), and twice normal blood flow with one half normal arterial O_2 concentration caused by a reduced O_2 saturation. The simulation was then performed for two types of hypoxia: stagnant hypoxia and hypoxic hypoxia. Stagnant hypoxia was simulated by setting blood flow rate to one half normal while maintaining normal arterial O_2 concentration. Hypoxic hypoxia was simulated by setting arterial O_2 concentration to one half normal while maintaining normal blood flow rate. Other parameters of the model were the same as described in our previous model[3][4]. For example, the systemic hematocrit was set to normal value (45%) for all the above cases. The maximal metabolic rate and the Michaelis-Menten constant (the value of tissue Po_2 when metabolic rate declines to

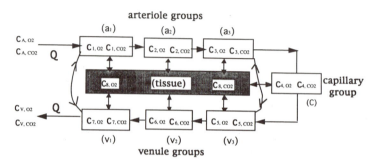

Figure 1. Block diagram of the multicompartmental model for O_2-CO_2 coupled transport in the microcirculation. (C: concentration, Q: blood flow rate, A: arterial, a: arteriole, c: capillary, v: venule, V: venous)

one half maximum) for the brain tissue were set to 0.00144 ml O_2/sec/ml and 5 mmHg. The CO_2/O_2 respiratory quotient was set to 0.8.

For each set of input data (blood flow rate and arterial Po_2), the model predicted the compartmental distribution of Po_2, Pco_2, O_2-Hb saturation, pH, O_2 concentration and CO_2 concentration. $\dot{D}o_2$ to the brain was then determined from the product of blood flow rate and arterial O_2 concentration; and $\dot{V}o_2$ was calculated from the product of blood flow rate and arteriovenous difference of O_2 concentration.

2.2. Animal Experiment

The effects of microcirculatory input variables on the cerebral $\dot{D}o_2$-$\dot{V}o_2$ relationship were examined in two rabbits under stagnant hypoxia and hypoxic hypoxia. The near-infrared spectroscopy (NIRS) technique developed by Jöbsis[7] was used to monitor the time course of cerebral tissue oxygen level.

Two female New Zealand White Rabbits weighing 2.8 and 3.2 kg were initially sedated by intramuscular injection of 20 mg/kg ketamine and 8 mg/kg xylazine. A lateral ear vein was cannulated for intravenous injection of a similar mixture for additional and continuing anesthesia. The rabbit was restrained in dorsal recumbency. An incision was made in the ventral midline of the neck for about 2" craniad from the manubrium sterni. An angular incision was made in the trachea and a "Y" cannula was inserted into the trachea distad and the other arms of this cannula were connected to a small animal volume controlled respirator (Harvard piston type). The respiratory parameters were initially adjusted to 15 ml volume and 40 per minute rate. During the entire experiment, the respiratory rate was controlled to maintain a normal arterial CO_2 level unless additional CO_2 is intentionally imposed.

The neck incision was extended distally to the midpoint of the sternum. The thymus tissue was dissected free so as to expose the origins of the common carotid artery (source of both external carotids and the right vertebral artery) on the right; as well as the left subclavian artery (source of the left vertebral artery) extending to the left and dorsally. Vascular occluding slings were passed around these last two vessels. This eliminated blood flow to the brain through the vertebral path, permitting control of cerebral blood flow through the carotid artery. The pericardium was opened to facilitate dissection and visulization of the vessels.

The femoral artery was cannulated for blood sampling. Using a GEM-STAT blood-gas analyzer (Mallinckrodt), blood samples were used to measure systemic hematocrit and O_2 and CO_2 partial pressures (Po_2a, Pco_2a) in the femoral artery. An electromagnetic flow-probe (BL-613) was placed around the exposed carotid artery. Both pulsatile and mean flow (Qp and Qm) were recorded using a chart recorder. The two optrodes of the NIRS instrument (Niroscope™ Monitor, Vander Corp., Durham, NC) were attached to the skin at both temples using a stereotaxic head-holder. Changes in cytochrome a,a3 redox state (aa3) representing space-averaged cerebral tissue PO_2, quantities of the reduced hemoglobin (Hb) and oxyhemoglobin (HbO_2), and total volume of cerebral blood (BV) were monitored by the Niroscope™ and recorded both by a chart recorder and by a IBM-compatible computer.

Blood samples were withdrawn and all data were recorded under "control" condition. Stagnant hypoxia was produced by lifting up a constriction sling around the common segment of the left and right carotid arteries so that mean blood flow rate was reduced by 50%. Thus, the O_2 delivery rate was decreased to 50% of normal. The time course of the monitored parameters was recorded and blood was sampled when a steady state was reached. The sling was then released. After all parameters stabilized, a gas mixture of 9.7% O_2 and 90.3% N_2 was used to replace the room air for the ventilator. Following the initial insult, the sling was used to narrow the carotid diameter in order to compensate for the effects of cerebral autoregulation and to maintain the same carotid blood flow rate. During this run, the O_2 delivery rate was decreased to 47% of normal. The time course of the monitored parameters was recorded and blood was sampled when a steady state was reached. The O_2-N_2 mixture was then replaced by room air. A rapid and complete carotid occlusion was then performed for 3 minutes using the constriction sling and all variables were recorded. At the completion of the experiments, an extra anesthetic dose was provided and the rabbits were euthanized using 100% N_2 while monitoring heart rate and arterial blood pressure.

3. RESULTS

3.1. Model Simulation

Figure 2 compares the compartmental Po_2 distributions of the two different cases with the same normal cerebral oxygen delivery rate (0.13 ml O_2/sec). Note that cerebral tissue Po_2 under conditions of twice normal blood flow with one half normal arterial O_2 concentration (8.4 mmHg) was apparently lower than that in the case of normal blood flow rate with normal arterial O_2 concentration (28.9 mmHg). The resultant oxygen extraction ratio ($\dot{V}o_2/\dot{D}o_2$) was 0.39 and 0.59 for each combination, respectively. Figure 3 compares the compartmental Po_2 distributions under stagnant hypoxia and hypoxic hypoxia with the same reduced oxygen delivery rate (0.066 ml O_2/sec). Note that cerebral tissue Po_2 under hypoxic hypoxia (6.6 mmHg) was lower than that under stagnant hypoxia (17.0 mmHg). The resultant O_2 extraction ratio was 0.71 and 0.96 for each combination, respectively.

3.2. Animal Experiment

Figure 4 depicts the time course of the Niroscope™ output variables after a step carotid occlusion. Note the decrease in HbO_2, the increase in Hb, and the rapid decrease in total blood volume and oxidized aa3. Also note that aa3 approached its baseline about 25 seconds after the occlusion, suggesting that cerebral tissue PO_2 dropped to a very low level at that time. Figure 5a shows that there was only a slight decrease in the aa3 level when carotid blood flow was reduced by 50% from its normal value. Figure 5b reveals

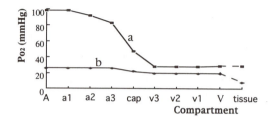

Figure 2. Compartmental Po_2 distributions predicted by the O_2-CO_2 coupled model for two different combinations of blood flow rate Q and arterial O_2 concentration but with the same normal cerebral O_2 delivery rate (0.13 ml O_2/sec). **a**: normal blood flow rate (0.68 ml/sec) with normal arterial O_2 concentration (corresponding to a partial pressure of 98.5 mmHg under the Pco_2A value of 40 mmHg); **b**: twice normal blood flow rate with one half normal arterial O_2 concentration (due to reduced arterial O_2 saturation). In the figure, A represents the input artery, a1, a_2 and a3 represent arteriole compartments, cap represents the capillary compartment, v3, v2 and v1 represent venule compartments, V represents the vein, and tissue represents the tissue compartment.

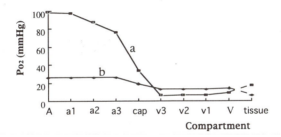

Figure 3. Compartmental Po_2 distributions predicted by the O_2-CO_2 coupled model under stagnant hypoxia and hypoxic hypoxia with the same reduced cerebral O_2 delivery rate (0.066 ml O_2/sec). **a**: stagnant hypoxia (one half normal blood flow rate with normal arterial O_2 concentration); **b**: hypoxic hypoxia (normal blood flow rate with one half normal arterial O_2 concentration).

that there was, however, a significant drop in the aa3 level after room air was replaced by a gas mixture of 9.7% O_2 and 90.3% N_2 (before blood flow adjustment). This result was not significantly changed when the blood flow rate was recovered by the sling.

4. DISCUSSION

Figure 2 suggests that, doubling the flow rate and halving arterial O_2 concentration resulted in lower $\dot{V}o_2$ even though $\dot{D}o_2$ was unchanged. In other words, restoring O_2 delivery rate from hypoxic hypoxia to normal by elevating blood flow rate is not as beneficial as restoring arterial So_2 level. Figure 3 suggests that $\dot{V}o_2$ under hypoxic hypoxia was lower than that under stagnant hypoxia. Therefore, the critical oxygen delivery for hypoxic hypoxia may be different from that for stagnant hypoxia. All above predictions are different from the conclusion of the biphasic concept.

The difference in compartmental Po_2 distribution between the two cases depicted in Figure 2 and Figure 3 reflects the effects of microcirculatory mechanisms in oxygen transport. In other words, $\dot{V}o_2$ may depend on not only the input variables, but also the mechanisms and parameters of microcirculatory gas transport which determine tissue Po_2.

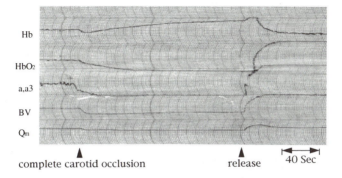

Figure 4. The responses of the Niroscope™ output variables to a step occlusion of carotid artery. (Hb: reduced hemoglobin; HbO_2: oxidized hemoglobin; aa3: oxidized cytochrome a,a3; BV: total blood volume; Qm: mean carotid blood flow rate.)

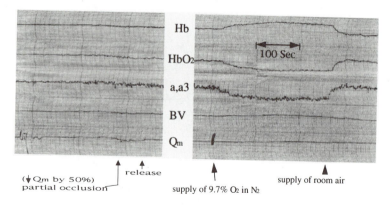

Figure 5. A comparison of the Niroscope™ output variables under reduced cerebral blood flow (a) and under reduced arterial O_2 saturation (b).

Figure 5 suggests that cerebral tissue PO_2 under hypoxic hypoxia was much lower than that under stagnant hypoxia, even though the amount of oxygen delivered under both conditions was similar. Oxygen consumption rate reflects tissue metabolism, and tissue metabolic rate is a function of tissue Po_2. Thus, our preliminary experiment appears to support the prediction of the model that stagnant hypoxia and hypoxic hypoxia may result in different cerebral oxygen consumption rate even though oxygen delivery rate is approximately the same. Both simulation and experimental results suggest significant change in cerebral tissue Po_2 when the combination of blood flow rate and arterial O_2 concentration changed but oxygen delivery rate was unchanged. The results demonstrated that $\dot{V}o_2$ is determined not only by $\dot{D}o_2$, but, at least, also by input variables such as arterial O_2 concentration and blood flow rate.

ACKNOWLEDGMENTS

This research was supported in part by the National Science Foundation under grant No. BES 9400329.

REFERENCES

1. Cain, S. M. Oxygen delivery and uptake in dogs during anemic and hypoxic hypoxia. *J. Appl. Physiol.* **42**, 228–234, 1977.
2. Samsel, R. W., and Schumacker, P. T. Oxygen delivery to tissue. *Eur. Respir. J.* **4**, 1258–1267, 1991.
3. Ye, G.-F., Moore, T. W., Buerk, D. G., and Jaron, D. A compartmental model for oxygen-carbon dioxide coupled transport in the microcirculation. *Ann. Biomed. Eng.* **22(5)**, 464–479, 1994.
4. Ye, G.-F., and Jaron, D. Regional delivery of oxygen and carbon dioxide in the microcirculation. in *Proc.16th Annual International Conf. of the IEEE Engineering in Medicine & Biology Society* , Baltimore, pp. 1166–1167, 1994.
5. Ye, G.-F., Moore, T. W., and Jaron, D. Contributions of oxygen dissociation and convection to the behavior of a compartmental oxygen transport model. *Microvas. Res.* **46**, 1–13, 1993.
6. Ye, G.-F., Buerk, D. G., and Jaron, D. Arteriolar contribution to microcirculatory CO2/O2 exchange, *Microvasc. Res.*, in press.
7. Jöbsis, F. F. Noninvasive, infrared monitoring of cerebral and myocardial oxygen sufficiency and circulatory parameters. *Science* **198**, 1264–1267, 1977.

42

MODIFICATION OF LOW DENSITY LIPOPROTEINS BY ERYTHROCYTES AND HEMOGLOBIN UNDER HYPOXIC CONDITIONS

C. Balagopalakrishna,[1] R. Nirmala,[1] J. M. Rifkind,[1] and S. Chatterjee[2]

[1]Laboratory of Cellular and Molecular Biology
National Institutes of Health, National Institute on Aging
4940 Eastern Avenue
Baltimore, Maryland
[2]Department of Pediatrics and Medicine
Lipid Research Atherosclerosis Unit
Johns Hopkins University School of Medicine
Baltimore, Maryland

ABSTRACT

Oxidation of low density lipoprotein (LDL) has been implicated in atherogenesis. It has also been suggested that modification of LDL in the presence of endothelial and smooth muscle cells is associated with the production of superoxide. Red cells and hemoglobin have been shown to be a source for enhanced superoxide production under hypoxic conditions. We now show that incubation of LDL with both hemoglobin and erythrocytes under hypoxic conditions produces the increased Relative Electrophoretic Mobility (REM) associated with LDL oxidation. With hypoxic hemoglobin, this reaction is over within 10 minutes, appreciably faster than other *in vitro* methods for LDL oxidation. The increased REM was found to be associated with partial deoxygenation of hemoglobin indicative of appreciable oxygen utilization and a more hypoxic state. At later times, the modified LDL was found to produce enhanced hemoglobin oxidation. The resultant modified LDL was shown to have elevated TBARS indicative of LDL oxidation. In addition, it was found to induce smooth muscle cell proliferation which is one of the biological factors thought to be associated with atherogenesis. The relatively rapid LDL modification detected with hypoxic erythrocytes and hemoglobin suggest that even under *in vivo* conditions with the antioxidants present in plasma, oxidation may still occur in the circulation with the associated vascular damage occurring as the blood containing elevated levels of oxidized LDL leave the pulmonary circulation.

1. INTRODUCTION

Until recently, detection of significant amounts of extracellular superoxide anion has been a phenomenon associated with the metabolism of activated phagocytes. We have shown recently[1] that under hypoxic conditions, erythrocytes are a source of increased flux of superoxide radicals due to the well known tendency of hemoglobin to autoxidize:

$$HbO_2 \quad \text{------------>} \quad Hb^+ \quad + \quad O^{2-.}$$

Oxyhemoglobin   methemoglobin   Superoxide

Autoxidation of hemoglobin is enhanced at reduced oxygen pressures, with maximum rate in oxidation seen when hemoglobin is 60–70 % oxygenated (Fig. 1). This increased oxidation under reduced O_2 pressures is due to a higher population of doubly and triply liganded states of oxyhemoglobin, which oxidize much more readily than fully liganded oxyhemoglobin.

In view of the proximity of the low density lipoproteins (LDL) to erythrocytes in circulation, we examined the possibility of oxidative modification of LDL by red cells and hemoglobin under hypoxic conditions. Oxidative modification of LDL has been suggested to play a major role in atherogenesis as well as in lesion propagation and pathogenesis as judged from the uptake of oxidized LDL by macrophages and the injury that is seen when cells in culture are exposed to oxidized LDL.[3] Oxidized LDL is also known to alter growth factor[4] and cytokine production,[5] to induce monocyte recruitment and adhesion to endothelium and alter cell migration and growth.[6] While several oxidants have been shown to modify LDL under *in vitro* conditions[7] viz., various cell lines, copper, iron, etc., the source of *in vivo* oxidants for LDL is still under debate. Using oxygenation levels of 60–70 % as found in the venous circulation, we found that LDL is more rapidly modified by red cells and hemoglobin under hypoxic conditions. In addition, the hypoxic modified LDL caused a greater proliferation of aortic smooth muscle cells than what is seen with LDL modified with $CuSO_4$.

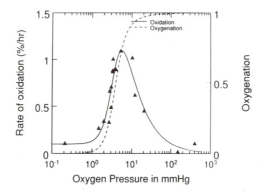

Figure 1. Rate of oxidation of purified human hemoglobin as a function of oxygen pressure, 0.05 M phosphate, pH 7.4, 0.1 mM NaCl, 0.1 mM EDTA, 25,000 U/ml catalase, and 75,000 U/ml superoxide dismutase (-▲-), oxidation; (—), oxygenation. (reproduced with permission from ref. 2)

2. EXPERIMENTAL PROCEDURES

2.1. Cells

Rabbit aorta smooth muscle cells were prepared from normolipedemic rabbits according to the procedure of Ross.[8]

2.2. LDL Isolation and Characterization

LDL was isolated from human blood plasma from healthy donors in the presence of EDTA by sequential ultracentrifugation. The LDL fraction was isolated between densities of 1.022–1.063 gm/ml. Total protein content of the LDL preparation was determined according to Lowry's procedure. The purity of the LDL preparation was determined by agarose gel electrophoresis and stained with red oil.

2.3. Preparation of Hypoxic Red Cells and Hemoglobin and LDL Oxidation

Fresh blood was obtained from the healthy participants of the Baltimore Longitudinal Studies on Aging (BLSA) and was freed from white cells by an initial percoll wash, followed by two washings with phosphate buffered saline, containing 0.1 mM EDTA, pH 7.4, at 4^0 C. By this procedure all the buffy coat and plasma were completely removed. The packed cells were then diluted to 5 % hematocrit and used for the experiments.

Hemoglobin samples were prepared from fresh erythrocyte lysates, obtained after centrifugation at 18000 rpm for 30 minutes to remove membranes. Hemoglobin A_0 was obtained from the Letterman Army Institute of Research at the presidio of San Francisco.

Hypoxic samples were obtained by deoxygenating red cells (5% HCT) and HbO_2 (A_0 or hemolysate, 0.5 mM) in a Labconco glove box to the desired P_{O2} (6 mm Hg that corresponds to 55–70 % oxygenation levels) and equilibrated by gentle rocking. The hypoxic modification of LDL was initiated by mixing erythrocytes or the hemoglobin solution with LDL [keeping the ratio of volumes of LDL:oxidant at 1:4] within the glove box. At various time points, aliquots from the reaction mixture were pipetted out into eppendorf tubes followed by addition of BHT (45 µm) which arrests further oxidation. The samples were stored at 4^0 C until analysis. Aliquots of the hypoxy samples (red cells and hemoglobin) were also transferred to specially designed spectroscopic cells with ground glass joints and provided with a side arm, for determining the oxy, deoxy, and methemoglobin levels and to spectrophotometrically follow the changes that occur when oxidants (heme proteins) are mixed with LDL in the side arm under the above pressures.

The fully-oxidized-LDL under normoxic conditions was obtained by dialyzing LDL against a 10 µm solution of $CuSO_4$ in phosphate buffered saline, overnight at 4^0 C. The oxidation was terminated with BHT.

2.4. Incubation of Smooth Muscle Cells with LDL Modified by Red Cells, Hemoglobin and $CUSO_4$

Confluent cultures of smooth muscle cells, within passage 3–5 were trypsinized and seeded (1 X 10^4) in 96 well microtiter plates. Such cells were incubated with Eagle's minimum essential medium, containing 10 % fetal calf serum, essential amino acids and glutamine. On the fourth day of the cell growth, medium was removed and cells were incubated for 2 hours with Ham's F-10 serum free medium. Both the hypoxic and copper modified LDL samples were then added to these cells at various concentrations (5, 10, 50 and 100 μg LDL/ml) and left overnight in the incubator.

2.5. Assay

2.5.1. Cell Proliferation. Proliferation of cells was assessed by incorporation of [³H] thymidine (2 μ C_i/ml F-10 medium) in the presence of 0.7 μg/ml thymidine, for 2 hours, at 37 degrees. The incorporation of [³H]thymidine into DNA was measured by radiocount.

2.5.2. Thiobarbituric Acid Reactive Substances (TBARS). The elevated levels of TBARS in oxidized LDL samples was estimated spectrophotometrically using malonaldehyde as a standard.[9]

3. RESULTS AND DISCUSSION

3.1. Relative Electrophoretic Migration (REM)

The hypoxic incubation of LDL with erythrocytes and hemoglobin at 6 mm Hg leads to rapid modification as evinced by complete absence of the usually detected "lag phase"[9] during the initial stages of the reaction. The REM behavior under hypoxia further shows a greater migration when compared with the behavior under normoxic conditions.[10] With erythrocytes, a 10 minute incubation produced a REM of 1.47 with an additional gradual increase in the electrophoretic migration to REM of 1.58 after 6 hours (Fig. 2a). For LDL incubated with partially oxygenated hemoglobin, the REM at 10 minutes was found to be 2.58 and it remained at this level for an additional 20 minutes. Afterwards, the REM decreased and after 6 hours it was 1.42 (Fig. 2b).

Under normoxic conditions, Paganga *et al*[10] observed REM of LDL to remain unchanged at 1 in the first two hours and then over the next 6 hours it gradually increases to a REM value of only 1.68. The lag phase that is usually observed in LDL modification, is actually taken to be a measure of the resistance exerted by β-carotene, and α-tocopherol (antioxidants present in LDL), to LDL modification by oxidants. The absence of such a lag phase under hypoxic conditions in the present study, indicates that both erythrocytes and hemoglobin under hypoxic conditions act as strong oxidants either by rapidly neutralizing the intrinsic antioxidants in LDL, or by bypassing the antioxidants, to cause substantial changes in the charge of the LDL.

3.2. TBARS

Increased amount of TBARS was seen during LDL oxidation. The concentration of TBARS (after 20 min incubation) follows the order LDL (modified with hypoxic hemoglobin) > LDL (modified with normoxic hemoglobin) > LDL (modified with hypoxic erythrocytes) (Fig. 3).

Further, the concentration of TBARS formed on LDL modified with hypoxic hemoglobin is nearly comparable to that seen when LDL was modified with $CuSO_4$ for 24 hours. As has been noted elsewhere,[11] when the concentration of lipid peroxides reach a threshold level of 40 nmoles/mg protein upon oxidative modification, LDL becomes cyto-

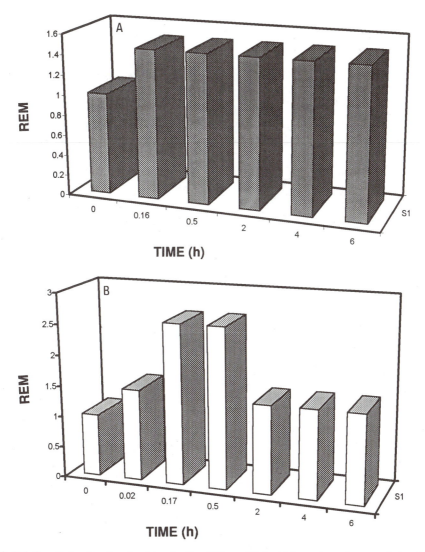

Figure 2. Relative electrophoretic migration of native LDL modified with hypoxic erythrocytes (2a) and hemoglobin (2b). The increased REM levels within the first one hour shows absence of "lag phase" in the hypoxic modification of LDL.

toxic, chemotactic and gets phagocytosed by macrophages. In the present case, such levels are observed in LDL modified with normoxic hemoglobin (62.55 nmoles/mg protein), hypoxic hemoglobin (71.34 nmoles/mg protein), and $CuSO_4$ (76.51 nmoles/mg protein) pointing to extensive oxidation.

3.3. Oxygen Consumption

During initial stages of the reaction with LDL, there was a rapid decrease in the oxygenation of oxyhemoglobin from 52 % to 34 %, i.e. LDL converts oxyhemoglobin to a

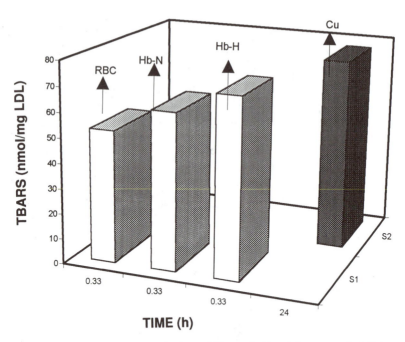

Figure 3. The concentration of TBARS determined on a LDL sample (5 mg/ml concentration) that was incubated with different oxidants, viz., hypoxic erythrocytes (5 % hct, 20 minutes, RBC), normoxic hemoglobin (0.5 mM, 20 minutes, Hb-N), hypoxic hemoglobin (0.5 mM, 20 minutes, Hb-H), and CuSO₄ (10 μM, 24 hours, Cu).

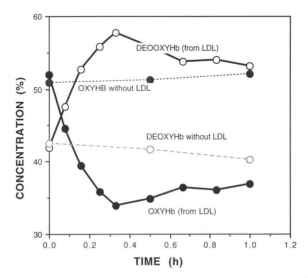

Figure 4. Deoxygenation of partially oxygenated hemoglobin in the first one hour of reaction of LDL with partially oxygenated hemoglobin. The percent oxy levels were calculated at different time intervals from visible spectrophotometry, by monitoring the spectral changes in the region 490–640 nm.

more deoxy form (Fig. 4). This decrease corresponds to an oxygen consumption in the range of 0.18 μm/mg. LDL. Presumably, this oxygen is used up for LDL oxidation.

3.4. Hemoglobin Oxidation

LDL incubation also results in an increase in hemoglobin oxidation. During the initial phase of the reaction, a 3.1 fold increase in the rate of oxidation was found. After this initial period, there is drop in the rate of oxidation with and without LDL. During this later period there is a 1.6 fold increase in the rate was seen which persists for 2 days (Fig. 5).

It is to be noted that oxidative reactions with LDL are known to involve peroxy, alkoxy, tocopheryl, and hydrocarbon radicals of different kinds that take part in many redox reactions. Hence it is not clear as to what factors lead to increased oxidation of hemoglobin.

3.5. Smooth Muscle Cell Proliferation

Proliferation of myointimal vascular smooth muscle cells is a prominent hallmark of atherosclerosis.[12,13] It is believed that injured endothelium produces growth factors that act on the neighboring smooth muscle cells to promote their proliferation.[14] The proliferation brought about by LDL that was modified by incubation with hypoxic hemoglobin (at 6 mm Hg) for 20 minutes, was compared with the effects produced by LDL that has been incubated with normoxic hemoglobin as well as with the LDL oxidized by $CuSO_4$ (Fig. 5). $CuSO_4$ oxidized LDL and LDL incubated with normoxic hemoglobin produced 2.7 fold proliferation of smooth muscle cells. On the other hand, hypoxic hemoglobin modified LDL produced a 4.8 fold proliferation of smooth muscle cells. In all cases while the proliferation dropped with higher doses of modified LDL, differences were distinct in each case. The $CuSO_4$ modified LDL became toxic when the dosage was in the region of 100 μg. At the same dosage, the hypoxic hemoglobin modified LDL continued to produce

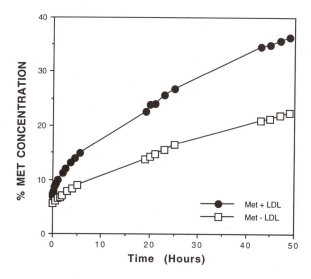

Figure 5. Oxidation of partially oxygenated hemoglobin in the first one hour of reaction of LDL with partially oxygenated hemoglobin. The percent met levels were calculated at different time intervals from visible spectrophotometry, by monitoring the spectral changes in the region 490–640 nm.

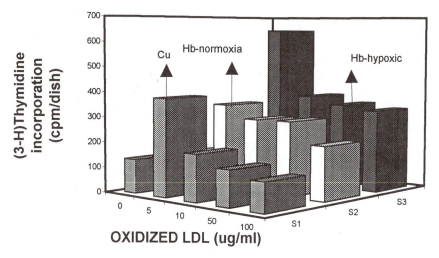

Figure 6. A comparison of the proliferation of smooth muscle cells seen when the cell culture was incubated with hypoxic, normoxic and CuSO$_4$ modified LDL at different concentrations (5, 10, 50, and 100 µg/ml). Proliferation seen (from radiocounting of incorporated ^{3}H-Thymidine) follows the order hypoxic hemoglobin modified LDL > normoxic hemoglobin modified LDL ~ CuSO$_4$ modified LDL.

smooth muscle cell proliferation at enhanced levels (2.4 fold). The normoxic hemoglobin modified LDL also continued to cause proliferation but at a lower rate (1.6 fold). It is important to note that even at 100 µg dosage (considered as toxic) of hypoxic hemoglobin modified LDL, the proliferation of smooth muscle cells is similar to the maximum proliferation seen with CuSO$_4$ modified LDL at 5 µg thereby indicating that hypoxic hemoglobin modified LDL is more potent than any other oxidant known thus far.

While it is known that aggregated platelets produce migration and proliferation factors that induce smooth muscle cells in the media to migrate into the intima and to proliferate there, our studies show for the first time that red cells and hemoglobin modified LDL can also bring about increase proliferation of aortic smooth muscle cells. While the significance of LDL modification by this pathway is not certain presently, it can be nevertheless assumed that in situations like restenosis or inflammations when erythrocyte lysis occurs, LDL modification by this pathway is certainly feasible as shown by these results.

4. CONCLUSIONS

Erythrocytes under hypoxic conditions is a source of superoxide radicals due to the enhanced tendency of hemoglobin to autoxidize under these conditions. Incubation of LDL with erythrocytes or hemoglobin under reduced oxygen pressures, leads to drastic changes when compared with the changes observed under normoxic conditions. High levels of REM, TBARS, oxygen consumption, hemoglobin oxidation, and smooth muscle cells proliferation, indicates that hemoglobin is a more potent oxidant than CuSO$_4$. This process is augmented *in vivo* under conditions such as inflammation or restenosis which result in erythrocyte lysis, thereby becoming a contributing factor to LDL oxidation. Further studies are underway to elucidate the mechanism of this oxidation under hypoxia and also any MAP kinase mediated signal transduction pathways in smooth muscle cell.

5. REFERENCES

1. Balagopalakrishna, C., Manoharan, P.T., Abugo, O.O., and Rifkind, J.M., 1995, The production of superoxide from hemoglobin bound oxygen under hypoxic conditions, *J. Biol. Chem.* (Submitted).
2. Rifkind, J.M., Abugo, O., Levy, A., Monticone, R., and Heim, J., 1993, Formation of free radicals under hypoxia, in *Surviving Hypoxia: Mechanisms of Control and Adaptation*, Ed. Hochachka, Lutz, P.L., Sick, T., Rosenthal, M., van den Thillart, G., CRC press, Ann Arbor, p. 509–539.
3. Hodis, H.N., Kramsch, D.M., Avogaro, P., 1994, Biochemical and cytotoxic characterestics of an *in vivo* circulating oxidized low density lipoprotein, *J. Lipid Res.*, 35: 669–677.
4. Auge, N., Pieraggi, M.T., Thiers, J.C., Negre-sawayre, and Salvayre, R., 1995, Proliferative and cytotoxic effects of mildly oxidized low-density lipoprotein on vascular smooth muscle cells, *Biochem. J.*, 309: 1015–1020.
5. Berliner, J.A., Schwartz, D.S., Territo, M.C., Andalibi, A., Almada, L., Lusis, A.J., and Quisimorio, D., 1994, Induction of chemotactic cytokines by minimally oxidized low density lipoprotein, *Adv. Expt. Med. Biol.*, 351:13–18.
6. Murugesan, G., Chisolm, G.M., and Fox, P.L., 1993, Oxidized low density lipoprotein inhibits the migration of aortic endothelial cells *in* vitro, *J. Cell. Biol.*, 120: 1011–1019.
7. Esterbauer, H., Gabicki, J., Puhl, H., and Jurgens, G., 1992, The role of lipid peroxidation and antioxidants in oxidative modification of low density lipoprotein, *Free Rad. Biol. Med.*, 13: 341–390.
8. Ross, R., 1971, The smooth muscle cells II. Growth of smooth muscle in culture and formation of elastic fibers, *J. Cell. Biol.*, 50: 172–186.
9. Fogelman, A.M., Shechter, I., Seager, J., Hokom, M., Childs, J.S., and Edwards, P.A., 1980, Malonaldehyde alteration of low density lipoprotein leads to cholesteryl ester accumulation in human monocyte-macrophages, *Proc. Natl. Acad. Sci. USA*, 77:2214–2218.
10. Paganga, G., Rice-Evans, C., Rule, R., and Leake, D., 1992, The interaction between ruptured erythrocytes and low-density lipoproteins, *FEBS* 303: 154–158.
11. Esterbauer, H., Dieber-Rotheneder, M., Waeg, G., Striegl, G., and Jurgens, G., 1990, Biochemical, structural, and functional properties of oxidized low-density lipoproteins, *Chem. Res. Toxicol.*, 3: 77–92.
12. Ross, R., *Nature* (London), 1993, The pathogenesis of atherosclerosis: A perspective for the 1990s, 362: 801–809.
13. Schwartz, S.M., Heimark, R.L., Majesky, M.W., *Physiol. Rev.*, 1990, Developmental mechanisms underlying the pathology of arteries, 70: 1177–1209.
14. Herman, I.M., *Haemostasis*, 1990, Endothelial cell matrices modulate smooth muscle cell growth, contractile phenotype, and sensitivity to heparin, 20 suppl. 1: 166–177.

43

WEAK SPOTS INSIDE THE MYOCARDIUM OF A LANGENDORFF RAT HEART OBSERVED BY NADH VIDEOFLUOROMETRY

O. Eerbeek[1] and C. Ince[1,2]

[1]Department of Physiology
[2]Department of Anesthesiology
Academic Medical Centre
University of Amsterdam,
the Netherlands

INTRODUCTION

Myocardial function is highly dependent on an aerobic metabolism and can only be maintained when the oxygen delivery is more than the oxygen demand. Dysoxia occurs when the demand of oxygen by the heart exceeds that being supplied through the myocardial vasculature. Hypoperfusion of the myocardium causes a marked heterogeneity of well and less well perfused areas. These areas have been shown to be anatomically defined by the properties of the myocardial microvasculature (King et al. 1985, Franzen et al. 1988, Ince et al. 1993, Rakusan et al. 1994, Duling 1994). The properties of these dysoxic areas under different physiological conditions have been most studied by NADH fluorescence imaging techniques (Barlow et al. 1976, Steenbergen et al. 1977, Ince et al. 1993, Vetterlein et al. 1995). The NADH fluorescence technique was introduced by Chance and makes use of the fluorescence properties of mitochondrial NADH for the measurement of mitochondrial energy state of tissue cells in situ (Chance et al. 1976). NADH is situated at the high-energy side of the respiratory chain and during dysoxia accumulates in concentration because less NADH is oxidised to NAD^+. Episodes of high cardiac oxygen consumption, as occurs during high work rates, causes reduction of NADH levels (Osbakken 1994, Ashruf et al. 1995). The optical properties of NADH and NAD^+ clearly differ. Upon excitation with UV-light (365 nm) NADH, unlike NAD^+, fluoresces at the 460 nm light (blue). Under borderline hypoxic conditions imaging the distribution of NADH in the heart surface shows a heterogeneous distribution of well, and less well perfused areas. The less well perfused areas we have termed as cardiac "weak spots" since they are first to become dysoxic when the heart becomes comprised such as occurs during severe tachycardia (Ince et al. 1993) or during severe vasoconstriction as occurs during nitric oxide synthesis inhibition in endotoxemic hearts (Avontuur et al.

1995). In their microscopic NADH fluorescence study of frozen biopsies from in vivo rat hearts, Vetterlein and co-workers found that non-hypoxic areas are located near the arterial portion of the capillary bed where oxygenation is favored during low-flow states (Vetterlein et al. 1995). This effect appears to contribute to the supply heterogeneity in the hypoperfused myocardium. By taking biopsies from rats in vivo this study also identified the presence of cardiac weak spots in vivo. In an NADH videofluorescence study in Langendorff rat hearts where observations were made of the dysoxic patterns evoked by embolization of different diameter vessels by different diameter microspheres, we identified cardiac weak spots as being determined by flow heterogeneities at the capillary level (Ince et al. 1993). Moreover, in this study the dysoxic areas identified by NADH fluorescence were found to correspond to low pO_2 areas identified by Pd porphine phosphorescence imaging. Cardiac hypertrophy and pH acidosis causes larger areas to become dysoxic (Steenbergen et al. 1977, Hulsmann et al. 1993). These findings in combination with our previous studies suggest that these larger dysoxic areas are most likely determined by arterioles instead of capillaries. Study of cardiac weak spots continuously in time, as can be accomplished by NADH videofluorometry, has so far only been accomplished on the epicardial surface of hearts. The advantage of continuous observation of the spatial and temporal properties of cardiac weak spots is that the dynamics of heterogeneity in the heart can be studied in time. The object of this study was to see whether cardiac weak spots can be observed continuously by NADH videofluorometry in the myocardium as well as in the epicardium. To this end Langendorff hearts with part of the left ventricle removed was studied with NADH videofluorometry during switches from normoxic to anoxic perfusion.

MATERIALS AND METHODS

The preparation: Male Wistar rats weighing between 250–300 g were anaesthetised with pentobarbital (50 mg/kg, intraperitoneally), heparinized (200 IU/kg, i.v.) and subsequently connected to an artificial respirator via a tube inserted into the trachea. After a thoracotomy, the heart and the aorta was dissected free. Then the heart was removed, cooled in cold perfusion medium and rapidly arranged for perfusion. Hearts were perfused according to the technique of Langendorff with the possibility of switching between two permanent available perfusates. The composition of the Tyrode for perfusion was 128 mM NaCl, 4.7 mM KCl, 1 mM $MgCl_2$, 0.4 mM NaH_2PO_4, 1.2 mM Na_2SO_4, 20.2 mM $NaHCO_3$, 1.3 mM $CaCl_2$, 11 mM glucose. Once mounted in the experimental set-up, a portion of the apex was excised by a sharp scissors thereby exposing a transection of the myocardium and enabling observation of part of the endocardium as well as part of the epicardium. NADH videofluorometric observations were made in whole and sectioned hearts before, during and after a step-wise change from normoxic perfusion to anoxic perfusion and back again to normoxic perfusion. Oxymetric changes in myocardial metabolism were achieved by switching the perfusate from oxygenated Tyrode saturated with 95% O_2 and 5% CO_2 to that saturated with 95% N_2 and 5% CO_2 and back again. The temperature of the perfusates was maintained at 37^0C. The perfusion pressure was fixed at 80 mm Hg and flow was measured by a Transonic flow probe. The hearts were paced at a frequency of 300 beats/min. A diagram of the experimental set-up is shown in Fig.1.

NADH fluorescence measurements: The videofluorometer and experimental set-up used has been described elsewhere in detail (Ince et al.1993). The 365 nm line from a 100W mercury lamp was selected by means of an UG-1 barrier filter to provide the light

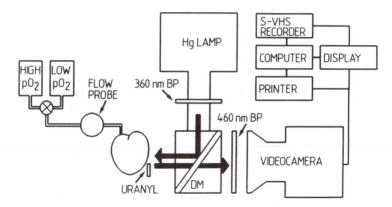

Figure 1. Experimental set-up for NADH videofluorometry consising of a Langendorff set-up with 2 reservoirs for Tyrode, one with oxygenated and one with de-oxygenated Tyrode. A small piece of uranyl fluorescence calibration glass is placed next to the heart as a fluorescence reference. An Hg arc lamp provides the 360-nm light needed for NADH excitation. CCD video camera detects 460-nm NADH fluorescence image. Dichroic mirror (DM) separated excitation and emission light at appropriate wavelengths. Signals were recorded on video recorder and analysed off-line.

needed for NADH excitation (Fig.1). A UV-sensitive image intensified CCD video camera fitted with a Micro-Nikkor 105 mm macro-lens was used to record NADH fluorescence images of the left ventricle of the heart. The NADH fluorescence signal was selected by means of a band pass filter centred around 470 "20 nm which was placed in the front of the camera. To enable correction of images for changes in the sensitivity of the videofluorometer and fluctuations in the intensity of the light source, a small piece of uranyl calibration glass was placed next to the heart within the excitation field. Images were recorded on a video recorder and computer analysed off-line. NADH fluorescence intensities are expressed in arbitrary units, which are defined as the ratio of NADH fluorescence intensity of myocardium and the fluorescence intensity of uranyl calibration glass.

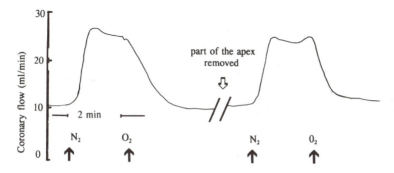

Figure 2. An example of a flow trace before and after sectioning during normoxia, anoxia and recovery from anoxia. After a period of normoxic perfusion, perfusate is switched to nitrogen-saturated Tyrode (N_2) and after back to oxygenated Tyrode (O_2) for the whole heart. Thereafter the same procedure was repeated for the apex dissected heart.

RESULTS AND DISCUSSION

To establish how the cross-sectioned myocardium recovers from an episode of anoxia, a step-wise change between normoxia and anoxia was first applied to Tyrode-perfused rat hearts after which normoxic perfusion was restored (n=4). Before removal of part of the apex to expose a cross-section of the myocardium step-wise change to anoxic perfusion and back again to normoxic perfusion was applied to the whole hearts to identify the location of the epicardial weak spots by observation with NADH videofluorometry. The mean normoxic flow for the whole heart before sectioning was 10 " 1.4 ml/min. Anoxic perfusion results in vasodilatation and hypoxic high flow. Maxima flow during perfusion with deoxygenated Tyrode was 26.7 " 1.2 ml/min. During restoration of normoxic perfusion the flow recovered to a mean value 10.1 " 2.3 ml/min. Next the heart apex was removed as shown in cartoon form in Fig. 3E and the same protocol as carried out in the whole heart was repeated again. An example of the flow trace of such a complete protocol is shown in Fig.2. The mean normoxic flow of these sectioned hearts was 10.1 " 2 ml/min, the maximum flow during anoxia was 27.8 " 1.4 ml/min and after recovery the mean flow returned to the original mean value of 10.7 " 3.1 ml/min. These results suggest that this manner of sectioning part of the apex has a marginal effect on global flow levels and the flow reactivity of the heart. An example of an NADH video fluorescence sequence associated with these manoeuvres in a sectioned heart is shown in Fig.3. Normoxic perfusion was associated with homogeneous low level of fluorescence (Fig.3A) and anoxic perfusion with homogeneous high fluorescence levels (Fig.3C). During recovery from anoxia patchy, strong fluorescent anoxic areas lagging behind normoxic areas were observed in the epicardium. NADH videofluorescence observation of the sectioned plane of the myocardium revealed similar patchy fluorescence areas as seen in the epicardium. During the normoxic phase (after total recovery) some small spots of tissue persisted in high fluorescence, probably because these areas were damaged during sectioning. Most of the cells in the section area recovered completely. In spite of removal of part

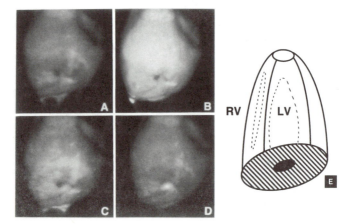

Figure 3. NADH fluorescence images of a cross-sected heart. A: weak fluorescence associated with normoxic perfusion. B: high fluorescence associated with full anoxia. C: patchy fluorescence image during restoration of normoxic perfusion after a hypoxic episode. D: same state as in A, after total restoration. E: A schematic drawing of cross-sected Langendorff rat heart.

of the apex, the presence of patchy high fluorescent areas associated with weak spots was found to occur not only on the surface of the heart but also in the muscle wall of all the hearts tested. NADH videofluorometry thus allows continuous observations of the temporal and spatial changes of these cardiac weak spots under different metabolic and hemodynamic conditions also in the endocardium and heart muscle wall.

REFERENCES

Ashruf, J.F., Coremans, J.M.C.C., Bruining, H.A. and Ince, C. 1995, Increase of cardiac work is associated with decrease of mitochondrial NADH, Am.J.Physiol., 269, H856-H862.

Avontuur, J.A.M., Bruining, H.A. and Ince, C. 1995, Inhibition of nitric oxide synthesis causes myocardial ischemia in endotoxemic rats, Circ.Res. 76, 418–425.

Barlow, C.H. and Chance, B., 1976, Ischemic areas in perfused rat hearts: measurements by NADH florescence photography, Science (Wash. DC) 193, 909–910.

Chance, B., 1976, Pyridine nucleotide as an indicator of oxygen requirements for energy-linked functions of mitochondria, Supp.1 Circ.Res. 38, 131–138.

Duling, B.R. 1994, Is red cell flow heterogeneity a critical variable in the regulation and limitation of oxygen transport to tissue? Adv.Exp.Med.Biol. 361, 237–247.

Franzen, D., Conway, R.S., Zhang, H., Sonnenblick, E.H. and Eng, C. 1988, Spatial heterogeneity of local blood flow and metabolite content in dog hearts, Am.J.Physiol. 254, H344-H353.

Hulsmann, W.C., Ashruf, J.F., Bruining, H.A. and Ince, C., 1993, Imminent ischemia in normal and hypertrophic Langendorff rat hearts; effects of fatty acids and superoxyde dismutase monitored by NADH surface fluorescence, Biochim.Biophys.Acta 1181, 273- 278.

Ince, C., Avontuur, J.A.M., Wieringa, P.A., Spaan, J.A.E. and Bruining, H.A., 1993, Heterogeneity of the hypoxic state in the rat heart is determined at capillary level, Am.J.Physiol. 264, H294-H301.

King, R.B., Bassingwaighte, J.B., Hales, J.R.S. and Rowell, L.B., 1985, Stability of myocardial blood flow in normal awake baboons, Circ.Res. 57, 285–295.

Osbakken, M.D., 1994, 1–2 Metabolic regulation of in vivo myocardial contractile function: multiparameter analysis, Mol. and Cell. Bioch.133/134, 13–37.

Rakusan , K., Batra, S. and Heron, M.I., 1994, A new approach for quantitative evaluation of coronary capillaries in longitudinal sections, Adv.Exp.Med.Biol. 361, 407–415.

Steenbergen, C., Deleeuw, G., Barlow, C., Chance, B. and Williamson, J.R., 1977, Heterogeneity of the hypoxic state in perfused rat heart, Circ. Res. 41, 606–615.

Steenbergen, C., Deleeuw, G., Rich, T. and Williamson, J.R., 1977, Effects of acidosis and ischemia on myocardial contractility and intracellular pH, Circ.Res. 41, 849–858.

Vetterlein, F. Prange, M., Lubrich, D., Penida, J. Neckel, M. and Schmidt, G., 1995, Capillary perfusion pattern and microvascular geometry in heterogeneous hypoxic areas of hypofused rat myocardium, Am.J.Physiol. 268, H2183-H2194.

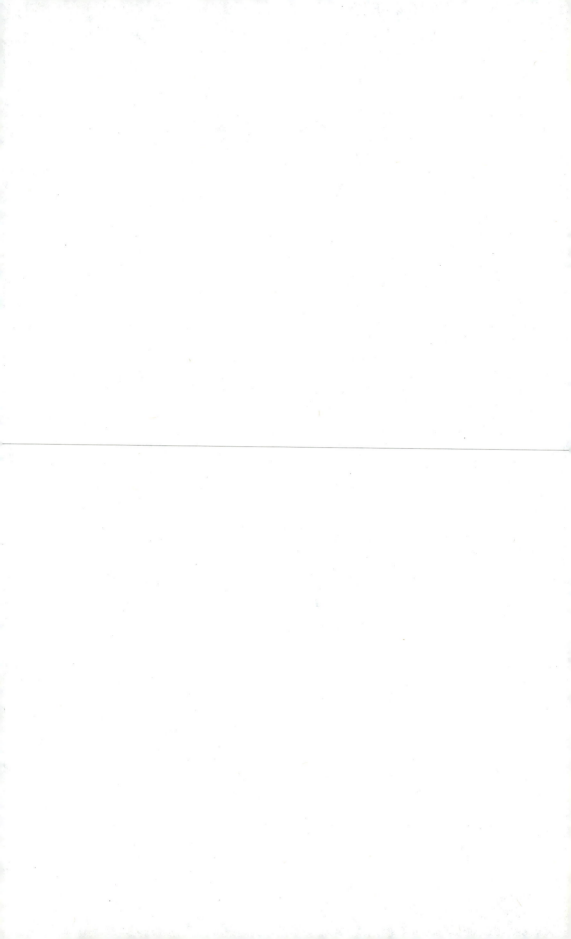

44

MICROVASCULAR GROWTH IN THE CHICKEN CHORIO-ALLANTOIC MEMBRANE

M. F. König, P. Schlatter, and P. H. Burri

Department of Anatomy
University of Berne, 3000 Berne 9
Switzerland

INTRODUCTION

The chorio-allantoic membrane (CAM) plays a vital role providing the chicken embryo with O_2. Its growth and in particular the growth of its capillary network has important implications for the development of the embryo. And yet, it still remains to be determined to what extent the capillary growth is affected on the one hand via vessel sprouting, and on the other hand by the insertion of transcapillary tissue pillars (posts) to form new intercapillary meshes (intussusceptive microvascular growth, IMG).

Quantitative morphometric analysis of the capillary growth in the CAM requires unequivocal identification of the whole vasculature. For lightmicroscopic work an appropriate marker for the safe identification of blood vessels is therefore necessary. Such a marker should clearly delimit the boundary between blood vessel and interstitium. To study structural changes with age, the label specificity should be independent of the developmental stage of the chicken embryo. In principle, there are three different ways to label the vascular bed: endothelial markers, red blood cell (RBC) labels and blood plasma tracers.

Endothelial markers such as alkaline phosphatase or dipeptidyl peptidase IV tend to diffuse into the interstitial tissue [1] thus masking small tissue areas such as tissue posts, commonly defined as meshes ≤2.5 μm in diameter [8].

Usually, CAM vessels are identified by staining RBCs with peroxidase (e.g. [11]). Evidently, however, this method does not stain blood vessels which do not contain RBCs. This might lead to an underestimation of the size of a capillary bed [9]. In addition, even at higher magnifications, the limits between capillary and interstitium cannot be clearly identified by this method.

The most common plasma tracers are fluorescently labeled macromolecules [2,10]. The disadvantages of this technique are, on the one hand, that the labeling intensity in larger capillaries might cover small tissue posts. On the other hand, the rapid loss in fluorescence intensity may require the immediate analysis of the tissue after the experiments, which is hardly feasible with a larger number of probes.

Oxygen Transport to Tissue XVIII, edited by Nemoto and LaManna
Plenum Press, New York, 1997

We recently developed a new plasma tracer to study pulmonary blood flow in rabbits [5]. This *in vivo* perfusion marker, consisting of highly concentrated albumin coated colloidal gold particles, turned out to label the capillary bed of the whole organism without the above drawbacks [6]. Even smallest capillaries were clearly identifiable on silver enhanced light microscopic paraffin sections. It was the aim of the current study to adapt this technique to the capillary network of the CAM of chicken embryos at light microscopic level with the goal to quantitatively analyze the intussusceptive growth of the capillary network.

METHODS

Preparation of Albumin Gold Complexes

Eight nm diameter gold particles were prepared as previously described [5]. One liter of gold solution was obtained by heating solution A (800 ml H_2O plus 10 ml 1% w/v $HAuCL_4$) to 60°C and quickly mixing it with solution B (150 ml H_2O, 40 ml 1% trisodium citrate, 2 ml 1% tannic acid (from Mallinckrodt Inc.)), also heated to 60°C. In a first concentration step, the gold colloid was gently boiled down to approximately 25% of its original volume (concentrated gold solution). To adjust the pH of the solution, 12 ml of 0.2 M sodium phosphate buffer (pH 6.1) was added to 250 ml of colloidal gold under rapid stirring. 19.5 mg of rabbit serum albumin dispersed in 10 mM sodium phosphate buffer were rapidly mixed with aliquots of 250 ml of the concentrated gold solution.

For further concentration, batches of the RSA-Gold suspension were centrifuged for 90 minutes at 35'000 g. The supernatant was discarded, and by a further centrifugation step at the same speed but for 150 minutes, the original gold quantity (corresponding to $\sim 1.5 \cdot 10^{16}$ particles [4]) was concentrated into 1 ml of solution. After dialysing against Ringer solution (pH 7.4), the gold solution was passed through 0.25 µm Millipore filters, frozen into liquid nitrogen and stored at -70°C.

Infusion of Gold Particles into Chicken Embryos

Thirty fertilized chicken eggs were incubated at 37°C. After three days of incubation (day 3), they were carefully opened and the contents transferred to Petri dishes and further bred in an incubator at 37°C until day 14. From day 5 onwards, the vascular bed of three animals per day was cannulated with a glass cannula (OD = 5 µm) by means of a micromanipulator under microscopic control. At the younger stages (day 5 to day 7) we selected the major vitelline vein, at the older stages (from day 8 onwards) a larger chorio-allantoic vein for cannulation. An age dependent amount between 0.03 ml (day 5) and 0.2 ml (day 14) of the highly concentrated colloidal gold suspension was then infused within 90 seconds into the blood stream of living chicken embryos. Then, the tracer was allowed to recirculate for another 210 seconds in order to obtain a total perfusion time of 5 minutes from the start of infusion until stop of blood flow by immersion fixation of the complete chicken embryo with half concentrated Karnovsky fixative.

Histological Procedure

After fixation for at least 24 h at 4°C, the complete CAM was carefully removed, and cut into two pieces of equal size. To visualize the colloidal gold particles by lightmicroscopy, one half of the CAM was randomly selected to perform the silver enhancement reaction. To this effect, the tissue was rinsed for 1 hour in distilled water and placed for 30 minutes into reducing buffer (0.5% wt/vol hydrochinone in citrate buffer pH 3.8) diluted 1:1 with double distilled water. Then the enhancement reaction was performed by transferring the CAM into the silver developer containing 1% (wt/vol) silver acetate in 0.25%(wt/vol) hydrochinone citrate buffer. After an exposure time of 30 to 60 minutes the specimen was briefly rinsed in distilled water and fixed for 5 minutes with Ilford paper fixer (diluted 1:9 in H_2O). After rinsing with tap water, the CAMs were counterstained with nuclear fast red. Following dehydration in ascending ethanol concentrations, they were transferred into xylol and mounted on glass slides.

For the study of the ultrastructural localization of gold particles, small pieces of the remaining CAM were cut and processed for electron microscopy [3,7]. Standard electron microscopic techniques were followed to dehydrate and embed the tissue in Epon resin. Sections were cut at 60 nm thickness and mounted on uncoated 200 mesh grids. To improve the visibility of the gold particles, the sections were only weakly counterstained with lead citrate (5 min) and uranyl acetate (5 min).

RESULTS

Due to the dark red stain of the colloidal gold solution, the *in vivo* distribution of tracer in the vascular bed of the CAM could be clearly followed up under the light microscope during tracer infusion. Complete perfusion of the arteries and veins occurred within approximately two minutes (day 6 to 14). In most CAM capillaries, the stain of our tracer could also be detected. After silver enhancement, the whole capillary bed was stained black (Fig. 1) with well defined contours allowing to recognize the intercapillary meshes standing out as white spots. It was remarkable, that the earlier stages of development (days 6–7) showed large tissue meshes (Fig. 2a), which became consistently smaller in later developmental stages (days 8–12, Fig. 2b). The latter not only showed smaller meshes, but also an increasing number of small tissue posts, defined as meshes ≤ 2.5 μm in diameter. From day 13 onwards, the number of tissue posts appeared to decrease. A morphometric study is in progress in order to provide a solid quantitative description of these changes, - data to be further used as a basis for growth regulation studies.

The electron microscopic sections allowed to study the gold particle distribution within the capillary bed. Gold particles were detected all over the plasma, even within the small space between RBCs and endothelial cell walls. Few particles were detected in endovesicles of endothelial cells and in the interstitial space, suggesting a transendothelial transport (Fig. 3).

DISCUSSION

The silver enhanced gold contrast technique used in the vascular system in the chicken embryo proved to be an adequate method for the visualization of a mainly two-dimensional capillary system in the light microscope. In such specimens it is possible in en face views to quantitatively assess the characteristics of the network structures by morphometric techniques. Electron microscopic examination confirmed that most gold particles were distributed within the blood plasma. Few gold particles were detected in the interstitial space. However, compared to the high gold concentration in the plasma, the interstitial gold concentration was negligibly small. Therefore, a bias towards artificial en-

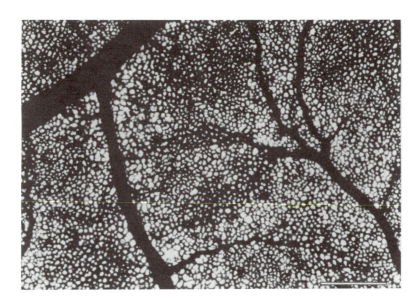

Figure 1. This low magnification allows to assess the degree of perfusion of CAM capillary network (day 7, scale marker 100 μm).

largement of the capillary profiles in silver enhanced sections can be excluded. An advantage of the method used is that it allows to examine practically the whole CAM on a single glass slide, which is ideally suited for quantitative growth assessment. By focussing through the capillary layer even the smallest tissue spots could clearly be recognized.

The present study also revealed that colloidal gold is an ideal tool to study *in vivo* capillary perfusion in the chicken CAM. All capillaries at all stages observed contained colloidal gold particles and were thus perfused after a circulation time of 5 minutes at least with plasma. This complete perfusion of the capillary bed by our tracer will enable us to quantitatively analyze the capillary growth in the CAM in future experiments. In contrast to our findings Spanel-Borowsky and co-workers [9] described an incomplete capillary network at day 10 after incubation. Since they used peroxidase as a marker, which is known to label exclusively RBCs, their finding might be explained by the presence of capillary areas devoid of RBCs.

From our preliminary quantitative observations, we assume that there are three phases of capillary growth in the CAM. The early days (6–7) showed only few posts, but large intercapillary meshes, which became smaller at days 8–12, a period marked by the presence of numerous small meshes and posts. At the later stages (days 13–14), we noticed again larger intercapillary meshes and fewer posts. These preliminary observations also indicate that at early stages of development, both sprouting and intussusceptive growth may be observed, whereas at later stages intussusceptive capillary growth seems to prevail. Evidently only a thorough quantitative analysis can clarify the question, at which stage sprouting and/or intussuceptive growth represent the predominant mode of capillary growth and what their quantitative contributions are with respect to total growth.

From our study we conclude that perfusion of colloidal gold particles and subsequent silver enhancement represents an optimal tool to label the capillary network of the chicken CAM for light microscopic analyses.

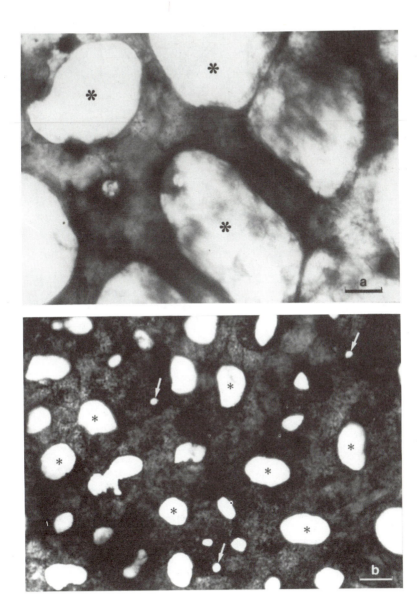

Figure 2. Comparison of capillary network structure in light micrographs at same magnification. **2a**: In early stages of development, large capillary meshes are predominant (*) and only few small tissue pillars can be detected (day 7, scale marker 10 μm). **2b**: At day 11 after incubation, the capillary meshes (*) are much smaller compared to day 7, the number of tissue pillars is markedly increased (arrows, scale marker 10 μm).

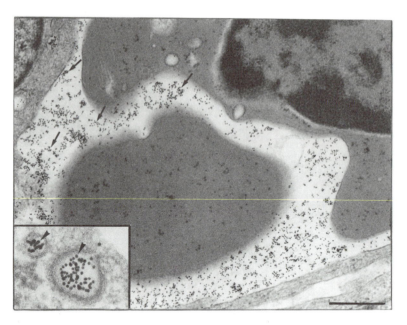

Figure 3. Electron micrograph showing that the gold particles are mainly located within the blood plasma (arrows). Particles are found in endothelial vesicles (arrowheads, scale marker 0.5 μm).

ACKNOWLEDGMENTS

The authors would like to thank Mrs. A. Lieglein, Mrs. B. de Breuyn, Mr. B. Hänni and Mr. K. Babl for their technical assistance.

REFERENCES

1. S. Batra and M.F. König, A novel method to demonstrate capillary geometry and perfusion patterns in rat brain from the same histological section. *Oxygen to Tissue Transport* in press:(1995).
2. U. Göbel, H. Theilen, and W. Kuschinsky, Congruence of total and perfused capillary network in rat brains, *Circ. Res.* 66:271–281 (1990).
3. H. Hoppeler, O. Mathieu, E.R. Weibel, R. Krauer, S.L. Lindstedt, and C.R. Taylor, Design of the mammalian respiratory system. VIII. Capillaries in skeletal muscles, *Respir. Physiol.* 44:129–150 (1981).
4. T. Kehle and V. Herzog, Interactions between protein-gold complexes and cell surfaces: a method for precise quantitation, *Eur. J. Cell Biol.* 45:80–87 (1987).
5. M.F. König, J.M. Lucocq, and E.R. Weibel, Demonstration of pulmonary vascular perfusion by electron and light microscopy, *J. Appl. Physiol.* 75:1–7 (1993).
6. M.F. König, E.R. Weibel, and S. Batra, Colloidal gold particles as an in vivo plasma marker in skeletal muscle and heart demonstrated by electron and light microscopy. *Am. J. Physiol.* submitted:(1995).
7. L. Mermod, H. Hoppeler, S.R. Kayar, R. Straub, and E.R. Weibel, Variability of fiber size, capillary density and capillary length related to horse muscle fixation procedures, *Acta Anat.* 133:89–95 (1988).
8. S. Patan, B. Haenni, and P.H. Burri, Evidence for intussusceptive capillary growth in the chicken chorio-allantoic membrane (CAM), *Anat. Embryol.* 187:121–130 (1993).
9. K. Spanel-Borowski, U. Schnapper, and B. Heymer, The chick chorioallantoic membrane assay in the assessment of angiogenetic factors. *Biomed. Res.* 9:253–260 (1988).
10. F. Vetterlein, U. Keitel, and G. Schmidt, Capillary filling kinetics in the rabbit heart during normoxemia and hypoxemia, *Am. J. Physiol.* 264:H287-H293 (1993).
11. J. Wilting, B. Christ, and M. Bokeloh, A modified chorioallantoic membrane (CAM) assay for qualitative and quantitative study of growth factors, *Anat. Embryol.* 183:259–271 (1991).

45

DIFFERENT ENZYME ACTIVITIES IN CORONARY CAPILLARY ENDOTHELIAL CELLS

T. Koyama,[1] M. Gao,[1] T. Ueda,[3] S. Batra,[2] K. Itoh,[1] T. Ushiki,[4] and K. Abe[4]

[1]Res Inst Electron Sc
[2]JSPS researcher to [1]
[3]Res Inst Immunol
[4]3rd Dept Anat
Medical School
Hokkaido University, 060 Sapporo
Japan

ABSTRACT

Differential distributions of alkaline phosphatase (AP) and dipeptydylpeptidase IV (DPPIV) were studied in coronary microvascular endothelial cells. Endothelial cells were obtained by the perfusion of coronary vessels with 0.1% trypsin PBS solution and cultured in uncoated culture dishes. Staining of cultured endothelial cells with AP- and DPPIV-sensitive reagents revealed blue or red staining, respectively. Most colonies showed cells of only one color, blue or red, even at the fifth passage. AP-sensitive cells, which were originally elongated, shortened and widened, proliferating to form monolayer colonies of cobble stone-like cells. AP-stainability became weak with repeated passages. DPPIV-sensitive endothelial cells remained elongated even after repeated passages. The cell shape and stainability seemed to be coupled and maintained through the five passages studied.

INTRODUCTION

The heterogeneity of microvascular endothelial cells makes it difficult to identify putative endothelial cells (Gerritsen et al. 1988). However, heterogeneity also seems to exist in the enzyme distribution between arteriolar and venular portions in coronary capillaries. Lojda (1979) reported that alkaline phosphatase (AP) is present only in arteriolar capillaries, and dipeptidylpeptidase IV (DPPIV) only in venular capillaries. Batra et al. (1989, 1991) utilized the staining of the two enzymes in studies of coronary capillary networks and obtained much information on the capillarity of the left ventricular wall and the

Oxygen Transport to Tissue XVIII, edited by Nemoto and LaManna
Plenum Press, New York, 1997

oxygen supply from the coronary system. The capillary domain area (CDA) is smaller in venular capillaries than in arteriolar capillaries, which seems reasonable from the view point of high oxygen tension in arteriolar and low oxygen tension in venular capillaries (Batra et al. 1991, 1992). Differences in adaptational changes in arteriolar and venular capillaries can also be examined in detail by this technique: the frequency of capillary branching differs between arteriolar and venular capillaries (Batra et al. 1991), and arteriolar capillaries increase in subendocardial tissues in the left ventricular wall of young rats subjected to 6 weeks of treadmill exercise (Gao et al. 1994). Differential staining has also been used in studies on the geometry of capillary networks in skeletal muscles (Mrazkowa et al. 1986) and cancer tissues (Longauer 1993).

The different enzyme activities, however, have never been investigated at the cellular level. Until the present study the question whether AP and DPPIV are expressed differentially in isolated coronary microvascular endothelial cells was unanswered and the stability of enzyme activity in isolated endothelial cells was unknown.

In the present work coronary endothelial cells were isolated from rat heart, cultured in plastic dishes, stained for AP and DPPIV, and studied morphologically.

METHODS

Cell Isolation and Culture

The abdomen was opened in nembutal-anesthetized male Wistar rats (6 weeks old, 145–150 g). A thin polyethylene tube was placed in the abdominal aorta and secured. The thorax was opened and the right atrium incised as an outlet for the perfusate. Phosphate-buffered saline (PBS) containing 0.1% heparin (10ml) was infused, to wash out blood from cardiac tissues. The polyethylene tube was advanced so that its tip was situated at the origin of the aorta, and sutured. PBS containing 0.1% trypsin was then infused for 3 minutes. The outflow of PBS from the right atrium was collected and centrifuged at 2000 rpm for 7 minutes at 4°C. Cells in the pellet obtained was quickly dispersed in the culture solution, RMPI supplemented with 10% fetal calf serum (RMPI+FCS), and plated on uncoated Falcon 60 mm tissue culture dishes. These dishes were incubated in an atmosphere of 5% CO_2, 95% air at 37°C with 90% humidity. The culture medium was replaced every 2 days.

Characterization

Low density lipoprotein (LDL) uptake which is specific to endothelial cells (Voyta et al.1984) was confirmed by application of acetylated LDL labeled with 1,1'-dioctadecyl-3,3,3',3'-tetramethylindocarbocyanine perchlorate (DiI) (Biomedical Technologies Inc., Stoughton, MA, USA). One ml of PBS-diluted DiI-Ac-LDL (10µl/mlPBS) was added to the tissue culture dishes when colonies of endothelial cells had formed in the primary culture. After 4 hour incubation at 37°C the fluorescent LDL solution was removed, and culture dishes were rinsed with PBS. Fluorescent light at 550nm emitted from cells excited by light at 514nm was observed under a fluorescence microscope. More than 95% cells emitted fluorescent light after 4 hour incubation with DiI-Ac-LDL. Rounded cells emitted stronger fluorescence than cells of an elongated, bamboo-leaflet shape. Cultures of endothelial cells were made without any selection at each passage.

Staining

Differential staining was done as described by Batra et al. (1989) with minor modifications as follows. Cells in the dishes were washed with PBS but not fixed with acetone. They were first treated with a reagent mixture specific to DPPIV consisting of 8mg glycyl-L-proline-4-methoxy-beta-naphthylamine dissolved in 1ml of NN- dimethylformamide, and 10mg fast blue B dissolved in 20ml of 0.1M acetate buffer (pH 7.4). One ml of the mixture was added to culture dishes and incubated for 90 or 180 minutes. This mixture was discarded and the cultures rinsed with PBS. Cultures were then incubated for 25 or 60 minutes with 1ml of reagent mixture specific to AP; this consisting of 20mg naphthol AS-Mx phosphate dissolved in 1ml NN dimethylformamide, and 20mg variamine blue salt RT dissolved in 10ml of 0.1 M Tris HCl buffer (pH9.2). After being rinsed with distilled water, cells were covered with crystal mount (Biomeda Corp, Foster City, CA) and dried at 70°C for 15 minutes. All reagents were purchased from Sigma Co if not otherwise mentioned, and were used without any further purification

To examine the localization of blue- and red-stained endothelial cells, colored microspheres with a diameter of 10μm (E-Z trac, Primech Inc. USA) were injected into the coronary artery of isolated and Langendorff-perfused rat hearts (Itoh et al. 1994). After injection the hearts were removed from the perfusion system, placed in OCT compound and frozen. The frozen left ventricular wall was sectioned with a cryotome and stained as described by Batra et al. (1989) but again without aceton fixation.

RESULTS

During the first two weeks of primary culture the proliferation of endothelial cells was slow. It took more than 15 days to get partial confluence. During the 2nd and 4th passages the proliferation rate was high and confluence was obtained by 5 days after passages; the proliferation rate was however, noticeably slowed down on the 5th passage.

The DPPIV and AP staining technique applied for the shorter incubation times given above red- and blue-stained cells, respectively; but the coloring was weak. On repetition of passages the blue stain for AP grew fainter. After 4 passages it could not be seen with the 25 minute incubation which was routinely used for tissue slices. Several combinations of reagent concentrations and incubation times were checked and simply prolonging the incubation time to 60 minutes proved satisfactory for AP staining. DPPIV staining did not decrease following passages, but incubation time was increased to 180 minutes to give stronger staining. During the first stage of the primary culture most cells were elongated. Their cytoplasm appeared thin and filmy. Blue-staining cells proliferated to give short roundish cells (Fig.1).

Red-staining cells also proliferated but remained rather elongated. Examples of colonies of round cells and elongated cells are shown in Fig.2. Often some cells in red staining colonies rose up in later stages, to form structures. The micrograph (Fig.3) shows a cross-section of a colony of red-stained cells. It seems probable that some material was excreted onto the surface of the culture dish. Usually colonies contained cells of only one color even on the fifth passage.

An example of a micrograph of colored microspheres in cardiac capillaries is shown in Fig.4. All microspheres stayed in the blue-stained capillaries. Thus, it can be concluded that blue-stained capillaries are situated on the arteriolar side and that blue-stained endo-

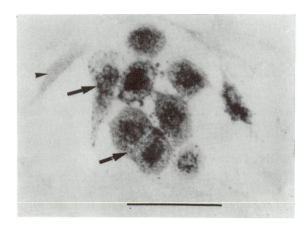

Figure 1. An example of capillary endothelial cells after primary cultur for one week, stained for alkaline phosphatase and dipeptidylpeptidase IV. Blue- and red-stained cells appear black (arrows) and grey (arrow heads), respectively. The horizontal bar represents 100μm.

thelial cells originate from the arteriolar portion of the capillary. Red-stained capillaries and red endothelial cells are considered to be from the venular side.

DISCUSSION

Since the trypsin solution was infused at the origin of the aorta, endothelial cells may have been isolated from the aorta and large coronary arteries as well as from the microvasculature. The total inner surface area of capillaries is, however, much greater than that of large blood vessels. Thus, most endothelial cells were probably isolated from microvessels. Experimental evidence supports this contention, since most cells initially showed the elongated shape typical of capillary endothelium (Folkman et al. 1979; Minakawa 1989).

Blue-staining endothelial cells were elongated during the first stage of primary culture, but the cells proliferating from them became shorter and wider. It seemed probable

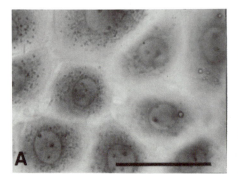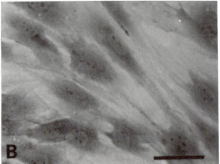

Figure 2. Examples of colonies of cobble stone-like cells (A) and elongated cells (B). The horizontal bars represent 50μm.

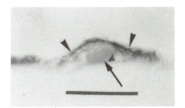

Figure 3. A micrograph of a cross-section of a monolayer colony of red-stained cells (arrow heads). Excreted material (arrow) under the corony can be seen. The horizontal bar represents 20μm.

that immediately after the isolation and settling on the culture dishes the endothelial cells 'remembered' the elongated shape in microvessels *in vivo*. Newly proliferated cells, however, lost their elongated shape and became rather round. The round cells retained their blue-stainability throughout the repetition of harvesting and passages.

On the other hand the red-staining elongated cells remained elongated after proliferation and continued to stain red. These results suggest that the differential distribution of the two enzymes was associated with different shapes of cultured cells. The different enzyme expression is maintained, coupled with the different shapes over the present five passages. The experiment with colored microspheres indicated a different *in vivo* localization of the enzymatically and morphologically different capillary endothelial cells.

The red-staining cells seemed to excrete some material from the lower side of the monolayer and formed folds, suggesting a stronger tendency to form structures than that in the blue-staining endothelial cells. This observation may be related to the angiogenic activity on the venular side (Ausprunk, Folkman 1977).

In conclusion endothelial cells which were isolated from coronary microvessels, and cultured in plastic dishes express either AP or DPPIV. AP-stained endothelial cells probably originate from arterioles and arteriolar portions of capillary networks, and DPPIV-stained cells from venules or venular portions. The cells retain their specific enzyme activity for five passages, although the AP activity gradually became weaker. Endothelial

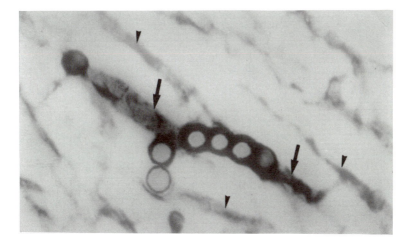

Figure 4. An example of colored microspheres (Φ=10μm) in cardiac capillaries. Blue and red staining appears black (arrows) and grey (arrow heads), respectively.

cells containing DPPIV showed an ability to form some structures in the monolayer colony even in uncoated plastic dishes.

REFERENCES

Ausprunk DH, Folkman J (1977), Migration and proliferation of endothelial cells in pre-formed and newly formed blood vessels during tumor angiogenesis. Microvasc Res 14: 53–65.

Batra S, Kuo C, Rakusan K (1989), Spatial distribution of coronary capillaries: A-V segment staggering. Adv Exp Med Biol 248: 241–246.

Batra S, Rakusan K, Campbell SE (1991), Geometry of capillary networks in hypertro-phied rat heart. Microvasc Res 41:29–40.

Batra S, Koyama T, Gao M, Horimoto M, Rakusan K (1992), Microvascular geometry of the rat heart arteriolar and venular capillary regions. Jap Heart J 33:817–828.

Folkman J, Haudenshild CC, Zetter BR (1979), Long-term culture of capillary endothe-lial cells. Proc Natl Acad Sci USA 76:5217–5221.

Gao M, Batra S, Koyama T (1994), Capillary geometry in the subendocardium of the left ventricle from young rats subjected to exercise training. In "Progress in microcirculation research" ed by Niimi H, Oda M, Sawada T, Xiu RJ, Pergamon Press, 187–191.

Gerritsen ME, Carley W, Milici AJ (1988), Microvascular endothelial cells:Isolation, identification, and cultivation. Advances in cell culture 6:35–66.

Itoh K, Batra S, Koyama T, Tamura M (1994), Local intracellular hypoxia induced by microembolization studied by myoglobin oxygen state. In "Progress in microcirculation research" ed by Niimi H, Oda M, Sawada T, Xiu RJ, Pergamon Press, 367–370.

Lojda Z (1979), Studies on dipeptidyl(amino)peptidase IV (glycylproline naphthylamidase). Histochem 59:153–166.

Longauer F, Bilcik P (1993), Enzymes in tumors of the breast. Histochemical study of the stroma in breast carcinomas. Bratisl Lek Listy 94:192–200.

Minakawa T (1989), Long-term culture of microvascular endothelial cells derived frommongolian gerbil brain. Stroke 20: 947–951.

Mrazkova O, Grim M, Carlson BM (1986), Enzymatic heterogeneity of the capillary bed of rat skeletal muscles. Amer J Anat 177:141–148.

Voyta JC, Via DP, Butterfield CE, Zetter BR (1984), Identification and isolation of endothelial cells based on the increased uptake of acetylated low density lipoprotein. J Cell Biol 99:2034–2040.

46

MYOCYTE HYPERTROPHY AND CAPILLARIZATION IN SPONTANEOUSLY HYPERTENSIVE STROKE-PRONE RATS

T. Koyama,[1] M. Gao,[1] S. Batra,[2] H. Togashi,[3] and H. Saito[3]

[1]Research Institute for Electronic Science
[2]JSPS Researcher to[1]
[3]1st Dept. of Pharmacology, Hokkaido University
060 Sapporo, Japan

ABSTRACT

Stroke-prone spontaneously hypertensive rats (SHRSP) are liable to suffer a stroke between 25 and 40 weeks of age. Left ventricular capillarity was studied in 40-week-old SHRSP to clarify the effects of hypertrophic changes in cardiomyocytes on oxygen transport capacity within the tissue. The innermost region of the left ventricular subendocardium at the level of the maximum diameter of the heart was investigated. Methods for sectioning and differential staining of arteriolar, intermediate and venular capillaries, and measurements for determining capillarity parameters were as previously described. Total capillary density decreased, while capillary domain areas increased along the whole capillary pathway. These changes in SHRSP seemed unfavorable for oxygen supply to ventricular tissues. To minimize the effects of the adverse changes, the ratio of the capillary to myocyte number increased markedly. The proportion of arteriolar capillaries increased and the venular proportion decreased.

INTRODUCTION

The decrement in capillary density that occurs during the development of cardiac hypertrophy in the spontaneously hypertensive rat is reversed as hypertrophy stabilizes. Capillary density is normalized by a proliferation of endothelial cells (Tomanek, Hovanec 1981). Wider and more variable intercapillary spacing, which may be disadvantageous to oxygen supply, was observed only in older hypertensive rats (Rakusan et al. 1984). We have found that, compared with WKY rats, spontaneously hypertensive rats (SHR) aged 11 weeks, showed increases in the capillary:myocyte number (C:M ratio) and the proportion of venular capillaries but no significant changes in the arteriolar and intermediate capillary domain areas in subendocardial left ventricular tissues (to be published). These results suggested that an adaptation in the capillarity occurs which reduces the disadvantageous effects of hyperterophic changes in cardiomyocytes. We were further interested in the question whether the capillarity of stroke prone rats (SHRSP) (Okamoto et al. 1974), which have higher blood pressure than SHR, could adapt to the hypertrophic changes. The systolic blood pressure of SHRSP was 219.9 mmHg in the aorta of anaesthetized rats (>25weeks old) (Minami et al. 1988), 230 mmHg at the tail of awake rats (Nagaoka et al. 1979). In the tail of SHR it was 208 mmHg at the age of seven months (Tomanek 1979). The highly increased blood pressure suggests that the myocytes are likely to become hypertrophic with an increase in their cross-sectional diameter. The diffusion path distance for oxygen would be increased, if capillary angiogenesis proceeds more slowly than the development of cardiomyocyte hypertrophy. Adaptational changes in cardiac capillarization in SHRSP are, therefore, of interest from the viewpoint of oxygen supply. Since the establishment of the SHRSP strain (Okamoto et al. 1974) these animals have attracted much attention because of the frequent incidence of stroke. Cerebral blood flow and therapeutic treatments (Yamori et al. 1979), humoral factors (Minami et al. 1988), and effects of steroids and thyroxine (Nagaoka et al, 1979, Akiguchi et al. 1979) have been investigated extensively in SHRSP. Cardiac capillarity, however, remains unstudied. In the present work ventricular capillarization in 40-week-old SHRSP was studied by the use of the differential staining method for arteriolar, intermediate and venular capillaries (Batra et al. 1989).

METHODS

SHRSP donated by Prof. Okamoto have been maintained for the last 10 years in the First Department of Pharmacology, Hokkaido University. Six 40-week-old specimens were used in the present study. Systolic blood pressure was measured with a tail cuff manometer. Rats were instantaneously sacrificed by decapitation. Hearts were quickly isolated, weighed, placed in O.C.T. solution and frozen in liquid nitrogen. Sectioning, differential staining and other procedures for capillarity measurements (capillary domain area, SDlog, capillary proportion) have been described previously (Batra et al. 1989, Gao et al. 1994). Measurements of myocyte cross-sectional area and capillarity parameters were made in the innermost region of the left ventricular subendocardium at the level of the maximum diameter of the heart.

RESULTS

The body weight (BW) of SHRSP was much lower than that of Wistar rats, but the heart and left ventricular weights (LVW) were larger. Values for the LVW:BW ratio and the systolic pressure of SHRSP were more than double those of Wistars. Despite the increased blood pressure the heart rate was higher in SHRSP than in Wistar rats (Table 1).

The average myocyte area and the C:M ratio were increased in SHRSP (Table 2), as were the capillary domain areas in the three capillary portions (Table 3). The degree of heterogeneity indicated by SDlog tended to be larger in SHRSP than in Wistars, the value for venular capillaries significantly exceeding that in Wistars (Table 3).

The proportions of arteriolar and intermediate capillaries increased but the proportion of venular capillaries decreased, resulting in a decrease in total capillary density (Table 4).

DISCUSSION

The high blood pressure in SHRSP aged 40-week-old caused hypertrophic changes in the left ventricles and individual cardiomyocytes. That neoangiogenesis of capillaries

Table 1. Basic data

	Age wks	BW g	HW mg	LVW mg	LVW/BW mg/g	BP mmHg	HR beats/min
Wistar n = 7	52	510±20	1021±49	792 ±40	1.55±0.05	120±18	360±30
SHRSP n = 6	40	312±24	1463±181	1213±80	3.91±0.47	240±30	420±41
Significance		p < 0.0001	p < 0.05	p < 0.05	p < 0.001	p < 0.0001	p < 0.0001

Values are means±SD, BW = body weight, HW = heart weight, LVW = left ventricle weight, LVW/BW = left ventricle weight to body weight, BP = systolic blood pressure at tail, HR = heart rate, Significance of difference was checked by Mann-Whitney's U-test, Wistar = Wistar rats, SHRSP = stroke-prone spontaneously hypertensive rats.

Table 2. Cardiomyocyte area and capillary to myocyte ratio (C:M)

	Myocyte area μm^2	C:M ratio
Wistar n = 7	620±269	1.09±0.05
SHRSP n = 6	1088±256	1.81±0.14
Significance	p< 0.05	p < 0.01

Values are means±SD.
Significance by Student's t-test.

Table 3. Capillary domain areas

	Capillary domain area(mm2)		SDlog	
	Wistar	SHRSP	Wistar	SHRSP
AC	647±55	772±267*	0.062±0.021	0.073±0.004
MID	565±64	676±260*	0.068±0.014	0.079±0.003
VC	538±38	685±294*	0.068±0.004	0.081±0.003*

Values are means±SD, AC=arteriolar capillary, MID= capillary between AC and VC. VC = venular capillary. *Significantly different from Wistar rats(p<0.05) by Student's t-test.

Table 4. Capillary distribution

	Capillary proportion No /mm^2		Capillary percentage %	
	Wistar	SHRSP	Wistar	SHRSP
AC	204 ± 61	345±74**	10.2±0.03	25.3±8.0**
MID	208 ± 83	543±127***	10.3±0.04	37.2±4.1***
VC	1600±168	597±185***	79.5±0.08	39.6±6.9***
Total	2012±204	1485±251***		

Values are means±SD.
Significantly different from Wistar by Student's t-test: **p < 0.01; ***p < 0.0001.

occurred is indicated by the increase in C:M ratio but it failed to keep pace with the hypertrophic changes. Capillary neoangiogenesis partly proceeds from the venular side (Folkman 1987): the decrease in the proportion of venular capillaries suggests a delay in this process. The total capillary density decreased with a resultant increase in the capillary domain area in all three types of capillary. The oxygen diffusion path length thus seems to be increased. In addition to venular neoangiogenesis capillaries can be arteriolized from the arteriolar side (Price et al.1994). In the present study the proportion of arteriolar capillaries increased. The large increase in arterial pressure probably caused an increase in the capillary pressure, which may have resulted in their progressive arterialisation. The increase in arteriolar capillaries which have a high partial pressure of oxygen may partially compensate for the low capillary density.

In conclusion, capillary angiogenesis occurs in SHRSP, as indicated by the increased capillary to myocyte ratio found in the inner most region of the left ventricle at 40 weeks. The cardiac hypertrophy, however, exceeds the capillary angiogenesis, so that the total capillary density is decreased. The oxygen diffusion distance is probably increased, which is disadvantageous for oxygen transport to cardiac tissues.

REFERENCES

Akiguchi I, Horie R, Yamori Y, Kameyama M (1979), Lethal course of stroke and thera-peutic effects in stroke-prone spontaneously hypertensive rats. In: Perspectives in cardiovascular research 4: Prophylactic approach to hypertensive diseases, ed Yamori et al., Raven Press, NY, 1979. 185–194.

Batra S, Kuo C, Rakusan K (1989), Spatial distribution of coronary capillaries: A-V segment staggering. Adv Exp Med Biol 248:241–246.

Folkman J, Klagsbrun M (1989), Angiogenic factors. Science 235:442–447.

Gao M, Batra S, Koyama T (1994), Capillary geometry in the subendocardium of the left ventricle from young rats subjected to exercise training. In: Progress in microcirculation research ed by Niimi H, Oda M, Sawada T, Xiu RJ, Pergamon Press, 187- 191.

Minami M, Sano M, Togashi H, Sakurai H, Saito H (1988), Stroke-related plasma nor- adrenaline, angiotensin II, arginine-vasopresin, and serotonin concentrations in stroke-prone spontaneously hypertensive rats. Progress in Hypertension, vol 1, ed. Saito et al. 89–114.

Nagaoka A, Shino A, Iwatsuka H (1979), Effects of dexamethasone and thyroxine on developments of severe hypertension and stroke-prone spontaneously hypertensive rats. In: Perspectives in cardiovascular research 4: Prophylactic approach to hypertensive diseases, ed Yamori et al., Raven Press, NY, 195–199.

Okamoto K, Yamori Y, Nagaoka A (1974): Establishment of the stroke-prone SHR. Circulation Research 34/35 (Suppl I): 143–153.

Price RJ, Owens GK, Skalak TC (1994) Immunohistochemical identification of arteriolar development using markers of smooth muscle differentiation. Evidence that capillary arterialization proceeds from terminal arterioles. Circulation Research 75:520–527.

Rakusan K, Hrdina PW, Turek Z, Lakatta EG, Spurgeon HA (1984), Cell size and capillary supply of the hypertensive rat heart: quantitative study. Basic Research in Cardiology 79:389–395.

Tomanek RJ (1979), The role of prevention or relief of pressure overload on the myocardial cell of the spontaneously hypertensive rat. A morphometric and stereologic study. Laboratory Investigation 40:83–91.

Tomanek RJ and Hovanec JM (1981) The effect of long term pressure-overload and aging on the myocardium. Journal of Molecular and Cellular Cardiology 13:471- 488.

Tomanek RJ, Searls JC, Lachen bruch PA (1982), Quantitative changes in the capillary bed during developing peak, and stabilized cardiac hypertrophy in the spontane ously hypertensive rat. Circulation Research 51:295–304.

Yamori Y, Horie R, Akiguchi I, Ohtaka M, Nara Y, Ooshima A: Pathophysiology and prevention of stroke in stroke-prone spontaneously hypertensive rats. In: Per spectives in cardiovascular research 4: Prophylactic approach to hypertensive diseases, ed Yamori et al., Raven Press, NY, 1979. 173–183.

47

ADEQUACY OF CEREBRAL VASCULAR REMODELING FOLLOWING THREE WEEKS OF HYPOBARIC HYPOXIA

Examined by an Integrated Composite Analytical Model

Karen L. Lauro[1,2] and Joseph C. LaManna[2]

[1]Department of Pulmonary and Critical Care Medicine
[2]Department of Neurology
Case Western Reserve University and School of Medicine
Cleveland, Ohio 44106

1. INTRODUCTION

Chronic exposure to moderate hypoxia is associated with considerable remodeling of the cerebral microvascular network. In rats exposed to hypobaric (0.5 ATM) hypoxia, cortical microvessel density increases to 171% of controls within the first week. Peak density is reached within two weeks. The increase in hematocrit follows a similar time course. Although the hemodynamic acclimation appears to complete after two weeks, levels of cortical metabolites, obtained after three weeks of exposure, suggest O_2 insufficiency at rest. Increased lactate and slightly decreased glycogen concentrations within the brain, along with increased glucose consumption are consistent with an increased dependence on anaerobic glycolysis for energy production. Whatever the production mechanisms, the restored ATP and phosphocreatine levels indicate the energy demand is being met.

Because of the current technical obstacles in directly measuring oxygen sufficiency in tissue and microrheological properties of non-superfical cerebral networks, an integrated composite analytical model was developed to address the following questions: Are the hemodynamic adaptations adequate to meet the oxygen demands of the tissue? Is the primary increase in capillary surface area due to sprouting, increasing parallel paths thereby reducing diffusion distance, or elongation of existing paths to allow longer unloading times? Is the high hematocrit a hemodynamic liability on the microvascular level?

The analytical model was developed by decomposing the problem into multiple physiological sub-domains, which in turn were decomposed according to the biological hierarchy of scale (tissue, cellular, and molecular). Three major issues emerged : 1) those that are biochemical (metabolic/acid-base balance model) and 2) those that are vascular (angioarchitecture/ hemodynamic model); 3) both of which are linked by exchange at the blood tissue interface (substrate blood/tissue transport, O_2 delivery model).

2. Methods

2.1. Animal Model

Male Wistar rats, housed in a hypobaric chamber, were exposed to one half atmosphere for a period of three weeks, (except for up to one hour a day when the pressure was returned to normal over a period of 10 minutes for cage cleaning, water, and food). Their littermates were used as controls.

2.2. Physiological and Stereological Measurements

2.2.1. Capillary Lumen Diameters. were measured on six μμ sections immunocytochemically stained for the blood-brain barrier glucose transporter, Glut-1. The rats were deeply anesthetized with ether, perfused through the heart with saline, and perfusion-fixed with an EM fixative and embedded in paraffin. The coronal sections were digitized using a microscope with a 40X objective, connected to a video camera and frame grabber. Luminal diameters were measured with a computerized ruler tool. Capillaries with diameters less than 2.9μm were considered to be plasmatic.

2.2.2. Capillary Tortuosity and Orientatiow. were measured in rats anesthetized with 4% chlorohydrate, perfused through the aorta with heprinized saline and reperfused with 7% gelatin containing FITC-dextran. Fluorescence images were obtained from 100 μm frozen sagittal sections with light and confocal microscopy.

Sub-networks of digitized capillary segments were manually traced as a series of straight line capillary fragments. Capillary segment length (L_{cs}) equals the sum of fragment lengths and the three dimensional tortuosity was estimated as (L_{cs})/(distance between capillary end points). Planar tortuosity and orientation correction factors are used to map the coronally measured microvessel density (N_{cap}) to the radius of the tissue exchange unit. The tortuosity factor corrects for the capillary segments which reentering the cut plane, preventing them from being multiply counted. It is estimated as the mean $\|\Sigma\Delta x\| - \Sigma\Delta x| / (L_{cs})$. The orientation correction was calculated as one plus the fraction of fragments oriented parallel to the coronal plane [i.e. $|\Delta x| \leq 1$ and $|\Delta y| \geq 5$].

2.2.3. Plasma β. OH-butyrate [LaManna and Lust, unpublished observation] chemically assayed using Sigma kit 310-A with the fluormetric procedure.

With the exception of P_{50},[2] the systemic physiological parameters listed in Table 1 were obtained during a previous study on awake rats[3]. The remaining data used in the model, Table 2, has been reported elsewhere[4,5,6]. The raw data was reanalyzed to combine the cortical regions.

2.3. Analytical Model

2.3.1 Metabolic Model. Chronically hypoxic rats initially lose weight, then regain it at a slower rate than their normoxic littermates. During starvation, elevated plasma ke-

Table 1. Effects of chronic hypobaric hypoxia on systemic physiological parameters

Parameter	Units	Control	Chronic hypoxia
Arterial PO_2 (P_aO_2)	Torr	101 ± 4.6	48 ± 3.1 [a]
Half saturation PO_2 (P_{50}) [(1)]	Torr	35	35
Arterial PCO_2 (P_aCO_2)	Torr	37 ± 3.3	26 ± 1.3 [a]
HCO_3	µMol*l⁻¹	22.3 ± 1.0	16 ± .9 [a]
Arterial pH	units	7.4 ± .03	7.41 ± .02
Hematocrit (Hct)	%	46 ± 2.29	63 ± 2.2 [a]
MAP	Torr	123 ± 6.5	115 ± 10.7
Body Temperature	°C	37.3 ± 1	37.0 ± .4
Body Weight	g	379 ± 14.3	317 ± 6.23[a]
Brain Weight	g	1.986 ± .08	1.872 ± .03[a]

Means ± S.E.M.　　(1) Baumann, 1971;　　a) P< 0.05

tones have been found to provide significant fuel for the brain[7]. Plasma β-OH-butyrate doubled in the hypoxic rats. Therefore, the ketones were assessed as a potential metabolic substrate.

Relative contributions of glycolytic and oxidative metabolism to energy production were estimated by solving the series of equations for conservation of mass of the metabolic substrates and products (i.e. ATP, glucose, β-OH-butyrate, acetoacetate), and the stoichiometry of glycolytic and oxidative metabolism. Since body temperature was experimentally maintained at 37°C with a heat lamp during the physiological measurements,

Table 2. Hemodynamic and metabolic indices to chronic hypobaric hypoxia acclimatization

Parameter	Units	Control	Chronic hypoxia	Method
Microvessel Density (N_{cap})[(1)]	N / mm²	397 ± 33	643 ± 37[a]	Alkaline phosphatase
Capillary Diameter	µm	4.88± 2.3	5.44 ± 2.05	Glut-1 transporter immunochemical stain
Plasmatic	%	8	4	Glut-1 transporter immunochemical stain
Capillary Segment Length[(2)]	µm	68	100[a]	Carbon black gel
Normoxic Capillary Path Length [(3)]	µm	422	~520	Epoxy vascular cast, computer model
Capillary Tortuosity	µm/µm	1.09 ± .2	1.24 ± .5	FITC-dextran gel
Capillary Orientation		1.06	1.13	FITC-dextran gel
Local Blood Flow[(1)]	ml*100g⁻¹*min⁻¹	124 ± 4.5	130 ± 14.5	Dual-label indicator fractionation, [C¹⁴]-butanol, [³H]-sucrose
Sucrose Space[(1)]	ml*100g⁻¹	2.1 ± .1	2.1 ± .1	[³H]-sucrose
ATP[(4)]	nMol / mg	12.1 ± .8	12.1 ± 1.1	Chemical assay
Phosphocreatine[(4)]	nMol / mg	18.0 ± 2.7	20.3 ± 2.2	Chemical assay
Lactate[(4)]	nMol / mg	10.1 ± 2.8	18.1 ± 3.7[a]	Chemical assay
Intracellular pH (pH_i)[(4)]	units	7.19 ± .06	7.25 ± .07	Neutral Red Histophotometry
Glucose Consumption[(4)]	µMol*100g⁻¹*min⁻¹	115.8 ± 3.2	159.5 ± 21.3[a]	[C¹⁴]-2-deoxyglucose autoradiography
Plasma β-OH-butyrate	mM	0.09	0.2	Chemical assay

Means ± S.E.M.　(1) LaManna, 1992; (2) Mironov, 1994; (3) Hudetz, 1989; (4) Harik, 1995;　a) P<.0.05

oxygen consumption was calculated based on the stoichiometry of consumption of the oxidative substrates assuming constant ATP production.

Intracellular phosphate and protein buffer systems are assumed to be unaltered by chronic hypoxia. Tissue acid-base balance was analyzed to consider metabolic effect of the hyperventilation induced hypocapnia according to the following equation :

$$\Delta \text{ [Buffer Base]} \cong \Delta \text{ [HCO}_3^-\text{]} = (\Delta \mathbf{PCO_2} * S * K1') / [H^+] = \Delta (\text{ [lactate}^-\text{]} + \Sigma \text{ [An}^-\text{]}) \cong \Delta \text{ [lactate}^-\text{]}$$

where S equals the CO_2 solubility coefficient , and K1' equals H_2CO_3 ionization coefficient.

2.3.2. Angioarchitecture and Hemodynamic Model. The hemodynamic model was used to define a "realistic" nominal capillary/tissue exchange unit based on measured regional morphological and physiological data, and analyze its hemodynamic characteristics and the rheological aspects of the blood flowing through it.

Initially, the capillary network was idealized as a series of parallel straight capillaries homogeneously distributed on the square grid, each supplying a hexagonal cylinder of tissue. A geometry correction converted the hexagon area to a cylinder. Using the orientation, tortuosity, and plasmatic correction factors defined above, the radius of the tissue exchange unit was approximated as:

$$\text{Radius}_{\text{Tissue}} = \frac{\text{geometry correction}}{2 * [N_{\text{cap}} * \text{orientation factor} * (1\text{- tortuosity}) * (1\text{-plasmatic})]^{1/2}}$$

Red blood cell velocity (υ_{RBC}) and capillary network mean path length (Path) are two critical parameters not accurately measurable in non-superficial cerebral networks today. Mean path lengths and transit times (MTT) for both the microcirculatory and capillary beds for the normoxic state were estimated by a computer simulation[6]. Hypoxic capillary path length was estimated by the normoxic path length scaled by the capillary segment length ratios determined experimentally. These path lengths are used as the length of the Krough cylinder.

υ_{RBC} was accurately measured down to a depth of 70 μm[8]. This was used as a starting value which was adjusted to give an oxygen tension histogram in agreement with the histogram measured by Lübbers[9] a PO_2 electrode in anesthetized guinea pigs[9].

The reduction of hematocrit with decreasing vessel radius noted by Fahraeus in larger vessels and its reversal at capillary diameters smaller than the RBC diameter, leads to a corresponding change in viscosity. Since the large vessel Fahraeus and small vessel reverse-Fahraeus blood viscosity effects are due to physically distinct phenomena, the marginal zone model [10] and the axial-train model[11] were combined by a weighed addition, where the weighting function was an unity sigmoid centered at the vessel diameter in which the transitions between the phenomena occur.

2.3.3 Oxygen Delivery Model. The O_2 delivery model is a steady-state transcapillary exchange model. It is based on Blum's[12] analytical solution for a single capillary Krough cylinder[12], which was extended to include oxyhemoglobin dissociation, Michaelis-Menten

O_2 consumption. Oxygen saturation was calculated using the Hill equation extended to correct for the Bohr and Root effect, as well as for temperature.

3. RESULTS AND DISCUSSION

The chronic reduction of one essential metabolic substrate has far reaching consequences. Hyperventilation increases O_2 uptake while decreasing arterial PCO_2, thereby altering blood and tissue acid base balance. Polycythemia, again increases O_2 carrying capacity of the blood, at the expense of blood viscosity and nutrient carrying capacity of the plasma. Remodeling of the microvascular system to increase capillary to tissue O_2 gradients must maintain the tissue/vessel balance between hydrostatic and osmotic pressures.

Minimum tissue PO_2 is often used as a criterion for accessing oxygen sufficiency. The calculated oxygen tensions profiles (Figure 1 A) and histograms (Figure 1 B) illustrate the model's prediction that the hemodynamic acclimatization to moderate hypoxia causes a flat O_2 field, providing significantly higher peripheral tissue PO_2 at rest, and a mean tissue PO_2 111% higher than normoxic (Table 3).

Musch[13] found arterial O_2 content, rather than PO_2, was a good index of tissue hypoxia after acclimatization. In his study, hypocapnia accounted for all of the lactate in moderate hypoxia (PaO_2:45 torr), and 40–60% of the increase in severe hypoxia (PaO_2:30 torr). Conversely, acute hypocapnic normoxemia led to increased cortical lactate of the same order of magnitude as we observed in chronic hypocapnic hypoxemia[14].

Modulation of intracellular metabolic acid concentrations has been proposed as a means of regulating intracellular pH independent of the Na^+ gradient, indirectly conserving ATP[14]. Change in metabolic acid production is due substantially to the pH dependence of ATP inhibition of phosphofructokinase (PFK) activity. The increased ventilatory rate

Table 3. Model results

Parameter	Units	Control	Chronic hypoxia	Hypoxic : Control Ratio
Oxidative ATP Production	% of Total	99.94	97.62	**0.98**
Arterial/Venous PCO_2	Torr	36.6 : 45.3	26.4 : 34.8	0.72 : 0.77
Arterial/**Venous** PO_2	Torr	100.8 : 37.9	47.7 : 37.7	0.47 : **0.99**
Max & Min Tissue Tension	Torr	100.8 : .71	47.7 : 18.7	0.47:26.34
Mean Tissue Tension	Torr	26.9	29.8	1.11
$CMRO_2$	ml O_2 *g^{-1}*sec^{-1}	2.5	2.44	**0.98**
O_2 Delivery	ml O_2 *g^{-1}*min^{-1}	248.7	274.8	1.10
Arterial/Venous O_2 Content	ml O_2 / ml Blood	200.5 :103.8	211.4 : 144.7	**1.05**:1.39
Tissue Cylinder Diameter	mm	57.8	44.2	0.76
Capillary Length	mm	422	520.3	1.23
Number of Paths	gm^{-1}	9.025E5	1.252E6	1.39
Local Blood Volume	ml*$100g^{-1}$	3.9	5.7	1.46
RBC Velocity	mm*sec^{-1}	1,256	1,128	0.9
Mean Transit Time	sec	0.34	0.47	1.38
Capillary Blood Viscosity	centipoise	1.8	1.78	**0.99**
Resistance	torr*sec*mm^{-3}	4.18E-4	3.23E-4	0.77
Capillary Flow	ml*sec^{-1}	2.35E-8	2.59E-8	1.10
Capillary Pressure Drop	torr	9.83	8.36	0.85
Pressure Drop / unit length	torr*mm^{-1}	0.02	0.02	0.80

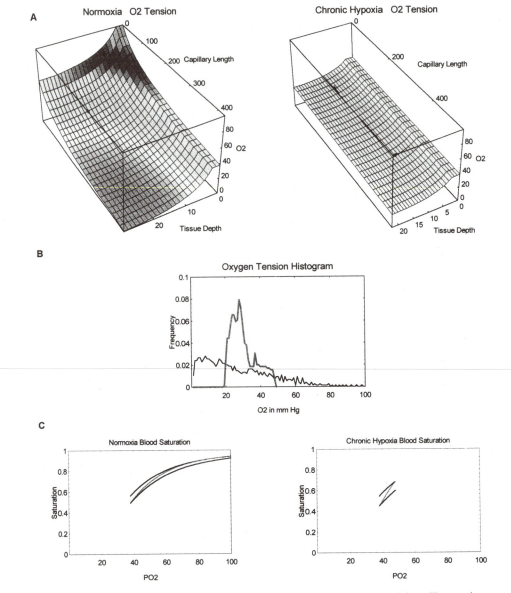

Figure 1. A) Oxygen tensions profiles and B) histograms [thick line: hypoxic] C) Arterial, capillary, and venous oxyhemoglobin dissociation curves.

observed in hypobaric hypoxia results in low tissue PCO_2. A decrease in tissue PCO_2 leads to an decrease in HCO_3^- and an increase in production of lactic and other metabolic acids. The lactic acid concentration is predominately effected. The calculated value of pH (7.26) based on the measured PCO_2 and cortical lactate concentration was less than 1% higher than the value measured. Conversely, the lactate level necessary to reestablish normal tissue pH was 30 nMol/mg dry weight as compared to the 18 measured. This would indicate a continued pH bias on PFK, and illustrates how glycolytic flux can be altered while maintaining an essentially constant rate of oxidative metabolism.

Dysoxia, rather than hypoxemia, requires an oxygen limited energy flux, independent of arterial PO_2. Oxidative metabolism of glucose and ketone bodies provides 98% of the ATP production in chronic hypoxia. Arterial O_2 content is more than restored by the increase in hematocrit. The decreased O_2 driving force is counterbalanced by an increase in mean transit times and decreased diffusion distances in the tissue, yielding an O_2 gradient sufficient to generate the flux necessary to support basal tissue O_2 consumption.

Acute normocapnic hypoxemic rats (PaO_2:41 torr) maintained control levels of $CMRO_2$[15]. Brief mild electrical stimulus of the cortex elicited transient increases in cytochrome a,a_3 oxidation in rats with $PaO_2 \geq 50$ torr, and transient increases in reduction of cytochrome a,a_3 and NADH with $PaO_2 \geq 40$ torr[16]. A graded response was observed with intermediate PaO_2. A partially reduced electron transport chain can maintain normal levels of ATP production with an increased concentration of substrates[17] [i.e.. ADP and NADH]. These studies indicate a lack of dysoxia with acute moderate hypoxemia. It is unlikely an acclimatization process would stop prematurely, providing a greater oxygen insufficiency than exists acutely.

The acclimatization strategy appears to be an increase in capillary volume due to a combination of increased capillary diameter, sprouting, and elongation. The diameters increase by 11%, decreasing blood viscosity and increasing blood flow. The model estimates a 39% increase in parallel paths thereby reducing diffusion distance. Existing paths are estimated to be elongated by 23% to allow longer unloading times.

The high hematocrit is usually thought to be a hemodynamic liability. However, blood viscosity is a function of both hematocrit and tube radius. As seen in Figure 2, the Fahraeus effect causes an equalization of viscosity at small vessel diameters. This combined with an increase in capillary diameter compensates for the increased hematocrit and capillary lengths. The resistance to blood flow in the capillary is less than normal, and the model predicts a slightly lower hydrostatic pressure drop along the capillary bed. This is supported by a restoration of local blood flow.

The changing oxygen affinity of the capillary blood during transit from the arterial to venous ends is illustrated in Figure 1 C. The limits of the capillary oxyhemoglobin dissociation curve is defined by the arterial and venous curves. In the normoxic state the capillary blood maintains near-arterial high affinity during half the transit, whereas the

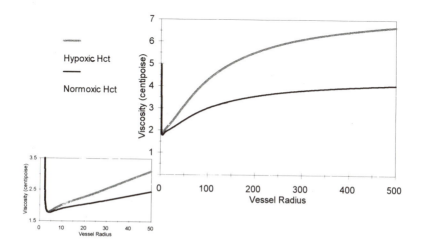

Figure 2. Blood viscosity as a function of vessel radius and hematocrit.

hypoxic affinity drops immediately. There is also a greater change in affinity from arterial to venous end, aiding in both the loading and unloading at the increased transit times.

   While the model could not answer the O_2 sufficiency question definitively, it was helpful in suggesting explanations for the conflicting experimental results. The possibility of acid-base balance as the source of increased anaerobic glycolysis had not been considered prior to the analysis of the oxygen delivery. The model predictions also suggest meaningful future experiments and modeling directions. Its use in our chronic hypoxia animal model illustrates how analytical modeling can provide insight as to the significance of individual physiological parameters. Most notable are the parameters which are returned to normal (bolded in Table 3), indicating these are physiologically important parameters the system seeks to control.

4. ACKNOWLEDGMENTS

This work was supported in part by NIH grants HL-02788 and NIH HL-42215

5. REFERENCES

1. Harik N., Harik S.I., LaManna J.C. On the Increased Cerebral Vascularity in Hypobaric Hypoxia: Time Course and Reversibity in Adult Rats. *JCBFM Vol 15, Suppl.* 1:S276, 1995.
2. Baumann R., Bauer C., and Bartels H. Influence of chronic and acute hypoxia on oxygen affinity and red cell 2,3 diphosphoglycerate of rats and guinea pigs, *Resp. Physiol.*, 11: 135–144, 1971.
3. Harik S.I., Lust W.D., Jones S.C., Lauro K.L., Pundik S., LaManna J.C., Brain glucose metabolism in hypobaric hypoxia, *J. Appl. Physiol.* 79:136–140, 1995.
4. LaManna, J.C., Vendel, L.M. and Farrell, R.M. Brain adaptation to chronic hypobaric hypoxia in rats. *J.Appl.Physiol.* 72:2238–2243, 1992.
5. Mironov, V., Hritz, M.A., LaManna, J.C., Hudetz, A.G. and Harik, S.I. Architectural alterations in rat cerebral microvessels after hypobaric hypoxia. *Brain Res.* 660:73–80, 1994.
6. Hudetz, A.G., Spaulding, J.G. and Kiani, M.F. Computer simulation of cerebral microhemodynamics. *Adv.Exp.Med.Biol.* 248:293–304, 1989.
7. Hawkins, R.A., Mans, A.M. and Davis, D.W. Regional ketone body utilization by rat brain in starvation and diabetes. *Am.J.Physiol.* 250:169–178, 1986.
8. Hudetz, A.G., Greene, A.S., Feher, G., Knuese, D.E. and Cowley, A.W.J. Imaging system for three-dimensional mapping of cerebrocortical capillary networks in vivo. *Microvasc.Res.* 46:293–309, 1993.
9. Lübbers, D.W. Oxygen Delivery and Microcirculation in the Brain. In: *Microcirculation in Circulatory Disorders*, edited by Manabe, Zweifach, and Messmer, Tokyo:Springer-Verlag, 1988,p. 33–50.
10. Haynes, R. Physical basis of the dependence of blood viscosity on tube radius. *Am.J.Physiol.* 198:1193–1200, 1960.
11. Whitmore, R. A theory of blood flow in small vessels. *J.Appl.Physiol.* 22:767–771, 1967.
12. Blum, J.J., Concentration profiles in and around capillaries. *Am.J.Physiol.* 198:991–998, 1960.
13. Musch, T.I., Dempsey, J.A., Smith, C.A., Mitchell, G.S. and Bateman, N.T. Metabolic acids and [H+] regulation in brain tissue during acclimatization to chronic hypoxia. *J.Appl.Physiol.* 55:1486–1495, 1983.
14. Siesjo, B.K. and Messeter, K. Factors determining intracellular pH. In: *Ion homeostasis of the brain*, edited by Siesjo, B.K. and Sorensen, S.C.,New York:Academic Press, 1970,p. 244–269.
15. Johannsson, H. and Siesjo, B.K. CBF and CMRO2 in hypoxia. *Acta Physiol.Scand.* 93:269–276, 1975.
16. LaManna, J.C., Light, A.I., Peretsman, S.J. and Rosenthal, M. Oxygen insufficiency during hypoxic hypoxia in rat brain cortex. *Brain Res.* 293:313–318, 1984.
17. Connett, R.J., Honig, C.R., Gayeski, T.E.J. and Brooks, G.A. Defining hypoxia: a systems view of VO2, glycolysis, energetics, and intracellular PO2. *J.Appl.Physiol.* 68:833–842, 1990.

48

USE OF A PFC-BASED OXYGEN CARRIER TO LOWER THE TRANSFUSION TRIGGER IN A CANINE MODEL OF HEMODILUTION AND SURGICAL BLOOD LOSS

S. Batra, P. E. Keipert, J. D. Bradley, N. S. Faithfull, and S. F. Flaim

Alliance Pharmaceutical Corp.
San Diego, California 92121

1. INTRODUCTION

Perfluorochemical (PFC) emulsions are inert compounds that demonstrate a high solubility for gases, and are being developed as temporary intravenous oxygen carriers for intraoperative use as an adjunct to surgical procedures involving autologous blood sparing techniques, i.e., predonation and acute normovolemic hemodilution (ANH).

ANH involves the removal of blood from a patient, just before or after the induction of anesthesia, and the simultaneous replacement of blood with a colloid or crystalloid plasma volume expander[1,2]. In this setting, a key question is whether PFC emulsions can maintain diffusive gradients for oxygen in the face of blood loss, thereby extending the limits of tolerable surgical anemia and delaying the initiation of blood transfusion.

The present study was designed to mimic the clinical scenario in which a PFC-based oxygen carrier is used in conjunction with autologous blood transfusion strategies. The hypothesis of this study was that PFC emulsion treated animals would be able to tolerate greater surgical blood loss compared to Control animals without compromising hemodynamics or systemic oxygenation.

2. METHODS

Sixteen purpose-bred beagles (13.1±0.3 kg [mean±SEM]) were anesthetized with isoflurane (1.5–2.5%), intubated and mechanically ventilated with a Siemens SV-900C servo ventilator (Siemens, Cerritos, CA). Animals were surgically instrumented to measure systemic and pulmonary pressures, heart rate and cardiac output (thermodilution), and to collect arterial and mixed venous blood samples. The spleen was surgically ligated to prevent autotransfusion of red blood cells. PFC emulsion formulation AF0144 (58% w/v

Oxygen Transport to Tissue XVIII, edited by Nemoto and LaManna
Plenum Press, New York, 1997

perflubron [perfluorooctyl bromide], 2% perfluorodecyl bromide with 3.6% egg yolk phospholipid; Alliance Pharmaceutical Corp.) was used in this study.

Under ventilation with room air, all animals were hemodiluted isovolemically to Hb=8.0 g/dL with *Hespan* (6% hydroxyethyl starch, Dupont). The autologous blood was collected in citrate, phosphate, dextrose-adenine (CPDA-1) collection packs (Baxter Fenwal, Deerfield, IL), centrifuged to form packed cells, and divided into units (defined as 10% of estimated blood volume) available for later transfusion. The fraction of inspired oxygen (FiO_2) was then increased to 100%, and animals were randomized to Controls (n=8) that were transfused with one "unit" of packed cells (Hct = 84±1%; 0.65±0.003 g Hb/kg), or PFC-treatment (n=8) that received a single dose of 1.35 g PFC/kg.

Following infusion of a unit of packed cells or PFC emulsion, animals were subjected to a period of volume-compensated blood loss using 1:1 *Hespan* replacement to maintain normovolemia. During blood loss, Controls were transfused each time they reached a Hb level of ~ 8.0 g/dL, whereas the PFC group was allowed to bleed to a lower hemoglobin level before the initiation of transfusion (~5 g/dL).

Following the blood loss period, both groups were transfused with all remaining autologous units. In Controls, this represented any remaining blood not transfused during the volume compensated blood loss. In PFC animals, all red blood cells collected during the initial intentional hemodilution period were still available for transfusion. A net loss of hemoglobin was defined as the within-group difference in total circulating Hb content from the start to the end of the study. Animals were then returned to room air ventilation for a final set of hemodynamic and blood gases measurements.

Data are expressed as means ± SEM. Differences within and between groups were determined by two-way analysis of variance (ANOVA) and Bonferroni post-hoc analysis as required using *Systat®* (Systat Inc., Evanston, IL). Statistical significance was accepted at $p<0.05$.

3. RESULTS

Transfusion of each "unit" of packed cells resulted in an increase in total Hb of ~1.0 g/dL. Hemodynamic parameters such as pulmonary, systemic and wedge pressures, heart rate cardiac output, were not notably different between groups. In response to hemodilution on room air, cardiac output increased by a mean of 77% in all animals (2.83 ± 0.23 to 5.02 ± 0.41 L/min). This increase was attributed to both an increase in heart rate and stroke volume. When the FiO_2 was increased to 1.0, cardiac output fell by 13% (to 4.38±0.41 L/min), and was essentially maintained at this level in both groups throughout the rest of the study.

Arterial PO_2 (PaO_2) increased from 89 ± 3 to 416 ± 7 mmHg when FiO_2 was increased to 1.0. There was a secondary 7% PaO_2 increase in response to PFC emulsion in the treated group. However, there was no difference in PaO_2 between PFC and Control animals for the remainder of the study. Mixed venous PO_2 ($P\bar{v}O_2$), a global indicator of systemic oxygenation, increased significantly by 18±3 mmHg (mean±SEM) in response to infusion of PFC emulsion (Fig. 1). In addition, $P\bar{v}O_2$ levels were consistently higher in PFC animals throughout the blood loss period (Fig. 2) despite the fact that total Hb levels were decreased to significantly lower values than in Controls ($p<0.05$).

After all autologous blood was transfused, there was a significant difference between groups in the total amount of Hb lost during the course of the study. This net loss of hemoglobin was significantly less for PFC-treated animals (Fig. 3, $p<0.05$). When ex-

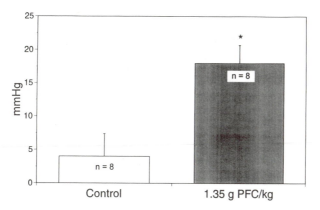

Figure 1. Increase in mixed venous PO_2 ($P\bar{v}O_2$) above the 100% oxygen ventilation post-hemodilution level. * = significant vs. Control (p<0.05). Data are means±SEM.

pressed according to our definition of a unit of packed cells, this difference represented a net savings of 1.5–2 units for PFC-treated animals.

4. DISCUSSION

The risks of allogeneic blood transfusion are well known, and the use of hemodilution techniques to reduce transfusion requirements have been noted[3,4]. The American College of Physicians have published a Guideline to consider elective transfusion with allogeneic blood as an outcome to be avoided[5].

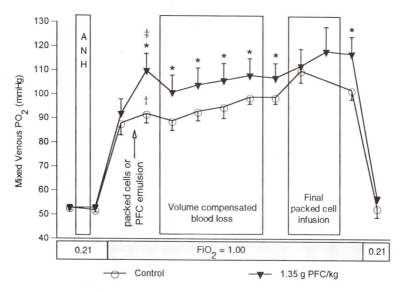

Figure 2. Mixed venous PO_2 ($P\bar{v}O_2$) over the course of the experimental protocol. * = significant difference between Control and PFC emulsion groups; † = significant effect of packed cells; ‡ = significant effect of PFC emulsion (p<0.05). Data are means±SEM.

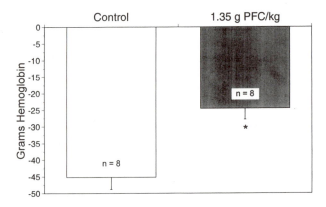

Figure 3. Net loss of hemoglobin over the course of the experimental protocol. * = significant vs. Control (p<0.05). Data are means±SEM.

The effects of acute normovolemic hemodilution on hemodynamics and oxygen transport have been studied extensively[6-8]. The basis for tolerance to moderate isovolemic hemodilution is that cardiac output increases, which compensates for the reduction in arterial oxygen content. Accordingly, oxygen delivery, the product of cardiac output and arterial oxygen content, is well maintained[9,10]. In the present study, the cardiac output response to isovolemic hemodilution was due to increases in both heart rate and stroke volume. Although in most studies in anesthetized dogs, the increase in cardiac output has been has been due augmentation of stroke volume, differences due to anesthesia have been noted. For a review see Spahn et al[11].

In hemodiluted patients undergoing surgery, the emerging benefits are that blood lost during surgery (post-hemodilution) will be more dilute, and further, a fresh source of autologous blood will be available for transfusion, as needed. The use of PFCs in this setting is designed to extend the degree of tolerable surgical anemia, thereby delaying the initiation of transfusion and sparing the limited supply of autologous blood.

By study design, following a single topload dose of PFC emulsion, treated animals were bled to significantly lower hemoglobin levels as compared to Control animals before the initiation of transfusion. Despite this ~3 g Hb/dL difference, hemodynamic parameters were well maintained, and systemic oxygenation, based upon PO₂ levels, was higher in animals treated with PFC emulsion.

5. CONCLUSION

By combining the use of a PFC-based oxygen carrier and surgical hemodilution, it may be feasible to safely lower the transfusion trigger. This strategy, when applied to a canine model of hemodilution and progressive surgical anemia due to volume-compensated blood loss, resulted in a significant net savings of 1.5–2 units of blood without any apparent compromise in hemodynamics or systemic oxygenation (based on $P\bar{v}O_2$ levels). Further studies are underway to look at oxygenation in a number of tissues when PFC-based oxygen carriers are used to partially compensate for acute surgical anemia.

REFERENCES

1. L. Stehling and H.L. Zauder, Acute normovolemic hemodilution, *Transfusion* 31:857–868 (1991).
2. K. Messmer, L. Sunder-Plassmann, W.P. Klovekorn, and K. Holper, Circulatory significance of hemodilution: rheological changes and limitations, *Adv. Microcirc.* 4:1–77 (1972).
3. P. Sejourne, A. Poirer, and J.L. Meakins, Effect of haemodilution on transfusion requirements in liver resection, *Lancet* 2:1380–1382 (1989).
4. P.M. Ness, D.L. Bourke, and P.C. Walsh, A randomized trial of perioperative hemodilution versus transfusion of preoperatively deposited autologous blood in elective surgery, *Transfusion* 32:226–230 (1992).
5. American College of Physicians, Practice strategies for elective red blood cell transfusion, *Ann. Int. Med.* 116:403–406 (1992).
6. H. Laks, R.N. Pilon, W.P. Klovekorn, W. Anderson, J.R. MacCallum, and N.E. O'Connor, Acute hemodilution: its effect on hemodynamics and oxygen transport in anesthetized man, *Ann. Surg.* 180:103–109 (1974).
7. K. Messmer, D.H. Lewis, L. Sunder-Plassmann, W.P. Klovekorn, N. Mendler, and K. Holper, Acute normovolemic hemodilution, *Europ. Surg. Res.* 4:55–70 (1972).
8. K. Messmer, L. Sunder-Plassmann, F. Jesch, L. Gornandt, E. Sinagowitz, M. Kessler, R. Pfeiffer, E. Horn, J. Hoper, and K. Joachimsmeier, Oxygen supply to the tissues during limited normovolemic hemodilution, *Res. Exp. Med.* 159:152–166 (1973).
9. C.K. Chapler and S.M. Cain, The physiologic reserve in oxygen carrying capacity: studies in experimental hemodilution, *Can. J. Physiol. Pharmacol.* 64:7–12 (1986).
10. A. Trouwborst, R. Tenbrinck, and E. van Woerkens, Blood gas analysis of mixed venous blood during normoxic acute isovolemic hemodilution in pigs, *Anesth.Analg.* 70:523–529 (1990).
11. D.R. Spahn, B.J. Leone, J.G. Reves, and T. Pasch, Cardiovascular and coronary physiology of acute isovolemic hemodilution: a review of nonoxygen-carrying and oxygen-carrying solutions, *Anesth.Analg.* 78:1000–1021 (1994).

49

EFFECT OF PERFLUOROCHEMICAL EMULSION ON HEMORHEOLOGY AND SHEAR INDUCED BLOOD TRAUMA

Possible Mechanisms and Future Applications

M. V. Kameneva, H. S. Borovetz, J. F. Antaki, P. Litwak, W. J. Federspiel, R. L. Kormos, and B. P. Griffith

University of Pittsburgh, Artificial Heart and Lung Center
Center for Biotechnology and Bioengineering
300 Technology Drive
Pittsburgh, Pennsylvania 15219

INTRODUCTION

Blood trauma has been recognized as one of the key problems associated with assisted circulation. Indeed, the main requirement for improved heart-assist devices is the reduction of blood cell damage. The extremely high shear forces and prolonged contact between blood and foreign surfaces can cause mechanical destruction of erythrocytes (hemolysis), activation of platelets, changes in mechanical properties of erythrocytes[1] and thus reduction of oxygen delivery. Even low level of hemolysis, in turn, drastically increases RBC aggregation at low shear conditions[2]. Additionally, plasma free hemoglobin can have a toxic effect on the cardiovascular system, probably because of hemoglobin vasoactivity, mediated by its property to bind nitric oxide (NO), an endothelium-derived relaxing factor[3]. Alternatively, NO might be destroyed by O_2 radicals formed in the presence of hemoglobin[3].

Clinical applications of heart-assist devices demonstrate some alteration of patient blood rheology[4-7]. It was found for example that mechanical circulatory support patients had an increased viscosity of blood and decreased RBC deformability.

Despite considerable investigation of blood trauma in heart-assist devices[8-13], there is very little information in the literature concerning pharmacological strategies to reduce hemolysis and ameliorate hemorheological alterations in these devices. Eicosapentaenoic Acid (EPA) which is known for its antiatherogenic and antithrombotic properties, was shown to reduce RBC destruction and aggregation in dogs during left heart bypass with a centrifugal pump[14,15]. The mechanism of EPA action has not been clarified.

Oxygen Transport to Tissue XVIII, edited by Nemoto and LaManna
Plenum Press, New York, 1997

We investigated *in-vitro* a new approach to reduce blood trauma and improve rheological properties of blood subjected to mechanical stress. For this we partially replaced blood plasma with perfluorocarbon (PFC) emulsion (Fluosol, Alpha Therapeutic Corp., Los Angeles, CA) with high gas solubility. Approximately 40 ml of O_2 can be dissolved in 100 ml of most liquid perfluorochemicals; carbon dioxide is about 2.5 times more soluble than oxygen[16]. FLUOSOL®, a 20% emulsion of two perfluorochemicals - perfluorodecalin and perfluorotri-n-propylaminecan, dissolves about 8 ml of O_2 per 100 ml of emulsion under oxygen partial pressure of 760 mm Hg[17]. For comparison, the oxygen capacity of blood is approximately 20 ml of O_2 per 100 ml of blood (1.39 ml O_2 / gm Hb)[18]. Indications for the Fluosol use are to protect myocardium during percutaneous transluminal coronary angioplasty (PTCA) in patients at high risk of ischemic complications of angioplasty[19]. Our *in-vitro* experiments aimed to investigate the effects of the PFC emulsion on rheological properties of blood and shear-induced blood trauma and the mechanisms of these effects.

MATERIALS AND METHODS

A mock circulatory loop (schematically shown in Figure 1) consisted of a centrifugal pump (Bio-Medicus, Bio-Medicus Co, Minneapolis, MN), PVC tubing, a water bath for maintaining temperature near 37° C (not shown in the picture), and a collapsible blood reservoir to avoid blood contact with air. Flow was determined by an in-line Bio-Medicus flow probe, and pressure was measured by a Statham pressure transducer (Viggo-Spectramed, Oxnard, CA). Each test of two hours duration included a "baseline" period (one hour duration) and a "fluosol" (one hour duration) period. For the latter, 20% of plasma volume was replaced with fluosol. Fluosol solution was prepared according to instruction, but was not oxygenated, since we did not plan to investigate the additional effect of oxygenation on studied parameters. In control experiments, blood was circulated for two hours without replacement of plasma volume with PFC. During each experiment the speed of the pump was not altered (2725±150 rpm and 3000 ± 60 rpm for PFC and control experiments, respectively). The volume flow and pressure at point "P" (see Fig. 1) were 3.0±0.4 L/min

Test Circuit

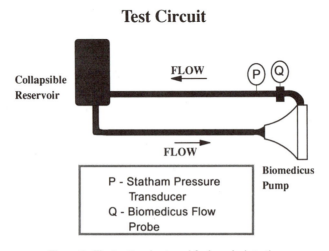

Figure 1. The *in vitro* circut used for hemolysis testing.

and 117±20 mm Hg for PFC experiments, and 3.1±0.3 L/min and 138±14 mm Hg for control.

A total of ten experiments were performed of which four served as controls. A 250 cc sample of animal blood (ovine or bovine) was used for each test. Hematocrit was determined in a microhematocrit centrifuge (TRIAC centrifuge, Clay Adams Division of Becton, Dickinson and Co.). Plasma free hemoglobin was measured prior to, one hour following the initiation of blood pumping, after partial replacement of plasma volume with PFC, and one hour following the pumping of blood with PFC. Hemolysis was characterized by the following Index of Hemolysis[20] (IH):

$$IH = \frac{\Delta Hb \cdot V \cdot (1 - Ht) \cdot 100}{Q}$$

ΔHb is the rate of increase of plasma free hemoglobin level (g/L-min), V - the total loop volume (L), Ht - whole blood hematocrit, and Q - the mean volumetric flow rate (L/min). Plasma free hemoglobin was measured by Gilford Spectrophotometer 240 (Gilford Instrument Laboratories Inc., Oberlin, OH).

RBC mechanical fragility was determined by the modified method described in (21). Three ml of blood or blood with PFC were placed into a 7 cc vacutainer with five 1/8" diameter metal shot added. The vacutainers were rocked on a standard rocker (Thermolyne Speci-Mix, Barnstead/Thermolyne, Dubuque, IA) and liberated plasma free hemoglobin was determined after one hour of rocking. A Mechanical Fragility Index was calculated as:

$$MFI = \frac{Hb_{final} - Hb_{base}}{Hb_{w.bl.} - Hb_{base}} \times 100$$

where Hb_{final} - plasma free hemoglobin (mg%) in blood sample exposed rocking, Hb_{base} - plasma free hemoglobin (mg%) in blood sample which was not rocked, $Hb_{w.bl}$ - hemoglobin concentration in whole blood (mg%). A total of ten experiments (six - human blood and four - ovine blood) were performed to study the effect of PFC replacement (20% of plasma volume) on RBC mechanical fragility. Mechanical fragility measurements were performed at room temperature (22-23°C).

In addition to hemolysis and RBC mechanical fragility, hemorheological parameters studied included whole blood viscosity and erythrocyte aggregation. They were determined in six samples of human blood with and without 20% replacement of plasma volume with PFC. Blood viscosity was measured by a Couette rheometer[22] (Contraves Low Shear 30, Contraves, Cincinnati, OH) over shear rates ($\dot{\gamma}$) from 0.277 to 128.5 sec^{-1}. Asymptotic blood viscosity was measured by a capillary viscometer[22] (Cannon Instrument Co., State College, PA) at a shear rate of approximately 600 sec^{-1}. RBC aggregation was estimated indirectly by measurement of the erythrocyte sedimentation rate[22] (ESR) and blood viscosity at low shear rate[23] ($\dot{\gamma}$=0.277 sec^{-1}). ESR rate was determined in disposable Wintrobe tubes with inner diameter 3 mm and length 115 mm (Wintrobe method). The sedimentation, i.e. the interface between the RBC column and plasma, was recorded after 1 hour. All rheological experiments were performed at room temperature[24] (22–23°C).

To study the effect of PFC particles on the near-wall concentration of RBCs, we pierced a tygon tube in the low pressure region of the circulatory loop with a hypodermic needle (size - 25 G) and collected the seeping blood directly into microhematocrit capillary. Blood flow rate through this small opening in a tube wall was approximately 10^5 times less than the flow rate through the tube. The near-wall hematocrit was compared to bulk hematocrit measured in a blood sample which was withdrawn through the port in a tube.

For examining the viscoelastic response to applied stress, we used the same circulation loop with some modifications. The outflow tygon tube was replaced with a long straight glass tube and blood reservoir was opened to atmosphere. Pressure drop (ΔP) along the glass tube and flow rate (Q) were recorded and Blasius friction factor $\lambda=(\Delta P/Q^2)(d^5\pi^2/8L\rho)$ and Reynolds number Re=$4Q/\pi dv$ (d, L - diameter and length of glass tube, ρ and v - density and kinematic viscosity of liquid) were calculated. These flow characteristics of PFC solutions were compared to the theoretical and experimental data for water and for polymer (Polyox WSR-301) solution which is known to have a very pronounced drag reducing effect.

Data were analyzed as follows. A mean value and standard deviation for each of the parameters were calculated for "baseline" and "fluosol" samples. Since each parameter was observed before and after exposure to a single pharmacologic treatment, we used the paired Student's t-test to test significance[25].

RESULTS

The results of our experimental study are summarized in Table 1. The replacement of 20% plasma volume with PFC reduced hemolysis (plasma free hemoglobin) by approximately 40% compared to "baseline" (p<0.02), during *in-vitro* pumping of ovine and bovine blood with a centrifugal pump. The Index of Hemolysis decreased from 0.019 ± 0.005 for "baseline" to 0.012 ± 0.005 for the "fluosol" group (p=0.015). In control experiments the Index of Hemolysis was 0.024 ± 0.002 during the first hour and 0.026 ± 0.006 for the second hour of blood circulation (p=0.340). The difference of Index of Hemolysis between "baseline" and first hour of control experiments was not statistically significant (p=0.105). In contradiction, the difference of Index of Hemolysis between "PFC" group and second hour of control experiments was statistically significant (p=0.003). The replacement of 20% plasma volume with PFC caused a significant (p<0.001) 30% reduction in the mechanical fragility of human RBCs and a statistically nonsignificant, but notable drop in the mechanical fragility of ovine blood. As regards the effect of PFC on blood viscosity, a 20% replacement of plasma volume with PFC emulsion in human blood remark-

Table 1. Effect of PFC on hemolysis, RBC mechanical fragility and rheological parameters of blood (each value represents mean ± SD)

	Baseline n=6	Fluosoln=6	Level of significance (p)
Hemolysis Index	0.019±0.005	0.012±0.005	p<0.02
Mechanical Fragility Index, Human blood	0.47 ± 0.06	0.33 ± 0.04	p<0.001
Mechanical Fragility Index, Ovine blood*	0.55 ± 0.07	0.40 ± 0.04	p=0.054
Low Shear Whole Blood Viscosity, cP $\dot\gamma$ =0.277 sec^{-1}	31.9 ± 6.1	18.2 ± 4.8	p<0.001
Erythrocyte Sedimentation Rate, mm/hour	16.7 ± 9.2	3.1 ± 3.0	p<0.005

*For these measures, n=4 for both groups.

ably reduced low shear blood viscosity by over 40% for shear rate $\dot{\gamma}=0.277$ sec^{-1}. Low shear viscosity decreased from 31.9 ± 6.1 cP for the baseline group to 18.2 ± 4.8 cP for samples with PFC, p<0.001. ESR fell by approximately 80% from 16.7 ± 9.2 mm/hour for baseline samples to 3.1 ± 3.0 mm/hour for PFC samples, p<0.005. The decrease of both low shear blood viscosity and ESR indicates a reduction in RBC aggregation. Asymptotic blood viscosity slightly increased by approximately 3% after 20% replacement of plasma volume with PFC (p=0.01). Hematocrit of blood samples was not affected by PFC.

The replacement of 20% plasma volume with PFC caused a statistically significant (p<0.001) reduction of near-wall hematocrit of flowing blood (Figure 2).

Blasius friction factor of PFC solution was found to be approximately 30% lower than that of water (Figure 3), i.e. flow characteristics of PFC solution are similar to drag reducing polymer solution.

DISCUSSION

Mechanical trauma of flowing blood has been investigated intensively *in-vivo* and *in-vitro* for at least 30 years. The most often studied aspect of the blood trauma problem is shear-induced hemolysis, and, particularly, critical values of shear stress and exposure time at threshold levels of hemolysis[26,27].

As mentioned earlier, there is very little available information concerning attempts to reduce hemolysis and ameliorate rheological properties of blood pumped by circulatory assist devices with pharmacological agents. Our study showed that partial replacement of blood plasma with PFC significantly reduced hemolysis in blood circulated *in-vitro*. PFC also significantly reduced the mechanical fragility of RBCs. Since we did not oxygenate PFC before use, these effects can only be attributed to the presence of PFC in blood and not its oxygen carrying capability.

The study of possible mechanisms of PFC effects demonstrated that partial replacement of plasma with PFC emulsion caused small but statistically significant decrease in the concentration of RBCs in the near-wall space. This result supports our hypothesis that PFC emulsion particles (a few hundred per single erythrocyte in our study) compete with

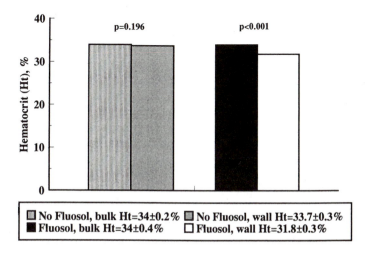

Figure 2. Effect of partial plasma replacement with Fluosol on near-wall concentration of RBC's.

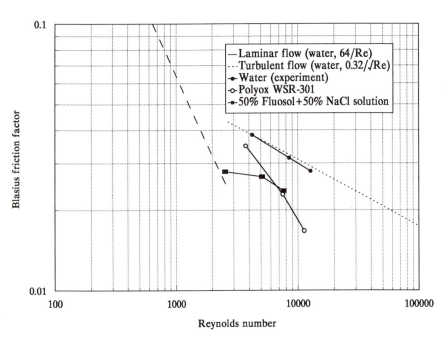

Figure 3. Flow characteristics of diluted fluosol emulsion, water , and solution of drag reducing polymer Polyox WSR-301 (concentration C=10 ppm).

RBCs for the near wall space and reduce RBC contact with wall surface. Our other finding that PFC emulsion demonstrated drag reducing effect, supports another possible mechanism of PFC effect on blood trauma. "Drag reduction" is a property of some special polymers and particles which increase flow at constant driving pressure in the presence of various complex flow regimes, due to reduction in the intensity of turbulent frequencies and elongational strains with accompanying reduction in wall shear stress[28]. The reduction in wall shear stress can decrease the trauma of blood cells.

Our other key finding is that 20% replacement of plasma with PFC significantly reduced low shear blood viscosity and ESR, and thus the RBC aggregation. This effect can be partially explained by the reduction of the plasma protein concentration, particularly fibrinogen. Additionally, PFC particles may obstruct the RBC bridging with fibrinogen. The decrease of RBC aggregation has immense clinical importance, since most cardiovascular patients have pathologically high aggregation of RBCs[22]. Our previous data (unpublished) showed a remarkable increase of RBC aggregation (low shear blood viscosity and ESR) in blood of cardiomyopathy patients and patients with assisted circulation as compared to healthy donors. Greatly enhanced RBC aggregation causes pathological elevation of capillary pressure and flow resistance[29].

Mechanisms involved in reducing blood trauma and RBC aggregation and mechanical fragility caused by PFC are not completely understood. Particularly, the effect of RBC redistribution in a flow stream due to PFC particles and its relevance to the well known Eckstein effect of increase in the near-wall concentration of small particles added to blood during flow in capillaries[30], need further investigation. It is not clear what kind of interaction between RBCs and PFC particles may lead to reduction in RBC aggregation and mechanical fragility.

Based on the results of the present study, PFC may offer the potential to improve rheological properties and to decrease hemolysis in blood exposed to mechanical stress. Our results indicate that PFCs may be successfully utilized not only to increase the oxygen supply but also to improve hemorheology and hemodynamics in patients with heart and lung assist devices.

ACKNOWLEDGMENT

The authors are deeply grateful to McGowan foundation, generous benefactor to the University of Pittsburgh for Artificial Heart and Lung Research.

REFERENCES

1. Schima H., Müller M.R., Papantonis D., Schlusche C., Huber L., Scmidt C., Trubel W., Thoma H., Losert U., and Wolner E. Minimization of hemolysis in centrifugal blood pumps: influence of different geometries. *The International Journal of Artificial Organs* **16**, 7, 521–529, 1993.
2. Seiyama A., Suzuki Y., Tateshi N., and Maeda N. Viscous properties of partially hemolyzed erythrocyte suspension. *Biorheology* **28**, 452, 1991
3. Winslow R.M., Vandergriff K.D., and Motterlini R. Mechanism of hemoglobin toxicity. *Annals of Biomedical Engineering* **21**, Suppl.1, 16, 1993.
4. Kormos R.L., Borovetz H.S., Griffith B.P., and Hung T.-C. Rheologic Abnormalities in Patient with the Jarvik-7 Total Artificial Heart. *Transaction of American Society for Artificial Internal Organs* **10** (3), 413–417, 1987
5. Hung T.-C., Butter D.B., Yie C.L., Sun Z., Borovetz H.S., Kormos R.L., Griffith B.P. and Hardesty R.L. Interim use of Jarvik-7 and Novacor artificial heart: blood rheology and transient ischemic attacks (TIA's). *Biorheology* **28**, 9–25, 1991.
6. Kamada T., McMillan D.E., Sternliev J.J., Bjork V.O., and Otsuji S. Erythrocyte crenation induced by free fatty acids in patients undergoing extracorporeal circulation. *Lancet* **2** (8563), 818–21, 1987.
7. Frattini P.L., Wachter C., Hung T.C., Kormos R.L., Griffith B.P., and Borovetz H.S. Erythrocyte deformability in patients on left ventricular assist systems. *Transactions of the American Society for Artificial Internal Organs* **35**, 3, 733–735, 1989.
8. Yarborough K.A., Mockros L.F., and Lewis F.J. Hydrodynamic hemolysis in extracorporeal machines. *Journal of Thoracic and Cardiovascular Surgery* **52**, 4, 550–557, 1966.
9. Oku T., Harasaki H., Smith W., and Nosé, Y. Hemolysis. A comparative Study of Four Nonpulsatile Pumps. *Transactions of the American Society for Artificial Internal Organs* **34**, 500–504, 1988.
10. Qian KUN-XI. Experience in reducing the hemolysis of an impeller assist heart. *Transactions of the American Society for Artificial Internal Organs* **35**, 46–53, 1989.
11. Qian KUN-XI. Haemodynamic approach to reducing thrombosis and haemolysis in an impeller pump. *Journal of Biomedical Engineering* **12**, 533–535, 1990.
12. Wurrsinger L.J. and Opitz R. (1991). Hematological principles of hemolysis and thrombosis with special reference to rotary blood pumps. *Proceeding of the International Workshop on Rotary Blood Pumps*. Edited by H. Schima, H. Thoma, G. Weiselthaler, and E. Wolner, Vienna, ISBN 3–900928–00–2, pp. 19–25.
13. Schima H., Schlusche C., Jeremejev B.V., Schor I., Geihseder, Müller M.R., and Losert U. Influence of centrifugal blood pump on the elasticity of erythrocytes. *Transactions of the American Society for Artificial Internal Organs* **37**, 658–661, 1991.
14. Sugiki M., Murakami A., Koton K., Takadou S., and Ueyama T. Effect of eicosapentaenoic acid on erythro-aggregometry in left heart bypass by centrifugal pump. *Japanese Journal of Artificial Organs* **21** (2), 575–580, 1992.
15. Sugiki M., Murakami A., Koton K., Ueyama T., Takadou S., Watanabe G., and Misaki T. Effect of eicosapentaenoic acid on erythrocyte aggregation in left heart bypass by centrifugal pump. *Artificial Organs* **17** (6), 561, 1993.
16. Geyer R.P. Perfluorochemicals as oxygen transport vehicles. *Biomat., Art. Cell, Art. Org.*, **16**, 31–49, 1988.
17. Lowe K.C. Synthetic Oxygen Transport Fluids Based on Perfluorochemicals: Applications in Medicine and Biology. *Vox Sang* **60**, 129–140, 1991.

18. Reeder G.D. *The Biochemistry and Physiology of Hemoglobin.* Reston, Virginia, American Society of Extra-Corporeal Technology, 1986, p. 4–15.
19. Kern M.J. The use of Fluosol during PTCA in patient at risk for ischemic complications. *The Journal of Invasive Cardiology*, **5** (Suppl. A), 1A, 1993
20. Naito K., Mizuguchi K., and Nosé, Y. The need for standardizing of hemolysis. *Artificial Organs* **18** (1), 7–10, 1994.
21. E.F. Bernstein, R.A. Indeglia, M.A. Shea, and R.I. Varco. Sublethal damage to the red cell from pumping. *Circulation* 35(4 Suppl):1226–33, 1967.
22. Lowe G.D.O., editor. *Clinical Blood Rheology.* CRC Press, Inc. Boca Raton, Florida, 1988.
23. Stuard J. and Nash G.B. Technological advances in blood rheology. *Critical Reviews in Clinical Laboratory Sciences* **28** (1), 61–93, 1990.
24. International Committee for Standardization in Haematology. Guidelines for measurement of blood viscosity and erythrocyte deformability. *Clinical Hemorheology* **6**, 439–53, 1986.
25. Glanz S.A. *Primer of Biostatistics.* 2-d edition. McGraw-Hill Information Services Company, Health Professions Division, 1987.
26. Sutera S.P. Flow induced trauma to blood cells. *Circulation Research* **41** (1), 2–8, 1977.
27. Leverett L.B., Hellums J.D., Alfrey C.P., and Lynch E.C. Red blood cell damage by shear stress. *Biophysical Journal* **12**, 3, 257–273, 1972.
28. Greene H.L. and Madan S.R. The role of fluid viscoelastisity during *in-vitro* destruction of erythrocytes. *Biorheology* 12:377–382, 1975.
29. Somer T. and Meiselman H.J. Disorders of blood viscosity. *Annals of Medicine* **25**, 31–39, 1993.
30. Eckstein E.C., Tilles A.W., and Millero III F.J. Conditions for the occurrence of large near-wall excesses of small particles during blood flow. *Microvascular Research* 36:31–39, 1988.

50

LONGITUDINAL STUDIES ON THE INTERACTION OF PERFLUOROCHEMICALS WITH LIVER CYTOCHROMES P-450 BY MEANS OF TESTING THE RATE OF DETOXIFICATION OF PENTOBARBITAL

J. Lutz[1] and M. P. Krafft[2]

[1]Department of Physiology
University of Würzburg
Röntgenring 9, D-97070 Würzburg
[2]Unité de Chimie Moléculaire
Université de Nice
F 06108 Nice Cedex 2, France

INTRODUCTION

Perfluorochemicals (PFCs), used as artificial oxygen carriers or diagnostic agents, accumulate for certain time periods within cells of the reticuloendothelial system, before they are eliminated through the lungs by expiration. However, hepatocytes also show an effect of the presence of this foreign material, though it is not metabolized and seems to act only in a catalytic way. This means that the active centers of some cytochrome P-450 isoenzymes are influenced (e.g. causing enzyme induction), but the response can also be a retardation of reactions by competitive inhibition of substrates and uncoupling of monooxygenation. Therefore, we studied the long-time effect of changes in pentobarbital detoxification by the cytochrome P-450 system after administration of different PFCs. This was done by measuring the pentobarbital sleeping time until reappearance of the righting reflex.

MATERIALS AND METHODS

Male Wistar rats of 210 - 350 g body weight, kept in macrolon cages and fed a standard diet (Altromin, Lage, Germany) with access to food and water *ad libitum,* received i.v. doses of 4.5 g/kg b.wt. of (in some cases differently emulsified) PFCs of the following compounds: bis-[F-butyl]ethene (F-44E), perfluorocyclohexylmorpholine (PFCHM), perfluorodecalin (PFD), and perfluorooctylbromide (PFOB). F-44E was emul-

Oxygen Transport to Tissue XVIII, edited by Nemoto and LaManna
Plenum Press, New York, 1997

sified either with a "dowel" (a mixed fluorocarbon-hydrocarbon molecule) of 1.4% F6H10E [1] and 2% egg yolk phospholipids or with 5.94% pluronic F-68 and 1.78% glycerol. PFCHM was emulsified with 2.5% egg yolk phospolipids and 0.5% perfluoroperhydrophenanthrene as a "higher boiling point oil" [2,3]. PFD was emulsified with 2.5% pluronic, 0.5% perfluoroperhydrophenanthrene and 0.5% egg yolk phospholipids. PFOB was emulsified with 4% egg yolk phospholipids and in a second trial together with 1.4% of the dowel F6H10E. The emulsions of F-44E and PFOB were produced in the Unité de Chimie Moléculaire, Nice, by M.P. Krafft et al. [1]; those of PFD and PFCHM in the Dept. of Chemistry of Biocompatible Compounds, Ulm, by H. Meinert et al. [3].

Six to 24 hours after administration of PFC to groups of 4 – 6 animals, the rats received a first injection (i.p.) of 30 mg/kg b.wt. of pentobarbital. The same was done with two control groups who had received only saline instead of PFC. The animals were positioned on their sides and the time to reestablish the righting reflex was determined. This is an indirect, but non-invasive measurement of the decrease in the intravascular concentration of pentobarbital. The measurements were repeated in the same rats in a nearly geometric line of days for up to 1–3 months. Since pentobarbital injections per se are not followed by enzyme induction, repeated use is suitable for testing the detoxification capacity in longitudinal studies.

RESULTS

In all experiments with a final acceleration of the detoxifying response, this event was preceded by a certain degree of inhibition, indicated by a statistically significant prolongation of the sleeping time. This remained below 130% of controls for F-44E and PFCHM, but exceeded 180% for PFD and 250% for PFOB. If F-44E was emulsified with pluronic F-68 instead of phospholipids, the sleeping time also rose above 200% of controls. The maxima were seen within the first 1–2 days after PFC injection.

After the initial prolongation of the sleeping time, in all but one group a final decrease of the pentobarbital induced sleeping time occurred. This was missed only for PFOB; in the other cases the depression of the sleeping time remained closely below 35 % for F-44E and PFCHM, but amounted to 65% in case of PFD. The largest depressions of sleeping time occurred between the 8th and 32nd day after the PFC injection; but the period of significantly abbreviated sleeping time persisted until the 48th day (Fig.1).

DISCUSSION

Hepatocytes show an indirect effect after the infusion of PFCs, although no metabolism occurs. Ullrich and Diehl [4] found an uncoupling of the microsomal monooxygenation system in phenobarbital treated rats after PFC administration. In 1984 we described that after administration of Fluosol-DA a prolongation of the sleeping time after pentobarbital anesthesia occurred, measured as the time to reappearance of the righting reflex in rats [5]. As mentioned above, pentobarbital injections are not followed by enzyme induction, so repeated injections can be used as control values for PFC treated animals. In these former experiments a prolongation up to 155% of the control sleeping times occurred. After 4 and 8 days the control values were reached. However, following extended studies of an induction of cytochrome P-450, as published by Obraztsov et al. [6] and others [7,8], a decrease of the sleeping time should be expected. This was confirmed by Lowe and Arm-

Relation of sleeping time after PFD 4.5 g/kg versus controls

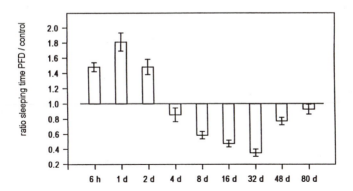

Figure 1. Results of a longitudinal study on pentobarbital detoxification, measured as the time to reappearance of the righting reflex, after a PFD emulsion. The ratio of the sleeping time in PFD treated rats compared to control rats is given; the size of groups was 4 animals. All values besides those of the 4th and 80th day are significantly different from 1.0.

strong [9] in experiments examining rats 4 days after administration of a perfluorodecalin emulsion. We repeated our experiments with a similar decalin emulsion and made long-time studies on the effect of this PFC on the sleeping time. Again, we found initially a prolongation of the sleep duration, however, followed by a long-lasting period of short-ened sleeping time. The initial increase in the sleeping time of 180% was followed by a decrease down to 35% of the control. This inductive effect lasted about two months. With F-44E and PCHM we found a similar reaction, first a prolongation, later a shortened of the sleeping time. When the F-44E emulsion was improved by a dowel, a distinct reduction of the changes in sleeping time could be noted. However, this is only a quantitative effect, since the same dowel was not able to convert the sleep prolongation of PFOB to an abbre-viation, that means no change to an enzyme induction as seen predominantly with FDC. This is in accordance with other results concerning the interaction of PFOB with cyto-chrome P-450 dependent monooxygenases of liver microsomal membranes [10].

The outcome is in line with the idea of an initial inhibition, followed by a later in-duction of barbiturate detoxifying enzymes of the cytochrome P-450 system. In contrast, emulsions of PFOB showed only the prolongation phase of sleeping time up to 30 days. For this PFC there was no clear evidence for a predominance of the inductive effect over the substrate competition in any phase after the first time period.

CONCLUSION

Utilizing an extended test series of sleeping time measurements after pentobarbital injections, the process of interaction of PFCs with cytochrome P-450 dependent liver mi-crosomal monooxygenases can be evaluated in a non-invasive manner. Different kinds of emulsifiers of the same PFC can considerably alter the uptake by hepatocytes and thus change the detoxifying reaction. Longitudinal studies within the same animal are possible and revealed partially unexpected long-lasting effects. The results corroborate the concept, that PFCs, in spite of their chemical inertness, exhibit certain types of biological activity, although obvious effects on the health of the animals could not be detected.

ACKNOWLEDGMENTS

The help of Marcus Kettemann, Egon Bruch and Barbara Pux in performing sleeping time tests is gratefully acknowledged.

ABSTRACT

Four perfluorochemicals, Bis-[F-butyl]ethene, perfluorocyclohexylmorpholine, perfluorodecalin and perfluorooctylbromide were compared by their influence on the liver cytochrome P-450 system, measuring the pentobarbital sleeping time as defined by the time of loss of the righting reflex in rats. In all experiments first a prolongation of barbital detoxification was observed, which lasted at least 2 - 4 days. Thereafter a very long extended period of abbreviated sleeping time followed which was only missed after perfluoroctylbromide. Thus substrate competition, uncoupling of monooxygenation and enzyme induction determine the detoxifying processes in the liver that follow the administration of perfluorochemicals.

REFERENCES

1. Cornélus C, Krafft MP, Riess JG: Mixed fluorocarbon/hydrocarbon molecular dowels help protect concentrated fluorocarbon emulsions with large size droplets against coalescence. Art. Cells, Blood Subs. Immob. Biotech. *22*, 1267–1272 (1994).
2. Sharma SK, Bollands AD, Davis SS, Lowe KC: Emulsified perfluorochemicals as physiological oxygen-transport fluids: assessment of a novel formulation. Advanc. Exp. Med. Biol. *215*, 97–108 (1987)
3. Meinert H, Fackler R, Knoblich A, Mader J, Reuter P, Röhlke W: On the perfluorocarbon emulsions of second generation. Biomat. Art. Cells Immob. Biotech. *20*, 805–818 (1992)
4. Ullrich V, Diehl H: Uncoupling of monooxygenation and electron transport by fluorocarbons in liver microsomes. Europ. J. Biochem. *20*, 509–512 (1971)
5. Lutz J, Wagner M: Recovery from pentobarbital-induced sleep after administration of perfluorinated blood substitutes. Artificial Organs *8*, 41–43 (1984)
6. Obraztsov VV, Shekhtman DG, Sologub GR, Beloyartsev FF: Induction of microsomal cytochromes in the rat liver after intravenous injection of an emulsion of perfluoroorgannic compounds. Biokhimiya *50*, 1220–1227 (1985)
7. Huang R, Cooper DY, Sloviter A: Effects of intravenous emulsified perfluorochemicals on hepatic cytochrome P-450. Biochem. Pharmacol. *36*, 4331–4334 (1987)
8. Shrewsbury RP, Oliver SR, White LG: The effect of moderately severe hemodilution with Fluosol-DA on cytochrome P-450 mediated antipyrine metabolism. Biomat. Art. Cells Art. Organs *17*, 393–402 (1989)
9. Lowe KC, Armstrong FH: Biocompatibility studies with perfluochemical oxygen carriers. Biomat. Art. Cells Immob. Biotech. *20*, 993–999 (1992)
10. Obraztsov VV, Grishanova AY, Shekhtman DG, Sklifas AN, Makarov KN: Interaction of perfluorooctylbromide with liver microsomal monooxygenase. Biokhimiya *58*, 1234–1239 (1993). Translation by Plenum Pub. Corp. (1993)

51

HIGH OXYGEN PARTIAL PRESSURE IN TISSUE DELIVERED BY STABILIZED MICROBUBBLES

Theory

Hugh D. Van Liew and Mark E. Burkard

Department of Physiology
University at Buffalo, SUNY
Buffalo, New York 14214

1. INTRODUCTION

We contend (3, 24) that significant amounts of oxygen can be carried in blood inside of gas bubbles. Synthetic stabilized bubbles are in development for enhancement of ultrasonic contrast (4, 6, 9, 15, 19, 22, 23, 28, 29). These injectable bubbles are small enough to traverse capillary beds and persist much longer than simple bubbles of air (25, 26). If the stabilized bubbles are permeable, gaseous forms of O_2, CO_2, and N_2 inside will exchange with the physically-dissolved counterparts in the blood and tissue when the bubble encounters various hydrostatic pressures and various gas partial pressures in the different parts of the circulatory system. Use of bubbles to carry O_2 may be more efficient than other technologies; hyperbaric treatments depend on O_2 carried in physical solution (5), and most blood substitutes require injection, into the circulation, of substantial amounts of foreign material, such as perfluorochemicals (1).

2. THEORY

Bubbles or pockets of gas in the body are usually absorbed (17), as discussed in the next section. One way that bubbles can be stabilized is for them to contain a gas, designated gas X, which has low solubility so it permeates across a gas-liquid interface very slowly (15, 25, 26); dodecafluoropentane is an example (3, 15). The slowly-permeating gas dilutes the O_2, CO_2, and any other gases in the bubble, lowering their partial pressures. Therefore the partial pressures of permeant gases can be essentially the same inside a bubble and outside even though the total pressure inside the bubble may be above the sum of partial pressures in the blood. We have argued (26) that at least some kinds of bubbles that are stabilized by mechanical structures will exhibit behavior that is similar to behavior of bubbles containing slowly-permeating gas.

2.1. Mathematics of Stabilization

Two possibilities for stabilizers are a mechanical structure around the bubble and a slowly-permeating gas. Pressures exerted by these are included in a general equation: mechanical pressures on a bubble (left side of Eq. 1) are equated with the sum of partial pressures of gases inside (right side):

$$P_B + P_{bl} + P_\gamma + P_\Gamma = Pbub_{N2} + Pbub_{O2} + Pbub_{CO2} + Pbub_{H2O} + Pbub_X \qquad (1)$$

In Eq. 1, P_B is barometric pressure, P_{bl} is blood pressure, P_γ is pressure due to surface tension, P_Γ is pressure due to a mechanical stabilizer, and the Pbub symbols stand for partial pressures of various gases inside the bubble. The $Pbub_X$ denotes partial pressure exerted by a slowly-permeating gas.

First consider the case that the bubble is not stabilized: P_Γ and $Pbub_X$ are zero. Total hydrostatic pressure inside can be well above barometric pressure (positive P_γ and P_{bl}). The effect of surface tension is inversely proportional to radius (R) of a spherical bubble, as stated by the Laplace relation: $P_\gamma = 2\gamma/R$, where γ is surface tension of the liquid. For example, if γ is 50 dyne/cm and R is 1 μm, total pressure inside a bubble is elevated to twice the normal atmospheric pressure. The high hydrostatic pressure elevates the sum of partial pressures inside. In contrast, the sum of partial pressures of gases outside are usually equal to or below barometric pressure; when a bubble is in contact with tissues or venous blood, utilization of oxygen by metabolism gives rise to the phenomenon known as inherent unsaturation or the oxygen window (27).

The tendency of gases to diffuse out caused by differences of partial pressures between inside and outside of the bubble can be counteracted either by a negative P_Γ on the left side of Eq. 1 or by a positive $Pbub_X$ on the right side. A negative P_Γ would reduce internal total pressure and thereby reduce partial pressures of all constituent gases; a positive $Pbub_X$ would dilute the other gases inside, thereby also reducing their partial pressures.

2.2. Graphical Depiction of Stabilization

Figure 1 illustrates contending forces for a stabilized spherical bubble. The curve above the axis, drawn from the Laplace equation, shows the absorptive pressure due to surface tension. The particular P_Γ curve below the axis is related to the reciprocal of radius raised to the third power; it becomes strongly negative at small radii. Use of R^3 is appropriate either for a slowly-permeating gas or a surface film of the gaseous type (7). In using a surface-active film as an example of a mechanical stabilizer, we assume that the film can exert a hydrostatic pressure. The evidence that this assumption is valid is that stable bubbles can be produced with surface-active molecules (6, 12, 22, 31).

In Fig. 1, the Sum curve crosses the zero axis because the magnitude of P_Γ is greater than P_γ at low radii. The bubble is stable at a radius slightly below 2 μm (circle); surface tension pressure of about +50 kPa is opposed by stabilizer pressure of -50 kPa. The positive slope as the curve crosses the axis is an essential feature: a bubble smaller than the stable radius will have a negative ÆPabs inside that will cause gases dissolved in the sur-

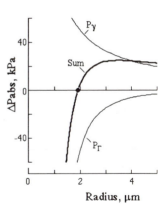

Figure 1. Mechanism of stabilization of a bubble (redrawn from (26)). Absorptive pressures as functions of radius (1 atm = 101.3 kPa). Thin curves: variables that affect growth or absorption, pressure caused by surface tension (P_γ) and a negative absorptive pressure due to a stabilizer (P_Γ). Heavy curve: the resultant sum of the two variables; a positive value corresponds to a pressure difference for causing diffusion of gas out of the bubble. Circle: stable radius where there is no pressure difference to cause diffusion.

roundings to diffuse in until the bubble reaches the stable radius. Conversely, a bubble larger than the stable radius will have a high ÆPabs so gases will diffuse out.

The behavior of a bubble depends on the sum of the pressures acting upon it. The Sum curve in Fig. 1 would be modified if there were a third pressure involved, such as the absorptive tendency due to the O_2 window (27), which is independent of bubble radius. With addition of this third pressure, the resultant of the three pressures would be higher than in Fig. 1 at all radii, and the stable radius would be smaller. The total pressure inside a mechanically-stabilized bubble would be below atmospheric pressure. Negative pressure generated by a mechanical stabilizer has been observed experimentally: Lategola implanted a rigid, permeable capsule in dogs' tissues (16); the pressure inside the capsule became about 6 kPa below atmospheric pressure, the value expected for the O_2 window.

The P_γ curve in Fig. 1 is a function of the aqueous medium around the bubble and does not vary from one case to another. However, the stabilizer curve can vary, so the Sum curve in Fig. 1 depends on the shape and position of the P_Γ curve. Behaviors of other types of mechanical structures will resemble behaviors of slowly-permeating gas or the gaseous type of surface film, but will not be identical insofar as their characteristics differ. Some stabilizers which resist growth as well as shrinkage may give a Sum curve that crosses the axis and proceeds strongly upward at the right rather than leveling off.

3. PREDICTIONS

Figure 2A shows our assumptions about the environmental changes faced by bubbles traversing the circulation. In the small upper graph, blood pressure is negligible in several parts of the circulation and highest in the systemic arterial tree (region SA). The main graph shows gas partial pressures in the blood; P_{N2} remains constant throughout the circulation and P_{O2} rises as the blood exchanges gas in the lung and falls during exchange with tissue.

For exploration of the O_2-carriage characteristics of the stabilized bubbles (3), we produced simulations of bubble contents computed by a previously-published system of equations (2). The numerically-solved system accounts for the major phenomena which determine bubble behavior, including diffusion of any number of gases across the gas/blood interface, surface tension, the oxygen window (27), and Boyle's law for pressure-dependence of gas volumes. Figure 2B shows the results of a simulation of a bubble going through the environments seen in Fig. 2A; the bubble is stabilized by slowly-perme-

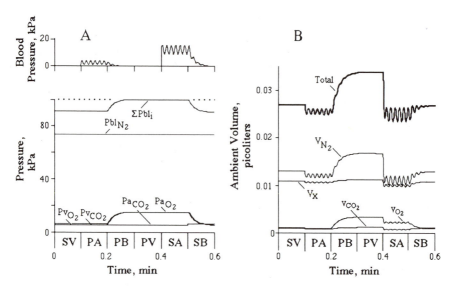

Figure 2. *In vivo* behavior of a bubble stabilized by a slowly-permeating gas in an air-breathing person (redrawn from (26)). A. Environmental variables that determine size and composition of a bubble at six locations in the circulation: SV = systemic vein, PA = pulmonary artery, PB = pulmonary small-vessel bed, PV = pulmonary vein, SA = systemic artery, and SB = systemic small-vessel bed. Small-vessel beds include arterioles, capillaries, and venules. Time spent in each location is arbitrarily set at 0.1 min. Top small graph is profile of blood pressure; main graph shows gas partial pressures, including the sum of partial pressures in blood (ΣPbl_i); dotted line is atmospheric pressure. B. Volumes of the bubble and the constituent gases.

ating gas X. In region PA, the blood pressure causes the total volume to shrink and to oscillate in size. Blood pressure affects V_{N2} more than V_X; both are compressed or decompressed by hydrostatic pressure changes, but N_2 also diffuses in and out. In PB, blood pressure is low and the blood becomes oxygenated; both cause bubble growth. The entering oxygen causes N_2 to enter to keep $Pbub_{N2}$ near Pbl_{N2}. In region SA, the high blood pressure compresses the bubble, causing O_2 and N_2 to leave. In SB, low tissue P_{O2} causes additional outward diffusion of O_2. It is evident that both N_2 and O_2 are picked up in the lungs and given off in the arteries and systemic small-vessel beds so there is transport from the lungs to arterial vessels and ultimately to tissues.

Figure 3 shows a larger bubble (6 μ m diameter in the pulmonary vein instead of the 4 μ m diameter in Fig. 2) in a person who begins to breathe pure O_2 at normal pressure. The high P_{O2} in lungs causes a large change of O_2 volume: the drop of ambient volume of O_2 between arteries and the systemic bed in Fig. 3B is about 0.085 picoliters. Conversion to standard pressure gives 0.11 picoliters (surface tension compressed the bubble contents). Although the O_2 is about 70% of their volume, bubbles can carry about 90 ml of usable O_2 (standard pressure) per 100 ml of bubble volume (ambient pressure). At 0.11 picoliters of O_2 per bubble, transport of 5 vol% of O_2 requires 4.6×10^8 bubbles/ml and volume fraction of gas in bubbles would be 0.07 (7 ml of gas per 100 ml of blood) in the lungs and 0.02 in the systemic small-vessel bed. In one protocol for hyperbaric oxygen therapy, the patient is compressed to 284 kPa (2.8 atm abs) for 90 min, breathing pure O_2. Our simulations for this situation showed that a pressurized bubble of 6 μm diameter can transport about 0.26 picoliters of O_2, expressed at standard pressure. Thus 5 vol% O_2 can

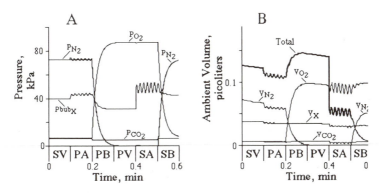

Figure 3. *In vivo* behavior of a bubble stabilized by a slowly-permeating gas in a person breathing pure O_2 (redrawn from (3)). A. Partial pressures in blood and the bubble; $Pbl_x = 0$; P_{O2} and P_{CO2} indicate these gases in both blood and bubble. B. Volumes of the bubble and the constituent gases.

be carried by 2×10^8 bubbles/ml, less than half of the number required if O_2 is breathed at 1 atm.

It is seen in Fig. 3B that N_2 is being carried out of the tissue as O_2 is being carried in; this residual N_2 buffers the changes brought about by fluxes of O_2 in and out of the bubble. As denitrogenation of the tissue proceeds, there will be much larger size fluctuations of the bubble and larger pressures exerted by the stabilizer mechanism (26).

4. UNLOADING OF O_2 IN TISSUE

There are two aspects to unloading of O_2 from bubbles (3, 24): there is release of O_2 as P_{O2} in the bubble equilibrates with tissue P_{O2} outside, but also there is additional release due to the decrease of bubble volume. These two phenomena give greater extraction, for a given change of P_{O2}, than either alone, and conversely, for a given amount extracted, the P_{O2} drop is less. Therefore, bubbles deliver O_2 at a higher P_{O2} than from a liquid containing physically-dissolved O_2, such as a perfluorochemical, in which the P_{O2} fall is directly proportional to the amount extracted. Bubbles will also deliver O_2 at a higher P_{O2} than is usual with blood, in which unloading occurs in the steep part of the Hb-O_2 curve.

For our simulations, we adopted two simplifications that may make the amounts of O_2 transported per bubble less than our simulations show. First, we simulated isolated bubbles, but the increased P_{O2} that might occur if large numbers of bubbles are present would exert a back pressure to curtail additional exit of O_2. Second, the quantities of transported O_2 may be overestimates if effective exchange times in small-vessel beds are shorter than the 6 sec allowed by our simulations or if exchanges between bubble and the surroundings are actually slower than predicted by the physical constants we used.

It remains to be seen whether O_2 transport by bubbles can become a practical clinical tool. Bubbles could provide a rapid but temporary increase in O_2 transport, or could be infused continuously for long-term oxygenation. The danger of embolization is greatest in the lung, where some emboli can probably be tolerated; in systemic small vessels, the danger is mitigated because bubbles will shrink if an embolus lowers P_{O2} by interfering with O_2 delivery. Observations have generally shown stabilized bubbles to be innocuous (8, 13,

14, 20, 30), but relatively large, unstabilized bubbles are known to cause damage (10, 11, 18, 21).

5. REFERENCES

1. Braun, R.D., R.A. Linsenmeier, and T.K. Goldstick. New perfluorocarbon emulsion improves tissue oxygenation in cat retina. J. Appl. Physiol. 72: 1960–1968, 1992.
2. Burkard, M.E., and H.D. Van Liew. Simulation of exchanges of multiple gases in bubbles in the body. Respir. Physiol. 95: 131–145, 1994.
3. Burkard, M.E., and H.D. Van Liew. Oxygen transport to tissue by persistent bubbles: theory and simulations. J. Appl. Physiol. 77:2874–2878, 1994.
4. Carroll, B.A., R.J. Turner, E.G. Tickner, D.B. Boyle, and S.W. Young. Gelatin encapsulated nitrogen microbubbles as ultrasonic contrast agents. Invest. Radiol. 15: 260–266, 1980.
5. Clark, J.M. Therapeutic and toxic effects of hyperbaric oxygenation. In: The Lung: Scientific Foundations (vol. 2), edited by R.G. Crystal, J.B. West, P.J. Barnes, N.S. Cherniak, and E.R. Weibel. New York: Raven Press, Ltd., 1991, p. 2123–2131.
6. D'Arrigo, J.S., S.-Y. Ho, and R.H. Simon. Detection of experimental rat liver tumors by contrast-assisted ultrasonography. Invest. Radiol. 28: 218–222, 1993.
7. Davies, J.T., and E.K. Rideal. Interfacial Phenomena, Second Edition. New York: Academic Press, 1963, p. 227.
8. Feinstein, S.B., P.M. Shah, R.J. Bing, S. Meerbaum, E. Corday, B-L. Chang, G. Santillan, and Y. Fujibayashi. Microbubble dynamics visualized in the intact capillary circulation. J. Am. Coll. Cardiol. 4: 595–600, 1984.
9. Goldberg, B.B., J-B. Liu, and F. Forsberg. Ultrasound contrast agents: a review. Ultrasound in Med. Biol. 20: 319–333, 1994.
10. Helps, S.C., and D.F. Gorman. Air embolism of the brain in rabbits pretreated with mechlorethamine. Stroke 22:351–354, 1991.
11. Hills, B.A., and P.B. James. Microbubble damage to the blood-brain barrier: relevance to decompression sickness. Undersea and Hyperbaric Med. 18:111–116, 1991.
12. Johnson, B.D., and R.C. Cooke. Generation of stabilized microbubbles in seawater. Science 213: 209–211, 1981.
13. Keller, M.W., S.B. Feinstein, and D.D. Watson. Successful left ventricular opacification following peripheral venous injections of sonicated contrast agent: an experimental evaluation. Am. Heart. J. 114: 570–575, 1987.
14. Keller, M.W., W. Glasheen, T. Kuldeep, A. Gear, and S. Kaul. Myocardial contrast echocardiography without significant hemodynamic effects or reactive hyperemia: a major advantage in the imaging of regional myocardial perfusion. J. Am. Coll. Cardiol. 12:1039–1047, 1988.
15. Kenny, A., D.J. Sahn, T. Shiota, A. Passafini, G. Pantely, A. Arai, M. Jones, S. Ge, I. Yamada, and M.D. Reller. A new phase shift echo contrast agent: EchoGen® ; (Sonus Pharmaceuticals) becomes a gas in blood to produce left heart and quantifiable myocardial contrast after venous injection. Studies in sheep and monkeys (Abstract). J. Amer. Coll. Cardiol., Feb 1994; 21: 450A.
16. Lategola, M.T. Measurement of total pressure of dissolved gas in mammalian tissue in vivo. J. Appl. Physiol. 19: 322–324, 1964.
17. Loring, S.H., and J.P. Butler. Gas exchange in body cavities. In: Handbook of Physiology, Section 3: The Respiratory System, edited by L.E. Farhi and S.M. Tenney. Bethesda: American Physiological Society, 1987, p. 283–295.
18. Philp, R.B., M.J. Inwood, and B.A. Warren. Interactions between gas bubbles and components of the blood: implications in decompression sickness. Aerospace Med. 43:946–953, 1972.
19. Smith, M.D., J.L. Elion, R.R. McClure, O.L. Kwan, and A.N. DeMaria. Left heart opacification with peripheral venous injection of a new saccharide echocontrast agent in dogs. J. Am. Coll. Cardiol. 13:1622–1628, 1989.
20. Ten Cate, F.J., P. Widimsky, J.H. Cornel, D.J. Waldstein, P.W. Serruys, and A. Waaler. Intracoronary albunex: its effects on left ventricular hemodynamics, function, and coronary sinus flow in humans. Circulation 88 (Part 1): 2123–2127, 1993.
21. Thorsen, T., H. Klausen, R.T. Lie, and H. Holmsen. Bubble-induced aggregation of platelets: effects of gas species, proteins, and decompression. Undersea Hyperbaric Med. 20: 101–119, 1993.

22. Unger, E.C., P.J. Lund, D.-K. Shen, T.A. Fritz, D. Yellowhair, and T.E. New. Nitrogen-filled liposomes as a vascular US contrast agent: preliminary evaluation. Radiology 185: 453–456, 1992.

23. Unger, E., D-K. Shen, T. Fritz, P. Lund, G-L. Wu, B. Kulik, D. DeYoung, J. Standen, T. Ovitt, and T. Matsunaga. Gas-filled liposomes as echocardiographic contrast agents in rabbits with myocardial infarcts. Invest. Radiol. 28:1155–1159, 1993.

24. Van Liew, H.D., and M.E. Burkard. Bubbles in circulating blood: stabilization and simulations of cyclic changes of size and content. J. Appl. Physiol. 79: 1379–1385, 1995.

25. Van Liew, H.D., and M.E. Burkard. Behavior of bubbles of slowly permeating gas used for ultrasonic imaging contrast. Invest. Radiol. 30:315–321, 1995.

26. Van Liew, H.D. and M.E. Burkard. Relationship of oxygen content to PO_2 for stabilized bubbles in the ciculation: Theory. J. Appl. Physiol. 8, 1996 (in press).

27. Van Liew, H.D., J. Conkin, and M.E. Burkard. The oxygen window and decompression bubbles: estimates and significance. Aviat. Space Environ. Med. 64: 859–865, 1993.

28. Violante, M.R., R.B. Baggs, T. Tuthill, P. Dentinger, and K.J. Parker. Particle-stabilized bubbles for enhanced organ ultrasound imaging. Invest. Radiol. 26: S194-S197, 1991.

29. Wheatley, M., B. Schrope, and P. Shen. Contrast agents for diagnostic ultrasound: development and evaluation of polymer-coated microbubbles. Biomaterials 11: 713–717, 1990.

30. Wilson, B., K.K. Shung, B. Hete, H. Leven, and J.L. Barnhart. A feasibility study on quantitating myocardial perfusion with Albunex®, an ultrasonic contrast agent. Ultrasound in Med. Biol. 19:181–191, 1993.

31. Yount, D.E., T.D. Kunkle, J.S. DArrigo, F.W. Ingle, C.M. Yeung, and E.L. Beckman. Stabilization of gas cavitation nuclei by surface-active compounds. Aviat. Space Environ. Med. 48:185–191, 1977.

52

EFFECTS OF PERFLUBRON EMULSION AND 100% OXYGEN BREATHING ON LOCAL TISSUE PO$_2$ IN BRAIN CORTEX OF UNANAESTHETIZED RABBITS

K. van Rossem,[2] H. Vermariën,[1] N. S. Faithfull,[3] L. Wouters,[2] and K. Decuyper[1]

[1]Department of Physiology
University of Brussels VUB
Brussels, Belgium
[2]Janssen Research Foundation
Beerse, Belgium
[3]Alliance Pharmaceutical Corp.
San Diego, California 92121

1. INTRODUCTION

Concentrated perfluorocarbon emulsions are known to increase oxygen availability in various tissues, especially during oxygen breathing (for review, see Faithfull, 1992). With respect to the central nervous system, F-decalin and F-tributylamine have been shown to increase oxygen availability in rabbit brain cortex by more than 100 % when oxygen breathing is applied (Clark et al, 1989). In cat retina the increase in tissue partial pressure of oxygen (PO$_2$) during oxygen breathing is significantly enhanced after intravenous injection of perflubron emulsion (Braun et al, 1992). In both of the preceding studies PO$_2$ was measured polarographically in either tranquillized or anaesthetized animals at a certain location in the observed organ. The present study was conducted in order to evaluate the effects of intravenously administered perflubron emulsion on local tissue PO$_2$ at different adjacent locations of the brain cortex in unanaesthetized rabbits, steering clear of possible anaesthesia-induced alterations in cerebral metabolism and perfusion, cerebrovascular reactivity and electrode properties. The effects were studied during air breathing and 100 % oxygen breathing.

Oxygen Transport to Tissue XVIII, edited by Nemoto and LaManna
Plenum Press, New York, 1997

2. MATERIALS AND METHODS

2.1. PO$_2$ Measurement

Local tissue PO$_2$ was measured polarographically at three adjacent locations in rabbit brain cortex by means of chronically implanted platinum electrodes with a cylindrical measuring tip (length 1 mm, ø 120 µm) covered with a homogeneous cellulose acetate membrane (thickness 20 µm) (van Rossem et al., 1992a). With these electrodes mean local PO$_2$ is measured over a section of cortical tissue approximately 1 mm thick. They were polarized (- 600 mV) with respect to a common Ag/AgCl electrode (ø 10 mm) fixed to the animal's ear. All electrodes were calibrated in aerated and deoxygenated Ringer solution at 38 °C. In vitro sensitivity to oxygen was 7.4 ± 2.5 nA/kPa. Since the long-term stability of our electrodes is not optimal (van Rossem et al., 1992a) we choose to report absolute values of electrode current (iO$_2$) rather than PO$_2$. Nevertheless, given their permanent linear behaviour and good short-term stability, relative PO$_2$ changes within a measuring period of a few hours can be quantified. As in this study the residual current of the electrodes (iO$_2$ when PO$_2$ = 0) was not determined in the waking animals, the percentage increase in PO$_2$ (taken to be equal to the percentage increase in iO$_2$) was slightly underestimated. Since the mean residual current in vivo is only 3.5 nA (van Rossem et al., 1992b) the induced error was very small.

2.2. Animal Treatment and Preparation

Male Dutch rabbits (HSD/POC) weighing 1600 - 2400 g were used for the experiments. In each animal a polymethylmetacrylate frame (8 x 6 x 3 mm) containing three electrodes was implanted into the skull as described earlier (van Rossem et al., 1992b). The electrodes were positioned in the somatosensory cortex of the left hemisphere (Figure 1). The inter-electrode distance was 2 mm.

The unanaesthetized rabbits were subjected to the experimental protocol (schematic representation, Figure 2) 10 days after implantation. After a 15-min stabilisation period of air breathing the animals were subjected to 100 % oxygen breathing for 5 min by applying a canine anaesthesia mask with a flow rate of 1 l O$_2$/min. After a subsequent 5-min period of air breathing, either perflubron emulsion (90 % w/v) (n = 6) or emulsion-vehicle (n = 7) was injected into the lateral ear vein at a dose of 6 ml/kg. Oxygen breathing was commenced again 30 minutes later. In order to evaluate the reproducibility of the technique of

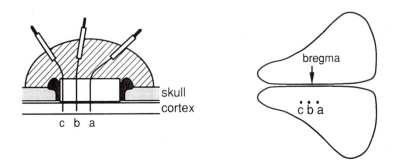

Figure 1. Schematic representation of the implanted frame and the location of the three oxygen electrodes. The inter-electrode distance is 2 mm.

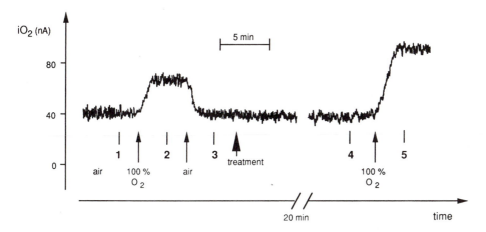

Figure 2. Schematic representation of the oxygen-breathing protocol. The time points when mean iO_2 was read off from the recording are indicated by numbers.

oxygen breathing a third group of rabbits (sham) was studied without injection of any substance (n = 5). iO_2 was monitored continuously throughout the experiment. To quantify the changes of PO_2 induced by treatment and oxygen breathing, mean iO_2 (determined by physiological fluctuations) was read off from the recording before and after each change of the composition of inspired gas (Figure 2).

Arterial blood gases, pH and haematocrit were determined from blood samples taken from the central artery of the ear at the beginning of the experiment and 5 min after onset of the second application of 100 % oxygen breathing.

The experiments were approved by the Medical Ethical Committee of the Belgian Fund for Medical Scientific Research.

2.3. Statistical Analysis

The effect of treatment during air breathing was evaluated by comparison of iO_2 at time points 3 and 4 (Figure 2). The effect of treatment during oxygen breathing was evaluated by calculation of the ratio of the percentage increase in PO_2 after treatment to the percentage increase before treatment. Mean values of the different measurement locations were taken for each animal. Data were analyzed after log transformation.

Groups of experiments were compared by either the Kruskal-Wallis one way analysis of variance (3-groups comparison) or the Wilcoxon-Mann-Whitney rank-sum test (comparison between perflubron- and vehicle-treated animals). Differences within groups were compared with the Wilcoxon signed-rank test. The level of significance was set at $p \leq 0.05$ (two-sided).

3. RESULTS

3.1. Local Tissue PO_2

In all animals normal physiological fluctuations of PO_2 with a frequency of 7 - 13/min were observed throughout the protocol.

In all animals oxygen breathing caused a rapid rise in local tissue PO_2. Stable values were reached within 2 min after the change of inspired gas mixture. The observed rise showed a marked variability not only between animals but also between adjacent locations in the same animal (see Table 1 for examples). In some animals the relative increase at a given location was more than 3-fold that recorded at a distance of 2 mm. On average, the effect of oxygen breathing prior to treatment (control) was comparable across groups (Figure 3). In the sham group the relative rise in local tissue PO_2 during the second PO_2 response was comparable to the first one (109 ± 19 % vs. 106 ± 25 %, mean $\pm$ SEM) indicating that the increase in tissue PO_2 in response to oxygen breathing was reproducible.

Injection of perflubron emulsion did not alter tissue PO_2 during air breathing, although, statistically, this lack of effect was significantly different from the slight decrease noticed in the vehicle group (p = 0.03).

The ratio of the percentage increase in PO_2 after treatment to that before treatment (Table 1) was significantly higher in the perflubron-treated than in the vehicle-treated group (2.6 ± 0.5 vs. 1.3 ± 0.1, p = 0.0082). The effect of perflubron emulsion varied amongst animals. Linear regression analysis did not reveal any correlation ($r^2 = 0.008$) between the percentage increase before treatment and the effect of perflubron emulsion. In the vehicle group the percentage increase after treatment was somewhat larger but not significantly different from the control value (p= 0.078).

Table 1. Local effects of 100 % oxygen breathing on cortical tissue PO_2

Perflubron		%increase in PO_2 before treatment	after treatment	ratio after/before	Vehicle		%increase in PO_2 before treatment	after treatment	ratio after/before
Rabbit 1	a	27	84	3.1	Rabbit 2	b	44	43	1.0
	b	25	123	4.9		c	31	21	0.7
	c	23	87	3.8	Rabbit 7	a	34	43	1.3
Rabbit 3	a	110	237	2.2		b	132	157	1.2
	b	86	193	2.2		c	43	62	1.5
	c	38	65	1.7	Rabbit 15	a	99	95	1.0
Rabbit 8	a	125	529	4.2		b	70	76	1.1
	b	200	738	3.7		c	68	81	1.2
	c	63	313	4.9	Rabbit 16	a	167	254	1.5
Rabbit 11	a	98	171	1.7		b	343	443	1.3
	b	58	126	2.2		c	228	248	1.1
	c	107	195	1.8	Rabbit 17	a	150	197	1.3
Rabbit 12	a	42	43	1.0		c	125	228	1.8
	b	126	248	2.0	Rabbit 18	a	66	71	1.1
	c	52	57	1.1		b	91	126	1.4
Rabbit 22	a	146	275	1.9		c	37	34	0.9
	b	137	210	1.5	Rabbit 23	a	89	109	1.2
	c	85	177	2.1		c	49	127	2.6
mean $\pm$ SEM*		86 ± 15	215 ± 65	2.6 ± 0.5	mean $\pm$ SEM*		101 ± 27	132 ± 37	1.3 ± 0.1

*For each animal the mean over the different locations (a, b, c) was used in the calculation of mean and SEM. The ratio in the perflubron group was significantly higher than in the vehicle group (Wilcoxon-Mann-Whitney rank-sum test, p = 0.0082)

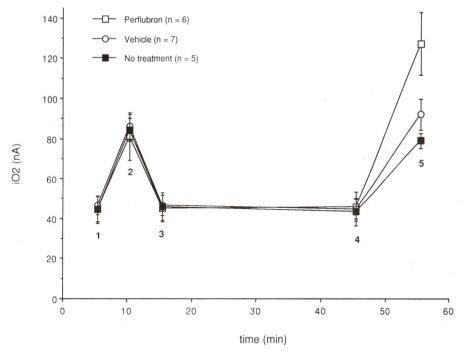

Figure 3. Time course of iO_2 during consequent periods of air breathing and oxygen breathing before and after treatment. Numbers refer to the respective time point when iO_2 was read off from the recording (see Figure 2). Bars indicate SEM.

3.2. Physiological Parameters

Physiological parameters are summarized in Table 2. No significant differences were noticed between groups at the onset of the experiment. Oxygen breathing induced a comparable rise in PaO_2 in all groups. Small changes in $PaCO_2$ and pH did not differ significantly between groups. In the perflubron-treated group the observed decrease in haematocrit was significantly different from the vehicle-treated and sham group (p = 0.035).

4. DISCUSSION

In this study the effects of perflubron treatment and 100 % oxygen breathing were studied at adjacent locations in the brain cortex of unanaesthetized rabbits. Anaesthetics may induce variable changes in local and regional cerebral blood flow and metabolism (Sokolof, 1959; Edvinsson et al., 1993), thereby influencing local oxygen availability and impeding standardized evaluation of cerebral microcirculation. Moreover, some anaesthetics such as halothane have been shown to induce errors in polarographic measurement of PO_2 (Severinghaus et al., 1971).

Perflubron emulsion did not significantly enhance cortical tissue PO_2 during air breathing. Although the small rise in tissue PO_2 (+ 1.7 %) was statistically significant from the small decrease (- 3.9 %) in the vehicle group, the clinical relevance of these

Table 2. Physiological parameters

		Perflubron	Vehicle	Sham
Before treatment, air breathing	Ht(%)	39.0 ± 0.5	39.3 ± 1.4	39.1 ± 2.4
	PaO_2 (kPa)	11.2 ± 1.0	11.2 ± 0.9	12.4 ± 2.4
	$PaCO_2$ (kPa)	5.3 ± 0.4	5.4 ± 0.3	5.4 ± 0.5
	pH	7.44 ± 0.04	7.44 ± 0.04	7.45 ± 0.02
After treatment, 100 % O_2 breathing	Ht (%)	36.5 ± 0.9	38.5 ± 2.3	39.0 ± 1.0
	PaO_2 (kPa)	73.7 ± 7.7	63.6 ± 10.7	68.1 ± 4.1
	$PaCO_2$ (kPa)	5.2 ± 0.5	5.8 ± 0.4	5.9 ± 0.6
	pH	7.39 ± 0.03	7.39 ± 0.02	7.39 ± 0.04

Values are expressed as mean ± SD

changes appears to be very limited. A small but significant rise in preretinal PO_2 (range 0.09 - 0.68 kPa) has been observed after intravenous injection of perflubron emulsion in cats (Braun et al., 1992). In our opinion it is appropriate to conclude that perflubron emulsion tends to improve tissue oxygenation in the central nervous system during air breathing. This effect may be enhanced in conditions of low baseline PO_2 as are seen in hypoxic tumours (Thomas et al., 1994).

Our results show that 100 % oxygen breathing on average doubles local tissue PO_2 in brain cortex but there is a marked variability between animals and even between adjacent locations in the cortex of the same animal. Perflubron emulsion significantly enhanced this increase but the effect was also variable. In some treated animals PO_2 at certain locations increased approximately 5 times more than it did without treatment, whereas in other animals the effect at some locations was limited. Electrode location relative to arterioles and local differences in tissue perfusion and vascular reactivity may explain this variability. Capillary flow and haematocrit may also differ and induce variable effects of perflubron emulsion and oxygen breathing in adjacent microvessels, but as we measure mean PO_2 over 1 mm of cortical tissue, such possible differences cannot fully explain our observations.

Enhancement of tissue oxygenation by first-generation perfluorocarbon emulsions during oxygen breathing was previously noted in rabbit brain by Clark et al. (1989). Increases of the PO_2 response comparable to our data were obtained only after repeated injections of large volumes of emulsion (20 ml/kg, equivalent to 2.0 g perfluorocarbon/kg). Relatively small volumes of concentrated perflubron emulsion appear to have at least the same efficacy. In cat retina, perflubron emulsion (3 g/kg i.v.) caused a 136 % increase in the PO_2 response to oxygen breathing (Braun et al., 1992), which is comparable to our data.

In conclusion, perflubron emulsion markedly enhances the increase of cerebrocortical tissue PO_2 induced by 100 % oxygen breathing. This effect may be therapeutically valuable in conditions of insufficient oxygen delivery and brain ischemia. It must be taken into account, however, that there is considerable effect variability across individuals and even at adjacent cortical locations in the same individual.

5. ACKNOWLEDGMENTS

This work was supported by FGWO contract 3.0023.91 (Belgian Fund for Medical Scientific Research) and by the OZR of the Free University of Brussels.

6. REFERENCES

Braun, R.D., Linsenmeier, R.A., and Goldstick, T.K., 1992, New perfluorocarbon emulsion improves tissue oxygenation in cat retina, *J. Appl. Physiol.*, 72(5): 1960–1968.

Clark, L.C. Jr., Spokane, R.B., Hoffmann, R.E., and Sudan, R., 1989, The nature of fluorocarbon enhanced cerebral oxygen transport, *Adv. Exp. Med. Biol.*, 248: 341–355.

Edvinsson, L., MacKenzie, E.T., and McCullogh, J., 1993, Vascular smooth muscle reactivity in vitro and in situ, in: *Cerebral Blood Flow and Metabolism*: 113–141, Ed. Edvinsson, L., New York, Raven Press.

Faithfull, N.S., 1992, Oxygen delivery from fluorocarbon emulsions - aspects of convective and diffusive transport, *Biomat. Art. Cells & Immob. Biotech.*, 20(2–4): 797–804.

Sokolof, L., 1959, The effects of drugs on the cerebral circulation, *Pharmacol. Rev.*, 11: 1–85.

Severinghaus, J.W., Weiskopf, R.B., Nishimura, M., and Bradley,A.F., 1971, Oxygen electrode errors due to polarographic reduction of halothane, *J. Appl. Physiol.*, 31: 640.

Thomas, C.D., Chavaudra, N., Martin, L., and Guichard, M., Correlation between radiosensitivity, percentage hypoxic cells and pO_2 in one rodent and two human tumor xenografts, 1994, *Radiat. Res.*, 139(1): 1–8.

van Rossem, K., Vermariën, H., and Bourgain, R.H., 1992a, Construction, calibration and evaluation of pO_2 electrodes for chronical implantation in the rabbit brain cortex, *Adv. Exp. Med. Biol.*, 316: 85–101.

van Rossem, K., Vermariën, H., Decuyper, K., Van Reempts, J., Laureys, M., and Bourgain, R.H., 1992b, Local tissue PO_2 during and after focal brain cortical infarction in rabbits, *Adv. Exp. Med. Biol.*, 317: 717–722.

53

CHROMATOGRAPHIC PROCESS IDENTIFICATION FOR PROTEIN C PURIFICATION USING FREQUENCY RESPONSE ANALYSIS

Mahesh V. Chaubal,[1] Kyung A. Kang,[1] Sriram S. Tadepalli,[1]
William N. Drohan,[2] and Duane F. Bruley[1]

[1]University of Maryland Baltimore County
5401 Wilkens Ave
Baltimore, Maryland 21228
[2]American Red Cross
15601 Crabbs Branch Way
Rockville, Maryland 20855

1. ABSTRACT

Frequency response analysis is applied for the analysis of liquid chromatography output of protein separation. Reduced data from simple chromatograms suggest that various Bode plot parameters, magnitude ratios, phase shift, the steady state gain, break frequency, and system order in the frequency domain, can be used to gain phenomenological insights on the system. Such an approach is advantageous because the validity of the model can be checked for two plots, the magnitude ratio vs. frequency and the phase shift vs. frequency, as compared to a single plot in the time domain. This approach also provides a useful empirical tool which can be quantifiably used for process validation and scale-up, especially for immunoaffinity and immobilized metal affinity chromatographic systems used for protein C purification.

2. INTRODUCTION

Protein C is a zymogen precursor of a serine protease present at a concentration of 4 mg/L in the human plasma. In its active form, this protein acts as a potent anticoagulant and hence its deficiency leads to thrombosis, which in turn decreases the supply of oxygen to tissues and therefore, may cause tissue necrosis, potential amputation and possibly death. Hence, in recent times, much effort has gone into the large scale production of Pro-

Oxygen Transport to Tissue XVIII, edited by Nemoto and LaManna
Plenum Press, New York, 1997

tein C from various sources including transgenic animal milk, animal cell cultures and human plasma. One important step in the large scale production is the purification process. Among the available alternatives, liquid chromatography has been proven to be the most successful technique for the purification of Protein C (Kang, et al., 1992). In the course of the development of a separation technique, various issues such as process identification, scale-up and process validation are the primary focus for quality assurance and production considerations. Moment theory is commonly used for the analysis of chromatographic pulse testing. However moment theory is difficult to use for the non-symmetric pulse outputs. Frequency response techniques have been successfully used for the analysis of different systems such as adiabatic humidifiers (Bruley and Prados, 1964) and physiological imaging in bio-photonics (Kang, et al., 1994). Initial studies with liquid chromatographic columns showed that this technique can be effective for the identification of liquid chromatographic columns (Dalton, et al., 1995). In this study we have examined the use of frequency response analysis for the pulse testing of liquid chromatographic columns, which can relate to the shapes of chromatograms with magnitude ratio and phase shift at various frequency values.

3. THEORY

The system response in the frequency domain is defined in terms of a transfer function as:

$$G(\omega) = \frac{Y(\omega)}{X(\omega)} = \frac{\int_0^{T_y} y(t)e^{-j\omega t}\,dt}{\int_0^{T_x} x(t)e^{-j\omega t}\,dt} \qquad [1]$$

where Tx and Ty represent the times when the input and output pulse values become zero, respectively; $x(t)$ and $y(t)$ are the time domain input pulse and output response, respectively; and where ω, t, and j denote the forcing frequency, time, and imaginary number, respectively. $X(\omega)$ and $Y(\omega)$ are the transformed input and output in the frequency domain, respectively.

The system response is then plotted in terms of the magnitude ratio (MR) and phase shift (ϕ) against the corresponding frequencies, wherein MR and ϕ are defined as:

$$\text{MR} = |G(\omega)| = \sqrt{\text{Re}^2(\omega) + \text{Im}^2(\omega)} \qquad [2]$$

$$\phi = \phi|_{G(\omega)} = \tan^{-1}[\frac{\text{Im}(\omega)}{\text{Re}(\omega)}] \qquad [3]$$

where $\text{Re}(\omega)$ and $\text{Im}(\omega)$ are the real and imaginary parts of the transfer function, $G(\omega)$, respectively. The computation of the product integral for data reduction from time to frequency domain is done using Filon's quadrature formula (Filon, 1928); (Bruley and Prados, 1964). The MR andϕ are then plotted against the forcing frequency, ω, as Bode plots. These Bode plots are then analyzed using the concepts of process control to obtain the individual system parameters such as steady state gain, break frequency, system order, and time constant (Coughanowr, 1991). Steady state gain is the magnitude ratio value at $\omega = 0$, break frequency is the frequency value at which the steady state horizontal line meets the decay curve for the magnitude ratio vs. frequency plot, and system order is the slope of the decaying curve above the break frequency, whereas the time constant is the inverse of break frequency (Kang et al., 1994).

Pulse testing involves the introduction of a pulse input to the system and recording the output in time domain. The pulse introduced should be large enough to invoke a discernible system response without forcing it into non-linear operation. In the case of a chromatographic system, the pulse would be a small aliquot of protein solution introduced at the top of the column which is assumed to be a Dirac Delta function.

4. RESULTS AND DISCUSSIONS

4.1. Theoretical Studies Using Probability Density Functions (pdfs)

In order to gain insights on how different chromatographic operational parameters affect the Bode plots, theoretical studies were performed, wherein the time domain chromatographic response to a dirac delta pulse input was assumed to be in the form of probability density functions (pdfs) as shown in Figure 1. The output from a particular chromatographic column depends on different phenomenological parameters such as the column matrix, dimensions and the elution conditions. In our studies, we examined the normal and log-normal shapes as system responses.

(1) Normal Density Function. As can be seen in Fig. 1a and 1b, this pdf assumes a symmetric chromatogram peak. Such a peak can be obtained under mild elution conditions, when the ligand molecules lose their affinities from the free state to the immobilized state (Kang et al.,1992). The equation used to generate a normally distributed peak is:

$$P(K) = \frac{1}{\sigma \sqrt{2\pi}} Exp[\frac{-(K - K0)^2}{2\sigma^2}]$$ [4]

where P(K) is the density function, K is the equilibrium coefficient between the protein and the ligand which is related to the retention time, K0 is the mode value for the density function peak which is related to the time when the peak is eluted, and σ is the standard deviation which is a measure of the peak spreading of elution profiles.

(2) Log-Normal Density Function. This pdf generates a chromatogram which is skewed towards the right hand side. Such a chromatogram could result when the buffer change is made abruptly from adsorption to elution (Kang et al., 1992). The equation for this type of distribution is:

$$P(K) = \frac{1}{\sigma K \sqrt{2\pi}} Exp[\frac{-\ln(K / K0) - \sigma^2}{2\sigma^2}]$$ [5]

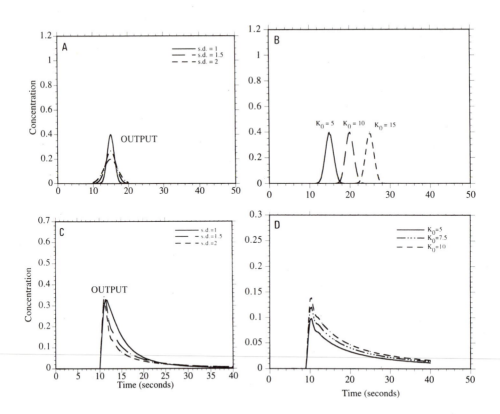

Figure 1. Chromatograms with the shape of normal and log-normal density function for varying standard deviations and mode values (K_0) for density function: (a) Concentration vs. time with varying standard deviation for a normally distributed chromatogram, (b) Concentration vs. time with varying mode values of the density function (retention time values) for a normally distributed chromatogram, (c) Concentration vs. time with varying standard deviation for a log-normally distributed chromatogram, and (d) Concentration vs. time with varying mode values of density function for a log-normally distributed chromatogram.

In both type of distributions, K0 (the mode of density function) and σ (the standard deviation) are the two parameters which would depend on the chromatographic system. A change in K and K0 values leads to a change in the retention time of the protein and can be caused by different phenomenological changes in the system such as: (1) change in transport delay; (2) change in gel matrix-protein interactions; or (3) the nature or concentration of the eluent. Similarly a change in the standard deviation which leads to peak spreading can be caused by (1) increased heterogeneity in the system, (2) increased non-equilibrium interactions between the solutes and ligands, etc.

To gain phenomenological insights on the system, we studied the effect of changing the mode of density function (K0) and standard deviation (σ) in the pdf equations (4) and (5) and observed the corresponding changes in the Bode plots. Figures 2a and 2b show the Bode plots obtained from reducing the pdf (4) into frequency domain for changing standard deviation. As can be seen from the Bode plots, with increased peak spreading, there is

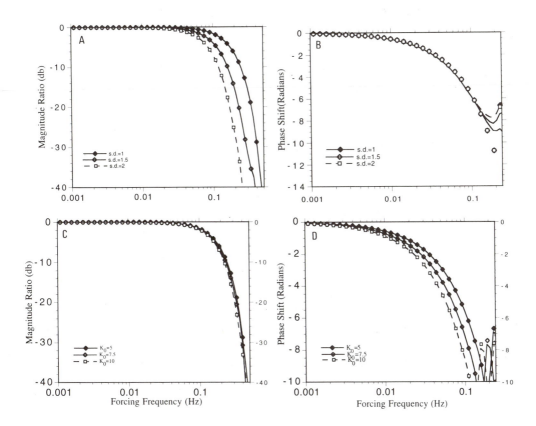

Figure 2. Bode plots obtained for normally distributed chromatograms: (a) Magnitude Ratio (MR) vs. forcing frequency for varying band spreading, (b) Phase shift (ϕ) vs. forcing frequency for varying band spreading, (c) Magnitude ratio (MR) vs. forcing frequency for changing retention time, (d) Phase shift (ϕ) vs. forcing frequency for changing retention time.

a tendency of the magnitude ratio to decrease (Fig. 3a) and break frequency to increase and a slight change in phase shift (Fig. 3b) unlike Fig. 2 where the magnitude ratios decrease considerably . There is a crossing over of curves in the higher frequency range in Fig. 3a. The system order in Fig. 3a is higher than that in Fig. 2a, while there is very little change in order in Fig. 2b and Fig. 3b. Further investigation is being carried out to explain this.

Figures 3c and 3d show the effect of the difference in retention times. There is a noticeable decrease of the magnitude ratios and the break frequencies with increase in retention time (Fig. 3c), while the phase shift shows a slight change (Fig. 3d). This is different from Fig. 2, where a considerable change in the phase shift is observed with a slight change in the magnitude ratio for increasing retention time.

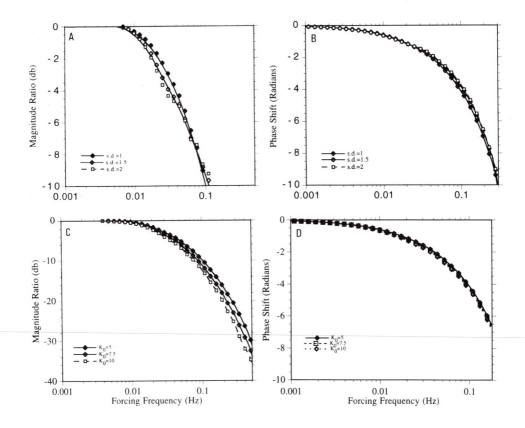

Figure 3. Bode plots obtained for a log-normally distributed chromatograms: (a) Magnitude ratio (MR) vs. forcing frequency, (b) Phase shift (ϕ) vs. forcing frequency for band spreading; (c) Magnitude ratio (MR) vs. forcing frequency for changing retention time, (d) Phase shift (ϕ) vs. forcing frequency for changing retention time.

The results indicate that the individual Bode plot parameters such as magnitude ratio, phase angle or break frequency are sensitive to phenomenological factors such as retention time, broadness of the peak, equilibrium coefficients, etc. Hence Bode plots can be used for the phenomenological modeling of the system.

4.2. Experimental Studies

Our next objective was to verify results obtained from our theoretical studies. For this purpose, chromatographic experiments were carried out using bovine serum albumin (BSA) (Sigma Chemicals, St. Louis, MO) as our model protein since its properties are most well documented. Pulse testing was carried out on a DEAE Sepharose fast flow gel (Pharmacia, Uppsala, Sweden). Chromatograms obtained from such experimental studies were slightly skewed to the right as in log-normal distribution. As can be seen in Fig. 4, when the chromato-

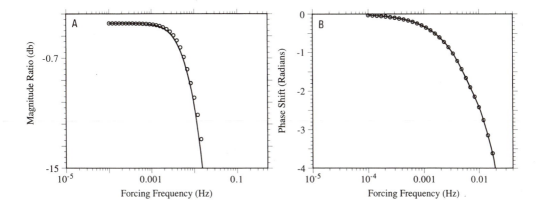

Figure 4. Bode plots obtained from BSA protein separation using a DEAE Sepharose fast flow gel: (a) Magnitude ratio (MR) vs. forcing frequency, (b) Phase shift (ϕ) vs. forcing frequency.

gram output was reduced to the frequency domain, a set of Bode diagrams representing this purification system was obtained. Transfer functions could be obtained for every system based on these parameters which serves as a finger-print for the system and can be used for system identification and serve as the phenomenological model.

5. CONCLUSIONS

Our studies show that pulse testing utilizing frequency response analysis tools can be useful for the phenomenological modeling of liquid chromatographic columns. Frequency response analysis can also be used as a quantifiable tool for the validation of column performance. This analysis would be useful since five control parameters (phase angle, magnitude ratio, steady state gain, break frequency, and system order) can be used for process identification. Future work would be done to further develop frequency response analysis via pulse testing for a thorough modeling of protein C purification, particularly for Immobilized Metal Affinity Chromatography (IMAC) and immunoaffinity chromatography. We also plan to study the use of this technique as an empirical tool that can be used for process scale-up.

6. ACKNOWLEDGMENTS

This work was partially supported by The Whitaker Foundation and the American Red Cross.

7. REFERENCES

Bruley, D.F.; Prados, J.W. 1964. Frequency Response Analysis of Wetted Wall Adiabatic Humidifier. *AIChE J.,* 11, 945–50.

Coughanowr, D.R. 1991. Process Systems Analysis and Control. 2nd Ed., McGraw Hill, New York.

Dalton, J.C.; Gupta S.; Bruley, M.D.; Kang, K.A.; Bruley, D.F. 1995. Chromatographic Process Identification via Pulse Testing For Column Standardization and Scale Up. *J. Chromatog*, In Press.

Kang, K.A.; Bruley D.F.; Londono, J.M.; Chance, B. 1994. Highly scattering optical system identification via frequency response analysis of NIR-TRS spectra. *Ann. of Biomed. Eng.*, 22, 240–252.

Kang, K.A.; Bruley D.F.; Ryu, D.D.R. 1992. Simulation of heterogeneous interaction between ligand and product biomolecules in affinity chromatography. *AIChE Symp. Ser.* 290 (88), 12–24.

Kang, K.A.; Ryu, D.; Drohan, W.D.; Orthner, C.L. 1992. Effect of matrices on the immunoaffinity purification of protein C. *Biotech. Bioeng.* 39 (11), 1086–1098.

54

SEPARATION OF RECOMBINANT HUMAN PROTEIN C FROM TRANSGENIC ANIMAL MILK USING IMMOBILIZED METAL AFFINITY CHROMATOGRAPHY

Joseph C. Dalton,[1] Duane F. Bruley,[1] Kyung A. Kang,[1] and William N. Drohan[2]

[1]Department of Chemical and Biochemical Engineering
University of Maryland Baltimore County (UMBC)
5401 Wilkens Ave. ECS 101
Baltimore, Maryland 21228
[2]American Red Cross
15601 Crabbs Branch Way
Rockville, Maryland 20855

1. ABSTRACT

Protein C is an important serine protease due to its ability to proteolytically cleave activated Factors V and VIII. Excess coagulation and blood agglutination can lead to plugged capillaries, thereby reducing oxygen transport to interstitial tissues. To treat patients with hereditary and acquired protein C deficiency would require a greater amount of Protein C than that available from human plasma. However, the potential demand for this protein could be met by the production of human protein C from transgenic animal mammary glands. Thus, research into inexpensive, efficient methods to purify proteins from transgenic animal milk will be a critical area of study for the large scale production of protein C.

Immobilized metal affinity chromatography (IMAC) is a novel method for the purification of protein C. A proposed method of purification is to take advantage of protein C's strong metal ion binding characteristics with IMAC to assist in the separation from transgenic animal milk. The separation procedure is benchmarked against current systems in use by the American Red Cross for purification of Protein C from transgenic porcine milk.

Common problems in developing separation schemes for new therapeutics are the initial availability of the product (protein), and time-to-market concerns. Extensive experimental tests for scaleable purification schemes are often cost and time prohibitive. In order to optimize an IMAC protocol with minimal waste of time and resources, total quality management tools have been adopted. Initial experiments were designed to choose buffer conditions, eluents, immobilized valence metals, and flow rates using Taguchi experimental design, which is a total quality management (TQM) tool. One of the values of Taguchi methods lies in the use of Latin orthogonal sets. Through the use of the orthogonal sets, the total number of experiments may be reduced, shortening the focus time on optimal conditions.

2. INTRODUCTION

2.1. Protein C

In human plasma, protein C circulates as an inactive zymogen (Figure 1). Protein C is converted to its active form at the endothelial cell surface by limited proteolysis with α-thrombin in complex with a cell surface membrane protein, thrombomodulin1,2,3. Activated protein C is a potent serine protease that regulates blood coagulation by inactivating Factors Va and VIIIa in the presence of calcium ions and phospholipids4,5,6,7,8,9,10. In addition to its anticoagulant function, activated protein C also enhances clot lysis11,12.

Protein C deficiency is normally inherited as an autosomal dominant trait with the adult onset of thrombophilia (also known as recurrent venous thrombosis). Heterozygous protein C deficiency has been difficult to measure, but is estimated to be 1/200 to 1/300 individuals in the U.S.A.13 Approximately 7% of heterozygotes with partial protein C deficiency have been found to have thromboembolic disease14. Homozygous protein C deficiency is more rare, and patients suffering this affliction do not survive infancy. In addition to inherited deficiencies of protein C, acquired deficiencies have been found in a variety of disease states15.

Research into the treatment of patients suffering from either hereditary or acquired protein C deficiency is ongoing. Protein C demand for prophylactic treatment of deficient patients will dictate that protein C be produced in large quantities at low cost. The treatment of just 100 homozygous protein C deficient patients, whose lifespan would be increased due to protein C replacement therapy, will require approximately one kilogram of protein C per year (unpublished data - the American Red Cross).

2.2. Protein C Sources

2.2.1. Blood Plasma. The human body contains approximately 4 liters of blood, at an average concentration of protein C at 4 µg/ml. While the separation of protein C from Fraction IV-1 paste of the Cohn fractionation process is technically feasible for large scale production, the supply of human blood is a limited resource, and cannot be expected to meet the increasing demand for protein C. Moreover, the risk of Hepatitis, AIDS or other transfusion transmitted diseases are inherent problems. Therefore, purified human protein C from plasma is used primarily as the model protein for recombinant protein C research.

2.2.2. Mammalian Cell Reactor Broth. Recombinant human protein C (rHPC) has been produced in mammalian cell lines16,17,18. The maximum production reported to date is approximately 1 mg/liter-cell-broth[17], from the adenovirus-transformed human kidney cell line 293 (ATCC product #CRL-1573). Unfortunately, the cell lines that give the greatest yield do not scale-up well. As cell density increases, post-translational modifica-

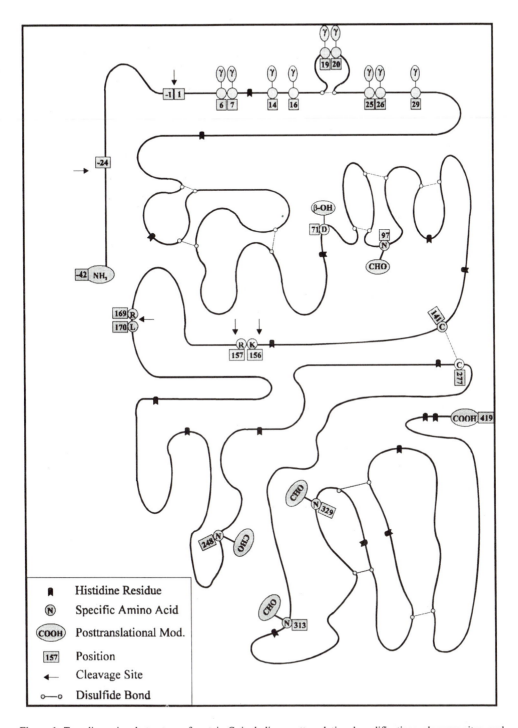

Figure 1. Two dimensional structure of protein C, including posttranslational modifications, cleavage sites, and histidine sites (based on protein structure provided by American Red Cross).

tions to the gla (region of 9 γ–carboxylated acid residues) domain become irregular[17,18]. Because the gla domain is essential for protein activity, large scale production using mammalian cell lines is not possible as yet.

2.2.3. Transgenic Animals. Transgenic pigs have been produced that generate protein C in their mammary glands[19,20]. Using techniques perfected in mice, a fusion gene consisting of human protein C cDNA inserted into the first exon of the mouse whey acidic protein gene was used as the gene construct (WAPPC-1). Transgenic porcine milk is collected by hand milking during the lactation period of the pig. The milk is skimmed to remove the fat and lower the fluid viscosity. Next, many of the milk proteins are removed through polyethylene glycol (PEG) precipitation. Protein C is released from casein micelles by solubilization in a sodium citrate and EDTA buffer. Again, PEG precipitation will separate the protein C from the caseins and further purify the solution. After a viral inactivation step, the γ-carboxylated proteins are separated using barium chloride precipitation. Protein C is then purified from residual contaminants using ion-exchange chromatography.[19]

Expression has been observed at up to 1g/liter milk19,20. Due to the success encountered with transgenic animals, and the comparable high production rates observed, it is believed that large scale production of protein C can be accomplished via this technology. The focus of this project will be to identify a method that could enhance, and improve the separation techniques presently in place.

3. TRANSGENIC ANIMAL MILK

3.1. Overall Protein Content

The contents of transgenic porcine milk include water, lipids, lactose, and minerals as well as a variety of proteins. The protein content is only 5.3 percent of the overall milk, and protein C is a much smaller percentage of that. Most of the protein content of animal milk is composed of members of the casein family, lactalbumins, and lactoglobulins.

3.2. Caseins Family

The casein family consists of α_{S1}, α_{S2}, β, γ, and κ variants (Table 1)21,22,23. The amino acid length ranges from 167 for κ casein to 220 for α_{S2} casein. Many caseins bind calcium ions and aggregate to form large micelles. In the process of forming these micelles, other proteins are bound within, including protein C.

Protein C is separated from micelles by chelating the calcium with EDTA, thus breaking apart the micelles. The protein C must then be separated from the caseins so that the micelles do not reform. Because of similar iso-electric points, and a shared affinity for calcium ions, traditional chromatographic methods (except immunoaffinity) cannot be utilized. Thus, PEG precipitation in tris-buffered-saline solution is used as the primary method for casein removal. It is thought that IMAC may be able to offer improvements in separation efficiency and purity over these methods presently in place.

Table 1. Casein distribution within milk[21,22,23]

Case in fraction	Casein distribution (g/l)	Percent of total casein	Percent of total milk protein
α-Casein	17.4	70	56
$\alpha_{s1\&2}$-Casein	~ 13.7	~ 55	~ 44
κ-Casein	~ 3.7	~ 15	~ 12
β-Casein	6.2	25	20
γ-Casein	1.2	5	4
Total	25	100%	80%

3.3. Histidine Content of Proteins

The histidine content of the proteins is critical to the adsorption of the proteins to the IMAC column. As displayed in Table 2, protein C has a higher number and greater percentage of histidines than nearly all other proteins in transgenic animal milk.[24,25,26,27] In addition to the high histidine content, are the two high affinity metal binding sites: the gla domain, and the β-hydroxyaspartic acid residue at position 71. It is therefore believed that protein C should display a high affinity for immobilized metals.

4. IMMOBILIZED METAL AFFINITY CHROMATOGRAPHY

Immobilized metal ion affinity chromatography (IMAC) has been in existence since 1975, with the pioneering work by Porath et al.28, under the name of metal chelate chromatography. In the following decade, the level of interest concerning IMAC did not increase sizably, but in the last 10 years interest has blossomed. Multiple review articles have been published29,30,31,32. Metal affinity separations exploit the affinities exhibited by functional groups on the surfaces of proteins with metal ions. Coordination between bound or chelated metals, and accessible metal binding residues on protein surfaces can approach the strength of "bio-specific" interaction, or even that between antigen and antibody. Even though the first demonstrations of IMAC were primarily low resolution group separations, recent examples show similar peptides fully resolved in high-performance IMAC with a pH gradient.

Table 2. Histidine content proteins[2,24,25,26,27]

Components	Number of histidines	Percentage of histidines / AA
Protein C	17	4.07
αs1-Casein	11	5.34
αs2-Casein	6	2.55
κ-Casein	3	1.6
β-Casein	5	2.16
α-lactalbumin	3	2.12
Serum Albumin	18	2.98
β-lactoglobulin	3	1.88

The overall contributing factor for protein binding is the number of accessible surface histidines33 (with tryptophan, cystein, and the carboxyl end contributing to a much lesser extent). The side chain of histidine dominates protein binding to chelated Ni^{2+}, Zn^{2+}, and Cu^{2+}. An N-terminus will also contribute to retention, although less than a surface histidyl. Other side chains and functional groups (such as cystein and tryptophan) make smaller contributions to a protein's apparent affinity for the chelated metal. Moreover, histidyl residues vary in their affinities for immobilized metal ions, which can be attributed to differences in histidyl pK_a's and steric accessibility of the imidazole nitrogens. Proteins with multiple accessible surface histidines can show heterogeneity in binding affinities[33,34]. This heterogeneity is caused by less than optimal binding to the support matrix, and is not an IMAC-specific problem. Non-specific binding on IMAC gels can be minimized at high salt concentrations.

5. EXPERIMENTAL FACTORS

The first step in examining protein C adsorption to IMAC columns is finding the operational factors that describe the system. The criteria is to maximize the ability to separate rHPC from contaminants at a specific point(s) of the overall separation processes. Presently used IMAC systems were benchmarked. Preliminary experiments were designed to find an operating system with the greatest potential for the separation of rHPC from caseins and albumin in transgenic animal milk.

The contributing factors to the experiments were identified (Table 3). Potential chelated metal ions were chosen as copper, nickel, and zinc. While PC shows at least two high affinity sites for calcium binding (the gla domain and the β-hydroxyaspartic acid), this metal forms micelles with caseins, and must not be re-introduced into the system. Another factor chosen was the amount of metal loading on the column. The amount of loading can affect the density of binding sites and metal ion transfer. Other factors such as the eluent method and conditions (protonation, competitor ligands, and chelating agents), ionic strength, flow rate, wash volume, and buffer composition are described in the experimental methods section.

The design of experiments was followed from Taguchi methods. To minimize experimentation, these factors (Table 3), at three levels, were used in conjunction with a Latin orthogonal matrix (L18) to design a set of 23 experiments. The success of these experiments are judged from the resolution and purity of separation. The overall results will

Table 3. Experimental factors chosen for the IMAC purification of protein C

Factor	Levels	Condition	1	2	3
8	3	Chelated metal ions (50 mM $MeCl_2$)	Cu^{2+}	Zn^{2+}	Ni^{2+}
7	3	Eluent condition	Isocratic	Slow Gradient	Fast Gradient
6	3	Flow rate (ml/hr)	10	20	30
5	3	Salt Level (M NaCl)	0.2	0.5	1
4	3	Eluent (elution method)	Protonation	Imidazole	EDTA
3	3	Volume of wash (CV)	2	4	6
2	3	Buffer Concentration (mM Buffer)	20 mM Acetate	50 mM PBS	40 mM TBS
1	2	Metal loading (percent maximum)	100	66	

allow quantification of the optimal combination of the system parameters to achieve separation of protein C from caseins and albumin.

6. MATERIALS AND EXPERIMENTAL METHODS

6.1. Proteins

Protein C and serum albumin was obtained from the American Red Cross, purified from blood plasma. Serum albumin and caseins were obtained from Sigma Chemicals (St. Louis, MI).

6.2. IMAC

Chromatography experiments were performed using a Pharmacia (Uppsala, Sweden) HiTrap 5 ml (2 cm inner diameter) Chelating Sepharose column. A Pharmacia FPLC system with a LCC-501 Plus liquid chromatography controller was used to program the separation methods. Buffering conditions chosen were 20 mM Sodium Acetate buffered saline, 50 mM phosphate buffered saline, and 40 mM Tris-HCl. Three experimental flow rates were used, 10, 20 and 30 ml/hr. Wash volume was ranged from 1 to 10 CV's, and determines the amount of washing the sample will undergo to minimize non-specific binding. The salt concentration was varied in experimentation from 0.2, 0.5, and 1.0 M sodium chloride. Elution conditions were varied from isocratic, fast gradient (10 CV), and a slow gradient (20 CV). For pH elution, the operational pH range was chosen from 7.4 to 4.2 (approximately the isoelectric point of protein C). Imidazole based elution used a 50 mM concentration of imidazole in the wash buffer (Tris-HCl or PBS). EDTA based elution used 10 mM EDTA in the wash buffer as the elution buffer. All chemicals used were purchased from Sigma.

6.3. Enzyme Linked Immuno-Sorption Assay (ELISA)

ELISA's were performed in Immunolon II 96 well flat bottom microtiter plates from Dynatech Laboratories, Inc. (Chantilly, VA). Buffers used for protein C polyclonal ELISA procedure include sample, blocking, and dilution buffer (12.5 mM Tris-HCl, 50 mM NaCl, pH= 7.2), and wash buffer (12.5 mM Tris-HCl, 50 mM NaCl, 0.05% Tween-20, pH= 7.2). The plates were coated at least one day in advance with rabbit anti-human protein C IgG's (Sigma, St. Louis, MI), and the detection antibody after sample injection was goat anti-human protein C IgG's (Sigma, St. Louis, MI).

6.4. SDS-Page

Fractions containing high concentrations of protein C were electrophoresed (Mini-PROTEAN II, Bio Rad, Melville, NY) under non-reduced and reduced conditions. Vertical slab mini-gels (7 x 8 cm) were run using a 10% resolving polyacrylamide gel and 4% stacking polyacrylamide gel containing 0.1% SDS under the method developed by Laemmli.35

7. RESULTS AND DISCUSSION

A sample of the experimental results is shown in Figure 2. The column was fully loaded with copper ions. A sample of 200 µl 25 µg/ml protein C, spiked with 25 µg/ml serum albumin and 100 µg/ml casein, was loaded onto the column. The sample was eluted using a pH gradient of 20 mM acetate buffer from 7.4 pH to 4.2 pH at a constant flow rate of 0.5 cm/min. Salt concentration, to minimize non-specific ion-exchange, was 1.0 M NaCl. Figure 2 displays the chromatogram with nonspecific adsorption of the eluent at 280 nm ultraviolet detection on the right-hand y-axis, and the ELISA based protein C concentration for the corresponding fractions on the left-hand y-axis. Matching peaks on the chromatogram with the ELISA correspond to fractions 3 and 7 (during wash), 15 (approximate 6.2 pH), and 17 (approximate 5.6 pH). Fractions containing protein C were run on SDS-PAGE (not shown) to determine protein content and purity.

While these experiments are still in progress, protein C separation from serum albumin and caseins using IMAC has demonstrated positive results. Presently, the system with the greatest potential was found using a pH gradient on zinc chelated columns. Using imidazole gradients less resolution has been achieved, with most proteins eluting in a single band. EDTA could not be used as a selective elution method, even in very low concentrations, as it non-selectively stripped the metal from the column. The EDTA would invariably strip the metal and proteins off the column in a non-selective manner.

After completion of each experimental run, the column was stripped and checked for residual protein C that did not elute. Overall protein C mass balances on the eluent, done by ELISA, typically showed approximately 10 percent total protein C recovery. This low total protein C recovery may be attributed to the low concentrations of protein C used in the samples, and the "sticky" nature of the molecule. Greater recovery is expected when using bio-equivalent concentrations of protein C from the transgenic animal milk purification process.

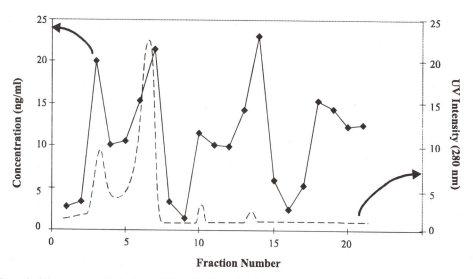

Figure 2. Chromatogram (dashed line, 280 nm UV intensity) for separation of a sample (200 µl, 25 µg/ml protein C and serum albumin, 100 µg/ml casein) and the ELISA based protein C concentrations (solid line, ng/ml) of collected fractions.

8. CONCLUSIONS

It is thought that the mechanism of binding between protein C and metal ions involves histidine sites on the surface of the molecule, but contributions from the β-hydroxyaspartic acid and gla domain may also be present. Protein C can be eluted from the IMAC column using a pH change, imidazole, or chelating agent gradient. In studies on separation from biological contaminants, the greatest purity of protein C has been achieved in later fractions, with most other proteins eluting early in the separation procedures.

From the results attained, it is believed that IMAC may be a valuable addition to the overall separation procedure to purify protein C from inherent contaminants in transgenic animal milk. A proposed area to fit IMAC into the overall purification processes would be after the breakup of the casein micelles using EDTA. The solution could then undergo a buffer change to remove the EDTA so that nonspecific chelation of the immobilized metals would not occur. The sample would then be loaded onto a scaled IMAC column and the protein C separated under optimal conditions.

Future work includes the completion of the design experiments, followed by verification on fractions from the actual transgenic animal milk purification process. Amidolytic and clotting assays will also be tested to verify the activity of the protein. Development of a mathematical model to study changes on experimental conditions is also underway.

9. ACKNOWLEDGMENTS

Special thanks go to the American Red Cross for their supply of proteins and technical expertise, and The Whitaker Foundation for their support of this project.

10. REFERENCES

1. Bruley D.F., Drohan, W.N. *Protein C and Related Anticoagulants*, Advances in Biotechnology Series, **11**, Gulf Publishing. Woodlands, Texas (1990)
2. Esmon N.L., Owen W.G., and Esmon C.T. (1982) *J. Biol. Chem.*, **257**, 859–864.
3. Esmon C.T, Owen W.G. (1981) *Proc. Natl. Acac. Sci U.S.A.*, **78**, 2249–2252
4. Walker F.J., Sexton P.W., and Esmon C.T. (1979) *Biochimica et Biophysica Acta*, **571**, 333–342.
5. Comp P.C., and Esmon C.T. (1979) *Blood*, **54**, no. 6, 1272–1281.
6. Dahlback B., and Stenflo J. (1980) *Eur. J. Biochem.*, **107**, 331–335.
7. Vehar G.A., and Davie E.W. (1980) *Biochemistry*, **19**, no. 3, 401–410.
8. Marlar R.A., Kleiss A.J., and Griffin J.H. (1982) Blood, **59**, no. 5, 1067–1072.
9. Suzuki J., Stenflo J., Dahlback B., and Theodorsson B. (1983) *J. Biol. Chem.*, **258**, no. 3, 1914–1920.
10. Fulcher C.A., Gardiner J.E., Griffin J.H., and Zimmerman T.S. (1984) *Blood*, **63**, no. 2, 486–489.
11. Taylor F.B., and Lockhart M.S. (1985) *Thromb. Res.*, **37**, 155–164.
12. deFouw N.J., Haverkate F., Bertina R.M., Koopman J., Wijngaarden A. and van Hinsbergh V.W.M. (1986) *Blood*, **67**, no. 4, 1189–1192.
13. Miletich J.P., and Broze G.J. (1986) *Circulation, Part II*, **74**, no. 4, 11–92.
14. Seligsohn U. (1987) *Report at the ISTH Subcommittee Meeting, Brussels*, July.
15. Kessler, C.M., and Strickland D.K. (1987) *CRC Reviews of Biochemistry*
16. Grinnell B.W., Berg D.T., Walls J., Yan S.B. (1987) *Bio/Technology*, **5**, 11, 1189–1192.
17. Yan S.C.B., Razzano P., Chao Y.B., Walls J.D., Berg D.T., McClure D.B., Grinnell B.W. (1990) *Bio/Technology*, **8**, 655–661.

18. Grinnell B.W., Walls J.D., Gerlitz G., Berg D.T., McClure D.B., Ehrlich H., Bang N.U., Yan S.B. (1990) *Protein C and Related Anti-Coagulants*. Gulf Publishing Company: 3, 29–63.
19. Velander W.H., Johnson J.L., Page R.L., Russell C.G., Subramanian A., Wilkins T.D., Gwazdauskas F.C., Pittius C., Drohan W.N. (1992) *Proc. Natl. Acad. Sci.*, 89, 12003–12007.
20. Morcol T., Velander W.H., Subramanian A., Page R.L., Drohan W.N. (1992) *Ph.D. Dissertation.*
21. Alexander L.J., Beattie C.W. (1992) *Anim. Genet.*, 23, 369–371.
22. Levine W.B., Alexander L.J., Hoganson G.E., Beattie C.W. (1992), *Anim. Genet.* 23, 361–363.
23. Chobert J.M., Mercier J.C., Bahy C., Haze G. (1976) *Febs Lett.* 72, 173–178.
24. Baldwin G., Weinstock J. (1988) *Nucleic Acids Res.* 16:9045–9045.
25. Bell K., McKenzie H. A., Shaw D. C. (1981) *Mol Cell Biochem* 35(2):103–11.
26. Alexander L. J., Das Gupta N. A., Beattie C. W. (1992) *Anim. Genet.* 23(4):365–7.
27. Levine W. B., Alexander L. J., Hoganson G. E., Beattie C. W. (1992) *Anim. Genet.* 23(4):361–3.
28. Porath J., Carlsson J., Olsson I., and Belfrage G. (1975) *Nature*, 258, 598–599.
29. Sulkowski E. (1985) *Trends in Biotechnology*, 3, 1–7.
30. Yip T., Hutchens T.W. (1992) *Methods in Molecular Biology.*, 2, 17–32.
31. Arnold F.H. (1991) *Bio/Tech*, 9, 152–156.
32. Porath J. (1992) *Protein Expression and Purification*, 3, 263–281.
33. Todd, R. (1993) Ph.D. Thesis, California Institute of Technology
34. Todd, R., Arnold, F.H. (1994) *Journal of Chromatography*, In Press
35. Laemmli, U.K. (1970) *Nature* (London) 227, 680–685.

55

PULMONARY DELIVERY OF HUMAN PROTEIN C AND FACTOR IX

Shalabh Gupta,[1] Francis Moussy,[1] Richard N. Dalby,[2] Shirley I. Miekka,[3] and Duane F. Bruley[1]

[1]Chemical and Biochemical Engineering Department
University of Maryland Baltimore County
Baltimore, Maryland 21228
[2]School of Pharmacy
University of Maryland at Baltimore
Baltimore, Maryland 21201
[3]Jerome H. Holland Laboratory
The American Red Cross
Rockville, Maryland 20855

1. INTRODUCTION

Recent advances in structural elucidation of numerous natural peptides and proteins[1], enhanced understanding of their role in several physiological processes, and the use of biotechnological techniques for their production have stimulated considerable interest in establishing peptides and proteins as therapeutic agents. A major problem, aside from proteolytic degradation and physical alteration of the protein molecule at the site of administration, is the slow rate of transport of macromolecules across membrane barriers into the systemic circulation.

Inhalation offers some exciting possibilities, since the route offers relatively short pathlength (0.4–1.0 μm) between the pulmonary epithelium and circulation coupled with the extensive absorptive surface and smaller airways of the alveoli (70 m^2 in man). This route of delivery has proven capable of delivering even large macromolecules with acceptable bioavailabilities. The objectives of this work were:

A) To Show that Aerosolization Can Potentially Destabilize Proteins. During jet nebulization denaturation may occur due to shear forces associated with the production of small droplets or the large air-water interface continuously being produced within the nebulizer[2]. Oxidation of proteins usually plays a minor role in overall deactivation.

B) To Demonstrate the Feasibility of Protein Delivery through the Lungs. A large alveolar surface area and a thin diffusion barrier makes the lungs a viable route of drug delivery for macromolecules such as Protein C and Factor IX. It avoids first pass hepatic metabolism while minimizing the opportunities for pulmonary metabolism due to relatively short residence time.

C) To Study a Delivery System that Can Serve as a Model for Delivery of Other Vitamin K Dependent Clotting Factors of Therapeutic Use. There are seven vitamin K dependent coagulation proteins (factors VII, IX, X and prothrombin and anticoagulant proteins, protein C and protein S) with similar structures (amino acid homology and molecular architecture) and physical properties. Information gained with Factor IX and Protein C may be applicable with little or no modification to the others.

1.1. Protein C and Factor IX as Model Proteins

These plasma proteins are produced by hepatocytes and need vitamin K for biosynthesis. They circulate in the blood in their inactive forms and are converted to active enzymes when blood coagulation is initiated. Factor IX (Christmas factor) is a single chain glycoprotein with a molecular weight of 56,800 kDa[3]. It occurs in blood plasma at concentrations of 4 μg/ml and has a half life ($t_{1/2}$) of 22 hrs. Hemophilia B patients are currently treated periodically with IV injections of Factor IX to control bleeding episodes. Episodic treatment is ineffective in preventing bleeding into the joints which results in joint degeneration and painful crippling deformities. A less invasive dosage regimen would enable the prophylactic maintenance of homeostatic control, which would prevent joint degeneration and greatly enhance the quality of life for the hemophilia B patient.

Protein C, unlike Factor IX is an anticoagulant and circulates as two polypeptide chains with an average molecular weight of 62 kDa. It occurs in blood plasma at 4 μg/ml and has a much shorter half life ($t_{1/2}$= 6–8 hrs) than Factor IX. In clinical situations, such as deep vein thrombosis (clot formation in vein), or pulmonary embolism, where a thrombus has already formed, rapid activation of the fibrinolytic systems by administration of anticoagulants is effective in diminishing the thrombus. The two major types of clinically useful anticoagulants, heparins and coumarins are associated with undesirable effects including thrombocytopenia, drug-drug interactions, bleeding, and skin necrosis[4]. Administration of a naturally occurring anticoagulant, like Protein C would potentially solve these problems while being therapeutically advantageous to the patient.

2. DELIVERY OPTIONS AND CONCERNS

Currently available options for the generation of inhalable aerosols include various types of nebulizers, propellant based systems (metered dose inhalers) and dry powder inhalers (DPI's). The critical issues in lung delivery of therapeutic peptides and proteins are shown in Table 1.

Formulation of proteins into MDI's and DPI's is a formidable task because dehydration and subsequent communion of proteins to produce powders in the size range suitable for inhalation may lead to loss of activity. In contrast there are numerous proteins

Table 1. Primary concerns during aerosol generation

1. Drug denaturation/Inactivation including aggregation and adsorption to device
2. Dispersibility(surface energetics, surfactant compatibility, propellant type)
3. Lung deposition efficiency(dose, particle size distribution)
4. Patient compliance, correlation of pharmacokinetic and pharmacodynamic data
5. Formulation issues and environmental impact of MDI propellants
6. Dose delivery efficiency and accuracy.

which can be nebulized, since they are invariably purified and initially formulated in aqueous solutions for parenteral administration. The air-blast nebulizer in its simplest form uses the Bernouilli effect to draw liquid up a concentric supply capillary that surrounds a narrow jet supplied with compressed air. More than 99% of the nebulized fluid is recirculated following impaction on internal baffles while only a small fraction of the aerosol escapes as inhalable aerosol.[5] Increased recycling promotes protein degradation. In this work we administered Factor IX using two types of nebulizers, a Side Stream disposable and the Pari LC jet Plus. In order for the protein to be absorbed systemically, the administration technique must maximize drug deposition in the pulmonary region. Stable aerosol systems with mass median aerodynamic diameters (MMAD) of less than 5 μm deposit about 70% of their discharged dose in the respiratory tract following slow oral inhalation.[6] Nebulized aqueous solutions, which deliver from 0% to 20% of their initial drug load are similar in efficiency to MDI's. Penetration of peripheral airways as opposed to tracheobronchial deposition appears to be more effective by nebulization of aqueous solutions, rather than with MDI's or Dry powder inhalers.

3. MATERIALS AND METHODS

Due to the high costs and limited availability of purified Protein C, our preliminary experiments were carried out using highly purified Factor IX . Purified human Factor IX was provided by the American Red Cross. Hence, the experimental procedures have been established with Factor IX, and experiments will be repeated with Protein C.

ELISA's were performed in Immunolon II, 96 well, flat bottom microtiter plates from Dynatek. Capture buffer (0.1M sodium bicarbonate, 1.0M sodium chloride, pH= 9.6), blocking buffer (0.05M monosodium phosphate, 0.1M sodium chloride, 10mg/ml BSA pH= 7.3) and wash buffer (0.05M monosodium phosphate, 0.1M sodium chloride, 0.05% Tween-20) are the three buffers used for Factor IX polyclonal ELISA procedure.

Capture antibody (Dako A300 Rabbit Anti-human Factor IX) used to coat the plates overnight, detection antibody (Boehringer mouse anti-human Factor IX) and labeled antibody (Dako P161 Rabbit anti-mouse IgG, HRP Labeled) were the three antibodies used for the Factor IX ELISA. NBS two component peroxidase from KPL labs was used as the substrate for the antibodies.

In order to evaluate the Factor IX activity a clotting assay was used. Congenital Factor IX deficient human plasma from universal reagents was mixed with the samples along with KONTACT APTT from pacific Hemostasis. Only active Factor IX reacts with the other clotting agents in the deficient plasma to form a clot. The rate of clot formation would suggest the amount of Factor IX active in our samples. Lancer Coagulyzer from CMS was used to study the clot times. The samples were diluted in BAT buffer (0.05M Imidazole, 0.1M NaCl, 0.1% (w/v) BSA AND 0.01% Tween-20).

3.1. Nebulizer Dryer Apparatus

The unit has four main components; air supply, heating system, nebulizer, and drying chamber. Fig. 1 shows a schematic of the apparatus. A nylon tube carries an 80 psig air supply to a pressure regulator. The air supply is split into two branches, each connected via a rotameter (Variable area flowmeters, 65 mm, Cole Parmer Instruments.) One branch directs air to a heating system. The second branch supplies pressurized air to the nebulizer. The air heating system consists of a fifty foot, one-half inch diameter, coiled copper tube wrapped with 2" x 8' silicone rubber heating tape (Barnstead/Thermolyne) connected to a proportional controller (Type 45500 Input Controller, Barnstead/Thermolyne). A nebulizer (Side stream disposable nebulizer or Pari LC Jet Plus nebulizer) generates droplets directly into the left side of the drying chamber via a "T" connector. One limb of the connector is blocked during experiments to drive all the aerosol into the drying chamber. As shown in the figure, the airtight drying chamber consists of a plexiglass cylinder 12 inches in height, with an internal diameter of 7 inches. The cylinder is divided vertically by a 0.25 inch plexiglass baffle to within 0.05 inch of the top. Drying air is fed into the bottom of the left side after passing through an expansion chamber approximately 1.5 inches in height and 3 inches in diameter. The nebulizer is attached through an orifice 3.5 inches above the base in the left side of the drying chamber. The copper exit tubing is located on the right side of the chamber at the base. This serves as an outlet for respirable size aerosol particles, which are bubbled into a buffer with a sparger or connected into a rat exposure chamber. Droplets exiting the nebulizer travel up the left side of the baffle, across, then down the right side of the drying chamber, carried by the drying air stream, before reaching the copper exit tube.

Advantages of this geometry include the impaction of excessively large droplets exiting the nebulizer on the central baffle, resulting in their removal from the product stream, while rapidly sedimenting droplets do not immediately contact a surface, and can thus be dried and reduced in size allowing them to remain entrained in the product stream.

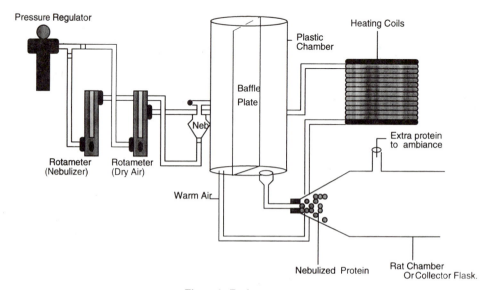

Figure 1. Equipment set up.

The drying chamber has a volume of 10.6 liters. leading to mean residence time 10.6 seconds at air flows of 60 liters/minute. Increased residence times (lower flow rates) lead to more complete drying and a higher concentration of inhalable aerosol particles (2–5 μm diameter), so long as the air stream does not become saturated with water. The experimental conditions for Factor IX delivery are given in Table 2.

4. RESULTS AND DISCUSSION

The data provided in this paper are for Factor IX. The in vitro experiments were performed using the Side Stream and the Pari LC jet plus nebulizers. The primary difference between the two is in their baffle design. Pari LC is a high output nebulizer producing more aerosol particles in the respirable range (2–5 μm diameter).

The objectives of the experiment were defined in terms of the following parameters:

- $\eta 1$= Fraction of the protein aerosolized.
- $\eta 2$= Fraction of the protein active after aerosolization.
- $\eta 3$= Fraction of the protein still active after exposure to nebulizer shear stress.

The primary objective was to maximize the amount of protein delivered from the nebulizer without deactivating it. Therefore the system efficiency (η_{sys}) could be expressed as:

$$\eta_{sys} = \eta_1 {}^* \eta_2$$

Initial experiments showed no protein collection due to failure of the impact sparger to the aerosol. To solve this problem we added a vacuum pump drawing 60 L/min additional make-up air to accelerate the particles and compare the collection efficiency. With this modification 19.8% of the aerosolized Factor IX was collected. Our objective was to collect respirable (2–5 μm) size particles using the drying chamber to provide enough residence time to reduce droplet size of the aerosol to the respirable range. Hence, the 19.8% efficiency represents a good estimate of respirable dose produced by the nebulizer. Unfortunately of this 20% none was active after collection. We hypothesized that in the process of aerosolization Factor IX was denatured due to shear forces imposed by the nebulizer or the large air water interface produced during the nebulization.

Table 2. Experimental conditions for Factor IX delivery

Compressed air pressure	50 psig.
Factor IX concentration in the nebulizers	40 μg/ml
Dry air flow rate to the chamber	10-12 liters/min.
Air flow rate to the chamber	3-5 liters/min.
Vacuum pump suction rate	60 liters/min.
Temperature in the drying chamber	45^0 C
Side stream nebulizer dose	10 ml or 400 μg/ml.
Side stream dosing time	75 mins.
Pari LC dose	8ml or 320 μg/ml.
Pari LC dosing time	15 mins.

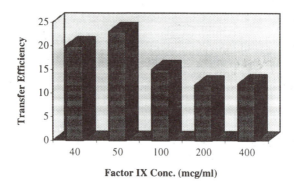

Figure 2. Optimal dose evaluation for Factor IX. Nebulizer flow rate: 3.4 L/min, compressure pressure: 50 psig.

To prevent protein denaturation bovine serum albumin (BSA) at 15 mg/ml, representing almost 400 times the Factor IX concentration was added. The proteins are surface active and tend to migrate to an air water interface. Their migration rate to the interface depends on their concentration in the formulation. Adding BSA at a much greater concentration not only helps in shielding the protein from air-water interface denaturation but also protects it from nebulizer shear stresses. Two control parameters, protein activity or nebulizer output were identified. Further improvement of the protein activity requires a thorough study of the protein's chemistry, which was considered a more formidable task than using a higher output nebulizer. The results clearly show that the system efficiency (η_{sys}) was doubled with the Pari LC jet nebulizer compared to the Side Stream nebulizer. Pari nebulizer also imposed more severe shear stresses on the protein and therefore denatured the protein by 35% showing itself to be more efficient in production of respirable size particles, at the expense of compromised protein stability. Therefore, a thorough study of protein deactivation due to device shear stresses is important while developing a potential protein aerosol delivery system.

Table 3. *In vitro* results for aerosol delivery of Factor IX

Experiment	Result	Conclusion
Factor IX solution (40μg/ml) nebulized in the Side Stream nebulizer	No protein was collected in the sparger collection flask.η_1= 0%.	Sparger flow rate increased to 60 L/min using a vacuum pump. η_{SYS} = 0%.
Factor IX solution (40 μg/ml) was again nebulized with the new set up.	Protein was collected completely deactivated.η_1= 21%, η_2= 0%,η_3=100%	Large air-water interface denaturation. BSA added at 15 mgs/ml.η_{sys}= 0%
Factor IX (40μg/ml) nebulized in the side stream nebulizer with the new formulation.(Factor IX + BSA)	η_1= 19.8%, η_2= 53%η_3= 100%	η_{sys} = $\eta_1*\eta_2$ = 10.5%10% of Factor IX can be effectively delivered.
Factor IX nebulized in the Pari LC Jet plus nebulizer with the new formulation(Factor IX + BSA)	η_1= 40%, η_2= 50%η_3= 65%	η_{sys}= $\eta_1*\eta_2$ = 20%This nebulizer has doubled the efficiency.

When attempting to maximize drug delivery, high protein concentration might not always lead to optimal results. Evaporation of droplets leads to increased protein concentration within the nebulizer reservoir and may ultimately destabilize the macromolecules depending on the rate of protein aggregation. At concentrations above the optimal value nebulizers may produce reduced respirable dose and thereby compromise on the nebulizer transfer efficiency. The plot below shows that 50 µg/ml is the optimal Factor IX concentration when using the following delivery parameters under the conditions indicated in the legend.

CONCLUSIONS

In the process of being aerosolized human Factor IX is 50% denatured at the air water interface. Pulmonary delivery optimization of proteins is a function of two parameters, device transfer efficiency and protein activity. An optimization of these control parameters is essential to develop a potential protein delivery system. Using Pari rather than the sidestream doubled the nebulization efficiency (η_1) but denatured 35% of the protein due to nebulizer shearing. The Side Stream nebulizer did not denature the protein due to shearing but generates a lower output of respirable particles. Thus high output nebulizers can cause denaturation of the protein due to their shearing. Bovine Serum Albumin (BSA) plays an important role in protecting the protein from interface deactivation. In vivo Factor IX delivery in rats to study the bioavailability and characterize its absorption from the lungs is in progress. On the basis of these results we shall then study the feasibility of Protein C delivery.

ACKNOWLEDGMENTS

This work was supported by the Special Opportunity award from The Whitaker Foundation and the American Red Cross.

REFERENCES

1. Vincent H. Lee: Changing needs in drug delivery in the era of peptide and protein drugs. *Peptide and Protein Drug Delivery.* Advances in Parenteral Sciences/4. (1991) 1–57.
2. Peter R. Byron: Determinants of drug and polypeptide bioavailability from aerosols delivered to the lung. *Advanced Drug Delivery Reviews,* 5 (1990) 107–132.
3. Ulla Hedner, Earl W. Davie: Introduction to Hemostasis and vitamin K dependent coagulation factors.. *Blood and blood forming tissue.* 2107–2133
4. J. Bryan Smith: Drugs affecting coagulation, fibrinolysis, and platelet aggregation. *Human Pharmacology, Molecular to Clinical.* (1995) 21.
5. Ralph W. Niven: Delivery of Biotherapeutics by Inhalation aerosols. Ralph W. Niven. *J. Pharmaceutical Technology* (July 1993) 72.
6. Peter R. Byron :Pulmonary targeting with aerosols. *J. Pharmaceutical Technology* (43). May 1987.

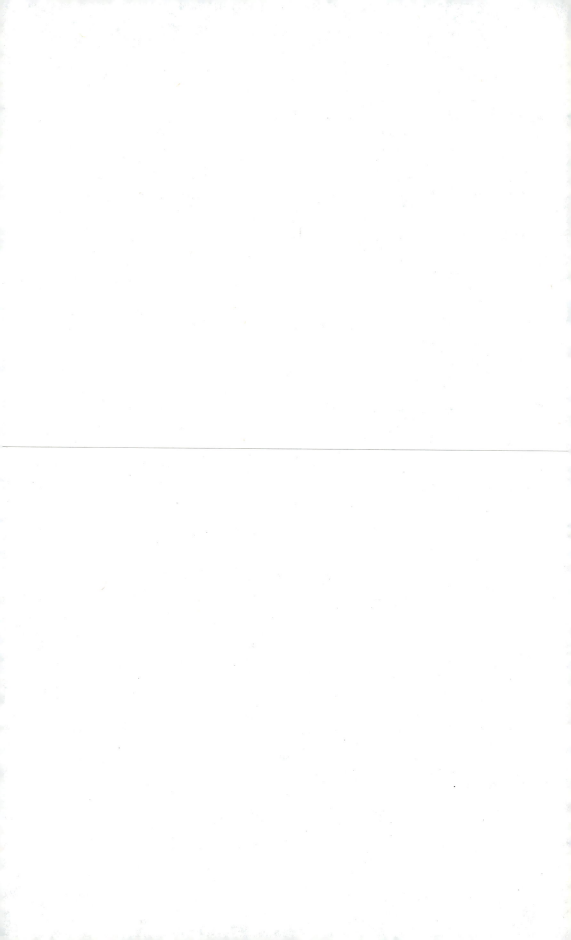

REUSABLE, REAL-TIME, IMMUNO-OPTICAL PROTEIN C BIOSENSOR

Kyung A. Kang,[1] Nabil A. Anis,[2] Mohee E. Eldefrawi,[2] William Drohan,[3] and Duane F. Bruley[1]

[1]Department of Chemical and Biochemical Engr.
University of Maryland Baltimore County (UMBC), 5401 Wilkens Ave.
Baltimore, Maryland 21228
[2]Department of Pharmacology and Experimental Therapeutics
School of Medicine
University of Maryland at Baltimore (UMAB)
[3]The American Red Cross

1. ABSTRACT

A Protein C (PC) biosensor can be used to diagnose PC deficiency, to monitor the PC level in the blood of PC deficient patients, and to measure the PC concentration in other PC-containing samples, such as PC producing animal cell culture broth or transgenic animal milk. A fully functional biosensor requires extremely high sensitivity and specificity, and real-time measurement. To satisfy these requirements, it is proposed to develop an immuno-optical fiber biosensor that utilizes PC-specific biomolecules (PC probes) tagged with fluorophores. The method involves immobilizing monoclonal antibody against PC (anti-PC) on the surface of an optical fiber. When PC in a sample is adsorbed to the anti-PC on the fiber, it can be reacted with the fluorophore tagged PC-probe. The intensity of light transported through the optical fiber, therefore, can be correlated with the concentration of PC in the sample. The sensor will be designed so it can be reused, following a simple elution step, thus reducing diagnostic expense. The preliminary study shows encouraging future for the real-time optical PC biosensor.

2. INTRODUCTION

2.1. Protein C

Protein C (PC), a vitamin K dependent plasma glycoprotein, is a potent anticoagulant and anti-thrombotic. Most vitamin K dependent proteins are coagulating factors (e.g.,

Factors II, VII, IX, and X) and PC is one of only a few anticoagulating factors. Therefore, most common treatments currently used for the patients with PC deficiency is blocking the biosynthetic pathway leading to the blood coagulating factors by structural analogs (antagonist) of vitamin K, such as cumarine. However, in this case, the liver stops producing not only the functionally normal blood clotting factors but also PC. At the same time, the patient's body becomes hemophiliac because of the lack of functional coagulating factors. Protein C is present in blood plasma as an inactive form (zymogen). In the presence of Protein S and phospholipids, when Ca^{+2} is attached to the 'gla' domain of its light chain, PC is activated thereby rendering the serine protease activity (Walker, 1981; Stenflo, 1984). The activated PC has potent anticoagulant properties due to its inhibitory action on coagulating factors, Factors V_a and VIII_a and its stimulatory effect on fibrinolysis by preventing the inhibition of plasminogen activator (Fig. 1; Esmon and Esmon, 1984).

2.2. Protein C Deficiency

Most PC deficiency is genetically inherited (Bertina et al., 1982; Boekman et al., 1983; Marciniak et al., 1985; Bruley and Drohan, 1990) or, sometimes, it is caused by liver disease. Because of PC's important functional properties in human body it is hypothesized that PC might be closely related to many other thrombo-embolic diseases. In homozygous PC deficient patients, the concentration of PC level is almost zero. Homozygous patients have a massive clotting problem, and without rapid blood transfusion or anticoagulant treatment, they die shortly after birth (Marciniak et. al., 1985; Marler, 1985). The frequency of homozygous PC deficient patients is 1:500,000. The heterozygous patients generally has a PC concentration at 30 - 60% of normal. The frequency of heterozygous deficiency with symptoms is 1:15,000 and that without symptoms is about 1:250, thus involving a large population. If not diagnosed and properly treated immediately, thrombo-embolic insults can occur in major organs, resulting in death, or in debilitating trauma to the extremities.

2.3. Need for a High-Sensitivity, High-Selectivity, Real-Time PC Biosensor

The average concentration of PC in normal human plasma is approximately 4 μg/ml. Since the concentration of PC is so low, existing protein assays, such as the Lowry

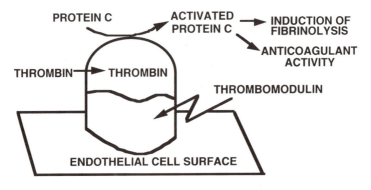

Figure 1. A schematic diagram of Protein C activation (based on Comp et.al., 1982).

method or spectro-photometer light absorption at 280 nm, are inappropriate for PC concentration measurement. Also, human plasma is composed of a large number of different proteins. The structure of many of these proteins is homologous to that of PC. To be fully functional, therefore, a PC biosensor has to be highly sensitive and specific to PC. Currently, PC concentration is mainly measured by ELISA, which takes at least two hours (usually one day). It is expensive, and the test kits cannot be reused. Therefore, the construction of a highly sensitive, highly specific, reusable, and real-time biosensor is urgently needed.

2.4. Proposed Immuno-Optical PC-Biosensor

The PC-biosensor proposed is composed of an anti-PC immobilized optical fiber and a reagent which contains a biochemical, highly specific to PC (PC-probe) and conjugated with a fluorophore. When PC in a sample is adsorbed to the fiber and reacted with the reagent, fluorescent light will be generated. The fluorescence intensity through the optical fiber will be correlated with the concentration of PC in the sample. Applying excitation input light at an appropriate wavelength to the fiber, fluorophores generate photons of another wavelength. The emitted light intensity can be correlated with the PC concentration in the sample. Since monoclonal antibodies are covalently immobilized on the fiber, the biosensor can be reused after the adsorbed PC molecules are washed off, using a proper elution buffer (Kang et al., 1992). The experimental procedure for PC concentration measurement (for both calibration and actual sample measurements) using the proposed immuno-optical PC biosensor is as follows:

1. Equilibrate the anti-PC immobilized optical fiber with the equilibration buffer.
2. Adsorb PC in the sample to anti-PC molecules on the optical fiber.
3. Wash the sensor with the first washing buffer.
4. Measure the baseline.
5. React the biosensor with the reagent containing the fluorophore tagged PC-probe.
6. Wash the fiber with the second washing buffer.
7. Apply the input light at the excitation wavelength and measure the emitted light intensity.
8. Elute the adsorbed PC with the elution buffer.
9. Regenerate the sensor using the regeneration buffer.
10. Re-equilibrate the fiber with the equilibration buffer.

3. PRELIMINARY STUDY

3.1. Materials, Instruments, and Methods

Protein C, Monoclonal Antibody Against Protein C. The University of Maryland Baltimore County (UMBC) has an on-going research project (Protein C Project), with the collaboration of the American Red Cross (ARC), Rockville, Maryland. The ARC has already developed a murine monoclonal anti-PC. It is produced by hybridoma and the isotype of the antibody is $IgG1_{ak}$. The ARC already have completed study on immuno-affinity purification of Protein C. Both Protein C and anti-PC have been supplied by ARC as needed.

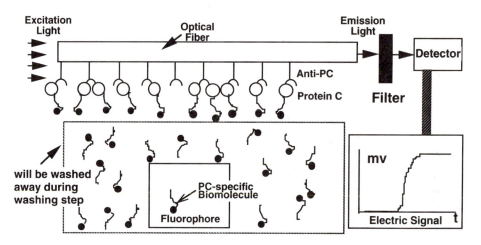

Figure 2. Schematic diagram of the basic principle of an immuno-optical Protein C biosensor.

Immobilization of Anti-PC on a Quartz Fiber. Anti-PC is immobilized on the quartz optical fiber by the method developed by Bhatia, et. al. (1989).

Conjugation of Fluorophore, FITC, to a PC Specific Biomolecules. The conjugation of the fluorophore, fluorosein isothiocyanate (FITC, Sigma, St. Louis, MO), to bio-molecules is performed by the method developed by Suszkiw and Ichiki (1976; Rinderknecht, 1960). For the preliminary study, equimolar concentrations of PC and 10% FITC on celite are mixed on 0.5 ml of 0.05M sodium bicarbonate buffer, pH 9.5, for 15 minutes at room temperature. After removing celite, the reaction mixture is passed through gel permeation chromatography to purify the biomolecule conjugated with FITC or dialyze the sample to remove free (unreacted) FITC molecules.

Fluorometer. The fluorometer used for PC sensor is designed and built by ORD, Inc. (North Salem, NH; Eldefrawi et al., 1992; Roger et al., 1991). The fiber used for this experiment is a quartz fiber, 1 mm diameter with polished ends (1 x 60 mm; Ord, Inc.). Before the actual measurement, anti-PC is immobilized on the surface of the fiber. An antibody-immobilized-fiber is placed in the flow cell and liquid samples are applied to the cell by a peristaltic pump. The flow cell allows the center 47 mm of 60 mm fiber to be immersed in a 46 ml chamber. The light source is a 10-W Welch Allyn quartz halogen lamp. Three lenses; a filter to select the excitation wavelength, 485/20 nm, for the excitation of the fluorophore, fluorosein isothiocyanate (FITC); and a beam splitter for guiding the input light to the cell, are placed between the lamp and the flow cell. Band pass filters, 510 LP and 530/30 nm, are placed to pass the emission light only and lenses transfer the emission light from the fiber in the cell to the detector. The emission light from the fiber is converted to electrical energy and amplified by a Hamamatsu S-1087 silicon detector and the output is recorded on a strip chart recorder.

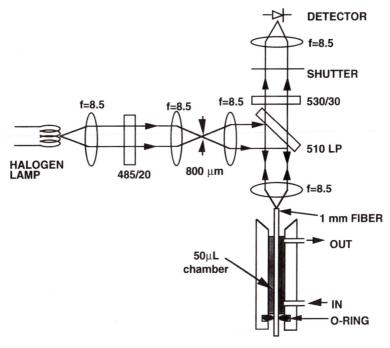

Figure 3. Schematic diagram of a Portable Fluorometer (Roger et al., 1989).

3.2. Preliminary Results and Discussion

Specific and Non-Specific Binding of PC to Anti-PC. To determine whether the signal intensity from a PC biosensor is above the noise level or not, an anti-PC-immobilized quartz fiber was reacted directly with PC (without PC-probe molecules proposed here) tagged with fluorophore, FITC, and the signal intensity from the biosensor was observed. Anti-PC was covalently immobilized onto quartz fibers. 70 μg (in 100 μl) of PC was adjusted to pH 9.5 with 1 M sodium carbonate to obtain a 50 mM carbonate buffer solution. The PC solution was mixed with approximately 500 μg of FITC on celite and incubated for 15 minutes at room temperature. The sample was briefly centrifuged to precipitate the celite and was loaded on a Sephadex size exclusion chromatography column (1 cm x 15 cm) and then was eluted with PBS. The fractions containing the conjugated PC was pooled and its protein content was determined. 2 ml of PC tagged with FITC (PC-FITC) was obtained at the concentration of 23 μg/ml. Protein C-FITC at various concentration was applied into the flow cell. As a control study, equimolar FITC solution alone was applied to the cell also. After the adsorption stage, the pump was switched off and the fiber was washed with PBS/BSA solution. The emitted light intensity was recorded from the beginning to the end of the experiment.

Figure 4 shows a comparison between (a) the light emission from the specific binding reaction between PC-FITC and anti-PC immobilized on the fiber and (b) that from the non-specific binding reaction between FITC and anti-PC. As can be seen in the figures, the specific adsorption of PC-FITC to anti-PC shows a fluorescent signal completely different from the non-specific reaction of FITC to anti-PC. While FITC only was removed by PBS/BSA completely PC-FITC remained on the fiber. Therefore, it was found that there would be no

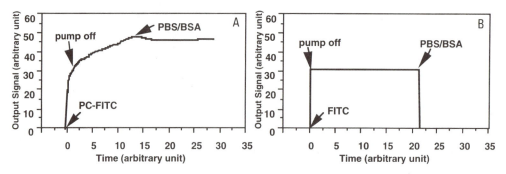

Figure 4. Fluorescent emissions representing the reaction between (a) specific reaction between PC and anti-PC on the fiber and (b) non- specific reaction between FITC alone and anti-PC (qualitative study).

major difficulty to differentiate the specific binding from the non-specific. The degree of non-specific binding to specific binding is proposed to be more thoroughly studied with PC-FITC.

Figure 5 describes the emission light intensity detected by a silicon detector when 2 μg/ml of PC-FITC was reacted with the anti-PC probe. Maximum voltage output for this reaction is shown to be 55 mV. The resulting photon intensity appears to be satisfactory, although the sensitivity needs to be improved since the lowest value of our measurement range is decided to be only 0.5 μg/ml (approximately 1/8 of normal PC concentration in plasma). The sensitivity study is proposed to be performed more systematically with PC-probe-FITC molecules.

4. FUTURE WORK: DEVELOPMENT OF PC-PROBE

An antibody binding domain is a portion of an antibody F_{ab} part, which actually three-dimensionally fits to a specific antigen. Molecular weight of this section is approximately 25,000, much smaller than the entire IgG (MW=150,000) or IgM (MW=970,000) and, therefore, an antibody binding domain generates less steric hindrance (Fig. 6). *In vitro* generation of random combinations of antibody binding domain libraries avoids immunization, and the subsequent display of the combinations on the surface of a bacteriophage allows the generated binding domains to be screened for specific properties (Huse, et al., 1989).

For the PC-biosensor development proposed here, the isolated antibody binding domain libraries against PC have more advantages to be used as PC-probe than regular monoclonal antibody because of it lower molecular weight, which generates less steric

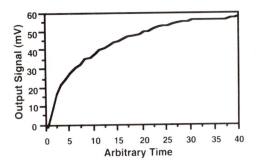

Figure 5. Kinetics of fluorophore-tagged-PC molecules reacting with monoclonal antibody on the the surface of optical fiber, in terms of voltage generated by the photons detected by a silicon detector.

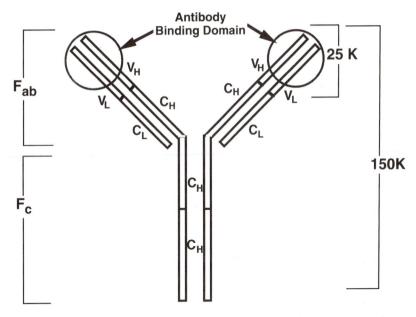

Figure 6. Artificially generated antibody binding domain libraries: Protein C-Probe.

hindrance and its lower production cost. However, the molecular weight of this domain is large enough to react with fluorophore at a high ratio. Also, the property of the PC-probe can be custom designed, e.g., selection of libraries with various binding affinity at specific reaction conditions. These domains can be obtained much cheaper than regular monoclonal antibodies because they can be produced by *E. coli*.

The basic principles for producing antibodies binding domain for a biomolecule are:

1. Reproduce the genetic library of human antibody binding domains *in vitro* using polymerase chain reaction technology.
2. Express the genetic library as individual proteins on the surface of a bacteriophage.
3. Quickly and efficiently screen the expressed protein library for antibodies possessing specific binding properties.
4. The isolated antibody binding domain can be produced in bulk and attached to a solid support as affinity gel matrices or optical fibers for biosensors.

5. CONCLUSIONS

The user for this PC-biosensor research is 'a *Lab Technician* who will analyze blood samples'. A fully developed PC-biosensor will facilitate the progress on other sub-projects under the Protein C Project at UMBC. Real-time accurate measurement of PC concentration in human blood plasma is critical for the fast diagnosis and appropriate monitoring of pathological conditions for PC-deficient patients. When PC is administered a sensor is essential to maintain appropriate PC blood levels in a cost effective and efficient manner. Currently, there is a lack of real-time biosensors for clotting and anti-clotting factors in human plasma, as well as Protein C, despite the large population of patients with conditions related to these factors. When PC immuno-optical biosensor development is completed, the same principles can be applied to measure other plasma factors for fast diagnosis of diseases related to the hemostasis. Exactly the same principles can be used also for the diagnosis of other diseases if proper probes for disease representing biomolecules, e.g. cancer representing molecules or pathogen, can be developed. The reusable biosensor will reduce the diagnostic and administration expense as well.

Preliminary results show high feasibility for developing a real-time biosensor that can accurately measure Protein-C concentration less than 1 µg/mL in various bio-samples.

6. ACKNOWLEDGMENTS

This research is partly supported by The Whitaker Foundation and The American Red Cross. The authors would like to thank to Dr. Michael Sierks for the research support of antibody domain against Protein C. The authors also would like to thank to the Internal and External Advisory Committee members for this Protein C Project at UMBC.

7. REFERENCES

Bertina, R., Broekmans, A., van der Linden I., and Mertens, K., "Protein C Deficiency in Dutch Family with Thrombotic Disease", *Thromb. Haemostasis* (Stuttgart), 48 (1), 1–5, 1982.
Bhatia, S.K., Shriver-Laker, L.C., Prior, K. J., Georger, J.H., Calvert, J.M., Bredehorst, R., and Ligler F.S., "Use of thiol-terminal silanes and heterobifunctional crosslinkers for immobilization of antibodies on silica surfaces," *Analytical Biochemistry*, 178, 408–413, 1989.
Boekman, A., Veltkamp, J., and Bertina, R., "Congenital Protein C Deficiency and Venous Thromboembolism", *New England Journal of Medicine*, 309 (6), 340–344, 1983.
Bruley, D.F. and Drohan, W.N., *Protein C and Related Anticoagulants - Advances in Applied Biotechnolgy Series*, 11, Gulf Publishing Company, Houston, 1990.
Comp, P. Jacocks, R., Ferrell, G., and Esmon, C., "Activation of Protein C *in vivo*", *J. Clin. Invest.*, 70, 127–134, 1982.
Eldefrawi, M.E., Eldefrawi, A.T., Roger, K.R., and Valdes, J.J., "Pharmaceutical Biosensors," in *Immunochemical Assays and Biosensor Technology for the 1990's* (Nakamura, R.M., Kasahara, Y., and Rechnitz, G.A., eds.), Am. Soc. Microbiol. Publ. Washington DC, 391–406, 1992.
Esmon, C. and Esmon, N., "Protein C Activation," *Seminars in Thrombosis and Hemostasis*, 10 (2), 122–130, 1984.
Huse, W.D., Sastry, L., Iverson, S., Kang, A. S., Alting-Mees, M., Burton, D.R., Benkovic, S.J., and Lerner, R.A., "Generation of a large combinatorial library of the immunoglobin repertoire in phase lambda," *Science*, 246, 1275–1281., 1989.
Kang, K.A., Ryu, D., Drohan, W.D., and Orthner, C.L. "Effect of Matrices on the Immunoaffinity Purification of Protein C", *Biotech. & Bioengr.*. 39(11), 1086–1098, 1992.
Marciniak, E., Wilson, D., and Marlar, R., "Neonatal Purpura Fulminans: A Genetic Disorder Related to the Absence of Protein C in Blood", *Blood*, 65 (1), 15–20, 1985.
Marlar, R., "Protein C in Thromboembolic Disease", *Seminars in Thrombosis and Hemostasis*, 11 (4), 1985.
Rinderknecht, H., "Ultra-Rapid Fluorescent Labeling of Protein," *Nature* 193 (4811), 167–168, 1962.
Roger, K.R., Eldefrawi M.E., Menking, D.E., Thompson, R.G., and Valdes, J.J., "Pharmacological specificity of a nicotinic acetylcholine receptor optical sensor," *Biosensors & Bioelectronics*, 6, pp. 507–516, 1991.
Stenflo, J., "Structure and Function of Protein C", *Seminars in Thrombosis and Hemostasis*, 10 (2), 109–121, 1984.
Suszkiw, J.B., and Ichiki, M., "Fluorescein conjugated a-Bungarotoxin: Its properties and interaction with acetylcholine receptors", *Analytical Biochemistry*.73, 109–114, 1976.
Walker, F., "Regulation of Activated Protein C by Protein S", *J. of Biological Chemistry*, 266 (21), 11128–11131, 1981.

57

EFFECT OF EXERCISE AND ISCHEMIA ON TISSUE OXIMETRY AND CYTOCHROME IN NORMAL SUBJECTS, PATIENTS WITH CHRONIC LIMB PAIN, AND PATIENTS WITH MITOCHONDRIAL MITOPATHIES

T. C. Chelimsky,[1] K. M. Mcneeley,[1] B. Comfort,[2] C. A. Piantadosi,[2] and J. C. LaManna[1]

[1]University Hospitals of Cleveland and School of Medicine
Case Western Reserve University
Cleveland, Ohio 44106
[2]Duke University Medical Center
Durham, North Carolina 27710

1. INTRODUCTION

Near-infrared spectrophotometry (NIR) is a non-invasive measure of tissue oxygen delivery and utilization[1]. Its use has been limited, with one notable exception[2], to subjects at rest under conditions of ischemia. It is not clear whether reproducible and accurate measures of hypoxia using this technique can be obtained during dynamic exercise in the upper extremity, because changes in optical path length can alter the signals. The technique's greatest potential power as a clinical diagnostic tool in abnormalities of oxygen transport and utilization lies in the responses to changes in oxygen consumption, i.e. exercise.

Bank and Chance[2] demonstrated specific abnormalities of oxygen utilization during exercise of the lower extremities in patients with cytochrome *c* oxidase deficiency, myophosphorylase deficiency, and phosphofructokinase deficiency. Less specific disorders of mitochondria, such as the Kearns-Sayre syndrome, a disorder of mitochondrial DNA duplication, as yet without a specific enzyme abnormality[3], have not been investigated.

Our interest in assessing muscle oxygen delivery and utilization by NIR during exercise also arose out of studies in another patient population. Patients with reflex sympathetic dystrophy, a type of limb pain accompanied by demonstrable abnormalities in the limb, such as swelling, and skin temperature and color changes, during exercise of the limb, demonstrated a reduction in forearm muscle blood flow as measured by plethys-

Oxygen Transport to Tissue XVIII, edited by Nemoto and LaManna
Plenum Press, New York, 1997

mography (personal observation). Thus, we wished to know whether this finding could be supported by abnormalities of oxygen metabolism.

We studied NIR with three goals in view:

1. Establish whether NIR can reproducibly measure oxygen delivery and utilization in an intermittently exercising forearm, and determine the physiologic effect of this exercise, in comparison to the effect of ischemia.
2. Evaluate oxygen delivery and utilization in a group of patients with the reflex sympathetic dystrophy syndrome (RSD).
3. Investigate the abnormalities in patients with a relatively non-specific disorder of mitochondria, Kearns-Sayre syndrome (KSS).

2. METHODS

(1) Subjects. We studied six healthy volunteers, aged 18–40 years, without history of any neurologic illness, any illness requiring on-going care, and off all medications of any kind. Brief neurologic examination was normal. Five mitochondrial mitopathy patients with Kearns-Sayre syndrome were studied. Three patients had biopsy-proven disease, and two were strongly suspected by clinical phenotype. Three patients with reflex sympathetic dystrophy were studied. All had pain, allodynia, swelling and vasomotor changes in one upper extremity.

(2) Exercise/Ischemia Protocol. Maximum grip strength was determined for each hand. Subjects were then asked to exercise the stronger hand at 50% of its maximum for 2 seconds every 4 seconds over a 30 second period, followed by a 90 second rest period. This step was repeated. After the second 90 second rest, complete ischemia was initiated by rapid automatic inflation of a blood pressure cuff around the arm to 240 mm Hg. A third identical 30 second exercise period occurred 150 seconds into the ischemia. The cuff was released at 240 seconds, and the study continued until all measurements returned to baseline. The entire protocol was repeated for the weaker hand at 50% of its maximum, and for the stronger hand at 50% of the maximum of the weaker hand.

(3) NIR Measurements. These were performed as previously reported[1] using four solid state GaAlAs lasers calibrated at 775, 810, 870, and 904 nm, each firing every 400 usecs for 100 usecs through a fiberoptic cable attached on the surface of the skin just lateral to the extensor carpi radialis. A fiberoptic photoreceptor was placed 2.5 cm away medially, and covered with foil. NIR signals were analyzed using published trend monitoring algorithms[4]. Measurements were continuous throughout the protocol.

(4) Data Analysis. For each condition and measured parameter, the maximum change in the amplitude of the signal, and the slope of the change were calculated by manual measurement, off the recorded strip. The most linear portion of any rise or fall was taken as the slope. During ischemia, the change induced by exercise was estimated by continuing the ischemic curve visually, and subtracting the difference associated with the duration of exercise. Thus, for each subject, there were 5 conditions (exercise 1, 2, ischemia, exercise during ischemia, and ischemia release), 4 parameters (hemoglobin, HbO2, volume, and cytochrome), and 3 runs (strong limb, weak limb, and strong limb at

the weak strength), or 120 measurements. All numbers were entered into a spreadsheet where statistical analysis was performed, generally using a two-tailed Student's t-test.

3. RESULTS

3.1. Normals and Trends across All Subjects

Results in normals are summarized in the table. Figure 1 shows the actual data in a normal subject. As shown here, and in graphic form in the two subsequent figures, both exercise and ischemia produced a drop in oxyhemoglobin and a rise in deoxyhemoglobin in all subjects and patients. The changes due to ischemia were approximately twice those due to exercise at 50% maximum force. Blood volume (fourth figure) decreased during ischemia, as well as during all 3 periods of exercise. All findings were highly reproducible between the first and second exercise periods.

The rate of change during exercise was generally greater than that during ischemia for both deoxyhemoglobin (2.34±.84 vs 1.57±.59) and oxyhemoglobin (-2.09±.8 vs -1.48±.43) in normals. The largest slope, however, was seen during recovery from ischemia, with values in normals being -3.51± 1.7 (Hb) and 3.75 ± 2.33 (HbO$_2$). In normals, the stronger hand, weaker hand, and stronger hand done at 50% of the weak hand's capacity were similar in their hemo-

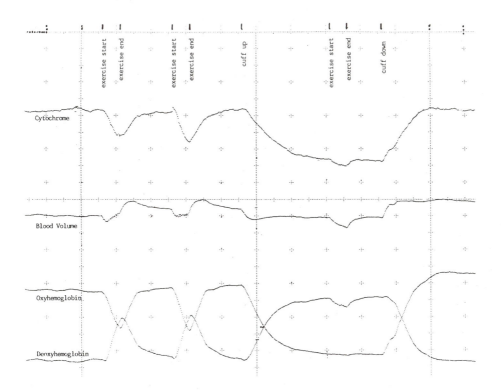

Figure 1. Data as originally recorded in a normal subject. The time between each cross-hair is 1 minute, and between the dividing lines, 5 minutes. Blood volume trace represents the addition of oxyhemoglobin and deoxyhemoglobin.

globin responses but, as expected, there was a strong trend for a greater drop in cytochrome oxidation state with increasing exercise.

3.2. Patients with RSD

Interestingly, these patients also showed little difference between painful and non-painful extremities. Patients with RSD differed from normals in both the strong and weak hands in several respects:

1. There was clearly less decrease in oxyhemoglobin during exercise, despite an indistinguishable drop during ischemia (figure 2) and a similar drop in cytochrome during exercise.
2. Despite this, the increase in deoxyhemoglobin with exercise was not significantly different in RSD patients compared to normals, the trend even being in the direction of a smaller decrement with exercise. The drop during ischemia, and ischemic exercise was identical to that in normals (figure 3).
3. Patients with RSD tended to exhibit a lower total labile signal in both the involved and uninvolved extremities for all parameters (figure 4). As expected, slopes were also smaller, though time to maximum change was not clearly different.
4. The post-ischemic overshoot in cytochrome oxidation was largest in the RSD group (figure 5), suggesting that their baseline may be closer to ischemia. Also, the normal gradient in cytochrome reduction with increasing exercise level was not seen.

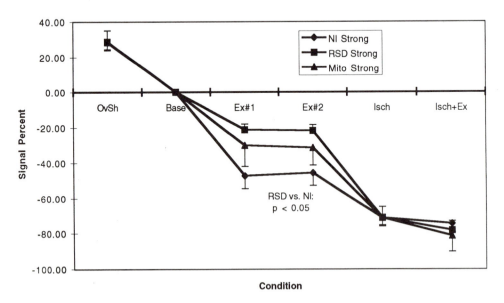

Figure 2. Change from baseline in oxyhemoglobin with each condition of the protocol. The average change is expressed as a percentage of total labile signal (TLS) from ischemia to overshoot and averaged for all subjects. OvSh: post-ischemic overshoot; Base: baseline, defined as 0; Ex#1 and #2: first and second non-ischemic exercise periods; Isch: ischmia; Isch+Ex: exercise during the ischemic period; Nl: Normal subjects; Mito: subjects with mitochondrial disorder; RSD: subjects with reflex sympathetic dystrophy.

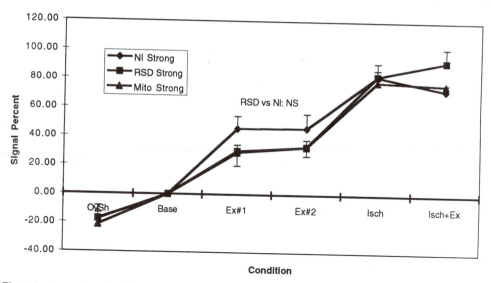

Figure 3. Change from baseline in deoxyhemoglobin with each condition of the protocol. Calculations and abbreviations are identical to figure 2.

3.3. Patients with KSS

In many respects, the findings in KSS were intermediate between normals and RSD patients. The drop in oxyhemoglobin was lower than normals and higher than RSD pa-

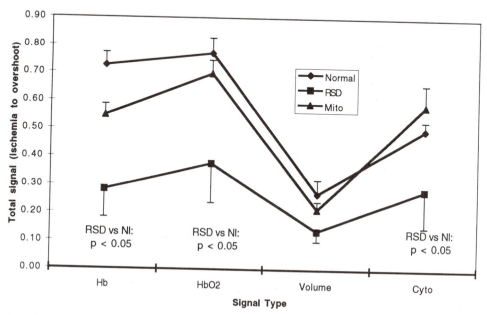

Figure 4. Total labile signal (arbitrary units) for each of the recorded signals, averaged for all subjects. Hb: deoxyhemoglobin; HbO2: oxyhemoglobin; Cyto: cytochrome a,a_3.

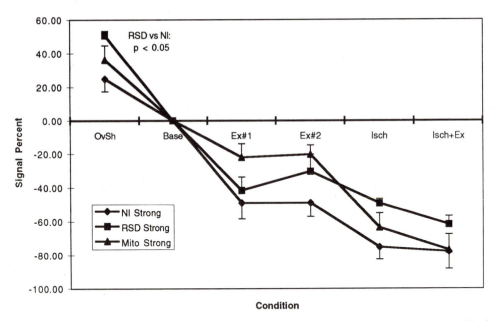

Figure 5. Change in cytochrome a,a_3 for each condition in the protocol. Calculations and abbreviations are identical to figure 2.

tients, but not significantly different from either group. The increase in deoxyhemoglobin was identical to the RSD group, and lower than normal. Total labile signal did not differ from normal.

Unique to patients with KSS was a lower ratio of the drop in cytochrome oxidation state with exercise to the drop with ischemia, though this was seen mainly in the strong hand, with only a trend present in the weak hand, and no difference when the strong hand exercised at 50% of the weak hand's maximal force.

4. DISCUSSION

This study demonstrates that near-infrared oximetry can reliably and reproducibly measure the shift from oxyhemoglobin to deoxyhemoglobin as well as the drop in cytochrome oxidation state in muscle during intermittent upper extremity exercise, both with and without ischemia. Our results for exercise are in agreement with those of Bank and Chance[2] for the lower extremity, who also found a decrease in blood volume, and the expected changes in hemoglobin.

We also find that exercise alone decreases muscle oxygenation supply faster than does ischemia alone, implying either that exercising muscle outstrips its blood supply, or that some of the signal originates in myoglobin. The similarity between strong and weak hands for nearly every parameter in subjects and patients is surprising, and suggests that workload is only a partial determinant of the findings.

Other factors such as sympathetic tone may impact on oxyhemoglobin supply, and may explain the differences seen in the RSD patients. These changes include the reduction in total labile signal, and the apparent proximity of the baseline to an ischemic state (reflected by the larger post-ischemic overshoot in cytochrome), which could account for some of their pain. An increase in total flow would explain how the changes in *both* oxy and deoxy-hemoglobin can be less than normal with aerobic exercise, yet be similar to normal during ischemic exercise (once flow is cut off). The symmetry of the findings, similar to skin blood flow[5] suggests an abnormality of blood flow control in the nervous system, rather than at the tissue level.

The lower exercise/ischemia cytochrome drop in patients with KSS, as well as the absence of any gradient with exercise level suggests that these patients may have inefficient utilization of O_2 by cytochrome a,a_3. Further studies using differing levels of exertion in these patients and in normal subjects will clarify many of these questions.

5. REFERENCES

1. Hampson NB and Piantadosi CA: NIR monitoring of human skeletal muscle oxygenation during forearm ischemia. J Appl Physiol 1988; 64:2449–2457.
2. Bank W and Chance B: An Oxidative Defect in Metabolic Myopathies: Diagnosis by Noninvasive Tissue Oxymetry. Ann Neurol 1994; 36:830–837.
3. Duplications of Mitochondrial DNA Kearns-Sayre Syndrome. Muscle & Nerve 1995; Supplement 3:S154–158.
4. Duhaylongsod FG, Griebel JA, Bacon DS, Piantadosi CA: Effects of muscle contraction on cytochrome a,a_3 redox state. J Appl Physiol 1993; 75(2):790–797.
5. Bej M and Schwartzman R. Abnormalities of cutaneous blood flow regulation in patients with reflex sympathetic dystrophy as measured by laser doppler fluxmetry. Arch Neurol 1991; 48:912–915.

58

MEASUREMENT OF CEREBRAL VENOUS SATURATION IN ADULTS USING NEAR INFRARED SPECTROSCOPY

C. E. Elwell,[1] S. J. Matcher,[1] L. Tyszczuk,[2] J. H. Meek,[2] and D. T. Delpy[1]

[1]Department of Medical Physics and Bioengineering
[2]Department of Paediatrics
University College London
United Kingdom

INTRODUCTION

Saturation measurements have long been used to provide information about oxygenation levels within tissue in the form of a single percentage value. Whilst the measurement of peripheral arterial oxygen saturation (SaO_2) provides useful information about the delivery of oxygen to the brain, a measure of the actual level of cerebral oxygen consumption and uptake would be a more useful guide for the direction of therapies. Oxygen consumption is the product of cerebral blood flow (CBF) and the difference between arterial and venous oxygen content. Measurements of cerebral venous saturation can therefore be used as an indicator of oxygen consumption and have been shown to be a useful clinical parameter in the management of patients with compromised cerebral haemodynamics (Garlick et al., 1987, Cruz et al., 1991).

In adults undergoing intensive care, continuous jugular bulb oximetry is currently used as a method of assessing cerebral oxygenation. However this is an invasive method requiring regular calibration against blood samples and careful positioning of the sampling catheter which can be sensitive to movement artefact (Dearden et al., 1993).

Near infrared spectroscopy (NIRS) allows the non invasive measurement of changes in the concentration of oxy and deoxyhaemoglobin (HbO_2 and Hb). Although in its current form NIRS cannot measure absolute chromophore concentrations, it can be used in conjunction with specific physiological manoeuvres to estimate various haemodynamic parameters including blood flow and blood volume (Edwards et al., 1988, Wyatt et al., 1990, Elwell et al., 1994). Groups investigating neonatal cerebral haemodynamics have used head tilting to reduce venous return in order to measure cerebral venous saturation (SvO_2) (Wyatt et al., 1986, Skov et al., 1993). Yoxall et al. (Yoxall et al., 1995) have recently described a method in which SvO_2 is measured from the blood volume changes induced by partial occlusion of the jugular vein. Measurements made on a group of neonates and children agreed well with those from co-oximetry of jugular bulb blood.

The purpose of the present study was to determine if the same jugular occlusion technique could be used to measure SvO_2 in the adult, and to observe the effects of hypoxia on SvO_2 in a group of healthy adult volunteers to assess the clinical applicability of the method. In addition, measurements of mean cerebral saturation made using a novel multisite NIRS monitor are presented as preliminary results and compared to the SvO_2 data.

THEORY

NIRS

The theoretical details of NIRS have been given elsewhere (Cope et al., 1988, Cope, 1991). The technique relies upon using a modified Beer-Lambert law, which describes optical attenuation in a highly scattering medium such as biological tissue, to quantify the changes in concentration of the chromophores oxy and deoxyhaemoglobin and oxidised cytochrome oxidase (CytOx) (Delpy et al., 1988b). Since the degree of light scattering is dependent upon, among other factors, the type of tissue interrogated, a scaling factor called the differential pathlength factor (DPF) is incorporated in order to quantify the chromophore changes in units of µmol of chromophore per litre of tissue ($\mu mol.L^{-1}$). DPF has recently been measured in the heads of a group of 100 adults using the phase resolved spectroscopy technique, and a mean (±SD) value of 6.26 ± 0.88 at 807nm was obtained (Duncan et al., 1995). It is important to note that since the absolute concentration of chromophore is unknown, all measurements are expressed as absolute concentration *changes* from an arbitrary zero baseline at the start of the measurement period. The NIRS system used in this study therefore quantifies *changes* in tissue concentration of Hb and HbO_2 from an arbitrary baseline.

A NIRS system which provides an absolute measurement of tissue haemoglobin saturation (SO_2) has also recently been described (Matcher et al., 1995). The spatially resolved spectrometer (SRS), incorporates several detectors housed in a single probe which is placed 5–6 cms from the source. Combining these multi distance measurements of optical attenuation with the usual multi wavelength spectroscopy data, it is possible in principle to calculate the relative concentrations of Hb and HbO_2 in the illuminated tissue and hence to estimate mean tissue haemoglobin saturation. Preliminary studies with this and other tissue saturation monitors working on different principles have shown that trends in saturation can be measured, although the absolute saturation values appear to be lower than expected from arterial and venous saturation measurements (Lui et al., 1995, Miwa et al., 1995). Data from a prototype SRS was available on some of the subjects in this study enabling the time course of the changes in tissue saturation to be observed.

In this paper the term $[Hb_{diff}]$ will be used to represent the difference between the $[HbO_2]$ and $[Hb]$ concentrations and the term $[Hb.T]$ will be used to represent their sum.

Physiology

Since changes in chromophore concentration can be quantified absolutely using NIRS, the technique lends itself to saturation measurements. When a small change in blood volume is induced, as in the jugular occlusion method, the resulting increase in

HbO$_2$ and Hb.T can be quantified and SvO$_2$ can be estimated from a simple ratio calculation;

$$SvO_2 \ (\%) \ = \ \frac{\Delta HbO_2}{\Delta HbO_2 \ + \ \Delta Hb} \ x \ 100 \ = \ \frac{\Delta HbO_2}{\Delta Hb.T} \ x \ 100 \tag{1}$$

NIRS does not differentiate between light absorbed by blood in the arterial, venous or capillary compartments, so an assumption is made in these measurements that the increase in blood volume detected (ΔHb.T) is purely venous blood retained in the field of view. It is the mean saturation of this total blood pool which is calculated. Changes in oxygen consumption and CBF will affect the validity of this assumption, but it is assumed that when the duration of the occlusion is less than ten seconds these effects are minimal.

The SRS system provides a continuous measurement of SO$_2$ without the need for any manipulations or physiological manoeuvres. Again, since the exact tissue volume illuminated is a combination of arterial, venous and capillary vascular compartments the tissue saturation measured by this instrument will be referred to as mean cerebral saturation (SmcO$_2$).

METHOD

The subjects for this study were 11 healthy adults (age range 23 - 32 years, median 29 years, three female) with no known respiratory or cardiovascular disorders. The study was approved by the University College London Faculty of Clinical Science Committee on the Ethics of Clinical Investigation and informed written consent was obtained from the subjects prior to the investigation.

Instrumentation

The optodes from an NIR spectrometer (NIRO 500, Hamamatsu Photonics KK, Japan) were housed in a custom-made holder with fixed interoptode spacing of 4 cm and this was placed high on the left side of the forehead beneath the hairline. Pulsed laser diodes produced light at four wavelengths (779, 819, 849, 908 nm) and a photomultiplier tube was employed for detection of transmitted light. Data were collected every 0.5 second and the changes in concentration of HbO$_2$ and Hb were calculated using a previously established algorithm (Cope, 1991, Essenpreis et al., 1993, Duncan et al., 1995).

Arterial oxygen saturation (SaO$_2$) and heart rate (HRT) were monitored using a pulse oximetry probe positioned on the finger (Novametrix 520A, Wallingford, USA). End tidal carbon dioxide tension (EtCO$_2$) was recorded using an optical sensor in the expiratory line of the breathing circuit (Novametrix 7000A, Wallingford USA). The analogue outputs of both the pulse oximeter and capnograph were linked directly to the NIRO 500 for real time display and storage along with the NIRS data.

The optodes from the SRS system (when available) were placed on the right side of the forehead and fixed in position at a spacing of 5 cm. Care was taken to maximise the distance on the head between the emitting optode of the SRS system and the detector of the NIRO 500 system in order to avoid signal interference. The SRS system sampled data every 2 seconds and event markers were used to synchronise the signals from the two spectrometry systems.

An automated gas blending system (Elwell et al., 1995) was used to supply a controlled mixture of oxygen and nitrogen to the subject via a Waters bag and mouthpiece. The inspired oxygen fraction (FiO_2) was continuously monitored using an oxygen analyser (Model 5550, Hudson, Temecula, CA) upstream of the Waters bag. Subjects wore a nose clip to ensure that the inspired oxygen concentration was well controlled and a one way valve vented expired gas to prevent rebreathing.

Procedure

Subjects lay supine breathing a normoxic gas mixture from the circuit. Once comfortable, gentle pressure was then applied to one or both of the jugular veins to produce partial occlusion of the vessel. Each occlusion lasted approximately 5 seconds and was repeated at least ten times. FiO_2 in the breathing circuit was then slowly reduced to approximately 0.14 to produce a decrease in SaO_2 of less than 10%. Once a stable baseline had been achieved, the partial jugular occlusions were repeated. Throughout the study the beginning of each occlusion was marked as an event on the NIRO 500. SaO_2, HRT and $EtCO_2$ were continuously recorded throughout.

DATA ANALYSIS

On sections of NIRS data during which jugular occlusions were performed a regression of ΔHbO_2 against $\Delta Hb.T$ was performed. SvO_2 was then estimated from the slope of the regression line using equation 1. Occlusions producing a regression with the correlation coefficient (r) ≤ 0.85 were not used in further analysis, resulting in a mean ($\pm SD$) of 9 $\pm$ 3 occlusions being used for each subject at normoxia and hypoxia. On the same data sections the mean values of SaO_2, HRT and $EtCO_2$ were also calculated. The mean values for SvO_2, SaO_2, $EtCO_2$ and HRT were calculated for each subject under normoxic and hypoxic conditions. Using analysis of variance (ANOVA) statistics with subject number as a dummy variable to take into account the intersubject variation (Bland et al., 1995), the measured SvO_2 values were compared with SaO_2 and $EtCO_2$ values. In addition the mean change in Hb.T between the normoxic and hypoxic states was calculated. In one subject the calculated SvO_2 values were superimposed on the $SmcO_2$ data from the SRS system.

RESULTS

Figure 1(a) shows the NIRS data collected during a typical jugular occlusion at normoxia with the resulting regression, from which SvO_2 is calculated, shown in Figure 1(b). The mean ($\pm SD$) SvO_2 measured at normoxia ($SaO_2 = 96.0 \pm 0.8\%$) was $70.1 \pm 3.5\%$ which reduced to $60.7 \pm 4.2\%$ during hypoxia ($SaO_2 = 89.9 \pm 1.1\%$).

Figure 2 demonstrates the relation between the SaO_2 (x) and SvO_2 (y) data in the form of paired points for each subject. The relationship is described by the line $y = 1.48x - 72.04$, where $r = 0.9$ (95% confidence intervals of slope = 0.97 to 1.99). ANOVA showed no significant correlation between SvO_2 and $EtCO_2$.

The intersubject coefficient of variation on the SvO_2 measurements was 5% at normoxia and 7% at hypoxia and the intrasubject coefficient of variation was 8% normoxia and 10% at hypoxia. Using the statistical method described above, the arterial-venous dif-

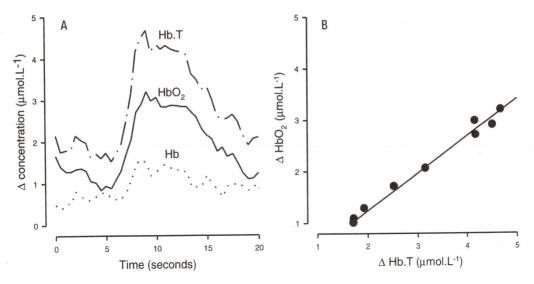

Figure 1. (a) NIRS data collected during a jugular occlusion at normoxia showing the parallel rise in Hb.T and HbO$_2$ and (b) the resulting regression from which SvO$_2$ is calculated.

ference (SaO$_2$-SvO$_2$) was shown to be correlated to SaO$_2$ (p < 0.05). The mean (± SD) change in Hb.T between the normoxic and hypoxic states was 1.9 ± 1.2 μmol.L^{-1}.

Figure 3 shows the superimposed plot of SvO$_2$ data together with a continuous SRS SmcO$_2$ recording. The SaO$_2$ data is also included to indicate the onset of hypoxia.

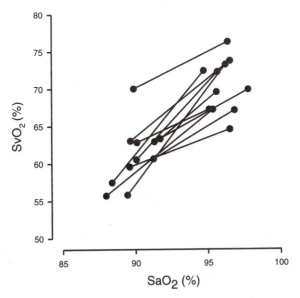

Figure 2. Mean SvO$_2$ values measured at hypoxia and normoxia with lines joining the paired points for each of the 11 subjects.

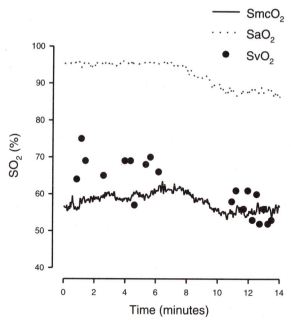

Figure 3. SmcO$_2$ data (measured by SRS), SvO$_2$ values (measured from jugular occlusion) and SaO$_2$ data (measured from pulse oximetry) on a single subject during normoxia and hypoxia.

DISCUSSION

This paper presents evidence that the measurements of SvO$_2$ from the changes in HbO$_2$ and Hb.T during jugular venous occlusion in adults is possible. The mean SvO$_2$ value measured using the venous occlusion at normoxia method agrees well with published values for cerebral mixed venous saturation measured at the jugular bulb in normal adults (Gibbs et al., 1942).

The data presented show the expected correlation between SaO$_2$ and SvO$_2$ although the slope of the regression is not unity. It would be expected that in conditions where CBF, oxygen consumption and cerebral blood volume (CBV) remain constant any change in SaO$_2$ should produce an equal change in all vascular compartments (i.e. SvO$_2$ and SmcO$_2$). Several reasons for this discrepancy may be considered.

It is likely that as a response to hypoxia CBF and CBV would increase. In these studies a small (<2%) increase on Hb.T was observed indicating a negligible increase in CBV. If CBF increased significantly in response to hypoxia this would cause a decrease in the arterial-venous difference and produce an SvO$_2$/SaO$_2$ slope of less than unity. If a change in oxygen consumption is responsible for the discrepancy, this would have to be in the order of a 20% increase from the baseline value. This would seem an unlikely response to a small change SaO$_2$ in normal individuals studied at rest. Since SvO$_2$ is calculated from a ratio of chromophore changes, optical pathlength does not in principle influence the exact calculations. However, if optical pathlength were to be affected by hypoxia this may affect the validity of comparing measurements at different levels of SaO$_2$. Previous studies have shown that even during large changes in optical attenuation such as those produced by total forearm cuff ischaemia (Ferrari et al., 1993) and severe hypercapnia challenges in the rat (Delpy et al.,

1988a) the change in DPF is less than 15%. The changes in attenuation due to mild hypoxia are therefore highly unlikely to produce a significant alteration in DPF during this phase.

The calculated slope depends upon the accuracy of both the SvO_2 and SaO_2 measurements at different levels of oxygenation. In a previous study on newborn infants, a mean difference of 1.7% was demonstrated between SvO_2 measured using the above occlusion method and co-oximetry of jugular bulb blood. A mean accuracy of ±2% is quoted for the SaO_2 measurements between 80–100% (Novametrix, Wallingford, USA). Assuming that SaO_2 data becomes less reliable at lower oxygenation levels, the SvO_2/SaO_2 regression analysis was repeated excluding the two subjects where SaO_2 dropped below 89%. The SvO_2/SaO_2 slope was reduced, however the change was not significant.

One possible explanation for an SvO_2/SaO_2 slope of greater than unity is that during hypoxia the illuminated volume may shift more towards the venous field. This requires further investigation which may take the form of a study comparing SvO_2 from venous occlusion measurements with those using jugular bulb oximetry at different levels of SaO_2 during graded hypoxia together with an independent measure of CBF (and if possible CBV).

The occlusion manoeuvre itself is simple to perform in adults once the jugular vein has been located, a task which is more difficult in subjects with more muscular necks. A series of 10 occlusions took less than two minutes and caused minimal, if any discomfort to the subjects. The mean increase in blood volume during an occlusion was equivalent to a rise in CBV of approximately 4%.

The intrasubject coefficient of variation seen in this study was comparable to those quoted by Yoxall (Yoxall et al., 1995). As already demonstrated in a previous study (Elwell et al., 1994), at lowered levels of FiO_2 oscillations in SaO_2 which are related to respiratory rate are evident. This phenomenon is again evident as a higher coefficient of variation on the SaO_2 measurements at hypoxia compared to normoxia. This may also account for the increased coefficient of variation in the SvO_2 at lowered FiO_2.

The validity of the use of NIRS for the interrogation of the adult brain has often been questioned due to the unknown contribution of the significant layers of extra cerebral tissue within the illuminated area. In the measurement of SvO_2 the pathlength factor is not used, since the calculation is purely a ratio.

The preliminary SRS data presented here confirms that the instrument follows trends in oxygenation. Work is currently in progress to determine the likely cause of the underestimation in absolute mean tissue saturation measured by this technique.

CONCLUSION

We conclude that the venous occlusion method may be used to measure SvO_2 in the adult and that the values obtained are related to those of SaO_2. At normoxia the measured SvO_2 values compare well with those quoted in the literature. Given the coefficient of variation on the measurements, several occlusions may be necessary to produce clinically reliable data. Further work needs to be done to fully validate the technique over a range of oxygenation states.

ACKNOWLEDGMENTS

This work has been supported by grants from the United Kingdom Medical Research Council, the Welcome Trust and Hamamatsu Photonics KK.

REFERENCES

Bland, J.M., Altman, D.G., 1995. Calculating correlation coefficients with repeated observations: Part 1 - correlation within subjects. *BMJ* 310:446.

Cope, M. 1991. The development of a near infrared spectroscopy system and its application for non invasive monitoring of cerebral blood and tissue oxygenation in the newborn infant. *Ph.D. Thesis, University College London*

Cope, M., Delpy, D.T., 1988. A system for the long term measurement of cerebral blood and tissue oxygenation in newborn infants by near infrared transillumination. *Med. Biol. Eng. & Comp.* 26(3):289–294.

Cruz, J., Miner, M.E., Allen, S.J., Alves, W.M., Gennarelli, T.A., 1991. Continuous monitoring of cerebral oxygenation in acute brain injury: assessment of cerebral hemodynamic reserve. *Neurosurgery* 29:743–749.

Dearden, N.M., Midgley, S., 1993. Technical considerations in continuous jugular venous oxygen saturation measurement. *Acta. Neurochir.* 59:91–97.

Delpy, D.T., Arridge, S.R., Cope, M., Edwards, A.D., Reynolds, E.O.R., Richardson, C.E., Wray, S., Wyatt, J.S., van der Zee, P., 1988a. Quantitation of pathlength in optical spectroscopy. *Adv. Exp. Med. & Biol.* 248:41–46.

Delpy, D.T., Cope, M., van der Zee, P., Arridge, S.R., Wray, S., Wyatt, J.S., 1988b. Estimation of optical pathlength through tissue from direct time of flight measurement. *Phys. Med. Biol.* 33(12):1433–1442.

Duncan, A., Meek, J.H., Clemence, M., Elwell, C.E., Tyszczuk, L., Cope, M., Delpy, D.T., 1995. Optical pathlength measurements on adult head, calf and forearm and the head of the newborn infant using phase resolved optical spectroscopy. *Phys. Med. Biol.* 40:295–304.

Edwards, A.D., Wyatt, J.S., Richardson, C., Delpy, D.T., Cope, M., Reynolds, E.O.R., 1988. Cotside measurement of cerebral blood flow in ill newborn infants by near infrared spectroscopy. *Lancet* 2:770–771.

Elwell, C.E., Cope, M., Edwards, A.D., Wyatt, J.S., Delpy, D.T., Reynolds, E.O.R., 1994. Quantification of adult cerebral haemodynamics by near infrared spectroscopy. *J. Applied Physiol.* 77:2753–2760.

Elwell, C.E., Cope, M., Kirkby, D., Owen-Reece, H., Cooper, C.E., Reynolds, E.O.R., Delpy, D.T., 1995. An automated system for the measurement of the response of cerebral blood volume and cerebral blood flow to changes in arterial carbon dioxide tension using near infrared spectroscopy. *Adv. Exp. Med. & Biol.* 361:143–155.

Essenpreis, M., Elwell, C.E., Cope, M., van der Zee, P., Arridge, S.R., Delpy, D.T., 1993. Spectral dependence of temporal point spread functions in human tissues. *Appl. Opt.* 32(4):418–425.

Ferrari, M., Wei, Q., De Blasi, R.A., Quaresima, V., Zaccanti, G., 1993. Variability of human brain and muscle optical pathlength in different experimental conditions. *Proc. SPIE* 1888:466–472.

Garlick, R., Bihari, D., 1987. The use of intermittent and continuous recordings of jugular venous bulb oxygen saturation in the unconscious patient. *Scand. J. Clin. Lab. Invest.* 47 [Suppl 188]:47–52.

Gibbs, E.L., Lennox, W.G., Nims, L.F., Gibbs, F.A., 1942. Arterial and cerebral venous blood. Arterial differences in man. *J. Biol. Chem.* 144:325–332.

Lui, H., Hielscher, H., Kurth, C.D., Jacques, S.L., Chance, B., 1995. Time-resolved photon migration in a heterogeneous tissue-vessel model. *Proc. SPIE* 2389:150–156.

Matcher, S.J., Kirkpatrick, P., Nahid, K., Cope, M., Delpy, D.T., 1995. Absolute quantification methods in tissue near infrared spectroscopy. *Proc. SPIE* 2389:486–495.

Miwa, M., Ueda, Y., Chance, B., 1995. Development of time resolved spectroscopy system for quantitative non-invasive tissue measurement. *Proc. SPIE* 2389:142–149.

Skov, L., Pryds, O., Greisen, G., Lou, H., 1993. Estimation of cerebral venous saturation in newborn infants by near infrared spectroscopy. *Pediatr. Res.* 33(1):52–55.

Wyatt, J.S., Cope, M., Delpy, D.T., Edwards, A.D., Wray, S.C., Reynolds, E.O.R., 1986. Quantification of cerebral oxygenation and haemodynamics in sick newborn infants by near infrared spectrophotometry. *Lancet* ii:1063–1066.

Wyatt, J.S., Cope, M., Delpy, D.T., Richardson, C.E., Edwards, A.D., Wray, S., Reynolds, E.O.R., 1990. Quantitation of cerebral blood volume in human infants by near-infrared spectroscopy. *J. Applied Physiol.* 68:1086–1091.

Yoxall, C.W., Weindling, A.M., Dawani, N.H., Peart, I., 1995. Measurement of cerebral venous oxyhaemoglobin saturation in children by near infra red spectroscopy and partial jugular venous occlusion. *Pediatr. Res.* 38:319–323.

59

SIMULTANEOUS ASSESSMENT OF CEREBRAL OXYGENATION AND HEMODYNAMICS DURING A MOTOR TASK

A Combined Near Infrared and Transcranial Doppler Sonography Study

Christina Hirth, Hellmuth Obrig, José Valdueza, Ulrich Dirnagl, and
Arno Villringer

Department of Neurology
Charité Humboldt-University Berlin
Schumannstr. 20/21
10098 Berlin

ABSTRACT

During performance of a sequential finger opposition task we measured changes in regional cerebral blood oxygenation (rCBO) over the motor cortex and blood flow velocity changes (CBFV) in the middle cerebral artery in a combined near-infrared spectroscopy (NIRS) and transcranial Doppler Sonography (TCD) study. Stimulus duration was 60 s followed by a 90 s rest period. During performance of the motor task we observed an increase in [oxy-Hb] a decrease in [deoxy-Hb] and an increase in MCA flow velocity. These changes were significantly more pronounced contralaterally than ipsilaterally to the moving hand. The time course of changes in [oxy-Hb] and CBFV were strikingly similar, showing a pronounced initial over-shoot.

This study proves the feasibility of a simultaneous assessment of microcirculatory hemodynamics and cerebral oxygenation at high temporal resolution.

INTRODUCTION

Near infrared spectroscopy (NIRS) is an optical method that allows continuous non-invasive assessment of intravascular and tissue oxygenation (Jöbsis 1977). The relative signal contribution of extra- and intracerebral tissue is still unclear; however, it has been shown that using this method it is possible to measure oxygenation changes corresponding to functional brain activation (Hoshi and Tamura 1993, Kato et al. 1993, Villringer et al. 1993, Obrig et al. 1996). In the present study we compared NIRS findings during functional brain activation to simultaneously performed measurements of middle cerebral artery blood flow velocity. The aims of the present study were: 1) to supply further evidence of the intracerebral origin of the NIRS signal, and 2) to establish a model for the simultaneous assessment of microcirculatory hemodynamics and regional cerebral oxygenation.

METHODS

Subjects

Experiments were performed in 13 healthy right-handed male and female volunteers, mean age 27 (range 22–45) years.

Activation Paradigm

A sequential finger opposition task was used to induce functional brain activation. The subjects were advised to alternately move the thumb of each finger as accurate and as fast as possible.

Near Infrared Spectroscopy

The method and theory of NIRS has been explained in detail elsewhere (Jöbsis 1977, Cope et al. 1988, Chance 1991). We used a NIRO 500 monitor (Hamamatsu Photonics K.K.) with four different wavelengths (775, 825, 850, 904 nm). The near infrared light emitted by a pulsed laser source was guided to the subjects head through a fibre-optic bundle called the optode. The light penetrates biological tissue and is strongly scattered. Thus, some of the reflected light can be received by a second optode placed a few centimeters apart from the light emitting optode. Photons are counted by a photomultiplier tube. Light attenuation was measured at each wavelength. Under the assumption that scattering properties do not change profoundly during the experimental period, changes in optical density can be attributed to changes in light absorption by the three chromophores oxy-Hb, deoxy-Hb and Cyt-O_2. Each of these chromophores has characteristic absorption spectra in the near infrared region. Concentration changes of oxy-Hb, deoxy-Hb and Cyt-O_2 can thus be calculated from absorption changes according to a modified Lambert Beer Law. Measurements were performed continuously with a sampling time of 1 s [Total-Hb] was calculated as a sum of [oxy-Hb] and [deoxy-Hb]. Concentration changes are expressed in arbitrary units (AU). Assuming a differential path length factor (DPF) of 5.93 (van der Zee et al. 1992) these AU would correspond to Δ µM. If true DPF is different these measurement in AU would have to be scaled accordingly in order to correspond to Δ µM. Measurements were taken with an interoptode distance of 3.5 cm. Concentration changes are believed to stem from a semicircular volume between the two optodes. Penetration depth is controversial, but it is very likely that cortical grey matter lies within the sample volume (Liu et al. 1996, Okada et al. 1995).

Transcranial Doppler Sonography

Continuous recordings of cerebral blood velocity (CBFV) of the left middle cerebral artery (MCA) were carried out with a computer-assisted transcranial ultrasound doppler device (Multidop X DWL, Sipplingen, Germany) using a 2 MHz pulsed ultrasound transducer. Left MCA was insonated transtemporally at a depth of 50 mm. After localization of optimal insonation position, the Doppler probe was secured with a head band to ensure continuous insonation without observer interaction at a relatively constant insonation angle. The envelope curve of the Fourier transformation spectra was digitally stored on the hard disk of a personal computer. CNFV was calculated from the envelope curve of the fourier spectra. To smooth systolic/diastolic fluctuations, data were low-pass filtered with a frequency of 0.7 Hz (Aaslid 1992).

Experimental Set-up and Protocol

The NIRS optodes were placed over the left hemisphere at C3 position according to the international EEG 10/20 system. According to MRI-based comparison of external landmarks and underlying brain structures, this region corresponds to the location of the motor hand area with low interindividual variation (Steinmetz et al. 1989). Measurements of cerebral blood flow velocity (CBFV) were simultaneously obtained from the left middle cerebral artery (MCA). During the whole experiment subjects lay quietly in a dimmed room with closed eyes. They were instructed not to move of speak. Regional oxygenation changes and CBFV changes were measured continuously and simultaneously throughout the whole experiment. The experimental protocol consisted of 60 s finger movement periods alternating with 90 s of rest. The motor task was performed either contralaterally (right hand) or ipsilaterally to optode position (left hand). Ten trials of each condition were performed in an alternating fashion.

Data Analysis

Data of ten cycles were averaged time-locked to movement onset for each subject and each condition. Grand average curves were obtained by averaging over all subjects with a task-related response in both methods. Individual average curves were set to zero related to 10 s baseline preceding the stimulation period and were smoothed over 5 data points with a smoothing average procedure. Mean peak values for first and second maximum during early and late phase of stimulation were calculated for each parameter using the following fixed time windows (8–13 s and 57–67 s after onset of stimulation for deoxy-Hb; 7–12 s and 55–65 s after onset of stimulation for all other parameters). All values are given as mean ± standard deviation. Comparison between mean peak values during ipsi- versus contralateral finger movement were performed using the paired Student's t-test. A different of $P< 0.05$ was considered to be statistically significant.

RESULTS

An increase in CBFV was accompanied by regional cerebral oxygenation changes in 8 out ot 13 subjects. Two subjects showed task-related changes in TCD measurements without changes in NIRS measurements. Three subjects revealed no task-related changes in either method. The 5 subjects without task-related changes in either one or both methods were excluded from further analysis. Figure 1 gives the time course of regional oxygenation changes and changes of blood flow velocity in the left MCA during ipsi- and contralateral motor stimulation as a grand average across the 8 remaining subjects. The NIRS response was characterized by an increase of [oxy-Hb] and [total-Hb] and a decrease of [deoxy-Hb]. TCB measurements elicited an increase in CBFV in the left middle cerebral artery. Both methods demonstrated a characteristic biphasic temporal profile with a short-term rapid component during the initial phase and a long-lasting component with slow continuous changes during the late phase of stimulation.

RCBO Changes during Motor Activation

As shown in Fig. 1 [oxy-Hb] demonstrated an initial overshoot (0.42 ± 0.40 AU) peaking at 9.6 ± 2.0 s after onset of stimulation[*]. Following this transient overshoot [oxy-Hb] continuously increased again to reach a second maximum of (0.67 ± 0.46 AU) a few seconds after the end of the stimulation period. A poststimulus undershoot was seen in some subjects, but was not clearly present in the grand average curve (Fig 1).

Ipsilateral response showed a very similar time course; however, signal amplitude was significantly smaller ([oxy-Hb]): 0.15 ± 0.24 and 0.34 ± 0.37, [deoxy-Hb]: -0.01 ± 0.08 and -0.05 ± 0.05; [total-Hb]: 0.15 ± 0.25 and 0.29 ± 0.35 AU).

[Deoxy-Hb] demonstrated a biphasic decrease with a rapid initial drop (-0.13 ± 0.17 AU) peaking at 13.1 ± 3.9 s after onset of stimulation and a continuous negative slope (-0.20 ± 0.15 AU) subsequently. Thereafter a poststimulus overshoot was observed. In contrast to [oxy-Hb] the biphasic response pattern was less pronounced.

[Total-Hb] had an approximately similar response pattern as [oxy-Hb] (0.30 ± 0.46 and 0.49 ± 0.47 AU).

CBFV Changes during Motor Activation

A biphasic increase in CBFV within the left MCA was also observed during performance of the motor task. A fast initial rise (contralateral 3.6 ± 2.9, ipsilateral 0.5 ± 2.3 cm/s) within 8.5 ± 1.3 s[†] after onset of stimulation was followed by a decrease to near baseline values during contralateral finger movement and below that during ipsilateral finger movement. The subsequent slow continuous increase during the late phase of stimulation was only slightly higher than the initial peak and reached its maximum (contralateral 3.9 ± 1.9 ipsilateral 1.7 ± 2.5 cm/s) after the end of the stimulation period. The response was always followed by a poststimulus undershoot.

Comparison of Regional CBO Response and CBFV Response during Motor Activation

The task-related increase of CBFV within the left MCA was paralleled by an increase in [oxy-Hb] and [total-Hb] and a reverse response in [deoxy-Hb]. The time course of CBFV matched closely the response pattern of [oxy-Hb] and [total-Hb]. Despite the similarities in response characteristics we observed noteworthy time-variant differences. The relative amplitude of the first versus the second maximum differed between the two

---

[*] Note that NIRS and TCD measurements were not precisely synchronized, hence there may be an error of approximately 1 s when comparing the two methods.
[†] Note that TCD and NIRS measurements were not precisely synchronized, hence there may be an error.

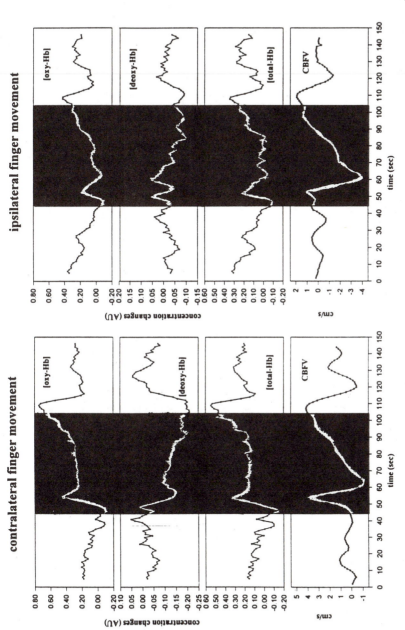

Figure 1. Grand average over 8 subjects demonstrating task-related changes in NIRS and TCD measurements during performance of sequential finger opposition task in the contralateral and ipsilateral hand. The time course is given of oxygenation changes ([oxy-Hb], [deoxy-Hb] and [total-Hb]) measured over the left hemisphere (C3 position according to international 10/20 system) and changes of CBFV within the left MCA (bottom). The dark area indicates the 60 s stimulation period. Oxygenation changes are given in AU corresponding to μmol if the assumed DPF of 5.93 is correct. Changes in [deoxy-Hb] are scaled differently to better visualize the smaller response.

modalities: For [oxy-Hb] the peak value of the initial overshoot was only approximately 2/3 of the second peak value (0.42 versus 0.67 AU). For CBFV the peak values were of similar size (3.6 versus 3.9 cm/s). Between the two peaks the signal returned to baseline for CBFV, whereas it was clearly above baseline for [oxy-Hb].

Ipsi-Contralateral Comparison

In both methods a smaller response was detected during ipsilateral finger movement than during movement of the contralateral hand. This difference was already statistically significant during the initial phase of stimulation for [oxy-Hb], [deoxy-Hb] and CBFV was more pronounced during the second half of the stimulation period. Whereas [total-Hb] changes became statistically significant different only during the late phase of stimulation (Fig 2).

DISCUSSION

In the present study oxygenation changes over the left C3 position, presumably corresponding to motor cortex, and changes of CBFV within the left middle cerebral artery during performance of 60 s finger opposition task were compared.

contralateral finger movement

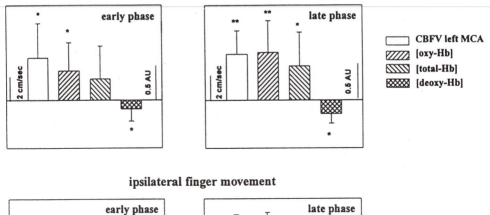

ipsilateral finger movement

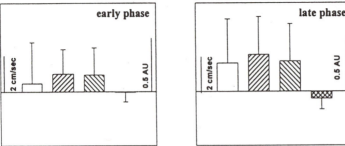

Figure 2. Mean peak values ± standard deviation (n=8) during the initial and late phase of stimulation are given for ipsi- and contralateral hand movement, respectively. Statistically significant side-to-side differences were seen for CBFV, [oxy-Hb] and [deoxy-Hb] during the initial phase of stimulation and for all measured parameters during the late phase of stimulation. * = < 0.05; ** = < 0.01.

Oxygenation Response

During performance of the motor task as we have previously described (Villringer et al. 1993, Obrig et al. 1996) the typical response consisted of an increase in [oxy-Hb] and [total-Hb] and a decrease in [deoxy-Hb]. During the 60 s stimulation period we observed an initial overshoot of these parameters which peaked after approximately 9[‡]s for [oxy-Hb] and 13 s for [deoxy-Hb]. This response was generally of higher amplitude contralaterally to the moving fingers. Hence these data indicate that NIRS measures a localized oxygenation response; however, there seems to be significant ipsilateral oxygenation changes too. Several studies have investigated the influence of extracerebral tissue to the NIRS signal. Although an exact measurement of extracerebral signal contribution has not been archived so far, it has been shown

that skin blood flow has only minor effects on the measured signal changes (Villringer et al. 1993, Smielewski et al. 1995, Kirkpatrick et al. 1995). In addition, it has been demonstrated that the portion of extracerebral contribution decreases with an increase of interoptode spacing (McCormick et al. 1992). In the present study interoptode distance was comparatively small. However, since we did not perform absolute concentration measurements, but rather measurements of changes during functional activation, signal contribution of extracerebral tissue should cancel out as long as there is no stimulus-correlated oxygenation change of extracerebral tissue. The fact that we measured a clear dominance of contralateral versus ipsilateral oxygenation changes supports the notion of an intracerebral origin of the signal. Whether the ipsilateral changes also arise from intra- rather than extracerebral sources, or whether they reflect a global extracerebral origin, we hoped to clarify somewhat by simultaneous TCD recordings.

MCA Blood Flow Velocity Response

CBFV increased during performance of the motor task. It showed an initial overshoot peaking after 8.5[‡] seconds. The response was more pronounced contralaterally but there was also clear ipsilateral response. These findings are in good agreement with TCD studies during performance of the same motor task (Sitzer et al. 1994).

Comparison of Oxygenation Response and Blood Flow Velocity Response

Both methods showed a response which was more pronounced contralaterally, but they also showed a clear ipsilateral task-related change. The time course of changes in [oxy-Hb] and [total Hb] were remarkably similar to the one of CBFV. [Deoxy-Hb] showed a reverse response and the timing of the initial overshoot seemed somewhat delayed.

The good agreement between the time course of the MCA velocity changes and NIRS parameters, as well as the contralaterally stronger response, support the intracerebral origin of the NIRS measurements. This is further supported by studies which showed correlation between PET and NIRS measurements (Hoshi et al. 1994, Villringer et al. 1994) as well as between fMRI and NIRS (Kleinschmidt et al. in press).

---

‡ Note that TCD and NIRS measurements were not precisely synchronized, hence there may be an error.

Despite the similarity in response pattern and time course we also found time-variant differences in CBFV and NIRS response. Whereas the initial peak in CBFV reaches almost the same level as the second peak, the changes in oxygenation parameters are less pronounced during the initial phase than during the late phase of stimulation. This difference is probably related to the fact that NIRS measurements reflect local oxygenation changes in a relatively small sample volume, whereas CBFV reflects hemodynamic changes in an artery supplying a much larger territory. Activation of additional brain areas during finger tapping task has been demonstrated previously by PET and fMRI studies (Kim et al. 1993, Deiber et al. 1991). It is therefore likely that hemodynamic changes in those additional brain areas cause a higher change in CBFV in the supplying MCA during the initial phase of stimulation. Another reason for a discrepancy between TCD and NIRS measurements may be a time-variant change in oxygen metabolism during ongoing stimulation, as has been suggested by Frahm et al. (Frahm et al. 1996).

Our findings are in general agreement with two recently performed TCD-NIRS studies during carotid endarterectomy and vasoreactivity testing (Kirkpatrick et al. 1995, Smielewski et al. 1995). These studies also demonstrated that rCBO changes parallel changes in CBFV during global alterations of cerebral blood flow.

In conclusion, we were able to demonstrate that changes in regional cerebral oxygenation induced by functional activation, parallel task-related changes in CBFV within the supplying intracerebral artery. The results provide evidence that NIRS measurements reflect intracerebral oxygenation changes during functional activation. The observed time-dependent quantitative differences in rCBO response and hemodynamic response in large vasculature might be explained by time-variant changes in the size of the activated territory, or changes in oxygen consumption over time.

REFERENCES

Aaslid R. Cerebral hemodynamics. In: Newell DW, Aaslid R eds. Transcranial doppler. New York, Raven Press, 49–55, 1992.

Chance B. Optical method. Annu Rev Biophys Chem 20:1–28, 1991.

Cope M, Delpy DT. System for long-term measurement of cerebral blood and tissue oxygenation on newborn infants by near infrared transillumination. Med Biol Eng Comput 26:289–294, 1988.

Deiber M-P, Passingham RE, Colebatch JG, Friston KJ, Nixon PD, Frackowiak RSJ. Cortical areas and the selection of movement: a study with positron emission tomography. Exp Brain Research 84:393–402, 1991.

Frahm J, Krüger G, Merboldt K-D, Kleinschmidt A. Dynamic uncoupling and recoupling of perfusion and oxidative metabolism during focal brain activation in man. MRM 36:143–148, 1996.

Hoshi Y, Onoe H, Watanabe Y, Anderson M, Bergstrom M, Lilja A, Langstrom B, Tamura M. Non-synchronous behavior of neuronal activity, oxidative metabolism and blood supply during mental tasks in man. Neurosci Lett 172:129–133, 1994.

Hoshi Y, Tamura M. Detection of dynamic changes in cerebral oxygenation coupled to neuronal function during metal work in man. Neurosci Lett 150:5–8, 1993.

Jöbsis FF. Noninvasive infrared monitoring of cerebral and myocardial oxygen sufficiency and circulatory parameters. Science 198:1264–1267, 1977.

Kato T, Kamei A, Takashima S, Ozaki T. Human visual cortical function during photic stimulation monitoring by means of near-infrared spectroscopy. J Cereb Blood Flow Metab 13:516–520, 1993.

Kim S-G, Ashe J, Hendrich K, Ellermann JM, Merkle H Ugurbil K, Georgopulos AP. Functional magnetic resonance imaging of motor cortex: hemispheric asymmetry and handedness. Science 261:613–617, 1993.

Lirkpatrick PJ, Smielewski P, Whitfield PC, Czosnyka M, Menon D, Pickard JD. An observational study of near-infrared spectroscopy during carotid endarterectomy. J Neurosurg 82:756–763, 1995.

Kleinschmidt A, Obrig H, Requardt M, Merboldt KD, Dirnagl U, Villringer A, Frahm J. Simultaneous recording of cerebral blood flow changes during human brain activation by magnetic resonance imaging and near infrared spectroscopy. JCBF, in press.

Liu H, Boas DA, Arjun GY, Chance B. Influence of clear cerebrospinal fluid on NIR brain imaging and cerebral oxygenation monitoring. Proceeding OSA Topical Meeting AWE3–1–33, 1996.

McCormick PW, Stewart M, Lewis G, Dujovny M, Ausman JL. Intracerebral penetration of infrared light. J Neurosurg 76: 89–97, 1992.

Obrig H, Hirth C, Junge-Hülsing J, Döge C, Wolf T, Dirnagl U, Villringer A. Cerebral oxygenation changes in response to motor stimulation. J Appl Physiol, submitted.

Okada E, Delpy DT. The effect of overlying tissue on NIR light propagation in neonatal brain. Proceedings DSA Topical Meeting AMB3–1–3–3, 1995.

Sitzer M, Knorr U, Seitz R. Cerebral hemodynamics during sensorimotor activation in humans. J Appl Physiol 77 (6):2804–2811, 1994.

Smielewski P, Kirkpatrick P, Minhas P, Pickard J, Czosnyka M. Can cerebrovascular reactivity be measured with near infrared spectroscopy? Stroke 26:2285–2292, 1995.

Steinmetz H, Fürst G, Meyer B-U. Craniocerebral topography within the international 10–20 system. Electroencephalogr Clin Neurophysiol 72:499–504, 1989.

Van der Zee P, Cope M, Arridge SR, Essenpreis M, Potter LA, Edwards AD, Wyatt JS, McCormick DC, Roth SC, Reynolds EO, et al. Experimentally measured optical pathlength for the adult head, calf and forearm and the head of the newborn infant as a function of inter optode spacing. Adv Exp Med Biol 316:143–153, 1992.

Villringer A, Planck J, Hock C, Schleinkofer L, Dirnagl U. Near infrared spectroscopy (NIRS): a new tool to study hemodynamic changes during activation of brain function in human adults. Neurosci Lett 154:101–104, 1993.

Villringer K, Villringer A, Minoshima S, Ziegler S, Herz M, Schuh-Hofer S, Obrig H, Hock C, Dirnagl U, Schwaiger M. Frontal brain activation in humans: a combined near infrared spectroscopy and positron emission tomography study. Soc Neurosci Abst 20:355, 1994.

60

LENGTH OF RESTING PERIOD BETWEEN STIMULATION CYCLES MODULATES HEMODYNAMIC RESPONSE TO A MOTOR STIMULUS

Hellmuth Obrig, Christina Hirth, Jan G. Junge-Hülsing, Claudia Döge, Rüdiger Wenzel, Tilo Wolf, Ulrich Dirnagl, and Arno Villringer

Department of Neurology
Charité, Humboldt-Universität zu Berlin
10098 Berlin-Mitte
Germany

ABSTRACT

The influence of different lengths of the pre-stimulation resting period on the magnitude of a hemodynamic response evoked by motor stimulation was examined in 10 subjects by means of near-infrared spectroscopy (NIRS). A motor stimulus was used which has been previously established as a model for functional activation studies with NIRS. Subjects performed a 20 s finger opposition task in the hand contralateral to NIRS probe localization over left sensorimotor area (C3', according to the 10–20 system). The duration of the pre-stimulation resting period was varied from 10s to 50s and response magnitude was assessed for each of the interstimulus intervals (10 s, 20 s, 30 s, 40 s and 50 s). Data analysis showed that response magnitude in oxygenated and deoxygenated haemoglobin concentration changed with different interstimulation intervals. Interestingly the greatest NIRS response was obtained with a resting period of 30 s prior to stimulation; shorter and longer resting periods resulted in smaller responses. The time course and the dependence of response magnitude on interstimulus interval differed between [oxy-Hb] and [deoxy-Hb] changes. For [oxy-Hb] the previously described fast initial increase ('overshoot') and the post-stimulation undershoot was more clearly seen with long pre-stimulation resting periods. Cytochromeoxidase oxygenation changes did not change significantly with different interstimulus intervals.

We conclude that comparisons between different functional activation studies with techniques relying on stimulus evoked changes in cerebral hemodynamics must take into account not only the quality of the experimental paradigm and the length of the stimula-

Oxygen Transport to Tissue XVIII, edited by Nemoto and LaManna
Plenum Press, New York, 1997

tion period, but also that the resting period between repetitive stimulations is important for the response amplitude and its time course.

INTRODUCTION

Near-infrared spectroscopy has been recently introduced for functional stimulation studies (Hoshi 1993, Hoshi 1994, Kato 1993, Villringer 1993, Obrig 1994c Okada 1993). The method provides information about local hemodynamic changes by monitoring concentration changes in oxygenated and deoxygenated haemoglobin ([oxy-Hb], [deoxy-Hb]). In previous studies we demonstrated that the typical response to a motor stimulus consists of an increase in [oxy-Hb] and a decrease in [deoxy-Hb]. We also showed, that different rates of task performance modulate the response elicited (Obrig 1995a). The results are shown in Figs. 1 and 2.

The present study was performed to investigate, whether the temporal protocol of the experiment is of importance for the hemodynamic response elicited, specifically whether the amplitude of the hemodynamic response is altered by the length of the preceding resting period. The question was addressed as functional hemodynamic studies (funtional MRI and PET) often use repetitive stimulations which are averaged to overcome signal-to-noise problems (Kwong 1992, Belliveau 1992, Frahm 1992, Deiber 1991, Grafton 1991). The expectation was that there might be an 'optimal' interstimulus resting period, which results in a maximal response.

The present study also reports on changes in cytochrome oxidase oxygenation, which are simultaneously assessed by NIRS. The signal-to-noise ratio is worse for this parameter than for [oxy-Hb] and [deoxy-Hb] changes. Also the exact physiological meaning of the changes is less well understood. The reason to report on the results is that results showed distinctly different response between parameters. These differences may help to

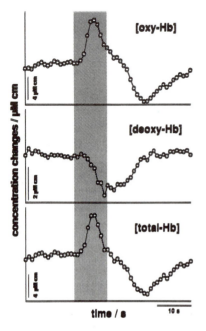

Figure 1. Grand average over 44 subjects performing a sequential motor task in the hand contralateral to probe positioning over C'3 position corresponding to sensorimotor area according to 10–20 system. Shaded area depicts the 10 s stimulation period. Changes are given in µM * cm. The scales for [oxy-Hb] and [deoxy-Hb] are different so as to better visualize the response, [deoxy-Hb] response has only one third of the magnitude of [oxy-Hb] response. Note different time course and amplitude of [oxy-Hb] and [deoxy-Hb] changes.

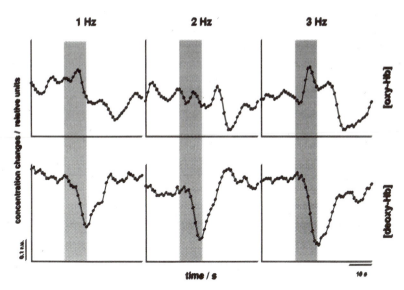

Figure 2. Average over [oxy-Hb] (upper row) and [deoxy-Hb] (lower row) response in all 12 subjects who performed the finger opposition task at different performance rates (1, 2 and 3 Hz corresponding to 1st, 2nd and 3rd column). Data were smoothed by a gliding average procedure over 4 seconds. Contralateral response at 3 Hz performance rate was normalized to 1 relative unit in each subject and parameter before averaging procedure (see fig. 1) hence response magnitude cannot be compared between parameters. Note the increase in amplitude with increasing performance rate.

differentiate the putative measure of tissue oxygenation from a vascular hemodynamic response.

METHODS

We used a NIRO-500 monitor to assess changes in cerebral oxygenation. The method, explained elsewhere in detail (Cope 1988), relies on the relative transparence of brain tissue for near-infrared light (700–1100). As haemoglobin and cytochromeoxidase are the principal biological absorbers in this spectral region, concentration changes can be calculated from changes in optical densities on the basis of a modified Beer's law. Technically, the light produced by a pulsed laser at four wavelengths (775, 825, 850 and 904 nm; pulse rate: 1.9 kHz/λ) is guided to the subject's head by a fibre optic bundle, a so-called optode. As the light is strongly scattered, part of the reflected light can be collected by a second optode fixed some centimeters apart from the light emitting probe. If scattering properties of the tissue are assumed to remain constant, changes in light attenuation can be ascribed to changes in absorbtion in a banana-like shaped volume connecting the two probes. Concentration changes in oxygenated, deoxygenated and total haemoglobin (Δ[oxy-Hb], Δ[deoxy-Hb] and Δ[total-Hb] = Δ[oxy-Hb] + Δ[deoxy-Hb]) as well as changes in redox state of cytochrome oxidase (Δ[Cyt-O$_2$]) are calculated according to an algorithm described by Cope and Delpy (Cope 1988, Delpy 1988).

We used an interoptode distance of 3.5 cm resulting in an acceptable signal-to-noise ratio over the hairy skull and still resulting in a sampling volume within cortical tissue according to theoretical considerations (van der Zee 1990, van der Zee 1992) and previous experimental results using the same setup (Obrig 1994c). Optodes were positioned over the left hemisphere, embracing C3' postion of the international 10–20 system, which corresponds to hand representation on the precentral gyrus with a 1 cm intersubject variability (Steinmetz 1989, Homan 1987). If no changes could be elicited during the first few stimulation cycles, optodes were repositioned until a stimulus associated decrease in [deoxy-Hb] or a clear increase in [oxy-Hb] could be seen. This procedure never required placement of the optodes more than approximately one centimeter away from C3'.

Subjects lay in a quiet, dimmed room and were asked to keep their eyes closed during the whole experiment to keep distraction at a minimum. Beginning and end of each stimulation period, during which subjects were to perform a sequential finger opposition task with their right hands, was announced by the examiner.

The stimulation protocol consisted of ten cycles with a fixed temporal protocol. After a longer resting period (> 60 s) subjects underwent 6 stimulation periods lasting 20 s each. The interstimulation resting periods were varied from 10 to 50 seconds (see fig. 3). Cycles contaminated by major movement artifacts or inconsistent with the exact temporal protocol were discarded as a whole and excluded from further analysis. The rate of the finger opposition was not externally controlled, but subjects were asked to perform the task as quickly and accurately as possible. This resulted in a opposition frequency of about 3 Hz. All subjects had no history of neurologic disease, gave informed consent, and were paid for their participation.

DATA ANALYSIS

Data were averaged over all ten cycles time-locked to first movement-onset in each subject. These individual averages served as a basis for further analyses. For a grand average (fig. 4) the 10 seconds preceding the first stimulation period were set to zero in the individual averages were normalized to 1 relative unit (difference between minimal and maximal value in each subject) and smoothed by a gliding average over 5 data points. To find out whether the changes in response amplitude seen in the grand average were statistically significant, MANOVAS for repeated measures with polynomial contrasts were performed. For this analysis response magnitude was assessed for each subject and each pre-stimulation resting period by calculating the difference between the minimal value during the 10 s preceding stimulus onset and the maximum during the stimulation. For [deoxy-Hb] which shows a stimulus-associated decrease difference between pre-stimulus maximum and minimal value during the stimulation period was assessed (see fig. 4). As the first stimulation period was preceded by different lengths of resting period (at least 60 s but in some cyles slightly longer) the analysis only relied on the 5 different interstimulus intervals ranging from 10 s to 50 s. In a single factorial model the influence of the interstimulus interval was tested in each parameter (see Table 1a), a two factorial model was

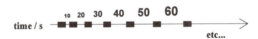

Figure 3. Stimulation protocol of 1 cycle. The interstimulation resting period between the 20 s stimulation periods was modulated from 10 s to 50 s. Black boxes denote stimulation periods. Each subject performed 10 cycles.

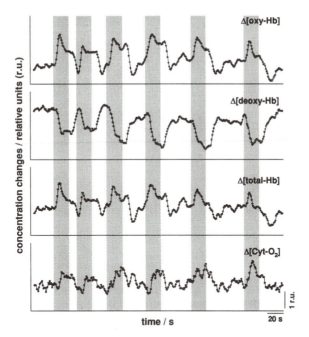

Figure 4. Grand average over all 10 subjects, showing the influence of different prestimulation resting periods on the magnitude of the NIRS response. The ten seconds prior to the first stimulation period were set to zero in each individual average, then individual averages were normalized to 1 relative unit for each parameter (difference of minimal and maximal value) and finally smoothed by a gliding average over 5 data points. A comparison of amplitudes is not valid between parameters due to nomalization; in absolute measures [deoxy-Hb] changes reach about a third of the magnitude of [oxy-Hb] changes.

Figure 5. Response magnitude for the different parameters as a function of prestimulation period length. The lighter shaded areas show means and standarddeviation for responses elicited after 10s, 20s, 30s, 40s and 50s. The darker bars show response magnitude of the first stimulation in each cycle preceded by a resting period of 60 and more seconds. For statistical analysis only the values of 10–50s prestimulation period were used. Comparison between parameters is not valid as data were normalized to 1 relative unit prior to averaging procedure (comp. Fig. 4)

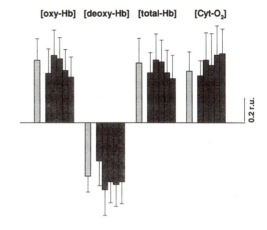

Table 1a. Influence of the interstimulus interval in a single factorial model

parameter	[oxy-Hb]	[deoxy-Hb]	[total-Hb]	[Cyt-O2]
F-value	2.71	4.03	2.27	1.95
significance	*0.032	**0.004	$0.063	n.s.

Table 1b. Influence of the interstimulus interval in a two factorial model

factors	P(parameter)	T(time)		PxT
F-value	0	3.76	2.52	
significance	n.s.	**0.006	*0.043	

used to find out whether the influence of interstimulus interval was different between the respective parameters (Table 1b).

RESULTS

Figure 4 shows the grand average across all subjects. The nature of the NIRS response confirms previously reported results with the same stimulation paradigm (Obrig 1994a, Obrig 1994b, Kleinschmidt 1995). The response consists of a stimulus associated increase in [oxy-Hb] and a decrease in [deoxy-Hb]. As data were normalized the greater response amplitude in [oxy-Hb] is reflected but by the changes in [total-Hb] which also increases during the stimulation. Oxygenation of cytochrome oxidase, a putative measure for tissue oxygenation, increases with a greater latency than the hyperoxygenation in the vascular compartment reflected by [oxy-Hb] increase and [deoxy-Hb] decrease.

Magnitude and time course of the response is altered by the different interstimulation intervals. The greatest response of [oxy-Hb] is seen with a preceding resting period of 30 s; for [deoxy-Hb] responses after 20 s and 30 s of rest are greatest. Interestingly response magnitude does not monotonously increase with greater interstimulation intervals, on the contrary, with resting periods longer than 30 s response magnitude decreases. The [oxy-Hb] response shows yet another feature. The time course differs from the [deoxy-Hb] response in that there is an initial fast overshoot and a post-stimulus undershoot. These specific features of the [oxy-Hb] response are much more pronounced with longer prestimulation resting-periods (compare response after 10 s (2nd shaded area) with the one after 50 s of rest (shaded area to the very right of figure 4)). [total-Hb] changes much resemble the [oxy-Hb] stressing that [deoxy-Hb] changes contribute much less to blood volume changes during the stimulation. For changes in cytochrome oxidase oxygenation response seems to increase with length of the pre-stimulation period. Response after 50s of rest is greatest, the response at the beginning of the cycle following at least 60 s of rest is, however, smaller than expected assuming a simple correlation.

Statistical analysis was performed to test two hypotheses. Firstly a single factorial MANOVA was used to test whether changes in response magnitude depending on the length of pre-stimulation resting period reached statistical significance. Table 1a gives the results of the analysis for each parameter. [oxy-Hb] and [deoxy-Hb] changes were significantly influenced by interstimulus interval. For [total-Hb] only a trend (p = 0.06) was seen and changes of [Cyt-O2] response seen in the grand average did not reach statistical significance. In a two-factorial model it was then tested, whether the changes in response magnitude differed between the two parameters, in which they had proven significant ([oxy-Hb] and [deoxy-Hb]). The analysis showed that [oxy-Hb] and [deoxy-Hb] respond differently to respective prestimulus resting period lengths (see crosscorrelation between 'T' (time) and 'P' (parameter)).

DISCUSSION

The present study demonstrates that

1. the length of the pre-stimulation resting period is of relevance for the magnitude and the time course of the hemodynamic response elicited by a motor stimulus.
2. an interstimulation interval of 30–40 s results in a maximal response of the vascular hemodynamic parameters ([oxy-Hb] and [deoxy-Hb]).
3. changes in [Cyt-O2], a putative measure of tissue oxygenation, differ in time course and modulatability from the parameters reflecting the vascular response.

In a previous study we have shown that the typical NIRS response to a motor stimulus consists of an increase in [oxy-Hb] and a decrease in [deoxy-Hb] during the stimulation period. This response is lateralized and localized. Our current understanding of the physiological relevance of this response is that the local hyperoxygenation is evidence of the tight coupling between cerebral hemodynamics and the underlying cortical neuronal activation. This understanding relates well to findings elicited by other functional techniques monitoring stimulus evoked changes in local cerebral hemodynamics. The comparison with functional magnetic resonance imaging (fMRI) (Kleinschmidt 1995, Obrig 1994a) has shown that the decreases in [deoxy-Hb] as monitored by NIRS corresponds well to the localized signal intensity increases using a blood oxygenation sensitive T2* fMRI technique. The result of the present study is, hence, of importance for many functional studies relying on regional hemodynamic changes to monitor cortical activity.

Changes in response by small alterations in a stimulation protocol have been reported for the motor stimulus used in the present study. In a fMRI study it was shown that response differs between paced and self-paced movements (Rao 1993). Also increases in response magnitude with higher performance rates have been reported for fMRI (Schlaug 1995) and NIRS (Obrig 1995) using the present motor stimulus. The fundamental difference from the response modulation reported here, is that for the present protocol the stimulus itself was not altered. Therefore, it is unlikely that an increase in response magnitude is caused either by the activation of additional cortical areas or by a different 'degree' of activation of the same cortical area. Rather, the differences between responses are to be explained by differences of the hemodynamic response itself.

Based on the concept of coupling (Villringer 1995, Fox 1986) between neuronal activation and hemodynamic response a different hemodynamic response to the same neuronal activation may be explained by the influence of two factors:

a. Baseline hemodynamics; i.e. hemodynamics during the resting period depend on its length.
b. Stimulation hemodynamics; i.e.stimulation induced hemodynamic changes in a cortical area depend on whether and at what latency the area has been stimulated before.

ad (a): As seen in figure 1 [oxy-Hb] and [deoxy-Hb] take some time after stimulus cessation to regain baseline values. As interstimulation intervals become smaller the prestimulation baseline may in fact rather reflect a post-stimulus hemodynamic change resulting in a local oxygenation different from that in previously unstimulated areas. The results of the present experiment did not demonstrate a major rise or fall of baseline oxygenation due to repetitive stimulation at short interstimulus intervals. An experiment more apt to answer this question will comprise a protocol with many cycles of stimulation repeated at a very short interval (10 s). Based on an experiment using fMRI of a visual stimulus it has been reported that there is an attenuation of event-related increase in signal intensity following azetazolamide administration (Bruhn 1994). Azetazolamide reduces basal cerebral vascular tone, thus increasing basal oxygen supply in all cortical areas. As localized neuronal activation results in a smaller response under this condition the response monitored may be seen as the difference between a basal oxygen supply subject to *modulation* and a level of local hyperoxygenation *required* by the task specific activation of neuronal cells. In order to solve this issue, quantification of the changes in oxygenation is necessary. In fact new NIRS techniques (time-resolved measurements, whole spectrum approaches) (Sevick 1991, Chance 1988, Matcher 1994) are able to provide quantitative values and may thus address this question on the mechanism of neurovascular coupling.

ad (b): A second factor to influence response magnitude in the present experiment is the time course of the hemodynamic response during the stimulation period itself. We have seen that during stimulation [oxy-Hb] and [deoxy-Hb] changes differ in time course (see Fig 4). A specific feature of the [oxy-Hb] response is a fast initial increase which yields in a lower plateau during later phases of the stimulation. This fast initial 'overshoot' during the stimulation period corresponds well to findings elicited by transcranial doppler sonography (TCD)(Sitzer 1989). The initial overshoot seen in TCD measurements is not lateralized and has been suggested to reflect a general arousal reaction. NIRS experiments (Obrig 1995) have shown that NIRS response reflects a rather localized change in oxygenation as seen in fMRI studies, but also the initially more generalized response as monitored by TCD in the large vasculature (Hirth 1995). The present experiment showed that the initial 'overshoot' in [oxy-Hb] measurements became more prominent with longer interstimulation intervals. Hence alterations of a more generalized less localized hemodynamic response in response to a functional stimulation may account for some of the modulatory effects of different interstimulation intervals. To address this issue a better spatial resolution of NIRS measurements is needed. Multichannel and NIRS imaging techniques have been proposed (Hoshi 1993, Benaron 1995, Shinohara 1993).

We conclude that the finding of a dependence of hemodynamic response magnitude depending on the length of the pre-stimulation period calls for further studies to understand its physiological basis, and may be of importance for functional techniques relying on the neuro-hemodynamic coupling.

As mentioned in the introduction, in this study we report on cytochrome-oxidase changes during motor stimulation. The questions concerning the spectral validity of the signal and even less those concerning the oxygenation behaviour during physiological neuronal activity cannot be answered by the present approach. Nonetheless, we believe it noteworthy that this parameter does not only show different temporal kinetics during the stimulation period but also differs as to its modulation in response to different temporal protocols. This finding makes a simple spillover of the haemoglobin signal unlikely and may reflect the generally different tissue oxygenation changes in response to functional neuronal activation.

REFERENCES

1. Belliveau, J. W., K. K. Kwong, D. N. Kennedy, J. R. Baker, C. E. Stern, R. Benson, D. A. Chesler, R. M. Weisskoff, M. S. Cohen, R. B. Tootell, and et al. Magnetic resonance imaging mapping of brain function. Human visual cortex. Invest. Radiol. 27 Suppl 2: S59-S65, 1992.
2. Benaron,D.A., W.F. Cheong, E.L. Kermit, D.K. Stevenson, A. Scwettman. Early results of Bedside Imaging of Brain Structure and Function Using Time-Resolved Tomographic Optical Scanning. ISOTT 1995 Book of abstracts (XII) 90, 1995.
3. Bruhn, H., A. Kleinschmidt, Boecker H., Merboldt K.D., Hänicke W., Frahm, J.. The effect of Acetazolamide on regional cerebral bloood oxygenation at rest and under stimulation as assessed by MRI. J Cereb Blood Flow Metab 14:742–8 1994.
4. Chance, B. , J. S. Leigh, H. Miyake, D. S. Smith, S. Nioka, R. Greenfeld, M. Finander, K. Kaufmann, W. Levy, M. Young, and et al. Comparison of time-resolved and -unresolved measurements of deoxyhemoglobin in brain. Proc. Natl. Acad. Sci. U. S. A. 85: 4971–4975, 1988.
5. Cope, M. and D. T. Delpy. System for long-term measurement of cerebral blood and tissue oxygenation on newborn infants by near infra-red transillumination. Med. Biol. Eng. Comput. 26: 289–294, 1988.
6. Deiber, M. P., R. E. Passingham, J. G. Colebatch, K. J. Friston, P. D. Nixon, and R. S. Frackowiak. Cortical areas and the selection of movement: a study with positron emission tomography. Exp. Brain Res. 84: 393–402, 1991.
7. Delpy, D. T., M. Cope, P. van der Zee, S. Arridge, S. Wray, and J. Wyatt. Estimation of optical pathlength through tissue from direct time of flight measurement. Phys. Med. Biol. 33: 1433–1442, 1988.
8. Fox, P. T. and M. E. Raichle. Focal physiological uncoupling of cerebral blood flow and oxidative metabolism during somatosensory stimulation in human subjects. Proc. Natl. Acad. Sci. U. S. A. 83: 1140–1144, 1986.
9. Frahm, J., h. Bruhn, K.D. Merboldt, W. Hänicke. Dynamic MR imaging of human brain oxygenation during rest and photic stimulation. J. Magn. Reson Imaging 2: 501–505, 1992.
10. Grafton, S. T., R. P. Woods, and J. C. Mazziotta. Within-arm somatotopy in human motor areas determined by positron emission tomography imaging of cerebral blood flow. Exp. Brain Res. 95: 172–176, 1993.
11. Grafton, S. T., R. P. Woods, J. C. Mazziotta, and M. E. Phelps. Somatotopic mapping of the primary motor cortex in humans: activation studies with cerebral blood flow and positron emission tomography. J. Neurophysiol. 66: 735–743, 1991.
12. Hirth C., H. Obrig , J.G. Junge-Hülsing, U. Weiner, C. Döge,U. Dirnagl, A. Villringer. ISOTT 1995 Book of abstracts XII, 92. 1995
13. Homan, R. W., J. Herman, and P. Purdy. Cerebral location of international 10–20 system electrode placement. Electroencephalogr. Clin. Neurophysiol. 66: 376–382, 1987.
14. Hoshi, Y. and M. Tamura. Dynamic multichannel near-infrared optical imaging of human brain activity. J. Appl. Physiol. 75: 1842–1846, 1993.
15. Hoshi, Y. , H. Onoe, Y. Watanabe, J. Andersson, M. Bergstrom, A. Lilja, B. Langstrom, and M. Tamura. Non-synchronous behavior of neuronal activity, oxidative metabolism and blood supply during mental tasks in man. Neurosci. Lett. 172: 129–133, 1994.
16. Kato, T. , A. Kamei, S. Takashima, and T. Ozaki. Human visual cortical function during photic stimulation monitoring by means of near-infrared spectroscopy. J. Cereb. Blood Flow Metab. 13: 516–520, 1993.
17. Kim, S. G., J. Ashe, K. Hendrich, J. M. Ellermann, H. Merkle, K. Ugurbil, and A. P. Georgopoulos. Functional magnetic resonance imaging of motor cortex: hemispheric asymmetry and handedness. Science 261: 615–617, 1993.
18. Kleinschmidt, A., H. Obrig, M. Requardt, K. D. Merboldt, U. Dirnagl, A. Villringer, J. Frahm. Simultaneous recording of cerebral blood oxygenation changes during human brain activation by magnetic resonance imaging and near-infrared spectroscopy. J. Cereb. Blood Flow Metab. 1995 in press.
19. Kwong, K. K., J. W. Belliveau, D. A. Chesler, I. E. Goldberg, R. M. Weisskoff, B. P. Poncelet, D. N. Kennedy, B. E. Hoppel, M. S. Cohen, R. Turner, T. Brady, B.R. Rosen. Dynamic magnetic resonance imaging of human brain activity during primary sensory stimulation. Proc. Natl. Acad. Sci. U. S. A. 89: 5675–5679, 1992.

20. Matcher, S. J., C. E. Cooper. Absolute quantification of deoxyhaemoglobin concentration in tissue near infrared spectroscopy. Phys. Med. Biol. 39: 1295–1312, 1994.

21. Obrig, H., A. Kleinschmidt , K.D. Merboldt, U. Dirnagl, J. Frahm, A. Villringer. Monitoring Cerebral Blood Oxgenation by Simultaneous High-Resolution MRI and Near-Infrared Spectroscopy. (1994a) Society of Magnetic Resonance, 2nd Meeting Book of Abstracts 67

22. Obrig, H., S. Brandt, B.U. Meyer, U. Dirnagl, A. Villringer. Vibratory, motor and transcranial magnetic stimulation in humans produce a localized change in cerebral oxygenation demonstrated with near-infrared spectroscopy. Society for Neuroscience (1994b) abstract.

23. Obrig, H., T Wolf, C. Döge, J. G. Junge Hülsing, U. Dirnagl, A. Villringer. Cerebral Oxygenation Changes during Motor and Somatosensory Stimulation in Humans, as measured by Near-Infrared Spectroscopy. (1994c) Oxygen Transport to Tissue XVII (Ince C, et al eds) Plenum Press NY (in press)

24. Obrig H., C. Hirth, J.G. Junge-Hülsing, C. Döge, T. Wolf, U. Dirnagl, A. Villringer. Cerbral oxygenation changes in response to motor stimulation. J Appl Physiol (submitted) 1995.

25. Okada, F. , Y. Tokumitsu, Y. Hoshi, and M. Tamura. Gender- and handedness-related differences of forebrain oxygenation and hemodynamics. Brain Res. 601: 337–342, 1993.

26. Rao, S. M., J. R. Binder, P.A. Bandettini, T.A. Hammeke, F.Z. Yetkin, A. Jesmanovicz, L. M. Lisk, G. L. Morris, W. M. Mueller, L. D. Estkowski, E. C. Wong, V. M. Haughton, J. S. Hyde. Functional magnetic resonance imaging of complex human movements. Neurology 43: 2311–2318, 1993.

27. Schlaug, G., J.N. Sanes, R.J. Seitz, V. Thangaraj, U. Knorr, D. Darby, H. Herzog, R.R. Edelman, S. Warach. Pattern and magnitude of cerebral blood flow changes are determined by movement rate. 'Brain Mapping ' Book of abstracts 1995.

28. Sevick, E. M., B. Chance, J. Leigh, S. Nioka, and M. Maris. Quantitation of time- and frequency-resolved optical spectra for the determination of tissue oxygenation. Anal. Biochem. 195: 330–351, 1991.

29. Shinohara, Y. , S. Takagi, N. Shinohara, F. Kawaguchi, Y. Itoh, Y. Yamashita, and A. Maki. Optical CT imaging of hemoglobin oxygen-saturation using dual-wavelength time gate technique. Adv. Exp. Med. Biol. 333: 43–46, 1993.

30. Sitzer, M. , U. Knorr, and R. J. Seitz. Cerebral hemodynamics during sensorimotor activation in humans. J. Appl. Physiol. 77: 2804–2811, 1994. Steinmetz, H. , G. Furst, and B. U. Meyer. Craniocerebral topography within the international 10–20 system. Electroencephalogr. Clin. Neurophysiol. 72: 499–506, 1989.

31. Steinmetz, H. , G. Furst, and B. U. Meyer. Craniocerebral topography within the international 10–20 system. Electroencephalogr. Clin. Neurophysiol. 72: 499–506, 1989.

32. van der Zee, P. , M. Cope, S. R. Arridge, M. Essenpreis, L. A. Potter, A. D. Edwards, J. S. Wyatt, D. C. McCormick, S. C. Roth, E. O. Reynolds, and et al. Experimentally measured optical pathlengths for the adult head, calf and forearm and the head of the newborn infant as a function of inter optode spacing. Adv. Exp. Med. Biol. 316: 143–153, 1992.

33. van der Zee, P. , S. R. Arridge, M. Cope, and D. T. Delpy. The effect of optode positioning on optical pathlength in near infrared spectroscopy of brain. Adv. Exp. Med. Biol. 277: 79–84, 1990.

34. Villringer, A. , J. Planck, C. Hock, L. Schleinkofer, and U. Dirnagl. Near infrared spectroscopy (NIRS): a new tool to study hemodynamic changes during activation of brain function in human adults. Neurosci. Lett. 154: 101–104, 1993.

35. Villringer, A., U. Dirnagl. Coupling of brain activity and cerebral blood flow - basis of functional neuroimaging. Cerebrovasc. Brain Metab. Rev. in press.

61

APPLICATIONS OF NIRS FOR MEASUREMENTS OF TISSUE OXYGENATION AND HAEMODYNAMICS DURING SURGERY

M. S. Thorniley,[1] S. Simpkin,[1] N. J. Barnett,[2] P. Wall,[2] K. S. Khaw,[3] C. Shurey,[1] J. S. Sinclair,[4] and C. J. Green[1]

[1]Department of Surgical Research
Northwick Park Institute for Medical Research
Northwick Park Hospital
Harrow, Middlesex, HA1, 3UJ
[2]Johnson and Johnson Medical
European Product Development Centre
Newport, Gwent, NP1 9UH
[3]Department of Anaesthetics and Plastic Surgery
Mount Vernon Hospital
Northwood, HA62RN
[4]Blond McIndoe Centre
Queen Victoria Hospital
East Grinstead, West Sussex, RH19 3DZ
United Kingdom

1. INTRODUCTION

Since 1977 when Jobsis described the first use of near infra-red spectroscopy (NIRS) for non-invasive monitoring of changes in cerebral oxyhaemoglobin (O_2Hb), deoxyhaemoglobin (HHb) and Caa_3 the field has undergone major transformations[1,2].

These have not only involved great improvements in instrumentation but also in the diversity of applications. The instruments have decreased dramatically in size from the early prototype versions[3] to more portable compact monitors[4]. Most instruments have had major advancements in hard and software which have generally led to an improved ease of use. Applications of NIRS are predominately for cerebral monitoring in particular in perinatology[5,6], although other measurements have been made during cardiac surgery[7,8] and hepatic transplantation[9]. However, several groups of researchers have realised that any tissue (organ) containing haemoglobin/myoglobin and which is at risk of hypoxia (ischaemia) would benefit from NIR monitoring[10–12]. The ability to measure changes in oxygenation and perfusion during harvesting and following transplantation or transfer of

Oxygen Transport to Tissue XVIII, edited by Nemoto and LaManna
Plenum Press, New York, 1997

free and pedicled flaps is potentially important in reconstructive surgery[13]. Rapid detection of a critical change in haemoglobin oxygen saturation could enable earlier and more successful intervention. For example, it would be beneficial if the onset and magnitude of the damaging effect of venous ischaemia could be detected and hence reduced[14].

It has been shown in a rabbit hind limb model that NIRS can detect and distinguish between various types of vascular compromise including arterial, venous or total obstruction (the latter most damaging post surgery)[11]. In addition to measuring haemodynamic variations, NIRS measures the oxidised form of Caa_3, the terminal enzyme of the respiratory chain. Changes in the redox state of Caa_3 are a function of pO_2, dependent upon oxygen delivery, and electron flow through the respiratory chain. The relative oxidation-reduction states of the individual respiratory chain components in mitochondrial extracts have been elegantly described by Chance and Williams, 1955[15]. In essence, in the *in vitro* situation with a low pO_2, Caa_3 is reduced and with a high pO_2 is oxidised, providing there is no limitation of electron flow via the respiratory chain.

Hence, if oxygen delivery is unlimited the redox state of Caa_3 can be altered by electron flow. For example, if the respiratory chain is damaged, then Caa_3 can become oxidised. This has been found to occur in several *in vivo* situations in which ischaemia followed by reperfusion resulted in damage to the respiratory chain[16,17]. The latter was assessed by *in vitro* measurements of the respiratory control indices and the activities of the individual respiratory chain complexes[16,17]; complex I of the respiratory chain has been found to be particularly sensitive to ischaemia reperfusion damage and these findings were correlated with non-invasive *in vivo* measurements of oxidation of Caa_3 as measured by NIRS[10,18–20].

Surgical procedures can invariably lead to some degree of vascular compromise and major surgery is frequently accompanied by haemorrhage. Even in the most well controlled of situations, systemic shock can arise; this results in poor perfusion, low tissue pO_2 and metabolic dysfunction.

The overall aim of these investigations was to test the ability of NIRS to detect disturbances in the vascular supply and metabolic state for application to the surgical situation.

In order to achieve our aim, models of 1) major surgery (hepatic transplant); 2) reconstructive surgery (myocutaneous flap); 3) haemorrhage; and 4) metabolic dysfunction (respiratory chain inhibitor) were developed.

1.1. Experimental Models

1.1.1. Model 1: Major Surgery-Hepatic Transplantation. We considered that if cerebral haemodynamics are compromised during transplantation and if this is exacerbated in animals following transplantation of livers which have been stored for long periods then NIRS should be able to detect differences in cerebral oxygenation and haemodynamics between minimally stored and longer preserved grafts. Cerebral measurements were made on 2 groups of rats in which the organs had been isografted either after flush with hypertonic citrate solution and minimal storage (25 min) at $1–2^0C$ (control, Group 1) or after 24 hr at $1–2^0C$ (Group 2). From our previous work in this experimental model, we would expect 100% survival in the recipients of minimally-stored livers, but only approximately 10% of the rats receiving 24 hr stored livers survive with good hepatic function[19].

1.1.2. Model 2: Reconstructive Surgery-Flap Model. We have developed a myocutaneous porcine flap model as a model for flap transfer whose design is ultimately intended for *ex-vivo* perfusion studies[4,13,21]. A flap was raised and tubed and the circulation allowed to readjust for 7–9 days. The effect of pedicle manipulations, venous, arterial and total occlusions on the flap oxygenation and haemodynamics was determined.

1.1.3. Model 3: Haemorrhage and Fluid Replacement. A rat model of haemorrhagic hypotension was developed in which NIRS cerebral measurements were made during removal of blood (approximately 10 min between each removal: 1 or 2 ml, to a maximum of 15 ml) with and without fluid replacement (Haemaccel[R], Behring, Behringwerke AG, Marburg) of 1 ml aliquots to a maximum of 4 ml via a femoral artery cannula.

1.1.4. Model 4: Metabolic Dysfunction. The use of sodium pentobarbitone (NaP), a specific inhibitor of complex I of the respiratory chain, provides a model of metabolic dysfunction. *In vitro* studies have shown that NaP results in complex I inhibition and in Caa$_3$ oxidation. *In vivo* administration of NaP causes a well established fall in metabolic rate and cerebral blood flow (CBF)[22].

2. METHODS

2.1.1. Animal Preparation and Surgical Procedures: Model 1. Male Lewis rats (200 – 300 g) were used in model 1 and male Lewis rats weighing 400–500 g in model 3. All animal procedures were carried out according to the Animals (Scientific Procedures) Act, 1986. Surgical anaesthesia was maintained using enflurane (1–2%) with O$_2$ delivered via a face mask at 0.5 l min^{-1}. Arterial oxygen saturation was maintained at 100% throughout the procedures (Ohmeda-Biox 3470). The temperature was controlled using a heating pad and generally monitored throughout using a rectal probe. Continuous FiO$_2$, EtCO$_2$ measurements and blood pCO$_2$ and pO$_2$ determinations were made throughout.

A Zeiss OPMI-6 operating microscope was used for all microsurgical procedures. Prior to hepatic surgery, donor rats were given 1 mg vit K i.v. and recipient rats 1 mg vit K i.v., 1 ml Haemaccel[R] i.v. (via the lingual vein) and 3 ml glucose subcutaneously. The surgical procedures were performed as previously described[19]. In the hepatic transplant model, hepatic isografts were perfused with hypertonic citrate solution with storage (1–2°C) for 25 min (Group 1, n=9) and 24 hr (Group 2, n=6).

2.1.2. Model 2. A tubed myocutaneous flap was then raised using the rectus abdominus muscle on its vascular pedicle in 9 female large White pigs (25–30 kg) and the flap circulation was allowed to adjust for 7–9 days[4,13,21]. The pigs were sedated with i.m, ketamine:xylazine (5:1 mg kg^{-1} body weight). Anaesthesia was induced with 2–4% halothane via an endotracheal tube and repirator. Arterial oxygen saturation was maintained at 100% throughout the procedures (Ohmeda-Biox 3470). The temperature was controlled using a heating pad and monitored throughout using a rectal probe. Continuous FiO$_2$, EtCO$_2$ measurements and blood pCO$_2$ and pO$_2$ determinations were made throughout.

2.1.3. Model 3. In this group male Lewis rats weighing 400–500 g were used. The femoral artery was cannulated and a portex catheter (flushed with heparinised saline 1000 U/50 ml) was used to facilitate either removal of blood, or fluid administration. NIRS cerebral measurements were made during removal of blood (n=10) (approximately 10 min between each removal: 1 or 2 ml, to a maximum of 15 ml) with and without fluid replacement Haemaccel[R] in 1 ml aliquots to a maximum of 4 ml.

2.1.4. Model 4. The femoral artery was cannulated and a portex catheter (flushed with heparinised saline 1000 U/50 ml) was used to facilitate pentobarbitone administration. NIRS measurements were made continuously following 3 mg additions (up to 36 mg) of a 60 mg ml⁻¹ pentobarbitone solution (n=6 rats). Termination was induced by sodium pentobarbitone infusion (60 mg).

2.2. NIRS Protocol

A CRITIKON* (* = Trademark) Cerebral Redox Research Model 2001 (Johnson & Johnson Medical, UK), NIRS instrument was used. A sensor with a 3.5 cm separation between emitter and detector was placed on the rat head. Following a 10 min period of stable baseline the abdomen was opened and the surgical procedures were performed as described. NIRS measurements were made for 10 min pre-laparotomy (baseline), during the harvesting of the recipient animal's liver, and throughout the transplantation procedure in model 1. NIRS measurements were made from induction of anaesthesia to termination in models 3 and 4.

In the flap model the same sensor was used. Flap measurements were made for 10 min (baseline) before occlusion; during the 2 min of occlusion (venous (n=12); arterial (n=9) or total (n=6) occlusions. Measurements were then continued up to 15 min post release of occlusions. Mean changes (± SEM) in NIRS parameters at the end of occlusion were determined and compared to baseline measurements.

2.2.1. NIRS Measurements and Theory. NIRS is based on Beer Lambert's Law which relates optical absorption to the concentration of light absorbing chromophores present in a measured volume of tissue. Beer Lambert's Law strictly applies only to a non-scattering medium, but the equation can be modified for measurements in scattering media such as biological tissue.

$$\text{Absorbance} = a.c.l.B. + G.$$

where a= molar extinction coefficient (mM⁻¹ cm⁻¹), c = concentration (mM), l = emitter-detection separation, cm, B = pathlength factor and G = geometry dependent factor.

It follows that by measuring changes in light absorption quantitated changes in chromophore concentration can be calculated, C = A/ c.l.B.

For a volume of tissue containing several chromophores, changes in absorption due to each component can be calculated by using multiple interrogating wavelengths applying the modified Beer Lambert's Law to each wavelength. Quantitated concentration changes for each chromophore are then calculated by solving the resulting set of simultaneous equations. The calculation of chromophore concentration uses a linear summation of absorption terms containing specific multiplication factors at each wavelength.

The CRITIKON* Cerebral Redox Research Monitor Model 2001 uses an algorithm based on published absorption spectra which have been obtained using isolated chromophores in non-scattering media. The haemoglobin and oxyhaemoglobin absorption spectra were obtained using haemolysed human blood[23]. The cytochrome difference absorption spectrum was obtained using purified cytochrome extracted from mitochondria[24]. The algorithm also incorporates wavelength dependent Differential Pathlength Factor data derived from "time of flight" studies[25].

Changes in the concentrations of O_2Hb, HHb and Caa_3 were calculated using the following table of multiplying factors:

Multiplying factors				
Wavelength (nm)	776.5	819	871.4	908.7
HHb	1.6436	-1.2510	-0.7075	0.6515
O₂Hb	-0.9384	-0.6945	0.5721	1.7344
Caa₃	-0.1398	0.9945	0.1664	-0.9715

Units: mM.cm absorption^{-1}. The calculated concentration change is expressed in μM multiplied by pathlength in cm.

Summation of changes in the concentrations of O_2Hb and HHb provides a measure of changes in the total tissue haemoglobin, (tHb), which reflect changes in tissue blood volume, hence giving an indication of perfusion. A further term, HbD or oxygenation index can be derived as: [HbD] = [O_2Hb]-[HHb]. This gives an indication of the net haemoglobin oxygenation status irrespective of any blood volume changes. This term is of great use following tissue transplantation in assessing the onset or recovery from venous congestion.

The instrument noise on the cytochrome and haemoglobin traces, measured with a sensor on a standard absorbing block and with the pathlength factor set to 1.0, is less than 0.05 and 0.5 μM respectively. A pathlength factor of 1 was used throughout.

2.3. Statistical Analysis

The mean changes in NIRS parameters at the end of the experimental period were determined and compared to baseline measurements. Data are presented as mean ± SEM. Statistical significance between groups was tested by an unpaired Student's t-test using two-way analysis of variance and were considered significant when $p < 0.05$. In the flap model, statistical significance was tested by a paired Student's t-test (considered significant if $p < 0.05$). The mean difference (± SEM) in parameters between the various types of occlusions was evaluated.

3. RESULTS

3.1. Model 1: Major Surgery-Hepatic Transplantation

The profound effects of hepatic transplantation on the cerebral haemoglobin oxygenation and perfusion level can be seen in Figs. 1 and 2. During the recipient stages of the transplantation procedures, the total haemoglobin, tHb (cerebral blood volume) decreased and the fall in the O_2Hb level was greater than the rise in the HHb level. The arrows represent the stage in the recipient phase when all the anastomoses were complete and the animal surviving on the new liver. Livers that had been stored for a minimal time (25 min) and transplanted resulted in the cerebral HHb level returning to baseline and recovery of the O_2Hb level over the 3 hours which correlates with 100% survival (Fig.1). However, isografting of livers which had been stored for 24 hr showed a continued divergence of the HHb and O_2Hb levels (Fig.2). There was no significant difference between the fall in cerebral blood volume between the two groups:-80.85±21.7 and -110.1±20.57 μM (Groups 1 and 2, respectively). However there was a highly significant difference between the cerebral haemoglobin oxygenation index HbD ([HbD]= [O_2Hb] -[HHb]), $p < 0.01$, measured in the two groups of animals after 2 hours; -97.8±20.02 and -277±40.6 μM (Groups 1 and 2, respectively). It was observed that whilst the cerebral Caa₃ remained

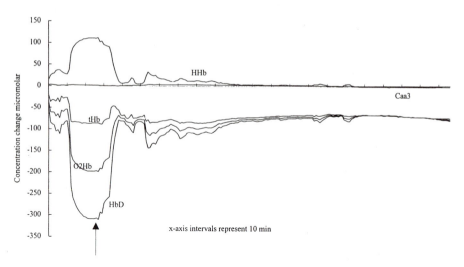

Figure 1. The effect of transplantation of a 25 min stored liver on cerebral NIRS measurements.

oxidised in minimally stored (25 min) graft recipients, cerebral Caa_3 became reduced following transplantation of prolonged (24 hr) stored livers.

3.2. Model 2: Reconstructive Surgery-Flap Model

The circulation in the raised, tubed myocutaneous flap was allowed to readjust and stabilise for one week before assessment. The NIRS parameters were continuously measured as the vascular responses of the flap were tested by performing arterial, venous or total occlusions followed by release of occlusion. Each type of occlusion had a characteristic response and the changes were highly significant compared to baseline. Venous occlusions (Fig. 3) resulted in increases in tHb 0.897 ± 0.18 μM and HHb 0.57 ± 0.11

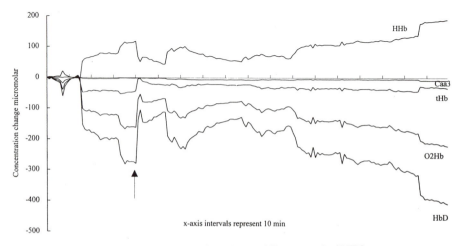

Figure 2. The effect of transplantation of a 24 hr stored liver on cerebral NIRS measurements.

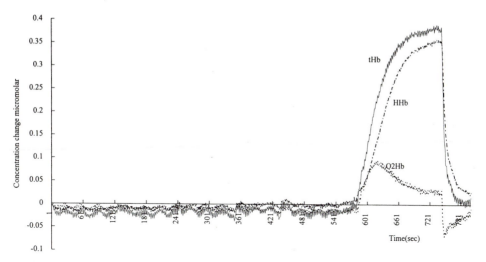

Figure 3. The effect of a venous occlusion on NIRS parameters.

µM. All arterial occlusions (Fig. 4) were characterised by decreases in tHb 0.352±0.047 µM and O₂Hb 0.41± 0.11 µM (unimpeded venous outflow). Total occlusion resulted in an increase in HHb 0.193±0.082 µM, fall in O₂Hb 0.151±0.044 µM but tHb was unchanged (Fig.5). A paired Student's t-test of the means showed that the differences between arterial and venous (p<0.01), and total and venous (p<0.02) occlusions were significant for all parameters.

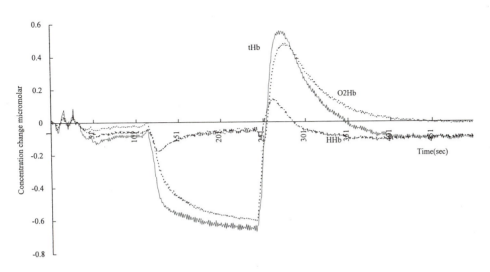

Figure 4. The effect of an arterial occlusion on NIRS parameters.

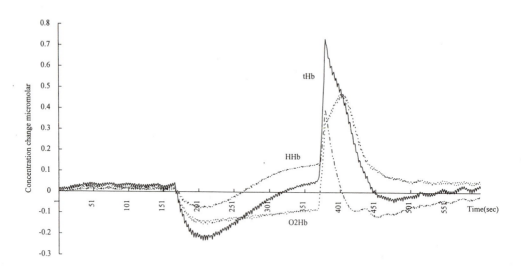

Figure 5. The effect of an arterial occlusion on NIRS parameters.

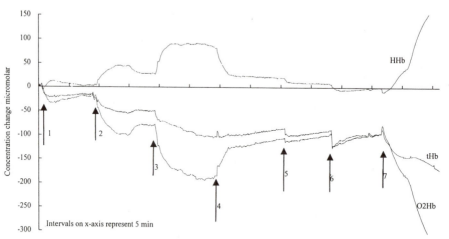

Figure 6. The arrows represent; 1. 1 ml exsanguination; 2. 1 ml exsanguination; 3. 2 ml exsanguination; 4. 1 ml Haemaccel[R]; 5. 1 ml Haemaccel[R]; 6. 2 ml Haemaccel[R]; and 8. 1 ml sodium pentobarbitone.

3.3. Model 3: Haemorrhage and Fluid Replacement

Slow withdrawal of blood (n=10 rats) resulted in a progressive fall in blood volume (tHb) and oxyhaemoglobin (O_2Hb) with an increase in deoxygenated haemoglobin (HHb)(Fig.6). Even at only 4% (1 ml) blood volume withdrawal the changes in the NIR parameters were significant compared to baseline (p<0.05). At approximately 4% blood volume depletion the total haemoglobin concentration fell by -17.71 µM; at 12% (3 ml) -70.83 µM, and at 36% withdrawal -193.33±33.4 µM (mean±SEM). As the tHb decreased the O_2Hb level fell, by -24.57, -114.0 and a maximum drop of -330.77 µM at 4, 12 and 36% blood volume depletion, respectively. Addition of 1 ml Haemaccel[R] (to a maximum of 4 ml, after 4 ml exsanguination) resulted in the level of HHb falling and a rise in the O_2Hb concentration.

3.4. Model 4: Metabolic Dysfunction

In this model we measured changes in cerebral Caa_3 and haemoglobin oxygenation induced by administration of sodium pentobarbitone. Figure 7 shows a NIRS plot of the effect of repetitive 3 mg doses of sodium pentobarbitone on rat cerebral NIRS parameters. There was an immediate oxidation of Caa_3, a fall in the oxyhaemoglobin and total haemoglobin concentration (cerebral blood volume). We found that infusion with sodium pentobarbitone (3 mg) resulted in oxidation of Caa_3 (2.98±0.89 µM), and a fall in the O_2Hb (-33.17±10.08 µM) and in the tHb (-28.83±7.91 µM) concentrations in all rats (n=6). All changes in NIRS parameters were highly significant compared to baseline and following small 3 or 6 mg doses of pentobarbitone returned to baseline after approximately 10 min. Terminal doses of pentobarbitone resulted in desaturation with a divergence of the O_2Hb (-317.7±10.91 µM), and HHb (+197.67±11.74 µM) signals, a large drop in tHb (-120.33±14.96 µM), and a biphasic response of Caa_3, an initial fast oxidation followed by a slow reduction.

4. DISCUSSION

Cerebral NIRS monitoring during hepatic transplantation showed clear changes in cerebral oxygenation and perfusion during the harvesting and recipient phases. There was a statistically significant difference in the cerebral haemoglobin oxygenation index between the two groups (p<0.01). This suggests that decreased cerebral haemoglobin oxygenation relative to utilisation is a major problem in these hepatic transplantation procedures. The lack of recovery of the cerebral NIRS parameters in animals receiving 24 hr stored livers can only be speculated. Possibilities are hepatic venous congestion resulting in systemic flow or cerebral oedema resulting in poor cerebral blood flow and perfusion.

The method of NIRS was also found to be of value in detecting and distinguishing between microcirculatory changes occurring as a result of arterial, venous or total vascular occlusion in a tubed myocutaneous flap. Venous congestion indicated by raised levels of deoxygenated haemoglobin with a concomitant increase in blood volume and the presence and magnitude of reactive hyperaemia were both easily recognisable features by NIRS. We believe that NIRS provides a sensitive and reliable post-operative monitor of tissue viability following transfer of free and pedicled flaps. As far as we are aware, this is the first usage of a NIRS instrument to assess changes in oxygenation in a flap model which closely simulates the clinical situation[13,23,24]. In the hypovolaemia model the results showed that changes in cerebral O_2Hb, HHb and tHb can be measured by NIRS even in response to only moderate blood loss. These preliminary NIRS measurements also suggest that fluid replacement improves cerebral oxygenation and the technique would be useful in assessing the benefit of fluid replacement in the Intensive Care Unit setting.

Apart from the obvious use of NIRS in measuring changes in haemoglobin oxygenation and haemodynamics, its use in assessing mitochondrial dysfunction has become more apparent. In particular since in the last few years the respiratory chain complexes have been found to be sensitive to ischaemia and reperfusion[16,17,19]. Hence it is an enormous benefit to not only make predictions about oxygen supply as well as oxygen utilisation. The administration of sodium pentobarbitone, an inhibitor of mitochondrial complex 1, results in a simultaneous oxidation of Caa_3 accompanied by a fall in the concentration of O_2Hb. The latter is a result of decreased cerebral blood volume, a function of the reduction in cerebral metabolic rate and blood flow. It was found that after administration of terminal doses of pentobarbitone, Caa_3 became initially oxidised then reduced, whilst O_2Hb concentration fell.

These findings are in agreement with the expected effect of sodium pentobarbitone, namely inhibition of NADH dehydrogenase of complex 1 of the respiratory chain[10,18,25], inhibition of Krebs cycle and glycolysis. Barbiturates are also well known to produce a parallel dose-dependent reduction in the cerebral metabolic rate and cerebral blood flow[22]; the resultant decreased electron flux and metabolic rate would be expected to lead to a greater proportion of Caa_3 becoming oxidised. A major problem in the use of non-invasive techniques is the reliance on the instrument and the associated algorithms; this has been described in detail elsewhere[26,27]. Many workers have showed that small errors in the algorithms can lead to either under or over enhancement of the Caa_3 signal. In these studies we measured divergence of the O_2Hb and Caa_3 signals under non-lethal conditions. Hypovolaemia or terminal dosing with sodium pentobarbitone resulted in both parameters decreasing in a linear manner. The results demonstrate that NIRS measurements of Caa_3 respond as expected to the well established biochemical interventions. The fact that Caa_3 became oxidised and oxyhaemoglobin decreased simultaneously suggests that NIRS is able to discriminate between the different chromophores. These findings are in agreement with others who reported that cerebral Caa_3 became reduced as determined by *in vivo* reflectance spectrophotometry when rats were subjected to either haemorrhagic or hypoxic hypotensive insult[28,29].

Many major transplantation techniques require hypotensive anaesthesia and there is a critical balance between the degree to which the blood pressure has to be lowered to facilitate raising and transplantation of the graft and the return to normotensive conditions to ensure the graft is not underperfused. In the recovery phase the circulatory state of the graft can be compromised by haemorrhage. Tissue under perfusion or shock following severe haemorrhage results in local hypoxia and metabolic dysfunction and if uncorrected can be a trigger for sepsis syndrome.

NIRS is extremely easy to use, yielding reproducible continuous results and would be of great use in the intensive care unit in assessing the aforementioned problems. This could be

---

Figure 7. A.The effect of sodium pentobarbitone upon rat cerebral O_2Hb and Caa_3 measurements. The 15 mg dose was the terminal dose. Key ▵ = Caa_3, ▢ = O_2Hb. B.The effect of sodium pentobarbitone upon rat cerebral HHb and Caa_3 measurements. 12/06/96 3:00 PM Key ▵ = Caa_3, ◊ = HHb. C.The effect of sodium pentobarbitone upon rat cerebral tHb and Caa_3 measurements. Key ▵ = Caa_3, O = tHb

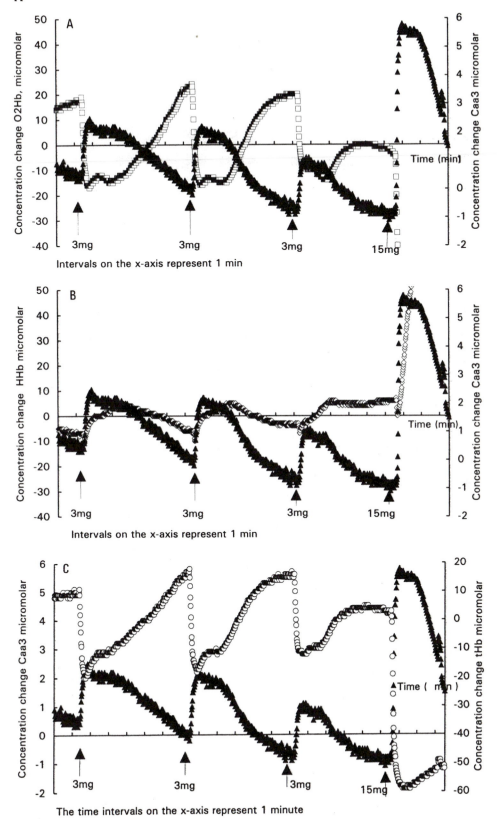

Intervals on the x-axis represent 1 min

Intervals on the x-axis represent 1 min

The time intervals on the x-axis represent 1 minute

of enormous benefit in assessing the balance between supply and utilisation of oxygen in tissues, especially in pathophysiological states such as sepsis or circulatory compromise.

5. ACKNOWLEDGMENTS

The authors would like to acknowledge the support provided by Dr IA Sammut, Ms Kate Rider and Mrs Angela Kidd and Johnson & Johnson Medical. We would like to gratefully thank Dr Caroline Dore for her invaluable statistical guidance.

6. REFERENCES

1. Jobsis F.F. (1977) Noninvasive infrared monitoring of cerebral and myocardial oxygen sufficiency and circulatory parameters *Science* **198**: 1264–1267.
2. Prough D.S. and Pollard V. (1995) Cerebral near infra-red spectroscopy; ready for prime time? *Crit Care Med* **23**: 1624–1626.
3. Cope M. and Delpy D.T. (1988) System for long-term measurement of cerebral blood and tissue oxygenation on newborn infants by near infra-red transillumination *Medical and Biological Engineering and Computing* **26**: 289–294.
4. Thorniley M.S., Sinclair S.J.& Green C.J. (1995) The use of a CRITIKON™ cerebral redox research monitor model 2001 for assessing flap viability during reconstructive surgery *Clin Sci* **89**: 32P.
5. Livera L.N., Spencer S.A., Thorniley M.S., Wickramasinghe Y.A.B.D., and Rolfe P. (1991) Effects of hypoxaemia and bradycardia on neonatal cerebral haemodynamics *Archives of Disease in Childhood* **66**: 376–380.
6. Livera L.N., Wickramasinghe Y.A.B.D., Spencer S.A., Rolfe P., and Thorniley M.S.(1992) Cyclical fluctuations in neonatal cerebral blood volume measured by near infra-red spectroscopy. *Arch Dis Childhood* **67**: 62–63.
7. du Pleiss A.J., Newburger J., Jonas R.A., Hickey P., Naruse H., Tsuji M., Walsh A., Walter G., Wypij D., and Volpe J.J (1995) Cerebral oxygen supply and utilisation during infant cardiac surgery *Ann Neurol* **37**: 488–497.
8. Levy W.J., Levin S., and Chance B. (1995) Near infra-red measurement of cerebral oxygenation:Correlation with Electroencephalographic ischaemia during ventricular fibrillation *Anaesthesiology* **83**: 738–746.
9. Thorniley M.S., Sammut i.A., Simpkin S., and Green C.J. (1995) An investigation into the effect of hepatic transplantation on cerebral oxygenation and haemodynamics *Biochem Soc Trans* **23**: 525–526.
10. Thorniley M.S., Lane N.J., Manek S., and Green C.J. (1994) Non-invasive measurement of respiratory chain dysfunction following hypothermic renal storage and transplantation *Kidney Int* **45**: 1489–1496.
11. Irwin M.S., Thorniley M.S., Dore C., and Green C.J. (1995) Near infra-red spectroscopy: a non-invasive monitor of perfusion and oxygenation within the microcirculation *British Journal of Plastic Surgery* **48**: 14–22.
12. Thorniley M.S., Lahiri A., Glenville B., Shurey C., Baker G., Ravel U., Crawley J., and Green C.J. (1995) Non invasive measurement of cardiac oxygenation and haemodynamics during transient episodes of coronary artery occlusion and reperfusion *Clin Sci* In Press
13. Thorniley M.S., Sinclair J.S., and Green C.J. (1995) The use of a CRITIKON™ cerebral redox research monitor model 2001 for assessing flap viability during reconstructive surgery *Br J Plast Surgery* (submitted)
14. Harrison D.H., Girling M., and Mott G.(1983) Methods of assessing the viability of free flap transfer during the post-operative period *Clin Plast Surg* **10**: 21–36.
15. Chance B. and Williams G.R. (1955) The respiratory chain and oxidative phosphorylation *J Biol Chem* **217**: 383–393.
16. Veitch K., Hombroeckx A., Caucheteux D., Pouleur H., and Hue L. (1992) Global ischaemia induces a biphasic response of the mitochondrial respiratory chain *Biochem J* **281**: 709–715.
17. Hardy L., Clark J.B., Darley-Usmar V.M., Smith D.R., and Stone D. (1991) Reoxygenation-dependent decrease in mitochondrial NADH: CoQ reductase (Complex I) activity in the hypoxic/reoxygenated rat heart *Biochem J* **274**: 133–137.

18. Lane N., Thorniley M.S., Manek S., Fuller B., and Green C.J. (1996) Secondary ischaemia and tissue damage in transplanted stored kidneys *Transplantation* In press

19. Thorniley M.S., Simpkin S., Fuller B., Jenabzadeh M.Z., and Green C.J. (1995) Monitoring of surface mitochondrial NADH levels as an indication of ischaemia during liver isograft transplantation *Hepatology* **21**: 1602–1609.

20. Schaefer C.F. and Biber B. (1993) Effects of endotoxaemia on the redox level of brain cytochrome a,a3 in rats *Circ shock* **40**(1): 1–8.

21. Sinclair J.S., Thorniley M.S.& Green C.J. (1994) A new tubed myocutaneous porcine flap for investigation of metabolic events following burn injury *Microsurgery* **15**: 213–214.

22. Scooper H.M. (1985) Barbiturates in brain ischaemia *Br J Anaesth* **57**: 82–951.

23. Wray S., Cope M., Delpy D.T., Wyatt J.S., and Reynolds E.O.R. (1988) Characterization of the near infrared absorption spectra of cytochrome *aa₃* and haemoglobin for the non-invasive monitoring of cerebral oxygenation *Biochimica et Biophysica Acta* **933**: 184–192.

24. Brunori M., Antonini E., and Wilson M.T. (1981) Metal Ions in Biological Systems XXIII Siegel H (Ed), Marcel Dekker, New York, pp 187–228.

25. Essenpries M., Cope M., Elwell C.E., Arridge S.R., Van Der Zee P., and Delpy D.T. (1993) Optical Imaging of Brain Function and Metabolism, Dirnagle U (Ed), Plenum Press, New York, pp 9–20.

26. Thorniley M.S., Sammut I.A., Simpkin S., and Green C.J. (1996) Non-invasive measurement of rat cerebral cytochrome oxidase using near infra-red spectroscopy: effect of pentobarbitone *Crit Care Medicine* (submitted)

27. Cope M., van der Zee P., Essenpreis M., Arridge S.R., and Delpy D.T. (1991) Data analysis methods for near infra-red spectroscopy of tissue:problems in determining the relative cytochrome aa₃ concentration SPIE 1991; **1431**: 251–261.

28. Proctor H.J., Cairns C., Fillipo D., and Jobsis-Vandervliet F.F. (1985) Near infrared spectrophotometry: potential role during increased intracranial pressure *Adv Exp Med Biol* **191**: 863–871.

29. Kariman K., Jobsis F.F., and Saltzman H.A. (1983) Cytochrome a,a3 reoxidation. Early indicator of metabolic recovery from hemorrhagic shock in rats *J Clin Invest* **72**: 180–191.

62

HOW TO EVALUATE SLOW OXYGENATION CHANGES TO ESTIMATE ABSOLUTE CEREBRAL HAEMOGLOBIN CONCENTRATION BY NEAR INFRARED SPECTROPHOTOMETRY IN NEONATES

M. Wolf, H.-U. Bucher, V. Dietz, M. Keel, K. von Siebenthal, and G. Duc

Clinic for Neonatology
University Hospital
8091 Zurich
Switzerland

1. INTRODUCTION

Brain injury is a major cause of long-term disability in newborn infants. Disturbed cerebral haemodynamics and oxygen supply may be important etiological factors, and these are currently investigated. Near infrared spectrophotometry (NIRS) in combination with pulse oxymetry is widely used to determine cerebral blood volume (CBV) in neonates. In a similar, but simpler way cerebral haemoglobin concentration (CHC), which is more relevant for cerebral oxygenation, can be obtained from the same measurements. It is better to use the CHC instead of the CBV because:

The haemoglobin content in blood does not have to be measured by drawing blood from the infant.

Furthermore we do not have to rely on a factor to convert the arterial or venous haemoglobin content into a capillary content.

We do not have to assume the haematocrit to be constant during a monitoring session.

The concentration of the oxygen carrier per tissue, the haemoglobin, is more important for the tissue oxygenation than the blood volume, because blood volume may be high, when haematocrit is low. Especially in newborn infants there is a wide variance of haemoglobin content in blood.

Under clinical conditions measurements are sometimes disturbed. The **aim** of this study was to find criteria to select valid slow oxygenation changes (SOC) measurements by optimising the test-retest variability (TRV) for two different methods to compute CHC.

Oxygen Transport to Tissue XVIII, edited by Nemoto and LaManna
Plenum Press, New York, 1997

2. THEORY

The principle of NIRS has been described extensively by Jobsis (1977), Wray (1988) and von Siebenthal (1992). NIRS measures quantitatively changes in oxygenated haemoglobin (O_2Hb in µmol/l), deoxygenated haemoglobin (HHb in µmol/l) and total haemoglobin (tHb in µmol/l) concentrations in the brain.

The measurement principle for cerebral blood volume was first described by Wyatt (1986 and 1990). A SOC is induced by altering the inspired oxygen fraction (FiO_2) of infants, who need additional oxygen. During this change the arterial oxygen saturation (SaO_2 in %) is measured by pulse oxymetry together with O_2Hb, HHb, tHb by NIRS. The SaO_2 is kept in a normal range between 85% and 95% (Figure 1).

Figure 1 shows a typical slow oxygenation change. Arterial oxygen saturation (SaO_2) and oxyhaemoglobin (O_2Hb) are decreasing and deoxyhaemoglobin (HHb) is increasing simultaneously during an alteration of FiO_2. The total haemoglobin (tHb), which corresponds to the sum of O_2Hb an HHb, remains constant.

Figure 2 shows an X-Y plot of the first 5.5 min of Figure 1. Arterial oxygen saturation (SaO_2) and oxyhaemoglobin O_2Hb correlate linearly.

The slope between O_2Hb and SaO_2 (Figure 2) is determined by a linear regression. The slope gives the amount of additional O_2Hb per % change in SaO_2. The CHC corresponds to the amount of additional O_2Hb for an extrapolated total (100%) change in SaO_2 (equation 1).

$$CHC = 100 * \frac{dO_2Hb}{dSaO_2} \left[\frac{\mu mol}{l} \right]$$

(1)

Assuming that tHb remains constant during the SOC, the HHb must react equal but opposite to the O_2Hb. Hence the signal to noise ratio can be improved by taking the oxygen index (OI) instead of O_2Hb (equation 2).

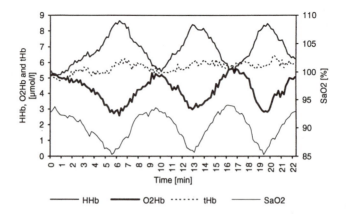

Figure 1. Typical slow oxygenation change. Arterial oxygen saturation (SaO_2) and oxyhaemoglobin (O_2Hb) are decreasing and deoxyhaemoglobin (HHb) is increasing simultaneously during an alteration of FiO_2. The total haemoglobin (tHb)), which corresponds to the sum of O_2Hb and HHb, remains constant.

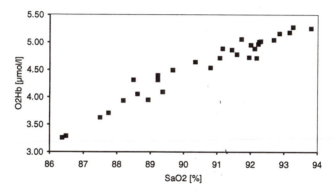

Figure 2. An X-Y plot of the first 5.5 min of Figure 1. Arterial oxygen saturation (SaO$_2$) and oxyhaemoglobin (O$_2$Hb) correlate linearly.

$$OI = \frac{O_2Hb - HHb}{2} \left[\frac{\mu mol}{l} \right]$$

(2)

The estimate of the slope can be further improved by applying two regressions, one using SaO$_2$ as x-variable and OI as y-variable and the other vice versa. Then the bisector of the angle between the two slopes is taken (equation 3). The noisier the data the further the two slopes are apart.

$$CHCr = 100 * \arctan\left(\frac{\tan\left(\frac{dOI_y}{dSaO_{2x}}\right) + \tan\left(\frac{dSaO_{2y}}{dOI_x}\right)}{2} \right) \left[\frac{\mu mol}{l} \right]$$

(3)

CHCr in equation 3 includes both improvements mentioned above. It is the first method to evaluate SOC.

CHCr is complicated to calculate. Therefore the simple method CHCm (equation 4), which just uses the minimum and maximum values of SaO$_2$ (SaO$_2$max, SaO$_2$min) and the synchronous OI values (OImax, OImin) to calculate the slope, was tested as well. CHCm can easily be estimated with a pocket calculator looking at a good graph.

$$CHCm = 100 * \frac{OI_{max} - OI_{min}}{SaO_{2max} - SaO_{2min}} \left[\frac{\mu mol}{l} \right]$$

(4)

Equations 3 and 4 are true under the following assumptions: a) The tHb remains constant during the SOC. b) The amount of oxygen consumed is constant. c) The SOC is slow enough, such that the cerebral oxygenation remains in steady state. d) There is a linear correlation between OI and SaO$_2$.

A SOC is never ideal with respect to these 4 assumptions, e.g.: the change in tHb during an SOC is never absolutely zero. What amount of change is still acceptable? To answer this question, quality criteria were defined, which quantify the change. Their influence on the TRV indicates how much change is acceptable.

3. DATA COLLECTION

3.1. Test-Retest Procedure

In clinically stable infants consecutive changes in FiO_2 produced SOC. The prerequisite for a true TRV is, that the actual CHC remains constant for all estimates during a session, which corresponds to one group of repeated measurements. This was considered to be fulfilled, if the total haemoglobin concentration (tHb) did not vary by more than ±1.5 µmol/l during a session.

3.2. Equipment

For the cerebral parameters a Critikon Cerebral RedOx Research Monitor 2001 was used. The differential pathlength factor for the quantification of the NIRS data was 4.4. Either a Hellige SMK 231 or a Nellcor N-200 pulse oxymeter measured the SaO_2 at the right hand of the infant. The data was recorded with a 0.56s sample interval.

3.3. Patients

Nine infants, who were either mechanically ventilated or had a nasal CPAP and needed additional oxygen, were included in this study. The infants had a median gestational age of 27 2/7 weeks (range: 26 1/7 weeks - 29 2/7 weeks), birthweight of 1030g (750g - 1290g) and postnatal age of 0.5 days (0 days - 8 days). 218 SOC measurements were recorded during 39 sessions. The sessions contained 3 to 12 SOC.

4. DATA PROCESSING

By averaging 18 samples the data were converted to an approximate 10s sample interval. CHCr and CHCm were calculated for all 218 SOC.

Figure 3 shows how the quality criteria were defined for the first 6 minutes of Figure 1. DUR corresponds to the duration of the slow oxygenation change. DOI refers to the change in oxygen index, DtHb to the change in total haemoglobin and $DSaO_2$ to the change of arterial oxygen saturation during that time.

4.1. Quality Criteria

As possible selection criteria the following variables were calculated for each SOC (Figure 3): The duration (DUR), the changes of SaO_2 ($DSaO_2$), tHb (DtHb), mean arterial blood pressure (DMAP), carbon dioxide (DCO_2), DtHb versus DOI (DtHb/DOI) during the SOC and the correlation coefficient (R^2, only for the regression).

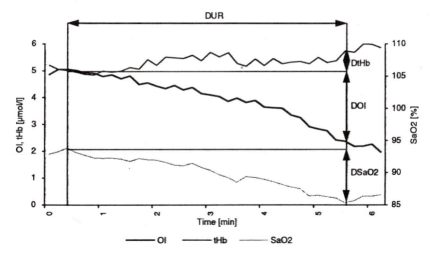

Figure 3. How the quality criteria were defined for the first 6 minutes of Figure 1. DUR corresponds to the duration of the slow oxygenation change. DOI refers to the change in oxygen index, DtHb to the change in total haemoglobin and DSaO$_2$ to the change of arterial oxygen saturation during that time.

4.2. Statistics

The CHCr and CHCm values were log-transformed to obtain homogeneity of variance. The TRV was determined according to equation 5:

$$TRV = \frac{\sqrt{\dfrac{\sum_{i=1}^{p}\sum_{v=1}^{n_i}(y_{iv}-y_{i.})^2}{N-p}}}{y_{..}} \qquad (5)$$

n_i = Number of measurements in the ith session
p = number of sessions
N = total number of measurements
y_{iv} = vth measurement in the ith session
$y_{i.}$ = mean of the ith session
$y_{..}$ = global mean

The 75 lowest TRV of all 16000 combinations of criteria at various levels of strictness were determined by a computer program. Because the TRV depends on the number of degrees of freedom remaining, after the acceptable measurements were selected, the program returned the lowest TRV for different minimum numbers of degrees of freedom

5. RESULTS

Table 1 shows the optimal quality criteria. Bot CHCr and CHCm are given for tetrameric haemoglobin.

Table 1. The resulting best quality criteria for each of the two methods of calculation
and their corresponding test retest variability (TRV) and mean cerebral
haemoglobin concentration (CHC)

Method	DUR	DSaO$_2$	DtHb/DOI	R^2	TRV	Mean CHC
CHCr	>1.2 min	>4%	<25% and >-25%	>0.85	17.3%	40.7µmol/l
CHCm	>1.5 min	>4%	<25% and >-25%		18.3%	38.7µmol/l

DUR, DSaO$_2$, DtHb/DOI and R^2 were found to be useful selection criteria (Table I).
CHCr and CHCm had a similar TRV (Table I). The proposed criteria rejected about 50%
of the measurements.

Table 2 shows how many measurements were rejected by each criterion.

6. DISCUSSION

The solutions shown in Table 1 were chosen out of the 75 returned by the computer
program according to three considerations: the optimum TRV, the lowest number of SOC
rejected and the reproducibility. A lower TRV of 13% can be achieved by using stricter
quality criteria and hence rejecting 75% of the SOC (e.g. by increasing $R^2>0.96$ for CHCr
in Table 1). If only 25% of the SOC are rejected, the TRV will increase to 23%. A reasonable balance between low TRV and high rejection was found in the solutions of Table 1.
The most important criteria to reduce the TRV were DtHb and R^2. DUR and DSaO$_2$ were
not critical for the TRV of our data, probably because most of our SOC were above a crucial limit. Nevertheless they were given in Table 1, because they may become important
for somebody trying to reproduce our data with lower DUR and DSaO$_2$.

DUR and DSaO$_2$ may be influenced by the operator during the measurement. These
numbers in Table 2 could therefore be reduced.

The assumptions indentified in the "theory" section are discussed below:

1. tHb is measured continuously and it therefore does not have to be assumed to be
   stable. In practice it shows that tHb is never absolutely stable and this poses the
   question of how much change of tHb is acceptable? The change of tHb is set in
   relation to the change in OI during the SOC, which corresponds to quality criterion DtHb/DOI, because the larger the change in OI the less an instability of tHb
   matters. This proved to be the best criterion among the ones pertaining to tHb
   (DtHb, DCO$_2$ and DMAP).
2. All changes in SaO$_2$ are small and in a normal range, i.e. the brain is well oxygenated. Hence it is unlikely, that a change in SaO$_2$ affects the oxygen consumption of the brain. Furthermore a change in cerebral oxygen metabolism will
   disturb the linear relationship between SaO$_2$ and OI, which is taken into account

Table 2. The percentage of rejection for each of the quality criteria

DUR > 1.2 min	DUR > 1.5 min	DSaO$_2$	DtHb/DOI	R^2
5.5%	14.7%	5.0%	32.6%	16.1%

by R^2. Still, small changes may not be totally excluded and may constitute part of the TRV.

3. That a change is slow enough is accounted for by DUR.

4. Movement artefacts may play a role during measurements. Again, they are likely to affect the linear relation between SaO_2 and OI, which is controlled by R^2.

Part of the TRV in the range of 18% may be explained by the small resolution of the pulse oxymeter of 1%.

Wyatt (1990) obtained a mean CBV value of 2.22±0.40 (SD) ml/100 g for healthy infants. For comparison we converted our CHCr and CHCm values into CBV and obtained 2.48±0.85 ml/100 g respectively 2.33±0.78 ml/100 g. Although the median gestational age and birthweight of our infants was lower by 1 5/7 weeks respectively 470 g, our CBV is in good agreement with Wyatt (1990).

7. CONCLUSIONS

A set of quantitative criteria determines the quality of the SOC measurement. Thus an acceptable TRV of 17.3% respectively 18.3% can be achieved. The CHCm method, which is much simpler to calculate, is almost as precise as the CHCr method.

8. ACKNOWLEDGMENTS

This work was funded in part by the Swiss Research Council and a Johnson & Johnson International Academic Support Award.

9. REFERENCES

Jobsis, Vander, Vliet, et al. Reflectance spectrophotometry of cytochrome aa3 in vivo. J Appl Physiol 1977;43(5):858–872.

von Siebenthal K, Bernert G, Casaer P. Near-infrared spectroscopy in newborn infants. Brain Dev 1992;14(135):135–143.

Wray S, Cope M, Delpy DT, Wyatt JS, Reynolds EO. Characterization of the near infrared absorption spectra of cytochrome aa3 and haemoglobin for the non-invasive monitoring of cerebral oxygenation. Biochim Biophys Acta 1988;933(184):184–192.

Wyatt JS, Cope M, Delpy DT, Wray S, Reynolds EO. Quantification of cerebral oxygenation and haemodynamics in sick newborn infants by near infrared spectrophotometry. Lancet 1986;2(1063):1063–1066.

Wyatt JS, Cope M, Delpy DT, et al. Quantitation of cerebral blood volume in human infants by near-infrared spectroscopy. J Appl Physiol 1990;68(1086):1086–1091.

63

EFFECT OF ANTIOXIDANTS ON HYPEROXIA-INDUCED ICAM-1 EXPRESSION IN HUMAN ENDOTHELIAL CELLS

Takuya Aoki,[1] Yukio Suzuki,[2] Kazumi Nishio,[1] Kouichi Suzuki,[1] Atsushi Miyata,[1] Yoshitaka Oyamada,[1] Masaaki Mori,[1] Hirofumi Fujita,[1] and Kazuhiro Yamaguchi[1]

[1]Department of Medicine
School of Medicine, Keio University
Tokyo, Japan
[2]Department of Internal Medicine
Kitasato Institute Hospital
Tokyo, Japan

1. ABSTRACT

The regulating mechanism of hyperoxia-induced ICAM-1 expression has not been elucidated. We studied the effect of antioxidants, including superoxide dismutase (SOD), catalase and N-acetylcysteine (NAC), on hyperoxia-induced ICAM-1 expression in human pulmonary artery endothelial cells (HPAEC) and human umbilical vein endothelial cells (HUVEC). Cells were cultured to confluence and exposed to either hyperoxic or normoxic gas with or without various kinds of antioxidants. The levels of ICAM-1 expression in the endothelial cells and the concentrations of reduced (GSH) and oxidized glutathione (GSSG) in the media were examined by flow cytometry and by spectrophotometry, respectively. After 48-hour exposure to hyperoxia, ICAM-1 expression was increased (HPAEC; 161 ± 21% and HUVEC; 163 ± 16%) and total glutathione concentration in the media was decreased as compared with normoxia. SOD did not change the GSH and GSSG concentrations in the media. Catalase dose-dependently decreased the supernatant GSSG concentration in both HPAEC and HUVEC, while the GSH concentration was nearly constant. NAC dose-dependently increased the supernatant GSH concentrations in both HPAEC and HUVEC. There was no difference in the supernatant GSSG concentrations between the NAC-treated HPAEC and HUVEC. There was no difference in ICAM-1 expression in either HPAEC or HUVEC with SOD treatment. ICAM-1 expressions in 100 U/ml (236 ± 20%) and 1,000 U/ml (315 ± 36%) of catalase were increased in HPAEC, and that in 1,000 U/ml (440 ± 209%) of catalase was increased in HUVEC. Five and 10 U/ml of NAC decreased ICAM-1 expression in HPAEC (141 ± 26% and 113 ± 11%) and

HUVEC (119 ± 23% and 106 ± 7%), respectively. These results suggest that extracellular glutathione may play a role in regulating hyperoxia-induced ICAM-1 expression in HPAEC and HUVEC.

2. INTRODUCTION

Adhesion molecules are thought to be indispensable for the accumulation of the inflammatory cells, which leads to tissue injury and remodeling. Elevated expression of intercellular adhesion molecule-1 (ICAM-1) on endothelium has been recognized in various inflammatory lung diseases including pulmonary fibrosis (1), asthma (2) and hyperoxic lung injury (3, 4). ICAM-1 is also considered to be important for neutrophil adherence to the endothelium, as well as eosinophil migration and airway hyperresponsiveness (2). Upregulation of ICAM-1 might promote these inflammatory processes. Oxidative stress may play an important role in induction of ICAM-1 expression. The mechanism regulating ICAM-1 expression has, however, been unclear. Recently, the expression of vascular cell adhesion molecule-1 (VCAM-1) expression has been reported to be regulated through an antioxidant-sensitive mechanism (5). However, there have been no systematic investigations aimed at determining whether ICAM-1 expression is regulated by a mechanism sensitive to antioxidants. Glutathione is known to be one of the most important oxidant scavengers. To investigate the regulating mechanism of hyperoxia-induced ICAM-1 expression, we studied the effects of superoxide dismutase (SOD), catalase and N-acetylcysteine (NAC) on hyperoxia-induced ICAM-1 expression in human pulmonary artery endothelial cells (HPAEC) and human umbilical vein endothelial cells (HUVEC).

3. MATERIALS AND METHODS

3.1. Antibodies and Reagents

Anti-human ICAM-1 monoclonal antibody and FITC-labeled goat anti-mouse IgG monoclonal antibody were purchased from Becton Dickinson (San Jose, CA). Human erythrocyte SOD, cell culture tested bovine erythrocyte SOD, bovine liver catalase and NAC were purchased from Sigma (St. Louis, MO). Human erythrocyte catalase was purchased from Athens Research and Technology (Athens, GA).

3.2. Endothelial Cell Culture

HPAEC and HUVEC (Kurabo, Osaka, Japan) were cultured in endothelial cell growth medium (EGM-UV; Kurabo) supplemented with 10% fetal calf serum, penicillin G (100 U/ml) and streptomycin (100 μg/ml; GIBCO, Grand Island, NY) at 37°C in a humidified incubator. The cells used for experiments were from the 5th to 12th passage. HPAEC and HUVEC were characterized by a pavement-like monolayer appearance, positive immunofluorescent staining with a specific anti-human von Willebrand factor antibody and high levels of angiotensin-converting enzyme activity in the culture media.

3.3. Oxygen Exposure Condition

The HPAEC and HUVEC were cultured to confluence in 25 cm^2 tissue culture flasks (Corning), and exposed to hyperoxia (90% O2, 5% CO2, 1 atm) for 48 hours at 37°C in a humidified multi-gas incubator (ASTEC, Tokyo, Japan). SOD, catalase and NAC were dissoloved in Dulbecco's phosphate buffered saline (D-PBS; GIBCO) and filtered. Various kinds and concentrations of SOD, catalase and NAC were added to the medium at the beginning of exposure to hyperoxia. Cells cultured under normoxic conditions (21% O$_2$, 5% CO$_2$, 1 atm) in a humidified incubator for 48-hours at 37°C without reagents served as the normoxic control. Data for each group represent the average of five cultures. After 48-hour exposure to hyperoxia, there was no significant difference in cell counts of HPAEC and HUVEC in all samples. Cell viabilities of HPAEC and HUVEC in all samples were assessed by trypan blue exclusion dye test. The viabilities of HPAEC and HUVEC in all samples exceeded 95% as determined by the trypan blue exclusion test. The endotoxin in media of HPAEC and HUVEC under all experimental conditions tested was measured by endospecy and toxicolor test, and was less than 15 ng/ml.

3.4. Flow Cytometric Analysis

The levels of ICAM-1 expression in HPAEC and HUVEC were determined by a flow cytometry. Cells were detached by treatment with 0.15 mM EDTA for 1 min at 37°C and washed with D-PBS. The suspended cells were incubated with anti-human ICAM-1 monoclonal antibody for 30 min at 4°C followed by FITC-labeled goat anti-mouse IgG monoclonal antibody. Cells were washed twice and fixed with 1% paraformaldehyde. The fluorescence and light-scattering properties of the cells were determined by using a FACScan flow cytometry system equipped with an argon laser (488-nm emission, 15-mW output; Becton Dickinson). Fluorescein isothiocyanate (FITC) green fluorescence was collected at 530 nm using a band-pass filter. In each sample, 10,000 cells were examined. The list mode was evaluated by the Lysis II system (Becton Dickinson). The results are expressed as percent intensity of fluorescence compared with the normoxic control (% control).

3.5. Preparation of Samples for Glutathione Assays

The concentration of total glutathione in each supernatant of HPAEC and HUVEC was assayed by using a modification of Tietze (6) and Owens (7) methods. A 600 µl of 0.6 N perchloric acid-0.001 M EDTA solution was added to a 600 µl of supernatant and centrifuged at 3,000 rpm for 10 min. The pH was adjusted to 7.0 with 3 M K$_2$CO$_3$. The samples were then centrifuged and used for the assay of total glutathione.

3.6. Masking of GSH

In order to measure the oxidized glutathione (GSSG) concentration, it is necessary to mask the GSH with N-ethylmaleimide (NEM). Masking of reduced glutathione (GSH) was due to a modification of Tietze (6) and Owens (7) methods. A 200 µl sample, 0.1 M phosphate-0.001 M EDTA buffer and 0.01 M NEM solution were mixed. After 10 minutes of mixing, 6 ml of diethylether was added to each sample, followed by vigorous shaking and centrifugation at 3,000 rpm for 10 min. The upper diethylether phase was discarded and the same extraction procedure with diethylether was repeated three times to remove excess NEM. Thereafter, diethylether was removed by bubbling nitrogen through the solution and the sample was used for the assay of GSSG. The GSH concentration was calculated by subtracting the GSSG concentration from the total glutathione concentration.

3.7. Glutathione Assays

The samples for the assay of total glutathione and GSSG described above were diluted ten-fold. A diluted 1 ml sample was mixed with 2 ml of 0.1 M phosphate-0.001 M EDTA buffer, followed by the addition of 50 µl of 10 mM 5–5'dithiobis (2 nitrobenzoic acid) (DTNB). After 5 minutes at room temperature, absorbance of nonglutathione sulfhydryl compounds, which react with DTNB to generate colored 5-thio-2 nitrobenzoic acid compounds, was measured. After this measurement, 4.8 mM NADPH and glutathione reductase were added to the samples and reacted for exactly 20 minutes. Absorbance at 412 nm was measured. Absorbance of nonglutathione sulfhydryl compounds was subtracted from sample absorbance, and glutathione concentration was calculated by the standard curve.

3.8. Statistical Analysis

The results are presented as means ± SD. All p values were determined using the one-way analysis of variance (ANOVA) followed by Fisher's paired least significant difference test (Stat View II; Brain Power, CA) to detect differences between groups. A $p < 0.05$ was considered statistically significant.

4. RESULTS

4.1. Expression of ICAM-1 under Hyperoxic Condition

The expression of ICAM-1 under hyperoxic conditions for 48 hours, in both HPAEC (161 ± 21%; $p < 0.01$) and HUVEC (163 ± 16%; $p < 0.01$), was increased as compared with normoxic conditions (HPAEC; 100 ± 14%, HUVEC; 100 ± 11%) (Figure 1).

4.2. Total Glutathione Concentration in the Media

After 48-hour exposure to hyperoxia, total glutathione concentration in the media of both HPAEC (0.747 ± 0.170 µg/ml; $p < 0.01$) and HUVEC (0.460 ± 0.089 µg/ml; $p < 0.01$) was decreased as compared with that of normoxia (HPAEC: 1.178 ± 0.310 µg/ml, HUVEC: 0.640 ± 0.025 µg/ml) (Figure 2). Total glutathione concentrations in the media of HPAEC were higher than that of HUVEC in both normoxic and hyperoxic conditions (Figure 2).

4.3. Effect of SOD on GSH and GSSG Concentrations

The concentrations of GSH and GSSG in media without cells were 0.062 ± 0.004 µg/ml and 0.134 ± 0.025 µg/ml, respectively. We studied the effect of SOD on supernatant GSH and GSSG concentrations (Table 1). There was no difference in the supernatant GSH and GSSG concentrations with the addition of SOD in either hyperoxia-exposed HPAEC or HUVEC.

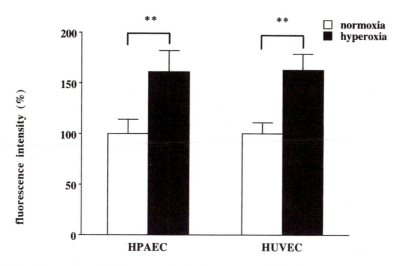

Figure 1. Effect of hyperoxia on ICAM-1 expression in HPAEC and HUVEC. The results are expressed as percent intensity against the normoxic control. The ICAM-1 expression in hyperoxia-exposed HPAEC or HUVEC was increased as compared with that in normoxic condition.

4.4. Effect of Catalase on GSH and GSSG Concentrations

The effect of bovine liver catalase on GSH and GSSG concentrations in the supernatant is shown in Table 2. Catalase at 100 and 1,000 U/ml decreased the supernatant GSSG concentration in HPAEC, and 1,000 U/ml catalase diminished the supernatant con-

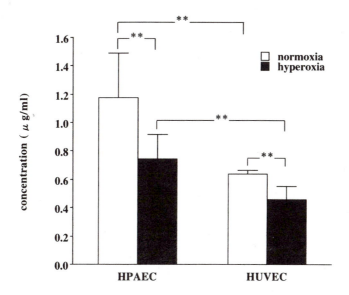

Figure 2. Effect of hyperoxia on total glutathione concentration in the supernatant of HPAEC and HUVEC. The concentration of total glutathione in hyperoxia-exposed HPAEC or HUVEC was decreased as compared with that of normoxic condition. Total glutathione concentration in the supernatant of HPAEC was higher than that of HUVEC under both normoxic and hyperoxic condition.

Table 1. Effect of SOD on extracellular GSH and GSSG concentrations

SOD (U/ml)	0	10	50	100
HPAEC				
GSH (μg/ml)	0.26 ± 0.03	0.31 ± 0.04	0.30 ± 0.02	0.24 ± 0.06
GSSG (μg/ml)	0.92 ± 0.24	0.94 ± 0.20	0.79 ± 0.13	0.94 ± 0.11
HUVEC				
GSH (μg/ml)	0.19 ± 0.05	0.21 ± 0.06	0.22 ± 0.04	0.17 ± 0.06
GSSG (μg/ml)	0.63 ± 0.11	0.65 ± 0.10	0.60 ± 0.07	0.58 ± 0.07

Data are presented as mean ± SD (n = 5).

centration of GSSG in HUVEC. The GSH concentration was nearly constant in cell supernatants. Human erythrocyte catalase had the same effect on GSH and GSSG concentrations.

4.5. Effect of NAC on the GSH and GSSG Concentrations

The effect of NAC on the GSH and GSSG concentrations in the supernatant is shown in Table 3. Five and 10 mM of NAC increased the supernatant GSH concentrations in both HPAEC and HUVEC as compared with the 0 mM of NAC. There was no difference in the supernatant GSSG concentrations between the NAC-treated HPAEC and HUVEC.

4.6. Effect of SOD, Catalase and NAC on Hyperoxic-Induced ICAM-1 Expression

There was no difference in ICAM-1 expression in either HPAEC or HUVEC with bovine erythrocyte SOD treatment. The effect on ICAM-1 expression by using human erythrocyte SOD showed the same results. ICAM-1 expressions in 100 U/ml (236 ± 20%; $p < 0.01$) and 1,000 U/ml (315 ± 36%; $p < 0.01$) of bovine liver catalase were increased in HPAEC, and that in 1,000 U/ml (440 ± 209%; $p < 0.05$) of the catalase was increased in HUVEC as compared with that in 0 U/ml of the catalase in HPAEC (161 ± 21%) or HUVEC (163 ± 16%). Human erythrocyte catalase showed the same effect on ICAM-1 expression. Five and 10 U/ml of NAC decreased ICAM-1 expression in HPAEC (141 ± 26% and 113 ± 11%) and HUVEC (119 ± 23% and 106 ± 7%), respectively.

Table 2. Effect of catalase on extracellular GSH and GSSG concentrations

catalase (U/ml)	0	10	100	1000
HPAEC				
GSH (μg/ml)	0.26 ± 0.03	0.30 ± 0.05	0.24 ± 0.04	0.17 ± 0.04
GSSG (μg/ml)	1.06 ± 0.18	1.08 ± 0.06	0.74 ± 0.06*	0.41 ± 0.102*
HUVEC				
GSH (μg/ml)	0.20 ± 0.04	0.17 ± 0.04	0.19 ± 0.05	0.17 ± 0.01
GSSG (μg/ml)	0.64 ± 0.13	0.66 ± 0.03	0.61 ± 0.11	0.31 ± 0.06*

Data are presented as mean ± SD (n = 5).
*p < 0.01 compared with the value of 0 U/ml catalase.

5. DISCUSSION

5.1. Extracellular GSH, GSSG and Total Glutathione Play a Key Role in Regulating Hyperoxia-Induced ICAM-1 Expression

Upregulation of ICAM-1 expression has been observed in various kinds of lung diseases, such as asthma (2, 8), pulmonary fibrosis (1, 9), pulmonary sarcoidosis (10) and pulmonary oxygen toxicity (3, 4). The mechanism of ICAM-1 expression in these diseases remains to be clarified. We demonstrated that decrease of extracellular glutathione level by the hyperoxic exposure was associated with increased ICAM-1 expression in both HPAEC and HUVEC, while increased glutathione by the addition of NAC decreased ICAM-1 expression (Figures 1 and 2, and Tables 2 and 3). On the other hand, administration of SOD, which did not alter the supernatant concentrations of GSH and GSSG (Table 1), did not change the levels of ICAM-1 expression in both HPAEC and HUVEC. These results suggest that extracellular GSH, GSSG and total glutathione play a key role in regulating hyperoxia-induced ICAM-1 expression in HPAEC and HUVEC.

5.2. Upregulation of ICAM-1 Expression in Inflammatory Lung Diseases May Be Associated with the Decrease in Glutathione Concentration

Glutathione is thought to be an important antioxidant in epithelial lining fluid (ELF), and total glutathione levels in normal human ELF were approximately 140-fold higher than plasma levels (11). The total glutathione concentration in ELF of patients with IPF is decreased (12). Therefore, the upregulation of ICAM-1 expression in IPF may be associated with the decrease in glutathione concentration. The expression of ICAM-1 is important for neutrophils (3, 4, 13, 14) and eosinophils (2, 8) to adhere to endothelium. Therefore, the increased ICAM-1 expression in IPF, asthma and other inflammatory lung disorders may induce recruitment of neutrophils or eosinophils. These cells are known to produce reactive oxygen species (ROS), and production of ROS result in GSH depletion. During progression of these diseases, there might be a vicious cycle that accumulation of neutrophils and eosinophils, which induced by increased ICAM-1 expression, release ROS and promote the GSH depletion. The GSH depletion elevated ICAM-1 expression, which promotes neutrophils and eosinophils to accumulate.

Table 3. Effect of NAC on extracellular GSH and GSSG concentrations

NAC (mM)	0	0.5	1	5	10
HPAEC					
GSH (µg/ml)	0.28 ± 0.01	0.27 ± 0.02	0.49 ± 0.11	3.10 ± 1.97*	5.07 ± 1.23*
GSSG(µg/ml)	0.86 ± 0.14	0.71 ± 0.02	0.69 ± 0.06	0.78 ± 0.09	0.75 ± 0.06
HUVEC					
GSH (µg/ml)	0.13 ± 0.04	0.07 ± 0.02	0.12 ± 0.02	2.12 ± 1.15*	4.15 ± 0.95*
GSSG(µg/ml)	0.29 ± 0.09	0.31 ± 0.04	0.24 ± 0.05	0.24 ± 0.0	0.20 ± 0.05

Data are presented as mean ± SD (n = 5).
*$p < 0.05$ and ** $p < 0.01$ compared with the value of 0 mM NAC.

5.3. Decreased GSSG by the Addition of Catalase Is Possibly Due to the Lower Rate of GSH Oxidation

Catalase and GSH peroxidase are located in different areas within cells. The former is found primarily in peroxisomes whereas the latter is in the cytoplasm and mitochondria. However, both are capable of reducing H_2O_2 and lipid peroxides (15). Hyperoxia increases H_2O_2 release from cells and the cytotoxicity of H_2O_2 is reported to be suppressed by the addition of 1,000 units/ml catalase (16). In our experiment, the addition of catalase decreased GSSG, but not GSH, in the extracellular media (Table 2). Catalase is known to scavenge H_2O_2 and reduced H_2O_2 might lower the rate of GSH oxidation, which might result in a decreased GSSG concentration.

5.4. Elevation of Extracellular GSH Is Due to Increased Efflux of GSH from Cells

The transport of GSH across the cell membrane is thought to be a one-way path. Intracellular GSH is reported to be released to the extracellular compartment in various tissues (17–19) and cells (20). On the other hand, influx of GSH is not known. Therefore the level of GSH may be determined by the GSH synthesis rate and the efflux rate (18, 19). Intracellular glutathione is present almost entirely (>96%) in its reduced form (GSH) and efflux of GSSG does not occur under physiologic conditions (21). NAC is known to elevate the intracellular glutathione level by increasing intracellular cysteine (22). The elevation of extracellular GSH by NAC might be due to increased efflux of GSH from cells secondary to GSH production inside the cells.

5.5. Protection Mechanism from High Oxidant Burden Might Exist in the Lung

Total glutathione concentration in the supernatant of HPAEC was higher than that of HUVEC under both normoxic and hyperoxic condition (Figure 2). As lung oxygen tension is higher than other organs, a protection mechanism from high oxidant burden might be needed.

6. CONCLUSION

In conclusion, 1) extracellular GSH, GSSG or total glutathione possibly works as one of the important factors to regulate ICAM-1 expression on hyperoxia-exposed endothelial cells. 2) Induction of ICAM-1 under a hyperoxic condition appears to be augmented as the glutathione concentration in the extracellular media is decreased, while increased glutathione decreased ICAM-1 expression.

7. REFERENCES

1. Van Dinther-Janssen, A.C.H.M., T. C. M. T. Van Maarsseveen, H. Eckert, W. Newman, and C. J. L. M. Meijer. 1993. Identical expression of ELAM-1, VCAM-1, and ICAM-1 in sarcoidosis and usual interstitial pneumonitis. *J. Pathol.* 170:157–164.

2. Wegner, C.D., R. H. Gundel, P. Reilly, N. Haynes, L. G. Letts, and R. Rothlein. 1990. Intercellular adhesion molecule-1 (ICAM-1) in the pathogenesis of asthma. *Science.* 247:456–459.

3. Wegner, C.D., W. W. Wolyniec, A. M. LaPlante, K. Marschman, K. Lubbe, N. Haynes, R. Rothlein, and L. G. Letts. 1992. Intercellular adhesion molecule-1 contributes to pulmonary oxygen toxicity in mice: role of leukocytes revised. *Lung.* 170:267–279.

4. Welty, S.E., J. L. Rivera, J. F. Elliston, C. V. Smith, T. Zeb, C. M. Ballantyne, C. A. Montgomery, and T. N. Hansen. 1993. Increases in lung tissue expression of intercellular adhesion molecule-1 are associated with hyperoxic lung injury and inflammation in mice. *Am. J. Respir. Cell. Mol. Biol.* 9:393–400.

5. Marui, N., M. K. Offermann, R. Swerlick, C. Kunsch, C. A. Rosen, M. Ahmad, R. W. Alexander, and R. M. Medford. 1993. Vascular cells adhesion molecule-1 (VCAM-1) gene transcription and expression are regulated through an antioxidant-sensitive mechanisim in human vascular endothelial cells. *J. Clin. Invest.* 92:1866–1874.

6. Tietze, F. 1969. Enzymic method for quantitative determination of nanogram amounts of total and oxidized glutathione. *Anal. Biochem.* 27:502–522.

7. Owens, C.W.I., and R. V. Belcher. 1965. A colorimetric micro-method for the determination of glutathione. *Biochem. J.* 94:705–711.

8. Bentley, A.M., S. R. Durham, D. S. Robinson, G. Menz, C. Storz, O. Cromwell, A. B. Kay, and A. J. Wardlaw. 1993. Expression of endothelial and leukocyte adhesion molecules intercellular adhesion monecule-1, E-selectin, and vascular cell adhesion molecule-1 in the bronchial mucosa in steady-state and allergen-induced asthma. *J. Allergy Clin. Immunol.* 92:857–868.

9. Shijubo, N., K. Imai, S. Aoki, M. Hirasawa, H. Sugawara, H. Koba, M. Tsujisaki, T. Sugiyama, Y. Hinoda, A. Yachi, M. Asakawa, and A. Suzuki. 1992. Circulating intercellular adhesion molecule-1 (ICAM-1) antigen in sera of patients with idiopathic pulmonary fibrosis. *Clin. Exp. Immunol.* 89:58–62.

10. Melis, M., M. Gjomarkaj, E. Pace, G. Malizia, and M. Spatafora. 1991. Increased expression of leukocyte function associated antigen-1 (LFA-1) and intercellular adhesion molecule-1 (ICAM-1) by alveolar macrophages of patients with pulmonary sarcoidosis. *Chest.* 100:910–916.

11. Cantin, A.M., S. L. North, R. C. Hubbard, and R. G. Crystal. 1987. Normal alveolar epithelial lining fluid contains high levels of glutathione. *J. Appl. Physiol.* 63:152–157.

12. Cantin, A.M., R. C. Hubbard, and R. G. Crystal. 1989. Glutathione deficiency in the epithelial lining fluid of the lower respiratory tract in idiopathic pulmonary fibrosis. *Am. Rev. Respir. Dis.* 139:370–372.

13. Barton, R.W., R. Rothlein, J. Ksiazek, and C. Kennedy. 1989. The effect of anti-intercellular adhesion molecule-1 on phorbol-ester-induced rabbit lung inflammation. *J. Immunol.* 143:1278–1282.

14. Lo, S.K., K. Janakidevi, L. Lai, and A. B. Malik. 1993. Hydrogen peroxide-induced increase in endothelial adhesiveness is dependent on ICAM-1 activation. *Am. J. Physiol.* 264: L406–12.

15. Chance, B., H. Sies, and A. Boveris. 1979. Hydroperoxide metabolism in mammalian organs. *Physiol. Rev.* 59:527–605.

16. Cantin, A.M., S. L. North, G. A. Fells, R. C. Hubbard, and R. G. Crystal. 1987. Oxidant-mediated epithelial cell injury in idiopathic pulmonary fibrosis. *J. Clin. Invest.* 79:1665–1673.

17. Bartoli, G.M., and H. Sies. 1978. Reduced and oxidized glutathione efflux from liver. *FEBS Lett.* 86:89–91.

18. Lauterburg, B.H., C. V. Smith, H. Hughes, and J. R. Mitchell. 1984. Biliary excretion of glutathione and glutathione disulfide in the rat: regulation and response to oxidative stress. *J. Clin. Invest.* 73:124–133.

19. Kaplowitz, N., D. E. Eberle, J. Petrini, J. Touloukian, M. C. Corvascue, and J. Kuhlenkamp. 1983. Factors influencing the efflux of hepatic glutathione into bile in rats. *J. Pharmacol. Exp. Ther.* 224:141–147.

20. Bannai, S., and H. Tsukeda. 1979. The export of glutathione from human diploid cells in culture. *J. Biol. Chem.* 254:3444–3450.

21. Bannai, S., and N. Tateishi. 1986. Role of membrane transport in metabolism and function of glutathione in mammals. *J. Memb. Biol.* 89:1–8.

22. Phelps, D.T., S. M. Deneke, D. L. Daley, and B. L. Fanburg. 1992. Elevation of glutathione levels in bovine pulmonary artery endothelial cells by N-Acetylcysteine. *Am. J. Respir. Cell. Mol. Biol.* 7:293–299.

64

LEUKOCYTE ADHESION IN PIAL CEREBRAL VENULES AFTER PMA STIMULATION AND ISCHEMIA/REPERFUSION *IN VIVO*

A. G. Hudetz,[1,2] J. A. Oliver,[5] J. D. Wood,[1] P. J. Newman,[3,4,5] and
J. P. Kampine[1,2]

[1]Department of Anesthesiology
[2]Department of Physiology
[3]Department of Cell Biology
[4]Department of Pharmacology
 Medical College of Wisconsin
[5]Blood Center of Southeastern Wisconsin
 Milwaukee, Wisconsin 53226

INTRODUCTION

Inflammatory stimulation of leukocyte adhesion in cerebral ischemia/reperfusion may result in vascular endothelial dysfunction, compromised microvascular blood flow and tissue oxygenation and neuronal death. Ischemia facilitates rolling and adhesion of leukocytes in mesenteric venules (Perry and Granger, 1992), however, this has not been demonstrated in the cerebral microcirculation. Nitric oxide has antiadhesion properties for leukocytes *in vivo* (Kurose et al, 1994) and may modulate leukocyte adhesion during cerebral ischemia/reperfusion.

Leukocyte rolling and adhesion can also be induced chemically, for example, using the chemotactic agent fMLP (Corvin et al, 1990) or the croton-oil derived phorbol ester, phorbol 12-myristate 13-acetate (PMA). PMA stimulates a variety of cells by direct activation of protein kinase C. In endothelial cells, this results in rapid degranulation of the Weibel-Palade bodies and expression of P-selectin on the cell surface (Geng et al, 1990). Interaction of P-selectin with its ligand on leukocytes is necessary for leukocytes to roll on the vessel wall under physiological shear stress (Moore et al, 1995). The effect of PMA on leukocyte-endothelial adhesion has not been demonstrated in the cerebral microcirculation *in vivo*.

Oxygen Transport to Tissue XVIII, edited by Nemoto and LaManna
Plenum Press, New York, 1997

In this work we examined if leukocyte adhesion in pial cerebral venules can be enhanced by stimulation with PMA or by ischemia and reperfusion with and without an inhibition of nitric oxide synthase.

METHODS

The cerebrocortical microcirculation was studied using intravital video-microscopy with techniques established in this laboratory (Hudetz et al, 1995). Adult male Sprague-Dawley rats were anesthetized with sodium pentobarbital (65 mg/kg) and underwent implantation of a closed cranial window with ports for perfusion and measurement of intracranial pressure (ICP) in the right parietal area. During the study the animals were anesthetized with halothane (0.5–1.0 MAC), paralyzed (80 mg Gallamine) and artificially ventilated with 25–30% O_2 in N_2. The end-tidal CO_2 was maintained at 33–35 mmHg. Core body temperature was controlled at 37°C. The left femoral artery and the right femoral vein were cannulated for measurement of blood pressure, and infusion of drugs and fluorescent dyes, respectively. The abdominal cavity was opened, and the spleen was either removed or tied off from the blood supply. To visualize circulating nucleated cells in microvessels, we infused either Acridine Orange (50 mg/ml, 1 ml/h) or Rhodamine 6-G (20 mg/ml, 0.1 ml/h) iv. We switched to Rhodamine 6G in the second series of experiments because we found that Rhodamine provided a higher image contrast than Acridine Orange and improved the differentiation of leukocytes from endothelial cells. Fluorescent images of leukocytes adhering to the endothelium of small pial veins are shown in Figure 1 as an example.

Observation was done using a modified Olympus epifluorescent video-microscope with 40X ultra long working distance lens. The video image of the microcirculation was monitored in real time as well as recorded on S-VHS tape for off-line analysis. Four random areas were chosen and recorded before infusion of the dye was begun. This protocol provided a means of distinguishing between auto-fluorescent objects and the adherent leukocytes.

To demonstrate leukocyte activation, the rats were treated with 5×10^{-6} M PMA which was superfused over the brain tissue under the cranial window. PMA was perfused at a rate of approximately 1.5 ml/hr for 30 minutes. Thirty-second long video recordings

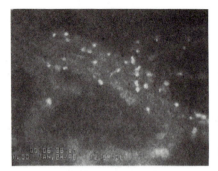 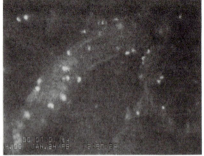

Figure 1. Fluorescently labeled leukocytes adhering to the endothelium of pial venules as seen through the cranial window using an intravital video-microscope. Two fields from the same experiments are shown. Fluorescent labeling is with Rhodamine 6G. Field width is 370 mm.

of each of the four areas were made at 10, 20, 30, 40, and 50 minutes following the beginning of the PMA exposure.

In a separate series of experiments, forebrain ischemia was induced by bilateral common carotid artery occlusion (BCO) followed by elevation of local ICP to 20 mmHg for 1 hour. The circulation was video-recorded at baseline, after BCO, BCO+ICP elevation at 5 and 60 minutes, and after reperfusion at 5 and 60 minutes. To determine if endogenous nitric oxide (NO) influenced leukocyte adherence in ischemia, a group of animals (N=10) was pretreated with N^w-nitro-L-arginine methyl ester (L-NAME), an inhibitor of nitric oxide synthase (NOS). L-NAME was infused at a dose of 20 mg/kg iv over a period of 10 minutes. A control group (N=4) was treated with the less active isomer D-NAME. At the end of the experiment, a micron grid was recorded at the appropriate magnification to allow determination of vessel length and diameter.

Data Analysis

The number of adhering leukocytes per endothelial surface of 15 to 80 mm venules and the duration of the interaction were measured off line, from the video recordings. Time periods analyzed were the control period prior to PMA superfusion and the period at 10 minutes exposure to PMA. Fluorescent objects present prior to infusion of acridine orange were mapped and eliminated from the analysis. All other fluorescent events were counted, and the length of time which elapsed between their entry into and exit from the microscopic field was determined for the 30-second recording period. The distance traveled by the cell was determined, and the velocity was calculated in mm/sec. Non-adhering leukocytes were used as markers of blood flow to yield blood flow velocity. Fluorescent events which were absent in the field prior to acridine orange infusion, but which were present for the entire 30-second recording period were scored as adherent for more than 30 seconds, and were referred to as long adherent events (LAE). In later analysis of the percentage of all leukocytes observed during the recording period which were defined as LAE, the criterion used for inclusion of a fluorescent event in this category was interaction with the vessel wall for at least 10 seconds. An estimate of more than 95% of all LAE defined using the 10-second interaction criterion were adherent for longer than 30 seconds. For determination of the percentage of total leukocytes observed which were defined as LAE (interacting with the vessel wall for longer than 10 seconds), all four areas were counted at all time points recorded. The total number of leukocytes in each vessel for the individual 30-second recording periods was calculated from the number observed in the first and last 5 seconds, multiplied by three. In the ischemic series, the number of leukocytes firmly adhering to the endothelium for at least 3 seconds were counted only. Most of these leukocytes adhered for the entire 30-second period and therefore these events usually qualified as LAE.

Statistics

Differences between experimental groups and treatments were analyzed by Analysis of Variance. LAE values were expressed as a percent of all fluorescent events within each observation period. Mean LAE for all animals was then normalized for background level of inflammation (percentage LAE observed during the control period before PMA superfusion) by subtracting the mean percent LAE at all time points before and after PMA exposure from the mean percent LAE at each time point. In the ischemia series, statistical tests were performed on firm adhesion events without normalization.

RESULTS AND DISCUSSION

PMA Stimulation

Before administration of PMA, very few labeled leukocytes were seen to roll along or adhere to the wall of venules. No leukocyte-endothelial interaction was observed in arterioles or capillaries. Increased rolling and adherence occurred as a result of exposure to 5×10^{-6} M PMA. In some instances, individual adherent leukocytes were observed for over 15 minutes, during which time they potentially extravasated. However, this was difficult to determine because of photobleaching of the fluorescent label.

The time of interaction of leukocytes with vascular endothelium and leukocyte velocity is associated with leukocyte rolling. As a measure of events which may be more closely associated with transendothelial migration, the cells which demonstrated longer adherence (LAE) were analyzed. Under control conditions, the number of adhering leukocytes was low, $5.4 \pm 2.3 \times 10^{-4}$ mm^{-2} (SD). PMA superfusion significantly increased leukocyte adhesion (LAE) at 10–30 min (Figure 2). This finding is similar to that of Corvin et al. (1990) who used the chemotactic agent fMLP to induce an approximately twofold increase in rolling and sticking of leukocytes to the endothelium of small cerebral venules *in vivo*.

We considered the possibility that PMA treatment would alter blood flow and shear rate in individual vessels through its effect on protein kinase C in vascular smooth muscle. PMA has been shown to decrease cerebral blood flow in rats (Uhl et al, 1993) and constrict pial arterioles when superfused over the brain surface of newborn pigs (Busija and Leffler, 1991). In our study, the change in flow velocity post-PMA was not statistically significant. Likewise, further analysis of flow velocity as a function of venule diameter (data not shown) did not reveal a significant effect of PMA on venular flow velocity (interaction term was not significant). Therefore, the increase in leukocyte adherence was ascribed to a direct, leukocyte activating effect of PMA.

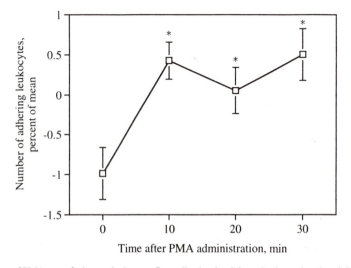

Figure 2. Effect of PMA superfusion on leukocyte firm adhesion in pial cerebral venules. *:p<0.05 vs. time zero.

Forebrain Ischemia. Before ischemia the number of leukocytes adhering for at least 3 seconds was 5.4 ± 2.3 (SD) $x10^{-4}$ mm^{-2} and increased significantly after BCO+ICP elevation to 7.9 and 11.3 $x10^{-4}$ mm^{-2} at 5 and 60 minutes, respectively. Leukocyte firm adhesion returned to the pre-ischemic baseline by 60 min of reperfusion (Figure 3). The latter finding is similar to that of Dirnagl et al. (1994) who demonstrated only a slight increase in the number of leukocytes rolling along or sticking to the venular endothelium in the cerebral cortex. However, the significant increase in leukocyte adhesion during cerebral ischemia has not been demonstrated before. Five of the ten L-NAME treated animals died after the initiation of cerebral ischemia but mortality in the D-NAME treated group was zero. There was no significant difference in leukocyte-endothelial adhesion between the surviving L-NAME treated and D-NAME treated animals. This appears to be consistent with the effect of L-NAME in the rat mesenteric preparation (Kurose et al, 1994) despite the clear antiadhesion effect of NO donors following ischemia/reperfusion. It is possible that leukocyte-endothelium interaction was indeed enhaced by L-NAME in some of the animals at the onset of ischemia, however, this could not be assessed due to the high rate of mortality. Pretreatment with L-NAME probably decreased cerebral blood flow before and at the onset of ischemia which would have confounded its direct effect on leukocyte adhesion. Thus, the presence of basal NO production may still be an important antiadhesion factor and influence the outcome of cerebral ischemia.

CONCLUSION

The results suggest that both PMA and forebrain ischemia stimulate leukocyte firm adhesion in small cerebral venules. Inhibition of NOS aggravates the outcome of focal cerebral ischemia and is consistent with the hypothesis that enhanced leukocyte-endothelial interaction may contribute to neuronal injury after stroke.

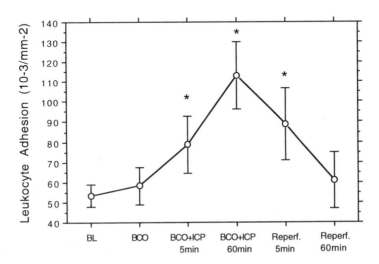

Figure 3. Effect of forebrain ischemia and reperfusion on leukocyte firm adhesion in cerebral venules *in vivo.* BL=baseline condition, BCO=bilateral carotid occlusion, ICP=intracranial pressure elevation, Reperf.=reperfusion (release of occlusion and lowering of intracranial pressure).

ACKNOWLEDGMENT

This work supported in part by the NSF Grant BES-9411631 and NIH Training Grant HL-07902.

REFERENCES

Busija, D.W., Leffler, C.W., 1991, Effects of phorbol esters in pial arteriolar diameter and brain production of prostanoids in piglets. *Circ. Res.* 69:1253–1258.

Corvin, S., Schürer, L., Abels, C., Kempski, O., Baethmann, A., 1990, Effect of stimulation of leukocyte chemotaxis by fMLP on white blood cell behavior in the microcirculation of rat brain. *Acta Neurochir. Suppl.* 51:55–57.

Dirnagl, U., Niwa, K, Sixt, G., Villringer, A., 1994, Cortical hypoperfusion after global forebrain ischemia in rats is not caused by microvascular leukocyte plugging. *Stroke* 25:1028–1038.

Geng, J.-G., Bevilacqua, M.P., Moore, K.L., McIntyre, T.M., Prescott, S.M., Kim, J.M., Bliss, G.A., Zimmerman, G.A., McEver, R.P., 1990, Rapid neutrophil adhesion to activated endothelium mediated by GMP-140. *Nature* 343:757–760.

Hudetz, A.G., Fehér, G., Weigle C.G.M., Knuese, D.E., Kampine J.P., 1995, Video microscopy of cerebrocortical capillary flow: response to hypotension and intracranial hypertension. *Am. J. Physiol.* 268:H2202-H2210.

Kurose, I., Wolf, R., Grisham, M.B., Granger, D.N., 1994, Modulation of ischemia/reperfusion-induced microvascular dysfunction by nitric oxide. *Circ. Res.* 74:376–382.

Moore, K.L., Patel, K.D., Bruehl, R.E., Li, F., Johnson, D.A., Lichenstein, H.S., Cummings, R.D., Bainton, D.F., McEver, R.P., 1995, P-selectin glycoprotein ligand-1 mediates rolling of human neutrophils on P-selectin. *J. Cell. Biol.* 128:661–671.

Perry, M.A., Granger D.N., 1992, Leukocyte adhesion in local versus hemorrhage-induced ischemia. *Am. J. Physiol.* 263:H810–815.

Uhl, M.W., Kochanek P.M., Schiding J.K., Nemoto E.M., 1993, Effect of phorbol myristate acetate on cerebral blood flow in normal and neutrophil-depleted rats. *Stroke* 24:1977–1982.

65

NITRIC OXIDE INHIBITS GROWTH OF VASCULAR SMOOTH MUSCLE CELLS *IN VITRO* BY MECHANISMS INDEPENDENT OF GUANYLATE CYCLASE

A. Sasse, G. Hoffmann, S. Birrenbach, and J. Grote

Department of Physiology
University of Bonn
Nussalle 11, D-53115 Bonn
Germany

1. INTRODUCTION

Nitric oxide (NO) is an important mediator molecule synthesized by several cell types including vascular smooth muscle cells (VSMC; Busse and Mülsch, 1990) and endothelial cells (EC; Rubanyi et al., 1986). It is generated by the conversion of L-arginine to L-citrulline, a reaction that is catalyzed by the enzyme nitric oxide synthase (NOS). NOS exists in at least three isoforms mainly classified to be either constitutive (cNOS) or inducible (iNOS). cNOS, as present in EC, is dependent on an increase in intracellular calcium concentration $[Ca^{2+}]_i$ and produces NO in the picomolar range. In contrast, iNOS, as present in VSMC, is independent of an increase in $[Ca^{2+}]_i$ and produces NO in the nanomolar range upon activation with endotoxins and cytokines. Recent studies have reported a growth inhibitory effect of nitric oxide in EC (Yang et al., 1994), cerebellar glial cells (Garg et al., 1992), and VSMC (Scott-Burden et al., 1993). Although it is not known whether endothelial derived NO exhibits any effects on VSMC growth in vivo, nitric oxide may play a role under conditions associated with endothelial cell damage and excessive VSMC proliferation, a feature characteristic of atherosclerotic blood vessel disease (Ross, 1993). A similar phenomenon also occurs after angioplasty as well as during hypertension and diabetes (Moncada et al., 1991). Hypertrophy of VSMC might at least in part be mediated by an inappropriate production and/or release of NO. The aim of the present study was to investigate the possible mechanism of NO-dependent inhibition of VSMC growth *in vitro*.

Oxygen Transport to Tissue XVIII, edited by Nemoto and LaManna
Plenum Press, New York, 1997

2. METHODS

2.1. Cell Culture

VSMC were isolated from the thoracic aorta of Wistar Kyoto rats by enzymatic dis-aggregation as previously described (Hoffmann et al., 1995). Cultured cells were main-tained in Dulbecco´s modified Eagle´s medium (DMEM, cc Pro, Karlsruhe, Germany) containing 50 µg/ml streptomycin, 50 U/ml penicillin, and 10% fetal calf serum (Gibco Life Tech., Eggenstein, Germany) in a humidified atmosphere of 95% air/5% CO_2. For experiments, passages 4 to 12 of subcultured cells were used.

2.2. RNA Isolation and Polymerase Chain Reaction

Following 12h and 48h incubation periods, total RNA was isolated by acid phenol-chloroform extraction, redissolved in water and its concentration determined photometri-cally at a wave length of 260 nm. One µg of total RNA was reverse-transcribed (RT) into first strand cDNA using oligo (dT)15 (Amersham Buchler, Braunschweig, Germany) as a primer for reverse trancriptase (M-MLRV superscript, Gibco Life Tech., Eggenstein, Ger-many). RT-generated cDNA encoding for rat iNOS and glyceraldehyde-3-phosphate de-hyxdrogenase (GAPDH) genes, respectively, were amplified using polymerase chain reaction (PCR). Expression of the housekeeping gene GAPDH served as control, RNA with no GAPDH band was excluded from further investigations. PCR was run for 30 cy-

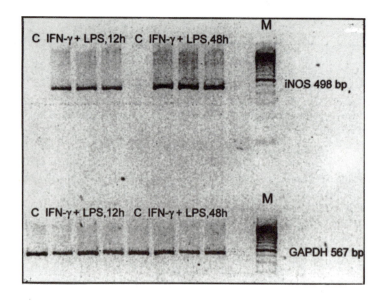

Figure 1. Qualitative analysis of iNOS mRNA expression detected as iNOS cDNA (length: 498 base pairs) fol-lowing 12h and 48h incubations of vascular smooth muscle cells with 100 U/ml interferon-γ (IFN-γ) + 5 µg/ml lipopolysaccharide (LPS). Lane C shows the control experiments in unstimulated cells, lane M indicates the mo-lecular marker. The lower part of the figure shows the corresponding GAPDH bands (length: 567 base pairs). Ex-pression of the housekeeping GAPDH gene served as internal control. Incubation experiments were performed in triplicate.

cles after an initial denaturation step at 94°C for 3 min with an amplification profile of each cycle consisting of denaturation for 1 min at 94°C, primer annealing for 1.5 min at 58°C and elongation for 3 min at 73°C.

2.3. Nitrite and Nitrate Assay

Synthesis of the stable the NO-metabolites nitrite and nitrate was determined in the cell-free culture supernatants incubated for 48h in L-arginine enriched medium DMEM without phenol red (Sigma Chemicals, Deisenhofen, Germany). Nitrate was reduced to nitrite by 0.1 U/ml nitrate reductase (Boehringer Mannheim, Germany) in the presence of 50 μM ß-NADPH and 5 μM FAD (Sigma Chemicals, Deisenhofen Germany). Total nitrite accumulation (NO_2^- + NO_3^-) was assayed by the Griess reaction. Nitrite concentrations were determined relative to a standard curve which holds for aqueous solutions of different sodium nitrite concentrations.

2.4. [³H]Thymidine Incorporation Assay

Prior to [³H]thymidine incorporation assay, cells plated on 24-well culture dishes were growth arrested by incubation in serum-free medium for 24h. The quiescent cells were incubated in DMEM containing or lacking experimental agents as indicated in Figure 2. In the last 4h of incubation, 1 μCi of methyl[³H]thymidine (Amersham Buchler, Braunschweig, Germany) was added to each well to determine DNA synthesis. The experiments were terminated by removing the media and washing the cells with phosphate-buffered saline. Acid insoluble material was precipitated with 10% trichloroacetic acid.

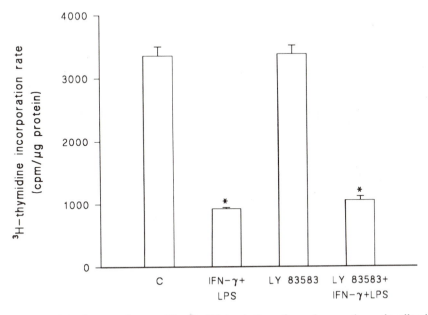

Figure 2. [³H]thymidine incorporation rate following 24h incubations of vascular smooth muscle cells with with 100 U/ml interferon-γ (IFN-γ) + 5 μg/ml lipopolysaccharide (LPS), 0.1 μM LY 83583, and 100 U/ml IFN-γ + 5 μg/ml LPS + 0.1 μM LY 83583, respectively. Data are given as means ± SEM of 3 separate experiments each performed in triplicate. *P<0.05 as compared to controls (C).

Wells were washed twice with ethanol and the remaining cell material was solubilized with 0.5 N NaOH. A 50 μl aliquot was removed from each well for protein determination (BioRAD protein assay, BioRAD Laboratories, München, Germany). 100 μl aliquots were transferred into scintillation vials and radioactivity incorporated into the DNA was measured by liquid scintillation counting. Data are given as counts per minute in relation to cell protein content.

2.5. Microculture Tetrazolium Assays

VSMC were grown on 96-well microtiter plates. Following treatment with serum-deprived medium for 24h subconfluent cells were incubated for 48h as indicated in Figures 3 and 4. At the end of each incubation period, mitochondrial dehydrogenase activity was determined photometrically at a wave length of 450 nm using tetratzolium formazan. Since mitochondrial dehydrogenases exhibit higher activities in proliferating cells, this assay is convenient for measurements of cell viability as well as proliferation efficiency.

2.6. Materials for Cell Incubation

Interferon-γ (IFN-γ) was purchased from IC Chemicals, Ismaning, Germany. Lipopolysaccharide (LPS) derived from Escherichia coli (Serotype 0111:B4), the exogenous nitric oxide donor sodium nitroprusside (SNP), and the stable cGMP analog 8-bromo-cyclic GMP were from Sigma Chemicals, Deisenhofen, Germany. The soluble guanylate cyclase inhibitor LY 83583 was obtained from Boehringer Mannheim, Germany.

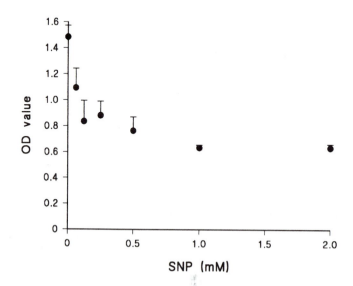

Figure 3. Mitochondrial dehydrogenase activity measured as optical density (OD) following 48h incubations of vascular smooth muscle cells with different concentrations of sodium nitroprusside (SNP). Data are given as means ± SEM, n=16.

2.7. Statistical Analysis

Results are expressed as means ± SEM; data were analyzed statistically by using the nonparametrical Mann-Whitney-U-test. P values < 0.05 were considered as significant.

3. RESULTS

As shown in Figure 1, coincubation of VSMC with 100 U/ml IFN-γ and 5 μg/ml LPS stimulated iNOS gene expression detected as iNOS cDNA 12h as well as 48h after the start of the treatments. [³H]thymidine incorporation rate was significantly lower in IFN-γ and LPS treated cells. Coincubation of VSMC with 0.1 μM LY 83583 did not affect this IFN-γ plus LPS induced inhibition of cell proliferation (Figure 2). iNOS gene expression was accompanied by an increase in the NO_2^- + NO_3^- concentration of cell-free culture supernatants thus indicating that VSMC were activated to produce NO (data not shown).

Mitochondrial dehydrogenase activity was significantly depressed in a dose-dependent manner when cells were exposed to SNP (Figure3). As depicted in Figure 4, the suppressive effect of SNP at a concentration of 1 mM (Optical density (OD) values 46% less than controls) was only in part antagonized by simultaneous application of 0.1 μM LY 83583 (OD values 20% less than controls). 8-bromo-cGMP (0.1 μM) treatment caused a decrease in mitochondrial dehydrogenase activity that was less pronounced than the effect induced by SNP (OD value 26% less than controls).

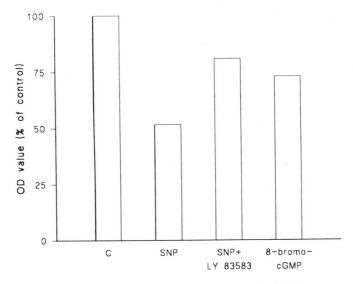

Figure 4. Mitochondrial dehydrogenase activity determined by optical density (OD) measurements following 48h incubations of vascular smooth muscle cells with sodium nitroprusside (SNP, 1 mM), SNP (1 mM) + LY 83583 (0.1 μM), and 8-bromo-cGMP (8-br-cGMP, 0.1 μM), respectively. Results are expressed as percent difference from controls (C).

4. DISCUSSION

The present study demonstrates that activation of the endogenous L-arginine-NO pathway as well as the application of an exogenous nitric oxide donor inhibits vascular smooth muscle cell growth *in vitro*. Thus, a constitutive production and release of NO from endothelial cells might be important for depression of medial cell growth and maintenance of cellular quiescence in vivo. In conditions associated with endothelial cell damage, insufficient NO generation may lead to excessive VSMC proliferation and, e.g., atherosclerotic blood vessel disease. Recent studies reported that the growth inhibitory effect of NO is present not only in VSMC, but also in endothelial cells (Yang et al., 1994), cerebellar glial cells (Garg et al., 1992), and Balb/c 3T3 fibroblasts (Garg and Hassid, 1990). However, the mechanisms whereby the NO generating pathway depresses cellular proliferation are still speculative. Since NO activates the cytosolic form of guanylate cyclase leading to an increase in intracellular cGMP concentration (Rapoport and Murad, 1983), an antiproliferative effect of cGMP is worth considering. Garg and Hassid (1989) could mimic the antimitogenic effect of exogenous NO donors by application of the stable cGMP analogue 8-bromo-cGMP. In contrast, a cGMP independent mechanism may also exist because Garg et al. (1990) have reported that exogenous NO-donors inhibit the proliferation of BALB/c 3T3 fibroblasts that lack soluble guanylate cyclase and are unresponsive to 8-bromo-cGMP. In our study, 8-bromo-cGMP caused a decrease in mitochondrial dehydrogenase activity but this effect was less pronounced than that induced by the exogenous NO donor SNP. Moreover, the growth-suppressive effect of SNP was only in part antagonized by simultaneous application of the soluble guanylate cyclase inhibitor LY 83583, and the antiproliferative action of the iNOS stimulators IFN-γ and LPS was completely unaffected by LY 83583. Therefore, the growth inhibitory effect of NO may at least in part be mediated by mechanisms independent of guanylate cyclase activation. It is possible that the antiproliferative effect of NO is due to its cytotxic effects as demonstrated for VSMC by Assender et al. (1991) or adenocarcinoma cells by Lepoivre et al. (1990). In our experiments, less than 1% of cells treated with SNP or IFN-γ + LPS stained with trypan blue. In addition, replating of cells did not result in different plating efficiency between cells exposed to exogenous NO donors and untreated cells. Thus, the growth inhibitory action of NO observed in our studies seems to be unrelated to its cytotoxic potential. Another possible mechanism by which VSMC respond to growth stimuli is an alteration in intracellular pH (Siffert and Düsing, 1995). It is tempting to speculate whether NO inhibits VSMC growth via changes in cytoplasmic pH. Studies on the influence of nitric oxide on the activity of pH regulatory systems are in progress in our laboratory.

ACKNOWLEDGMENTS

This study was supported by the "Finanzkommission der Medizinischen Fakultät", University of Bonn.

REFERENCES

Assender, J.W., Southgate, K.M., and Newby, A.C., 1991, Does nitric oxide inhibit smooth muscle proliferation? J. Cardiovasc. Pharmacol. 17 Su 3: S104-S107.

Busse, R., and Mulsch, A., 1990, Induction of nitric oxide synthase by cytokines in vascular smooth muscle cells. FEBS Lett. 275: 87–90.

Garg, U.C., and Hassid, A., 1989, Nitric oxide-generating vasodilators and 8-bromo-cyclic guanosine monophosphate inhibit mitogenesis and proliferation of cultured rat vascular smooth muscle cells. J. Clin. Invest. 83: 1774–1777.

Garg, U.C., and Hassid, A., 1990, Nitric oxide-generating vasodilators inhibit mitogenesis and proliferation of BALB/c 3T3 fibroblasts by a cGMP-independent mechanism. Biochem. Biophys. Res. Commun. 171: 474–479.

Garg, U.C., Devi, L., Turndorf, H., Goldfrank, L.R., and Bansinath, M., 1992, Effect of nitric oxide on mitogenesis and proliferation of cerebellar glial cells. Brain Res. 592: 208–212.

Hassid, A., Arabshahi, H., Bourcier, T., Dhaunsi, G.S., and Matthews, C., 1994, Nitric oxide selectively amplifies FGF-2-induced mitogenesis in primary rat aortic smooth muscle cells. Am. J. Physiol. 267: H1040-H1048.

Hoffmann, G., Ko, Y., Sachinidis, A., Göbel, B.O., Vetter, H., Rosskopf, D., Siffert, W., and Düsing, R., 1995, Kinetics of Na+/H+ exchange in vascular smooth muscle cells from WKY and SHR: effects of phorbol ester. Am. J. Physiol. 268: C14-C20.

Kariya, K.I., Kawahara, Y., Araki, S.I:, Fukuzaki, H., and Takai, Y., 1989, Antiproliferative action of cGMP-elevating vasodilators in cultured rabbit aortic smooth muscle cells. Atherosclerosis 80: 143–147.

Lepoivre, M., Chenais, B., Yapo, A., Lemaire, G., Thelander, L., and Tenu, J.P., 1990, Alterations of ribonucleotide reductase activity following induction of the nitrite-generating pathway in adenocarcinoma cells. J. Biol. Chem. 265: 14143–14149.

Moncada, S., Palmer, R.M., and Higgs, E.A., 1991, Nitric oxide: physiology, pathophysiology, and pharmacology. Pharmacol. Rev. 43: 109–142.

Nakaki, T., Nakayama, M., and Kato, R., 1990, Inhibition by nitric oxide and nitric oxide-producing vasodilators of DNA synthesis in vascular smooth muscle cells. Eur. J. Pharmacol. 189: 347- 353.

Rapoport, R.M. and Murad, F., 1983, Endothelium-dependent and nitrovasodilator-induced relaxation of vascular smooth muscle: role of cyclic GMP. J. Cyclic Neucl. Prot. Phosph. Res. 9: 281–296.

Ross, R., 1993, The pathogenesis of atherosclerosis: a perspective for the 1990s. Nature 362: 801- 809.

Rubanyi, G.M., Romero, J.C., and Vanhoutte, P.M., 1986, Flow-induced release of endothelium- derived relaxing factor. Am. J. Physiol. 250: H1145-H1149.

Scott-Burden, T., and Vanhoutte, P.M., 1993, The endothelium as a regulator of vascular smooth muscle proliferation. Circulation 87: V-51-V-55.

Siffert, W. and Düsing R., 1995, Sodium-proton exchange and primary hypertension. Hypertension 26: 649–655.

Yang, W., Ando, J., Korenaga, R., Toyo-oka, T., and Kamiya, A., 1994, Exogenous nitric oxide inhibits proliferation of cultured vascular endothelial cells. Biochem. Biophys. Res. Commun. 203: 1160–1167.

EFFECTS OF PUNCTURING ON THE MEASUREMENT OF LOCAL OXYGEN PRESSURE USING POLAROGRAPHIC MICROELECTRODES

H. Baumgärtl, W. Zimelka, and D. W. Lübbers

Max Planck Institut für molekulare Physiologie
Rheinlanddamm 201, 44139 Dortmund
Germany

INTRODUCTION

There are some reports in literature which document that methodological difficulties and errors may arise when polarographic needle electrodes are used to measure local pO_2 in semisolid media as, for example, organs, blood vessel walls, tissue homogenates, pellets of alginate or semisolid layers of polypeptides or polysaccharides. Different techniques of puncturing have been used to measure local pO_2 profiles within tissues. Earlier, mostly continuous punctures were used (see[1,2]). The electrode was mounted on a microscopic drive[3], on a micromanipulator moved manually or by a motor[4,5]. Measurements were performed mostly during insertion, but also during withdrawal[6–8]. Sometimes tissue was punctured first by a cannula and then, after withdrawal of the cannula, the pO_2 was measured within the puncturing channel[9]. It was observed with the insertion of the electrode, tissue was indented; thus, puncturing caused the structure of tissue to be changed. To reduce dimpling stepwise puncture by hand[10] or by a hydraulic microdrive was introduced, for example by using steps of a length of 50 or 100 μm[11,12] or of 10 μm[13]. Others proposed longitudinal vibration of the electrode, for example by 2 μm at 200–400 Hz[14]. There are now, for example, motor-driven stepping apparatus available (Nanostepper) which facilitate the application[2,15].

By puncturing 3% agar with a relatively large, glass insulated, recessed platinum electrode (tip diameter ca. 50 μm) using steps of 500 μm, Schuchhardt and Lösse (1973)[16] observed a variable pO_2 signal, mostly a decrease of the pO_2, although the pO_2 in the air equilibrated agar was constant. The variability of the signal could be reduced by inserting the electrode by smaller steps of 10 μm. The possible reason for such a variability of the signal was found by Baumgärtl et al. (1974)[17]. They showed that during continuous puncturing in concentrated agar solutions undissolved, microscopically visible particles were accumulating in front of the tip of the needle electrode. During accumulation the pO_2 signal decreased sharply, but when the tip penetrated the accumulated particles, the pO_2 signal increased suddenly to the expected value. It is well documented that filamental structures exist in gels (see[18]), which can influence the polarographically measured pO_2 signal[2,19–21].

To minimize the effect of accumulation of material and formation of a barrier in front of the tip of the electrode during insertion, a new technique of puncture was worked out: to release the pressure of puncturing the step of insertion was immediately followed by a step of withdrawal, for example: 2 steps of 50 μm "in" were followed by 1 step of 50 μm "out" (see[22]). Fleckenstein and Weiss (1984)[23] stressed that even an electrode with a relatively large outer diameter can be used if time of insertion and response time is short enough so that the pO_2 reading is obtained before any alterations can occur (see[24,25]).

Since our experiments with micro-needle electrodes had shown that in a medium containing polymeric substances the signal current of the pO_2 electrode can be influenced by the technique of puncture, we performed a series of experiments in gelatine gels of different concentrations and in tissue, comparing the results of continuous and stepwise puncturing with and without pressure release. Our results clearly show that the pucturing mode has a strong influence on the size of the local polarographic reduction current and that large artifacts can occur. To minimize artifacts an "optimal" technique of puncture has to be worked out for every special situation.

MATERIAL AND METHODS

1. Technique of pO_2 Measurements

All the pO_2 measurements in the following experiments were carried out using microcoaxial needle electrodes according to Baumgärtl and Lübbers[26,27]. The tip size of the needles, microscopically measured, was between 2 and 8 μm. The electrodes had a small recess filled with a double membrane of collodium and polystyrene. The tip of some electrodes was ground to an angle of 30 to 40° to facilitate the insertion into the medium to be measured (for more details see[2]).

The insertion of the calibrated electrode was done by an apparatus by which the electrode could be moved in short and quick perpendicular steps (Nanostepper. Bachhofer Reutlingen, Germany); the number and length of the steps as well as the velocity of insertion could be selected. To position the nanostepper it was fixed in a micromanipulator. The punctures were microscopically observed. The signal of the electrode was amplified and continuously recorded (30 mm/min, Servogor, Type SE 330).

2. Preparation of the Layer of Gelatine

For obtaining an appropriate layer of gelatine 3 to 6 foils of gelatine (Gelita, Deutsche Gelatine Fabriken Stoess AG, Ebersbach, Germany) were put in distilled water. After about 10 minutes the gelatine was transferred to boiling water and continuously stirred. Then, after 2 minutes of boiling the solution was filled into Petri dishes of glass or plastic so that a 15–20 mm thick layer was formed. The layers of gelatine looked completely clear, homogeneous and transparent. To investigate the structure the gelatine layer was sectioned by hand into ca. 300 μm thick slices. The slices were mounted on a slide and coloured by haematoxylin. For investigations with the scanning electron-microscope (Hitachi S-300) the slice was coated with a layer of 3 nm platinum and of 20 nm carbon.

3. Recording of pO_2 Profiles in the Lobe of Human Placenta during Dual *in Vitro* Perfusion

To study oxygen exchange processes in the human placenta the technique of dual invitro perfusion was applied (see[28,29]). pO_2 profiles were measured in 5 human placentae by puncturing the basal plate perpendicularly into the intervillous space (see Fig. 3). Puncturing was performed by stepwise penetration: 6 forward steps of 100 µm were immediately followed by 1 backward step of the same length. The time for the puncturing sequence was about 2 s. The next insertion followed after an interval of ca. 20 s. The electrode was withdrawn through the same channel in steps of 500 µm (5x100 µm).

4. Recording of pO_2 Profiles in the Brain

Tissue preparation and hemoglobin-free perfusion were done according to the technique of Heinrich et al. (1987)[30]. The tissue pO_2 was measured by puncturing the intact

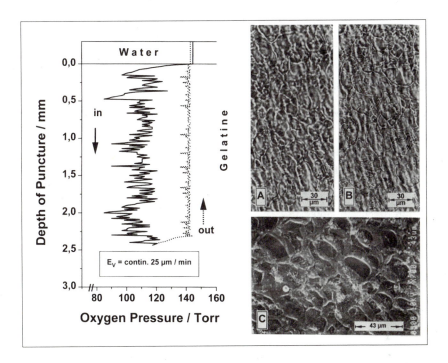

Figure 1. Polarographic signal of a pO_2 needle electrode during continuous puncturing of an air-equilibrated layer of 3% gelatine and the gelatine structure. Left side: Reduction currrent of the polarographic needle electrode (tip size: 2 µm) during continuous perpendicular insertion into a layer of 3% gelatine covered with water equilibrated with air (arrow in; solid line) as well as during continuous withdrawal of the electrode (arrow out; dotted line). E_v=speed of the movement of the electrode. Right side: gel structure of 3% gelatine dissolved in water. Microscopical (A, B) and scanning electron microscopical (C) pictures. The heterogeneity of the polarographic pO_2 signal during insertion was caused by the structural heterogeneity of the gelatine layer which was additionally changed by puncturing.

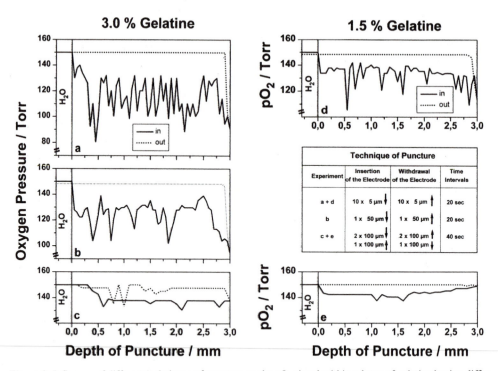

Figure 2. Influence of different techniques of puncture on the pO_2 signal within a layer of gelatine having different gelatine concentrations. The applied technique of puncture is documented in the table (right side). The measurements showed that by stepwise puncturing with pressure release the technique of puncture can be optimized.

dura of the left hemisphere of the blood-free perfused guinea pig brain (ca. 24°C) almost perpendicularly. The electrode was inserted by 2 steps of 100 μm and immediately withdrawn by 1 step of 100 μm to release the pressure. A step of 100 μm needed 10 ms. The penetration depth amounted to ca. 3 mm, whereby the electrode passed the gray matter and reached the white matter. Withdrawal of the electrode was carried out in steps of 100 μm. pO_2 readings were taken every 10 s. The measurement of a pO_2 profile over a distance of 3 mm needed about 5 min for insertion and another 5 min for withdrawal[31]. To record pO_2 profiles within the cortex of the normal blood-perfused brain the length of the steps of the puncture was only 50 μm (2 steps in, 1 step out). For technical details see Lübbers et al. (1994)[22].

RESULTS

1. pO_2 Measurements in Gelatine Layers

1.1. Continuous Insertion of the Polarographic Electrode. Figure 1 (left side) shows the pO_2 signal measured by a polarographic needle electrode during continuous vertical insertion (in) into a double layer of water and of 3% gelatine, as well as during continuous withdrawal (out). The speed of puncturing was E_v=25 μm/min. Every 12.5 μm a reading

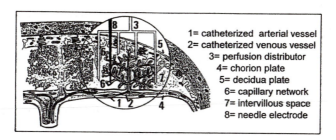

1= catheterized arterial vessel
2= catheterized venous vessel
3= perfusion distributor
4= chorion plate
5= decidua plate
6= capillary network
7= intervillous space
8= needle electrode

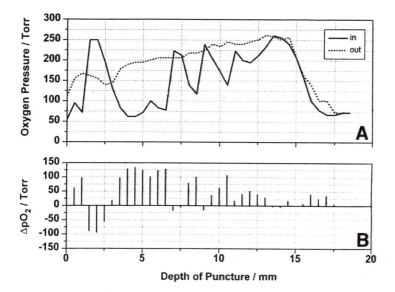

Figure 3. pO$_2$ profiles in the lobe of human placenta during dual in-vitro perfusion. Upper panel: Schematic drawing of a blood-free perfused human placenta. Middle panel: pO$_2$ profiles measured during insertion (in) and withdrawal (out) of the electrode. Heterogeneity is seen only during insertion. During withdrawal the pO$_2$ increases first similar to during insertion, but then remains distinctly larger and more homogeneous. Lower panel: pO$_2$ differences between the "in" and "out" traces.

was stored in a personel computer (measuring point). In the water layer the pO$_2$ signal remained constant; however, during insertion into the gelatine the polarographic signal distinctly decreased and became irregular. Over the whole distance of 2450 µm there were 53 peaks with rather large changes of local pO$_2$. For example, the steepest pO$_2$ increase between two measuring points was 32 Torr/12.5 µm and the steepest decrease 20 Torr/12.5 µm. The mean value measured in gelatine was 25% lower than in water (109±15 Torr as compared to 145.0 Torr).

When the electrode is withdrawn, it measures the pO$_2$ signal in the puncture. Within the channel the pO$_2$ signal increased and reached after 125 µm a rather stable value of 141±5 Torr which is close to the water value.

Figure 1 (right, A, B, C) shows microscopic pictures of the gelatine layer. In spite of the clear transparency of the gelatine there was a distinct network of fibers forming a heterogeneous structure. All the fibers had about the same diameters (3–6 μm), but different lengths. Distribution and concentration of the structural elements was very variable. Such a heterogeneous structure has a heterogeneous oxygen conductivity. Since the steepness of the calibration curve of the polarographic pO_2 electrode depends on the oxygen conductivity of the material to be measured, the pO_2 trace must mirror these local alterations of the oxygen transport during the insertion. Within the puncture channel, however, the remaining structural heterogeneity is rather small so that the pO_2 signal became almost constant during withdrawal.

A further question is whether the insertion itself could change the structure of the gelatine so that local heterogeneity increases. It was found that during continuous insertion local pressure does not remain constant, but increases gradually and then decreases, often suddenly. Although the tip of the electrode is small, during puncturing it collects several polymeric fibers forming a relative thick barrier in front of the penetrating electrode. During this process the puncturing pressure increases and reaches a value that is large enough to pierce the barrier. Since the forming of the barrier is connected with a change of the oxygen conductivity, this change becomes visible in the signal of the polarographic electrode.

Because of the strong interdependency between structure and puncturing technique, it was investigated in which way the profile of the pO_2 signal was influenced by changing the puncturing technique and by changing the structure by the concentration of the gelatine.

1.2. Stepwise Insertion. Because of the barrier formation the effect of different types of stepwise insertion was tested. In Fig. 2a the electrode was moved perpendicularly by 10 steps of 5 μm within 1 s followed by a pause of 20 s, and so on. The withdrawal in the puncturing channel occurred in the same way. In Fig. 2b the tip was moved in one step of 50 μm and in Fig. 2c in two steps of 100 μm. In Fig. 2c the puncturing pressure was released by withdrawing the electrode immediately by one step of 100 μm. As compared to continuous insertion, the irregularities of the pO_2 signal decreased by applying a stepwise insertion. Heterogeneity was additionally reduced by increasing the length of the steps. A further reduction occurred by releasing the puncturing pressure by a step backward, but this change of the moving direction can cause some irregularities during withdrawal of the electrode (Fig. 2c).

1.3. Changing the Structure. Since the density of the fibers within the gelatine gel can be changed by changing the concentration of gelatine (see[18]) pO_2 profiles in 1.5% gelatine were measured using the same puncturing techniques. Comparison of Fig. 2a with Fig. 2d and of Fig. 2c with Fig. 2e demonstrates that the signal traces were more homogeneous in 1.5% than in 3.0% gelatine.

The experiments show that

1. the mean pO_2 in the gelatine layer was always smaller than in the water layer, but during withdrawal the water value was approximated.
2. the mean pO_2 during insertion was always smaller than during withdrawal.
3. the difference between the mean pO_2 of water and of gelatine, as well as its variability, decreased by reduction of the gelatine concentration.
4. stepwise insertion with following pressure release and application of relative large steps reduced the variability of the mean pO_2.

2. pO$_2$ Measurements in Tissue

Since animal tissues always contain polymeric membranes, particles and networks of filaments it can be expected that measuring problems similar to those found in layers of gelatine occur when polarographic needles electrodes are used to measure local pO$_2$. Therefore, pO$_2$ profiles during insertion as well as during withdrawal were measured using the technique of stepwise puncturing with pressure release by immediate withdrawal of the electrode.

2.1. pO$_2$ Profiles in the Lobe of the Human Placenta. Figure 3 shows pO$_2$ profiles measured in the lobe of a human placenta during dual in-vitro hemoglobin-free perfusion. The cotyledon was prepared in such a way that the capillary network inside the villi was perfused via catheterized arterial and venous blood vessels (ca. 6 ml/min; schematic drawing within the circle, Fig. 3 upper panel). This network corresponds to the fetal blood flow compartment. The maternal blood circulates outside the villi in the so-called intervillous space. The intervillous space is perfused by a distributor having different catheters (empty tubes within the circle, Fig. 3 upper panel; ca. 20 ml/min). The perfusion medium of the fetal compartment was equilibrated with a gas mixture of 5% O$_2$+5% CO$_2$+90% N$_2$ and that of the maternal compartment with 95% O$_2$+5% CO$_2$. At the bottom, the intervillous space is closed by the chorion plate. Puncturing was performed by perpendicular, stepwise insertion of the electrode. The process of puncturing takes about 2 s; the new puncture follows after 20 s.

During the insertion (6 steps of 100 µm "in", 1 step of 100 µm "out") the pO$_2$ profile showed characteristic peaks and valleys (middle panel); however, during withdrawal it was more homogeneous. The pO$_2$ differences between the two traces are shown in the lower panel of Fig. 3. In Fig. 4 the measuring points of pO$_2$ profiles and the corresponding frequency histograms of 5 different placentae are drawn. The upper panel shows the values obtained during insertion, the lower panel the ones during withdrawal of the electrode. The solid line describes the mean pO$_2$ values calculated. The heterogeneity was always larger during insertion than during withdrawal. The mean pO$_2$ of 118±101 Torr measured during insertion was distinctly lower than the mean value of 163±116 Torr measured during withdrawal.

2.2. pO$_2$ Profiles within the Brain. By stepwise puncturing (2 steps of 100 µm "in", 1 step of 100 µm "out") 6 pO$_2$ profiles were measured in 6 hemoglobin-free perfused guinea brains (ca. 24°C). The perfusion medium was equilibrated with a gas mixture of 95% O$_2$+5% CO$_2$. Figure 5 shows the values measured during insertion and withdrawal. The solid line gives the mean pO$_2$ profiles. The frequency histogram of the values measured during the insertion showed the well known left-shifted pO$_2$ histogram; its mean pO$_2$ value is 139±76 Torr. During withdrawal the mean pO$_2$ value is larger and amounts to 196±112 Torr. The pO$_2$ distribution is less regular than during insertion.

In some cases it was observed that the trace "out" showed lower and more homogeneous pO$_2$ values than the corresponding trace "in". A careful check of the actual experimental situation revealed that in all these cases a pathological change of the brain had developed as, for example, brain edema (Fig. 6).

Since in blood-free perfused organs there is an artificially large pO$_2$ difference between inflowing arterial and outflowing venous pO$_2$ resulting in relatively large pO$_2$ gradients within the tissue (see Figs. 3 and 5) pO$_2$ profiles were also measured in normal blood-perfused brain (Fig. 7). The technique of puncture was slightly different: 2 steps of

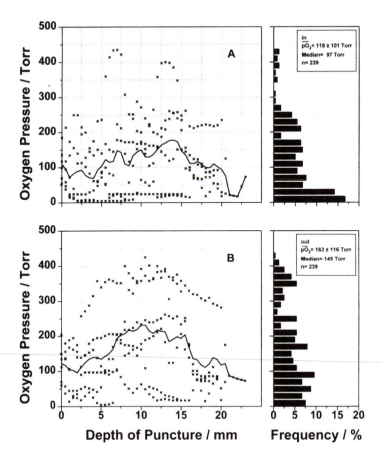

Figure 4. Pattern of local pO_2 distribution, pO_2 histograms and mean pO_2 profiles within the blood-free perfused human placenta measured during insertion and withdrawal of the electrode (dual perfusion). The measurements were performed in 5 human placentae using the same puncturing technique as in Fig. 3. The mean pO_2 as well as the mean pO_2 profile during insertion (upper panel) was smaller than during withdrawal (lower panel) of the electrode. Also, the number of values in the lower classes of the pO_2 histogram (class size 20 Torr) were larger during insertion than during withdrawal.

50 μm "in" were followed by 1 step of 50 μm "out". Also in the blood-perfused brain the trace "in" (Fig. 7A) showed a larger variability in the pO_2 values as compared to the values measured during withdrawal (Fig. 7B). Only at 10 locations (out of 60) was the pO_2 the same during insertion and withdrawal. Combining all measured pO_2 values and taking the local mean, a mean pO_2 profile was obtained (Fig. 7C) which looked somewhat similar to the profile of the insertion, but the amplitudes were smaller. The three frequency histograms demonstrate that in A, B and C a different distribution of pO_2 values was measured, although in all three cases the mean pO_2 was practically the same.

To compare the different results of the tissue measurements the cumulative histograms are displayed in Fig. 8. In normal blood-perfused brain (Fig. 8A) the trace "in" was rather similar to the trace "out" (pO_2 range 0–50 Torr) whereas in hemoglobin-free perfused brain (pO_2 range 0–500 Torr) the traces "in" and "out" were distinctly different, the

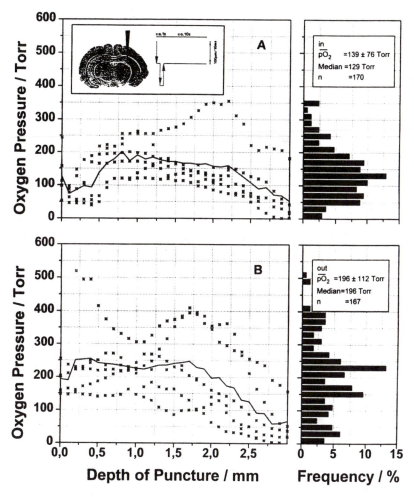

Figure 5. Pattern of local pO$_2$ distribution, pO$_2$ histograms and mean pO$_2$ profiles within the blood-free perfused guinea pig brain. The measurements were performed with pO$_2$ needle electrodes on 6 blood-free perfused guinea pig brains at 24°C. Technique of puncture: 2 steps of 100 μm "in", 1 step of 100 μm "out". The mean pO$_2$ as well as the mean pO$_2$ profile during insertion (upper panel) was smaller than during withdrawal (lower panel). During insertion the expected left-shifted pO$_2$ histogram was measured. The histogram during withdrawal showed a more irregular form.

"out" pO$_2$ values being larger, especially at higher pO$_2$ values (Fig. 8C). The pathological situation during a brain edema is shown in Fig. 8D. Also in the dual-perfused human placenta the "out" pO$_2$ values are larger than the "in" values (Fig. 8B). Both traces give valuable information about the oxygen supply of the tissue.

DISCUSSION AND CONCLUSION

The measurements in gelatine clearly demonstrated that the pO$_2$ signal of a rather thin, sharp polarographic needle electrode (tip diameter with reference electrode ca. 2–8

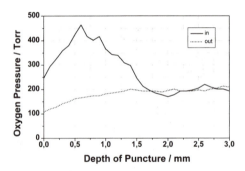

Figure 6. pO$_2$ profiles measured within a hemoglobin-free perfused guinea pig brain (18°C) during development of an edema. Same measuring technique as in Fig. 5. During the experiment an edema was developing. Under these conditions the mean pO$_2$ (181±26 Torr) and the pO$_2$ trace during withdrawal (dotted line) was smaller than the mean pO$_2$ (276±92 Torr) and the pO$_2$ trace (solid line) during insertion.

μm) was distunctly changed when the medium to be measured had a polymeric structure. By insertion the tip of the electrode can change the structure of the medium and form a barrier. Since this barrier can alter the oxygen exchange between electrode and medium, it changes the polarographic reduction current although the local pO$_2$ remains unchanged. Therefore, the measured pO$_2$ gradients are not real, but are "pseudo-pO$_2$ gradients". When the electrode penetrates the barrier it again reaches an environment with different diffusion conditions. These structural variations cause the large variations in the pO$_2$ signal. Such steep decreasing electrode currents followed by sudden increases have been observed by Baumgärtl et al (1974)[17] when the needle electrode was continuously advanced (150 μm/min) in different concentrated agar or agarose gel layers. It was remarkable that this phenomenon occurred at almost regular distances. After diminution of the gel concentration the intervals of the signal peaks were extended and at small concentrations the peaks were absent. During continuous puncturing these effects are the largest (Fig. 1). Similar pO$_2$ changes were reported when pellets of alginate were punctured[21]. The changes can be reduced by stepwise insertion (Fig. 2), but they did not disappear.

Klinowski et al. (1982)[32] found a continuously decreasing pO$_2$ signal when sterile gels of 1% or 2% agar were manually punctured by using steps of 35 μm in an angle of 45° (Transidyne electrode, tip size 3–7 μm). The authors explained their findings by an imbalance of the oxygen availability in the vicinity of the tip of the electrode and the oxygen consumption of the electrode. The polarographic electrode produces by its oxygen consumption an oxygen flux within the medium to be measured (see[17]). This O$_2$ flux causes a change of the local oxygen pressure; however the question is whether this effect is large enough to explain the measured profiles. It is interesting that a similar continuous decrease in air-equilibrated 3–5% alginate was found by Müller et al. (1994)[21] when alginate beads (3–5% concentration) were punctured by stepwise advancement of a needle electrode. Simultaneous microscopic observation, however, revealed that in this case during the insertion the alginate was compressed and accumulated in front of the electrode tip. This compression effect could be overcome by short withdrawals of the electrode. In all cases, however, the correct oxygen conductivity of the medium has to be known, i.e. the proper calibration curve, to obtain correct results.

Figures 1 and 2 show that in gelatine layers the comparison between the pO$_2$ trace obtained during insertion and withdrawal can be used to judge the quality of the measure-

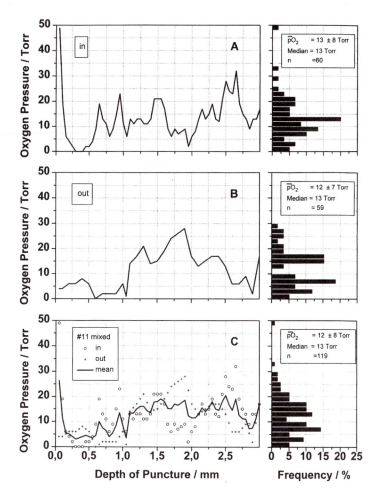

Figure 7. pO$_2$ profiles of a normal, blood perfused guinea pig brain with intact dura (37°C). Technique of puncture: 2 steps of 50 μm "in", 1 step of 50 μm "out". pO$_2$ histograms: class size 2 Torr. Upper panel: pO$_2$ profile and histogram during insertion of the electrode. Middle panel: pO$_2$ profile and histogram during withdrawal of the electrode. Lower panel: mean pO$_2$ profile calculated from the pO$_2$ values measured during insertion as well as during withdrawal. The heterogeneity during insertion was larger than during withdrawal. The mean pO$_2$ values were practically the same. The histograms were somewhat irregular, but the number of measuring values are small.

ment. Greenwood and Goodman (1967)[33], measuring pO$_2$ profiles in a yeast-agar model, found that the pO$_2$ during insertion was smaller than during withdrawal of the electrode. They explained the difference by assuming that the position of the electrode was different during insertion and withdrawal. Our experiments show that structural changes can also be responsible for such findings. Under some conditions the withdrawal trace mirrors the local pO$_2$ distribution without the artefacts caused by the insertion and, therefore, can be used as a check.

Measurements within the tissue are more difficult to judge. The pressure in front of the tip of the electrode which is necessary to penetrate the tissue is ca. $4 \times 10^7 Pa$[34]. This is sufficient to produce all the effects observed during puncturing the gelatine layers. Since it

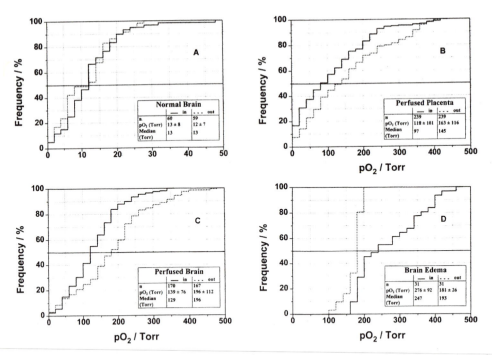

Figure 8. Cumulative pO_2 histograms measured by polarographic micro-needle electrodes during insertion and withdrawal of the electrode. Solid line (trace "in"): measuring values during insertion. Dotted line (trace "out"): measuring values during withdrawal. A: Normal blood-perfused guinea pig brain (Fig. 7). The trace "in" was similar to the trace "out". B: Hemoglobin-free perfused human placenta (Fig. 4). Similar traces in the lower pO_2 range, but large differences at higher pO_2 values. C: Hemoglobin-free perfused guinea pig brain (Fig. 5). Trace "in" and trace "out" were distinctly different. The trace "out" was moved to higher pO_2 values. D: Hemoglobin-free perfused guinea pig brain (Fig. 6). The trace "out" characterized a pathological situation: brain edema with low pO_2 values.

is well documented that large local pO_2 gradients occur within tissues the decision between real and pseudo-pO_2 gradients is sometimes difficult. Figure 3 shows the pO_2 profiles within the perfused human placenta. After penetration of the decidua plate the pO_2 increases penetrating the intervillous space (maternal compartment). Approaching the fetal compartment (capillary network) it decreases. During further insertion this pattern repeats. During withdrawal the pO_2 profile first equals the insertion pO_2, but then it remains larger and more constant, probably the tip of the electrode mostly being in the more uniform intervillous space. In Fig. 4 (profiles of 5 placentae) it can be seen that large differences are found not only during insertion, but also during withdrawal. The mean pO_2 measured during insertion is distinctly smaller than that during withdrawal (118 ± 101 Torr vs. 163 ± 116 Torr), however, the mean pO_2 profiles are similar. It demonstrates that for a real analysis a sufficient number of measurements are necessary[35].

Applying an appropriate puncturing technique, the pO_2 profiles and histograms measured within the blood-free perfused guinea pig brain ($24°C$) during insertion of the electrode (Fig. 5) corresponded well to values published in literature (see[36]). Because of the large, naturally occurring heterogeneity of local pO_2 it is difficult to judge whether compression effects and/or tissue damage had still affected the signal. To minimize tissue damage, slender electrodes with a tip size of about 1–3 μm should be used; but even such a small electrode produces a channel within the tissue. Because of the elasticity of the tissue the tip of the electrode, penetrating the interstitium, often displaces only cell bodies, capillaries or other structural elements without much damage. Then, during retraction of the electrode, the normal position is approximately restored so that this part of the channel is difficult to observe microscopically. But the compression and displacement of the tissue by the shaft of the electrode causes distinct and microscopically visible changes of the tissue structure. Such changes could also be documented by histological investigations[37–39] (see[1,2]). These changes increase with time and signs of inflammation can be seen[1]. Without compression effects and with only a small tissue damage the pO_2 profiles during insertion and withdrawal should be similar. Figure 5 shows that the mean pO_2 during insertion was smaller than during retraction, probably because tissue fluid could easier penetrate into the open electrode channel. The mean pO_2 profiles showed a similar structure, but by averaging part of the structural heterogeneity will be eliminated. The left-shifted histogram (A) measured during insertion became more irregular during withdrawal (B). We think that such similarities between "in" and "out" profiles can be used to check the functional state of the tissue. For example, when an edema had developed during perfusion the mean pO_2 was smaller during withdrawal and the pO_2 profile became more homogeneous (Fig. 6).

In principle, the situation of the normal blood-perfused brain (Fig. 7) is similar to that of the blood-free perfused brain, but the oxygen carrying capacity of blood reduces the range of the measured pO_2 values from 0-ca.500 Torr to 0-ca.50 Torr. The mean pO_2 values during insertion and withdrawal were practically the same. Consequently, the pO_2 gradients were smaller. The mean pO_2 profile which is obtained by combining "in" and "out" values (Fig. 7C) had —as expected— smaller amplitudes than profile A or B, but it lay within the normal range[22].

Our experiments show that the structure of the semisolid medium, or of the organ, does influence magnitude and dynamics of the measured local pO_2 values if the local pO_2 is measured during the insertion of the electrode, even if the tip has a diameter of only 1 to 5 μm. The best results were obtained when, before the reading, the pressure was released, e.g. by a step backward. The experiments with different concentrations of gelatine and different techniques of puncturing demonstrated clearly that the technique of puncture has to be adapted to the actual medium to obtain optimal results. The same holds for tissue measurements. An optimization can be achieved by choosing a sufficient speed of insertion, an appropriate length, as well as a suitable sequence of the steps. Sometimes, additionally, the angle of puncturing can be important. In many cases it is helpful to measure not only the pO_2 during the insertion, but also during withdrawal of the electrode.

REFERENCES

1. Silver, I A, Problems of the investigation of tissue oxygen microenvironment, *Adv Chem Ser* 118:343–351, (1973)
2. Baumgärtl, H, Systematic investigations of needle electrode properties in polarographic measurements of local tissue pO_2 , *in:* "Clinical Oxygen Pressure Measurement", A M Ehrly, J Hauss, R Huch,eds., Springer Verlag, Heidelberg New York, pp. 17–42, (1987)
3. Kunze, K, Die lokale, kontinuierliche Sauerstoffdruckmessung in der menschlichen Muskulatur, *Pflügers Arch* 292:151–160, (1966)
4. Leichtweiss, H-P, Lübbers, D W, Weiss, Ch, Baumgärtl, H, Reschke, W, The oxygen supply of the rat kidney: measurements of intrarenal pO_2, *Pflügers Arch* 309:328–349, (1969)
5. Erdmann, W, Microelectrode studies in the brain of fetal rats and new born rats, *Adv Exp Med. Biol* 94:455–461, (1978)

6. Cross, B A, Silver, I A, Some factors affecting oxygen tension in the brain and other organs, *Proc Roy Soc* 156:483–499, (1962)

7. Schröder, W, Die Messung des Sauerstoffdruckes in der Skelettmuskulatur - eine quantitative Methode zur Kontrolle der Sauerstoffversorgung und der Funktion der termninalen Muskelstrombahn, *Herz/Kreisl* 10(3): 146–153, (1978)

8. Baumgärtl, H, Ehrly, A M, Saeger-Lorenz, K, Lübbers, D W, Erste Ergebnisse intrakutaner Messungen von pO_2-Profilen, *in:* "Klinische Sauerstoffdruckmessung", A M Ehrly, J Hauss, R Huch, eds., Münchner Wissenschaftliche Publikation, München, pp 110–116, (1985)

9. Evans, N T S, Naylor, R F D, The effect of oxygen breathing and readiotherapy upon the tissue oxygen tension of some human tumors, *Br J Radiol* 34:418–425, (1963)

10. Schuchhardt, S, pO_2-Messung im Myocard des schlagenden Herzens, *Pflügers Arch* 322:83–94, (1971)

11. Nair, P, Whalen, W J, Buerk, D, pO_2 of cat cerebral cortex: response to breathing N_2 and 100% O_2, *Microvascular Research* 9:158–165, (1975)

12. Fuji, T, Baumgärtl, H, Lübbers, D W, Limiting section of guinea pig olfactory cortical slices studied from tissue pO_2 values and electrical activities, *Pflügers Arch* 393:83–87, (1982)

13. Smith, R H, Guilbeau, E J, The oxygen tension field within a discrete volume of cerebral cortex, *Microvascular Research* 13:233–240, (1977)

14. Kanabus, E W, Feldstein, C, Crawford, D W, Excursion of vibrating microelectrodes in tissue, *J Appl Physiol* 48:737–741, (1980)

15. Okada, Y, Mückenhoff, K, Holtermann, G, Acker, H, Scheid, P, Depth profiles of pH and pO_2 in the isolated brain stem-spinal cord of the neonatal rat, *Respiration Physiology* 93:315–326, (1993)

16. Schuchhardt, S, Loesse, B, Methodological problems when measuring with pO_2 needle electrodes in semisolid media, *in:* "Oxygen supply", M Kessler, D F Bruley, L C Clark, D W Lübbers, I A Silver, J Strauss, eds., Urban & Schwarzenberg, München-Berlin-Wien,pp. 108–109, (1973)

17. Baumgärtl, H, Grunewald, W, Lübbers, D W, Polarographic determination of the oxygen partial pressure field by Pt microelectrodes using the O_2 field in front of a Pt macroelectrode as a model, *Pflügers Arch* 347:49–61, (1974)

18. Bezrukov, M G, Die Bildung der Raumstruktur von Proteingelen, *Angew Chem* 91: 634–646, (1979)

19. Crawford, D W, Cole, M A, Performance evaluation of recessed microcathodes: criteria for tissue pO_2 measurement, *J Appl Physiol* 58(4):1400–1405, (1985)

20. Beunink, J, Baumgärtl, H, Zimelka, W, Rehm, H-J, Determination of oxygen gradients in single Ca-alginate beads by means of oxygen-microelectrodes, *Experientia* 45:1041–1047, (1989)

21. Müller, W, Winnefeld, A, Kohls, O, Scheper, T, Zimelka, W, Baumgärtl, H, Real and pseudo oxygen gradients in Ca-alginate beads monitored during polarographic pO_2-needle microelectrodes, *Biotechnology and Bioengineering* 44:617–625, (1994)

22. Lübbers, D W, Baumgärtl, H, Zimelka, W, Heterogeneity and stability of local pO_2 distribution within the brain tissue, *Adv Exp Med Biol* 345:567–574, (1994)

23. Fleckenstein, W, Weiss, Ch, A comparison of pO_2- histograms from rabbit hindlimb muscles obtained by simultaneous measurements with hypodermic needle electrodes and with surface electrons, *Adv Exp Med Biol* 169:447–455, (1985)

24. Fleckenstein, W, Die Entwicklung der Feinnadel-Gewebe-pO_2-Histographie zum klinisch eingesetzten Diagnoseverfahren, *Klinikum der freien Universität Berlin* 91–105, (1986)

25. Boekstegers, P, Fleckenstein, W, Rosport, A, Ruschewsky, W, Braun, U, Überwachung der Sauerstoffversorgung des Skelettmuskels und der Gesamtsauerstoffaufnahme bei koronarchirurgischen Eingriffen, *Anaesthesist* 37:287–296, (1988)

26. Baumgärtl, H, Lübbers, D W, Platinum needle electrode for polarographic measurement of oxygen and hydrogen, *in:* "Oxygen supply", M Kessler, D F Bruley, L C Clark, D W Lübbers, I A Silver, J Strauss, eds., Urban & Schwarzenberg, München-Berlin-Wien,pp. 130–136, (1973)

27. Baumgärtl, H, Lübbers, DW, Microcoaxial needle sensor for polarographic measurement of local O_2 pressure in the cellular range of living tissue. Its construction and properties, *in:* "Polarographic Oxygen Sensors", Gnaiger/Forstner, eds., Springer-Verlag, Berlin Heidelberg, 37–65, (1983)

28. Schneider, H, Huch, A, Dual in vitro perfusion of an isolated lobe of human placenta: method and instrumentation, *Contrib Gynecol Obstet* 13:40, (1985)

29. Baumgärtl, H, Schneider, H, Huch, R, Oxygen supply in isolated lobe of human placenta during dual in vitro perfusion with microcoxial needle electrodes, *in:* "Clinical Oxygen Pressure Measurement", A M Ehrly, W Fleckenstein, J Hauss, R Huch, Blackwell, eds., Ueberreuter Wissenschaft, Berlin, pp. 425–431, (1990)

30. Heinrich, U, Hoffmann, J, Baumgärtl, H, Yu B, Lübbers, D W, Oxygen supply of the blood-free perfused guinea pig brain at three different temperatures. *Adv Exp Med Bio.* 191:77–84, (1985)

31. Baumgärtl, H, Heinrich, U, Lübbers, D W, Oxygen supply of the blood-free perfused guinea-pig brain in normo- and hypothermia measured by the local distribution of oxygen pressure, *Pflügers Arch* 414:228–234, (1989)

32. Klinowski, J, Korsner, S E, Winlove, C P, Problems associated with the micropolarographic measurement of the arterial wall pO_2, *Cardiovasc Res* 16:448–456, (1982)

33. Greenwood, D J, Goodman,D, Direct measurements of the distribution of oxygen in soil aggregates and in columns of fine soil crumbs, *J Soil Sci* 18:182–196, (1967)

34. Himmelberg, H, Mechanisches Verhalten von Mikrostichelektroden zur Sauerstoffdruckmessung im Muskelgewebe, Dissertation, Münster (1983)

35. Grunewald, W A, Sowa, W, Capillary structures and O_2 supply to tissue: an analysis with a digital diffusion model as applied to the skeletal muscle, *Rev Physiol Biochem Pharmacol* 77:150–209, (1976)

36. Heinrich, U, Hoffmann, J, Lübbers, D W, Quantitative evaluation of optical reflection spectra of blood-free perfused guinea pig brain using a nonlinear multicomponent analysis, *Pflügers Arch* 409:152–157, (1987)

37. Schäfer, D, Höper, J, Alterations in rat liver cells and tissue caused by needle electrodes, *in:*" Ion and Enzyme Electrodes in Biology and Medicine", M Kessler, L C Clark Jr, D W Lübbers, I A Silver, W Simon, eds., Urban & Schwarzenberg, München, pp. 217–222, (1976)

38. Nair, M A, Spande, J I, Whalen, W J, Marking the tip location of pO_2 microelectrodes or glass micropipettes, *J Appl Physiol* 49: 916–918, (1980)

39. Cole, M A, Bernick, S, Warner, N E, Puffer, H W, Crawford, D E, Identification and evaluation of histopathology at microcathode puncture sites, *Microvasc Res* 25: 229, (1983)

67

COMPARISONS OF MEASUREMENTS OF pO_2 IN TISSUE *IN VIVO* BY EPR OXIMETRY AND MICRO-ELECTRODES

Fuminori Goda,[1,3] Julia A. O'Hara,[2] Ke Jian Liu,[1] Erik S. Rhodes,[2] Jeffrey F. Dunn,[1] and Harold M. Swartz[1]

[1]Department of Radiology
[2]Department of Medicine (Radiation oncology)
Dartmouth-Hitchcock Medical Center
Hanover, New Hampshire 03755
[3]The First Department of Surgery
Kagawa Medical School, 1750–1 Ikenobe Miki
Kagawa, 761–07 Japan

INTRODUCTION

Polarographic micro-electrode measurements are very useful for measuring pO_2 *in vivo*, especially for measurements of the variation of pO_2 within a tumor (1,2,8). This method has several advantages, including: it is the only direct method currently in extended use in the clinical setting; it can provide data on microscopic heterogeneity; and it is fairly widely available. While the micro-electrode method has become a type of "gold standard" for measurement of pO_2 in tissues, it has some limitations and disadvantages: it can be technically difficult; it has limited resolution at the very low levels of pO_2 that are important for many clinically relevant processes; and it can perturb the tissues significantly, especially when used in repeated studies to monitor pO_2 in tissues over time. Repeated measurements are especially desirable to follow the effect on tissue pO_2 after treatment with some drugs (e.g. anti-cancer drugs and anesthetics) and radiation, the effects of acute and chronic ischemia, and changes in respiratory factors. Electron paramagnetic resonance (EPR) oximetry appears to offer some complimentary advantages for such studies: it can monitor pO_2 continuously and/or repeatedly at the exactly the same localized area in tissue *in vivo* without the need for anesthesia; it can resolve small differences in pO_2 even at the very low levels that occur pathophysiologically; and it can be used in a variety of settings.

EPR oximetry is based on the effect of oxygen on EPR spectra of paramagnetic substances. We have investigated the physical properties, the biological and histological effects, and the safety of several oxygen sensitive EPR probes, such as fusinite, India ink, and lithium phthalocyanine (LiPc). They appear to have very suitable properties for measuring and monitoring pO_2 *in vivo* as described in detail in our previous publications (3–9). Briefly, the oxygen sensitive probes are paramagnetic materials which have EPR spectra whose peak-to-peak line widths are broadened only by paramagnetic gas, such as oxygen. These probes are calibrated using a Clark type micro-electrode and mixtures of gases (N_2 : O_2) of known pO_2. EPR spectra are obtained from the probe in implanted tissue using an *in vivo* EPR spectrometer. After line widths of EPR spectra are measured, the pO_2 values are obtained from the calibration curves.

In order to relate these two potentially complementary methods, it is important to compare pO_2 values in vivo measured by EPR oximetry, with pO_2 values measured at the same area by micro-electrodes. The purpose of this study is to obtain such data.

MATERIALS AND METHODS

Animals

These studies were carried out using three different tissues; muscle, tumor, and brain. Six-week old male BALB/C mice (Charles River, Wilmington, MA) were used to measure the pO_2 of femoral muscles. Transplanted mouse mammary adenocarcinoma (MTG-B) tumors, grown on 6-week old female C3H/HeJ mice (Jackson Laboratories, Bar Harbor, ME), were used to measure pO_2 of tumors. A subcutaneous injection (50 µl) of the tumor cell suspension (about 1.0×10^6 cells) in the right flank, resulted in tumors of approximately 7 to 8 mm in diameter 10 days post transplantation. For measurements of pO_2 of brains, we used male Wistar rats (175–200 g) (Charles River, Wilmington, MA).

EPR Oximetry and EPR Probes

A home-made EPR spectrometer equipped with a microwave bridge operating at 1.2 GHz (L-band) was used for all *in vivo* EPR measurements. Details on the extended loop resonator and L-band bridge are described in a previous publication (10). The EPR probes, India ink (Higgins 4485, Newark, NJ) or LiPc, were implanted in the tissue 12–24 h before making initial measurements of pO_2. Sterilized India ink particles (mean diameter < 1 mm) were suspended in isotonic saline and 20 µl of a suspension (100 mg/ml of India ink) was implanted into the femoral muscles or the tumors at a depth of 2 mm from the surface. An automatic injection device (Hamilton Co., Reno, Nevada) fitted with a 27 gauge needle was used for implantation. Three crystals of LiPc (diameter 100 µm) were implanted into the rat brain through the temporal bone using a 27 gauge needle.

Typical settings for the spectrometer were: magnetic field, 425 Gauss; modulation frequency, 27 KHz; modulation amplitude, one third or less of the line width, such as 0.20 - 0.50 Gauss (for India ink) or 0.030 Gauss (for LiPc); incident microwave power, 15 mW (for India ink) or 3 mW (for LiPc). The rats and mice were restrained in a plastic holder with a hole through which the leg, tumor, or head were exposed. The detecting EPR coil was positioned over the leg (for measurements in muscle), tumor or head (for brain measurement) and five spectra were recorded per animal (30 seconds or 60 seconds per spectrum, total measurement time was less than 10 min, including positioning of the animal and adjustment of the spectrometer). Spectral line widths of India ink were measured and the pO_2 values calculated from a calibration curve of line width at various pO_2.

The calibration curve of pO$_2$ vs. line width of India ink or LiPc was determined using a Bruker, ER 220D-SRC EPR spectrometer (9.6 GHz, X-band) and a commercial oxygen analyzer (Sensor Medics Co., Model OM-11, Anaheim CA). The calibration procedure was the same as described previously, including verification of its validity for 1.2 GHz studies (3,4,6,7).

Micro-Electrode

Clark style micro-electrodes with 25–75 mm outside tip diameters (Diamond General Corp., Ann Arbor, MI) were used to measure pO$_2$ and to compare with measurements made by EPR oximetry. Tissue measurements were made by making a small incision in the skin over the region of interest and inserting the electrode with a micromanipulator. Currents were recorded using a Keithley Model 485 picoammeter (Cleveland, OH). Calibration curves relating pAmps to pO$_2$ were obtained before and after each series of measurements (in air equilibrated saline and either N$_2$ or He bubbled, deoxygenated saline). Two-point *in vivo* calibrations also were performed following Dewhirst's procedure (11). Zero values were periodically checked by sacrificing the animal with the electrode in place and waiting for a stable tissue zero.

Since micro-electrode measurements of pO$_2$ in tissue generally require the use of anesthesia, the time dependent changes of pO$_2$ after anesthesia (90 mg/kg ketamine and 9 mg/kg xylazine, i.m.) were monitored using EPR oximetry. We used repeated EPR oximetry to determine the period in which pO2 was stable and made the comparison measurements of pO$_2$ using both techniques during that period. The electrode was inserted into the same region as the EPR probe either by retracing the path by which the probe was injected, or by using MRI to locate the position of the probe and guide the insertion of the electrode. We also monitored the respiratory rate and animal body temperature, the physiological factors that potentially could affect pO$_2$. Body temperature was monitored in the rectum at a depth of 10 mm using a YSI Model 511 Reusable Temperature probe (Yellow Springs Instruments, Yellow Springs, OH).

RESULTS AND DISCUSSION

To compare directly the pO$_2$ values in the tissues using these two techniques, we obtained data from the same site, under the same conditions. This required the use of anesthesia in order to insert the microelectrodes into the mice and, therefore, we needed to determine the effects of the anesthesia with the aim of establishing conditions where, if there were effects from the anesthesia, these effects would be stable during the time required to make measurements with the two methods. Using EPR oximetry, we were able to assess the time dependent effects on pO$_2$ of anesthesia and the changes of animal body temperature. Figure 1 shows the changes of pO$_2$ in the brain (rat) or skeletal muscle (mouse), respiratory rates, body temperatures in rats (A) and mice (B) after anesthesia with and without control of body temperature.

Rat Brain

The pO$_2$ decreased significantly 5 min after anesthesia, then these pO$_2$ values slightly decreased in the next 30 min, then there were no significant further changes during the next 30 min. Note animals in which the body temperature was controlled (mean

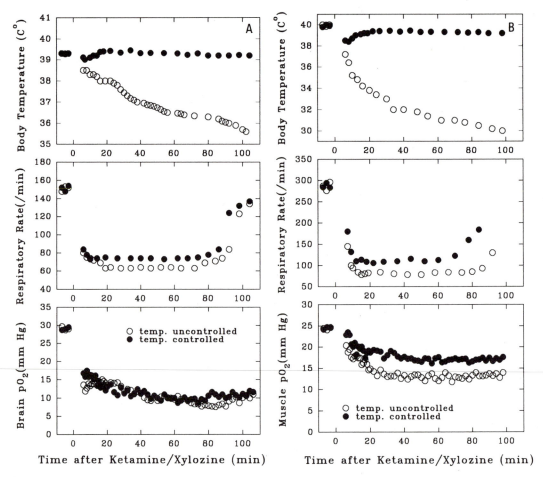

Figure 1. Changes of pO$_2$ in rat brain (A) and mouse muscle (B), body temperature, and respiratory rate after anesthesia with/without control of body temperature.

pO$_2$ value: 11.8 ± 0.3 mm Hg) had significantly higher (p < 0.05) pO$_2$ values and slightly slower reduction of pO$_2$ than animals in which the body temperature was uncontrolled (mean pO$_2$ values: 11.0 ± 0.3 mm Hg). These pO$_2$ values differed significantly (p<0.0001) from the pO$_2$ values of unanesthetized animals (mean pO$_2$ values: 29.8 ± 1.4 mm Hg).

Measurements of pO$_2$ in Muscle

Animals in which the body temperature was controlled (mean pO$_2$ value: 18.1 ± 0.4 mm Hg) had a significantly higher (p < 0.01) pO$_2$ value than that of animals whose body temperature was not controlled (mean pO$_2$ values: 14.3 ± 0.3 mm Hg) when the pO$_2$ was stable. These pO$_2$ values also were much lower than that of unanesthetized animals (mean pO$_2$ value: 24.2 ± 0.3 mm Hg). In the absence of procedures to control the body temperature, the anesthetic procedure led to a greater decrease of pO$_2$ in mice muscle.

Figure 2A shows the changes of pO$_2$ in individual tumors after anesthesia. Control animals received only saline. The average tumor volume was 128 mm^3 (7 days after trans-

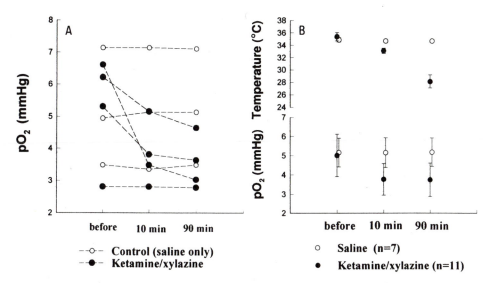

Figure 2. Changes of pO$_2$ in tumors (measured by EPR) and body temperature in mice after ketamine/xylazine anesthesia. A. Changes of pO$_2$ in representative individual animals; B. Average values of pO$_2$ in tumors and body temperature.

plantation). They had a variation of baseline pO$_2$ and/or pO$_2$ after anesthesia; this reflected a different local environment at the location of the EPR probes in the tumors. Some tumors had very low initial pO$_2$ values and these did not change after anesthesia. Figure 2B presents the average values of pO$_2$ in tumors (n=7) measured by EPR oximetry: 5.0 ± 1.1 mm Hg (before anesthesia), 3.8 ± 0.8 mm Hg (10 min after anesthesia) and 3.7 ± 0.9 mm Hg (90 min after anesthesia). The pO$_2$ decreased significantly ($p < 0.05$) 10 min after an-

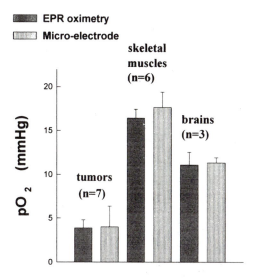

Figure 3. Comparison of pO$_2$ values in several organs measured by EPR oximetry and micro-electrodes. These measurements were performed under ketamine/xylazine anesthesia.

esthesia, but showed no significant further reduction during the next 90 min. The pO_2 in the unanesthetized group (received only saline) did not change during that period, irrespective of the pO_2 value prior to injection. The body temperature decreased significantly 10 min after anesthesia (from 38.8 ± 0.8 °C to 34.1 ± 1.4 °C) and decreased further to 28.1 ± 2.1 °C at 90 min after anesthesia, while the pO_2 did not decrease further (Figure 2(B)).

Figure 3 summarizes the data comparing measurements of pO_2 by EPR and microelectrodes. The times used to compare the pO_2 were chosen to occur during a period when the pO_2 was relatively stable. We measured with EPR at 30 min and with microelectrodes at 40 min after anesthesia in rat brain and mouse muscle. In tumors the measurements by EPR were made at 10 min and by micro-electrode at 30 min after anesthesia. The mean values of pO_2 measured by EPR oximetry vs. micro-electrode were 3.8 ± 0.8 vs. 4.0 ± 2.4 mm Hg (n=7) in tumors, 16.8 ± 1.0 vs. 17.2 ± 1.7 mm Hg (n=6) in muscles, 11.1 ± 1.4 vs. 11.3 ± 0.7 mm Hg (n=3) in brains. The values of pO_2 measured by EPR oximetry and micro-electrodes were not significantly different (paired t-test).

These data indicate that pO_2 measurements using EPR and micro-electrode methods produce comparable results in these three tissues. The mean values of pO_2 from the same sites in tissue under the same conditions after anesthesia measured by EPR oximetry and micro-electrode were essentially identical. Thus it seems feasible to select the method that is the most appropriate for the particular experimental needs. The positive aspects of EPR oximetry include its non-invasive nature (after insertion of the paramagnetic materials), accuracy, sensitivity, non-toxic and non-perturbing nature, and capability of providing continuous and/or repeated measurements from the same site. However, unlike the micro-electrodes, EPR cannot provide a histograph of variation of pO_2s over various regions of the tissue. There are likely to be some situations where it will be particularly advantageous to use both methods during the course of an experiment.

ACKNOWLEDGMENTS

This work was supported by ACS Grant BE-186 (JO'H), ACS IRG-1571 (JFD) from the NCCC, the Core Grant of the Norris Cotton Cancer Center CA23108, NIH Grant GM51630 (HMS) and used the facilities of the IERC at the Dartmouth supported by NIH grant RR-01811.

REFERENCE

1. Vaupel, P., Frinak, S., and O'Hara, M., Direct measurement of reoxygenation in malignant mammary tumors after a single large dose of irradiation. Adv. Exp. Med. Biol., *180:* 773–782, 1984.
2. Okunieff, P., Hoeckel, M., Dunphy, E. P., Schlenger, K., Knoop, C., and Vaupel, P., Oxygen tension distributions are sufficient to explain the local response of human breast tumors treated with radiation alone. Int. J. Radiat. Oncol. Biol. Phys., *26:* 631–636, 1993.
3. Swartz, H. M., Boyer, S., Brown, D., Chang, K., Gast, P., Glockner, J. F., Hu, H., Liu, K. J., Moussavi, M., Nilges, M., Norby, S. W., Smirnov, A., Vahidi, N., Walczak, T., Wu, M., and Clarkson, R. B., The use of EPR for the measurement of the concentration of oxygen in vivo in tissues under physiologically pertinent conditions and concentrations. Adv. Exp. Med. Biol., *317:* 221–228. 1992.
4. Liu, K. J., Gast, P., Moussavi, M., Norby, S. W., Vahidi, N., Walczak, T., Wu, M., and Swartz, H. M., Lithium phthalocyanine; a probe for electron paramagnetic resonance oximetry in viable biological systems. Proc. Natl. Acad. Sci. U S A, *90:* 5438–5442, 1993.
5. Bacic, G., Liu, K. J., O'Hara, J. A., Harris, R. D., Szybinski, K., Goda, F., and Swartz, H. M., Oxygen tension in a murine tumor: a combined EPR and MRI study. Magn. Reson. Med., *30:* 568–572, 1993.

6. Swartz, H. M., Liu, K. J., Goda, F., and Walczak, T., India ink: a potential clinically applicable EPR oximetry probe. Magn. Reson. Med., *31:* 229–232, 1994.

7. Goda, F., Liu, K. J., Walczak, T., O'Hara, J. A., Jiang, J., and Swartz, H. M., In vivo oximetry using EPR and India ink. Magn. Reson. Med., *33:* 237–245, 1995.

8. Goda, F., O'Hara, J. A., Rhodes, E. S., Liu, K. J., Dunn, J. F., Bacic, G., and Swartz, H. M., Changes of oxygen tension in experimental tumors after a single dose of X-ray irradiation. Cancer Research, *55:* 2249–2252, 1995.

9. O'Hara, J. A., Goda, F., Liu, K. J., Bacic, G., Hoopes, P. J., and Swartz, H. M., Oxygenation in a murine tumor following radiation; an in vivo electron paramagnetic resonance oximetry study. Radiation Research, 1995. *in press*

10. Nilges, M. J., Walczak, T., and Swartz, H. M., 1 GHz in vivo EPR spectrometer operating with a surface probe. Phys. Med., *5:* 195–201, 1989.

11. Dewhirst, M. W., Oliver, R., Tso, C. Y., Gustafson, C., Secomb, T., and Gross, J. F., Heterogeneity in tumor microvascular response to radiation. Int. J. Radiat. Oncol. Biol. Phys., *18:* 559–568, 1990.

68

CATCHMENT DEPTHS OF SURFACE ELECTRODES FOR H₂ AND O₂ IN TISSUE

D. K. Harrison

Vascular Laboratory, Directorate of Medical Physics
Ninewells Hospital and Medical School
Dundee, DD1 9SY, United Kingdom

1. INTRODUCTION

Polarographic electrodes have been used for many years to measure oxygen partial pressure (pO_2) in various organs and tissues, often in animal experiments, and have greatly contributed to the understanding of local mechanisms controlling tissue oxygen supply. Five years ago we reported the use of a hydrogen clearance technique using a multichannel electrode (Kessler & Lübbers, 1966, multiwire surface electrode, MDO) adapted to the detection of partial pressure of hydrogen (pH_2) in order to measure capillary blood flow in skeletal muscle (Harrison & Kessler, 1989a). This development meant that measurements of both blood flow and pO_2 could be made in similar volumes of tissue. Furthermore, methods were devised whereby local O_2 uptake rate could be calculated (Harrison *et al.* 1989; Harrison *et al.* 1990).

Apart from their application in blood gas analysers, the most widespread clinical application of the oxygen electrode has been the transcutaneous measurement of oxygen ($tcpO_2$) in neonates and in patients with peripheral vascular disease. Recently we have described a new transcutaneous hydrogen ($tcpH_2$) clearance technique for measuring capillary blood flow in human skin (Harrison *et al.* 1994).

In all of these applications, whether measuring H_2 or O_2, the question arises as to what part of the tissue is actually being interrogated. This is particularly important if these methods are being used in conjunction with optical techniques (Newton *et al.* 1994).

2. METHODS

A method for calculating the catchment depths of surface polarographic pH_2 and pO_2 sensors was used, based on the model of Grunewald (1970), which takes into account electrode properties such as anode/cathode diameter, membrane type and thickness, and diffusion conductivities for the gases in the tissues at the relevant temperature.

Oxygen Transport to Tissue XVIII, edited by Nemoto and LaManna
Plenum Press, New York, 1997

The diffusion conductivities for the gases are dependent upon the absolute temperature of the medium (van Krevelen, 1972; Harrison & Kessler, 1989b). The relationship for a given gas and PTFE (the material used for both types of electrode under consideration here) is described by:

$$\log K = C \times (1/T - 1/545) \tag{1}$$

where is K the diffusion conductivity, C a constant related to the gas constant, solubility, activation energy and molecular diameter of the gas, and T the absolute temperature. The resultant influence of T on K for PTFE is shown in Fig.1 for both H_2 and O_2.

According to Grunewald's analysis, the pressure, $p(r)$, in the diffusion field at a distance r perpendicular to the surface at the centre of a disk electrode is given by:

$$p(r) = p_c(1 - (r_0 + d_m)/r(1 + \delta)) \tag{2}$$

where p_c is the partial pressure of the gas in the medium, d_m the thickness of the membrane, r_0 the effective radius of the disk defined as $2R_0/\pi$ (R_0 being the true radius) and δ is given by:

$$d = K d_m / K_m r_0. \tag{3}$$

δ was defined originally as the "Diffusionsfehler" or "diffusion error" by Grunewald. However, this is a misnomer since it is not an "error" as such, but simply a term which accounts for the difference in diffusion conductivities between the medium (K) and membrane (K_m).

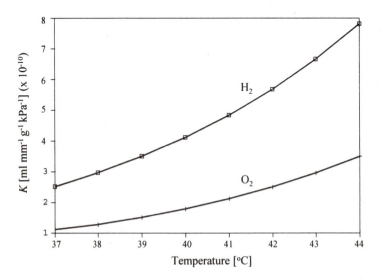

Figure 1. Influence of temperature on the diffusion conductivity K of PTFE for O_2 and H_2 within the relevant range.

If a composite membrane is used, for example in the case of the MDO, the "effective thickness", d'_m of the membrane should be used to calculate δ whereby the effective thickness of membrane (1) (eg cellophane), d'_1, is given by:

$$d'_1 = d_1(D_1/D_2)^{1/2} \qquad (4)$$

where d_1 is the real thickness of membrane (1) and D_1 and D_2 are the respective diffusion coefficients for the gas in the membranes. d'_1 is then added to the real thickness, d_2 of membrane (2) (PTFE) to give d'_m.

The given percentage catchment depth can thus be calculated from Eq.2 for appropriate ratios of $p(r)/p_c$, e.g. 0.95 or 0.98.

A two dimensional model was used to calculate the proportional contribution of the source of the electrode signal within the 95% catchment depth. This was done by weighting the mean diffusion gradient within 10° segments (e.g. ABCD) with the area of the segment (Fig.2). The relative diffusion gradient was calculated at the mid-point of the segment (e.g. P) outside the membrane. This was taken as being proportional to $dp(r)/dr$, i.e. $1/r^2$. The area of the segment, again outside the membrane, was also calculated and the two parameters multiplied in order to determine the weighting of the contribution of each segment to the electrode signal.

3. RESULTS

Catchment depths were calculated using the methods described above and the diffusion conductivities given in Table 1. d_m was 25 μm and r_0 4.8 μm. d'_mO_2 and d'_mH_2 for the MDO were calculated to be 18.7 μm and 20.2 μm, respectively.

Examples of relevant 95% catchment depths within the tissue are: 32 μm for H$_2$ and 8 μm for O$_2$ perpendicular to the centre of the electrode wire for the Kessler and Lübbers MDO electrode at 37°C in skeletal muscle. The equivalent 98% figures are 117 μm for H$_2$ and 57.5 μm for O$_2$. Values for the transcutaneous electrode (Dräger, Hemel Hemstead, UK) for H$_2$ and O$_2$ are given in Fig.3 for temperatures between 37 and 44°C.

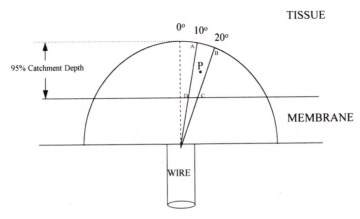

Figure 2. Diagram illustrating the weighting of segments for calculating the relative contribution to the electrode signal within the 95% catchment depth. For details see text.

Table 1. Values of diffusion conductivities for oxygen (KO_2) and hydrogen (KH_2) in the relevant media. All values are quoted for 37°C but were corrected where necessary. (Sources: Harrison & Kessler, 1989b; Harrison *et al.* 1994, van Krevelen, 1972.)

	KO_2 [ml mm^{-1} s^{-1} kPa^{-1}] × 10^{-10}	KH_2 [ml mm^{-1} s^{-1} kPa^{-1}] × 10^{-10}
PTFE	1.08	2.52
Muscle	3.65	4.67
Epidermis	4.40	5.59

Figures 4 and 5 show the shape of the catchment area, weighted for the proportion of contribution to the electrode current, for the MDO in muscle at 37°C and the transcutaneous electrode at 44°C in skin for H$_2$ and O$_2$.

4. DISCUSSION

The question of catchment depth is particularly important if such pH$_2$ and pO$_2$ measurements are combined simultaneously in order to derive further parameters such as oxygen uptake rate in muscle (Harrison *et al.* 1989). More recently, we have used transcutaneous electrode techniques simultaneously with optical techniques to measure both oxygen uptake rate and oxygen extraction (Newton *et al.* 1995) where knowledge of the relative catchment volumes of the techniques has been very important in interpreting the results obtained.

The present results show that both types of surface measurement, in both tissues, represent values obtained from a volume supplied by a single, or at the most three capillaries. The shape of the catchment depth derived from two dimensional calculations indicate that the larger proportion of the signal emanates from regions closer to the centre of

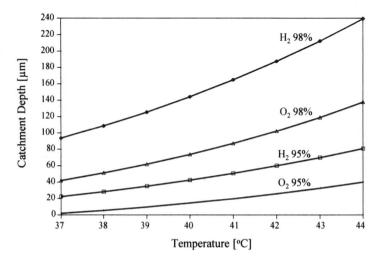

Figure 3. 95% and 98% catchment depths for the transcutaneous electrode for both O$_2$ and H$_2$ within the relevant temperature range in skin.

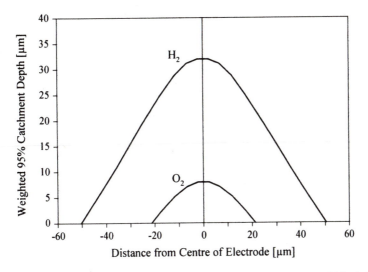

Figure 4. Shape of the weighted 95% catchment area of the MDO for H_2 and O_2 at 37°C in skeletal muscle.

the electrode (Figs. 4 and 5). However, further three dimensional calculations should be made in order to verify the shape of the catchment volume.

It has recently been shown that the properties of the electrode membrane are important when considering the consumption of an O_2 electrode (Grundmann & Lübbers, 1994). The present study shows that this is indeed also the case when considering catchment depth but that the influence of temperature is particularly strong and should always be taken into account.

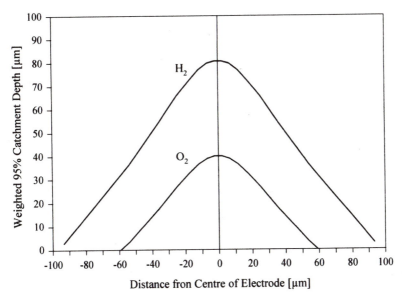

Figure 5. Shape of the weighted 95% catchment area of the transcutaneous electrode for H_2 and O_2 at 44°C in skin.

5. REFERENCES

Grundmann, A. and Lübbers, D.W., 1994, The determination of the O_2-consumption of the skin by the measurement of the decrease of the skin surface PO_2 after flow stop using an optical sensor without O_2-consumption. A theoretical analysis, *Funkt. biolog. Syst.* 22:265.

Grunewald, W., 1970, Diffusionsfehler und Eigenverbrauch der Pt-Elektrode bei pO_2 Messungen im steady state, *Pflüg. Arch. ges. Physiol.* 320:24.

Harrison, D.K. and Kessler, M., 1989a, Local hydrogen clearance as a method for the measurement of capillary blood flow, *Phys. Med. Biol.* 34:1413.

Harrison, D.K. and Kessler, M., 1989b, A multiwire hydrogen electrode for *in vivo* use, *Phys. Med. Biol.* 34:1397.

Harrison, D.K., Kessler M. and Knauf S.K., 1989, Regulation of capillary blood flow and oxygen supply in skeletal muscle in dogs during hypoxaemia, *J. Physiol.* 420:431.

Harrison, D.K., Birkenhake S., Knauf, S.K. and Kessler, M., 1990, Local oxygen supply and blood flow regulation in contracting muscle in dogs and rabbits, *J. Physiol.* 422:227.

Harrison, D.K, Abi Raad, R., Newton, D. and McCollum P.T., 1994, Transcutaneous hydrogen clearance — a new non-invasive technique for assessing blood flow in human skin, *Physiol. Meas.* 15:89.

Kessler, M. and Lübbers, D.W., 1966, Aufbau und Anwendungsmöglichkeiten verschiedener pO_2-Elektroden, *Pflüg. Arch. ges. Physiol.* 291:R82.

van Krevelen, D.W., 1972, "Properties of Polymers", Elsevier, Amsterdam.

Newton D.J., Harrison D.K., Delaney, C.D., Swanson Beck, J and McCollum P.T., 1994, Comparison of macro- and micro-lightguide spectrophotometric measurements of microvascular haemoglobin oxygenation in the tuberculin reaction in normal human skin, *Physiol. Meas.* 15:115.

Newton, D.J., Harrison D.K. and McCollum P.T., 1995, Oxygen extraction rates in inflamed human skin using the tuberculin reaction as a model, *J. Physiol.* submitted.

69

INTRARENAL pO$_2$ MEASURED BY EPR OXIMETRY AND THE EFFECTS OF BACTERIAL ENDOTOXIN

Philip E. James, Fuminori Goda, Oleg Y. Grinberg, Krzysztof G. Szybinski, and Harold M. Swartz

EPR Center, Department of Radiology
Dartmouth Medical School
Hanover, New Hampshire 03755

1. ABSTRACT

This study used Electron Paramagnetic Resonance (EPR) oximetry to detect the signal arising from oxygen-sensitive crystals of Lithium phthalocyanine (LiPC) implanted in the cortex and outer medulla of an isolated perfused rat kidney. Kidneys with implanted crystals were placed beneath the surface detector of an L-band spectrometer, and an additional gradient was induced between the poles of the magnet so as to separate the signals arising from each region, allowing simultaneous measurement of the partial pressure of oxygen (pO$_2$) at two locations within the same organ. In control kidneys, the pO$_2$ in the cortex was 96.9±7 and that of the outer medulla 11.0±4 mmHg. We found that perfusion pressure could be increased with little effect on the pO$_2$ of the outer medulla. At a critical point ($\approx$140 mmHg) however, pO$_2$ in this region was markedly increased and was accompanied by a decrease in vascular resistance. When kidneys treated in this way were then given L-NMMA (an inhibitor of nitric oxide synthase), the pO$_2$ in the outer medulla returned to baseline values, presumably by blocking nitric oxide-induced vasodilation. Inclusion of Lipopolysaccharide (LPS) into the perfusion media of control kidneys resulted in a decrease in the pO$_2$ in the cortical region and an increase in the outer medullary region. When L-NMMA was given prior to administration of LPS, the changes in pO$_2$ were prevented. Based on these results, we have developed a model which can account for these observations. It indicates that re-distribution of blood (and hence oxygen) within the kidney may have an important role in altering the solute (and oxygen) gradient early during the septic episode.

Oxygen Transport to Tissue XVIII, edited by Nemoto and LaManna
Plenum Press, New York, 1997

2. INTRODUCTION

Acute renal failure is a common characteristic of the septic state[1]. Although it has long been established that this is primarily caused by release of abnormal amounts of bacterial endotoxin (lipopolysaccharide, LPS)[2,3], its precise mechanism of action and its direct effect on renal tissue oxygen remain unclear.

In previous studies[4] we have measured the tissue pO_2 (partial pressure of oxygen) at several sites simultaneously within the same kidney *in vivo*. These results were in agreement with others[5] and depict a picture of the kidney in which the cortex is well supplied with oxygen from afferent arterioles, whereas pO_2 in the outer medulla is lower due to the fact that medullary blood is derived from efferent arterioles of the juxtamedullary glomeruli (in the cortex[6]), and the high metabolic turnover in medullary cells required to maintain an efficient urinary concentrating mechanism[7]. Furthermore, we demonstrated that within 5 minutes after intravenous injection of LPS, there is redistribution of blood within the kidney, resulting in decreased pO_2 in the renal cortex and increased pO_2 in the outer medulla region. Classical explanations for LPS-induced renal damage assign changes in oxygen utilization mechanisms (i.e mitochondrial dysfunction) later in the septic episode[8,9], and reduced oxygen supply due to systemic hypotension[10,11] as the main causes.

In the present study we directly measured pO_2 at several sites simultaneously within an isolated perfused kidney using Electron Paramagnetic Resonance (EPR) oximetry[12,13]. Using this system, we were able to control arterial flow and perfusion pressure, and monitor their influence on vascular resistance, tissue pO_2 and oxygen consumption. We then used these data in order to assess the effect of LPS directly on renal pO_2 without any LPS-induced effects on the systemic circulation. A model was developed which could account for the changes in pO_2 observed, and the potential role of LPS-induced nitric oxide (NO) in renal hemodynamics is discussed.

3. MATERIALS AND METHODS

3.1. Isolated Perfused Kidneys

Anesthesia was induced in male Wistar rats (300–400 g) by intra-muscular injection of a mixture of Xylazine/Ketamine (20 mg and 100 mg/Kg body weight) and the surgical procedure adapted from that used by other workers[14]. The descending aorta was cannulated with a 22 Gauge intravenous catheter and secured with surgical silk. In sequence, the ascending vena cava, right renal vein and artery, and aorta (just above the renal bifurcation) were ligated and cut distal to the ties. The ascending vena cava (lower portion) was cannulated using an 18 Gauge intravenous catheter and the kidney removed from the animal. Medium was perfused through the arterial catheter as soon as the upper aorta was ligated - ensuring that the period of no blood flow was kept to a minimum. For each perfusion, Krebs-Heinseleit solution was prepared containing albumin and amino acid supplements[15], and equilibrated with 95% O_2/5% CO_2. This was delivered into the thermostated perfusion system through a series of in-line Millipore filters (a pre-filter and a 0.45 µm-pore-diameter filter).

3.2. Perfusion Apparatus

An apparatus similar to that described by Gregg[16] was used for all experiments with slight modification; the kidney was placed within a plastic holder (similar to a funnel) which allowed removal and collection of the urine, and the arterial and venous cannulae were secured to the plastic mounting (see Fig.1). The perfusate was not re-circulated, and the pO$_2$ of the arterial (pO$_2^{in}$) and renal venous (pO$_2^{out}$) perfusate was measured continuously by two Clark-type electrodes (Yellow Spring Co.) which were enclosed in a specially fabricated gas-tight housing through which the entire media passed. The polypropylene membrane of the electrode formed one wall of the chamber. The arterial electrode was placed prior to the bubble trap; the renal venous electrode was attached to the outflow tube of the venous cannula. The current output of each electrode, at a polarizing voltage of 0.6–0.7 V, was measured with an ampmeter. These electrodes showed excellent linearity when calibrated with certified gas mixtures (Phoenix Distributors).

3.3. EPR

Lithium Phthalocyanine (LiPC) was used as the oxygen-sensitive probe. The linewidth of the EPR signal of this paramagnetic species shows linear dependence with pO$_2$, and is insensitive to changes in temperature or pH[13]. Crystals of LiPC were implanted into two regions of the kidney through the insertion of a 26 Gauge needle with a crystal within, and then extruding it with a fine wire. The needle was then removed from the kidney. At the end of each experiment, each kidney was dissected in order to verify the location of both crystals.

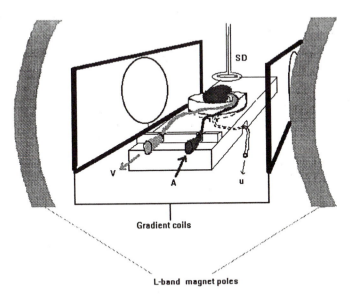

Figure 1. A diagram to show the perfusion apparatus and positioning of the kidney within the EPR magnet. The gradient coils produced a second magnetic field which separates the signal obtained from the different regions of the kidney. The kidney was perfused through the arterial cannula (A) and the outflow collected from the venous cannula (V) and ureter (u). Clark-type oxygen electrodes measured the pO$_2$ in *A* and *B*. The surface detector (SD) was placed immediately over the kidney allowing simultaneous measurement of the pO$_2$ of the cortex and outer medulla.

The apparatus was then placed between the poles of the magnet of a 1.1 GHz EPR spectrometer, and the kidney allowed to reach equilibrium for a further 10 mins. Perfusion pressure was monitored by a pressure transducer linked to a Hewlett-Packard monitor, and the flow rate from the peristaltic pump was adjusted so as to maintain a steady perfusion pressure, usually between 80–100 mmHg. A second pair of gradient coils was placed between the magnet poles; this separated the signal arising from each crystal and allowed simultaneous measurement of the pO_2 in the cortex (pO_2^c) and outer medulla (pO_2^m) (see Figures 1 and 2). EPR spectra were recorded every 20 seconds. Typical spectrometer settings were as follows: incident microwave power = 10 mW; modulation amplitude = 32 mGauss; scan range = 1 Gauss; time constant = 0.1 sec.

The linewidth was measured from the peak-to-peak separation (between maximum and minimum) of each EPR signal, and this was converted into a pO_2 value by comparison with a standard curve of LiPC linewidth against pO_2. This standard curve was calibrated using a Clark-type electrode and by varying the O_2:N_2 mix.

3.4. Cortex:Medulla Weight Ratio

This ratio was calculated by taking Nuclear Magnetic Resonance Images (MRI) of kidneys *in vivo* in two rats. An image sequence was used (T_2-weighted) which showed excellent contrast in the MRI signal intensity from each region of the kidney - cortex>inner medulla>outer medulla. Axial images were taken of 1.5 mm slices throughout each kidney, and the number of voxels within each kidney region was measured for each slice. These data were used to calculate a volume ratio between the three regions (cortex (40%) outer medulla (33%) and inner medulla (27%), and then converted into weight by measuring the wet weight of the kidney at the end of each experiment.

3.5. Experimental

Three types of experiments were performed using the system described above:-

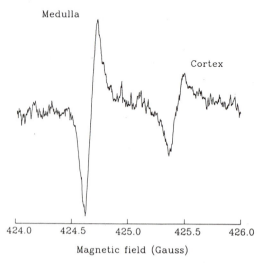

Figure 2. A typical spectrum obtained from two crystals of LiPC - one in the cortex, the other in the outer medulla.

3.5.1. pO$_2$ in Control Kidneys as a Function of Perfusion Pressure. Following the initial equilibration period, the flow was gradually increased. At each increment, perfusion pressure, urine flow, pO$_2$^{in} and pO$_2$^{out} were monitored, and renal pO$_2$^{c} and pO$_2$^{m} were recorded by repeated EPR spectra.

3.5.2. Influence of Endotoxin. The flow rate was gradually increased to obtain a perfusion pressure of 125 mmHg. Endotoxin (lipopolysaccharide, LPS; *E.coli* 0111B4, obtained from Sigma) was then included into the perfusion medium (2 mg/ml and 0.5 mg/ml;10 ml) and the EPR spectra recorded with time.

3.5.3. Influence of N^G-monomethyl-L-Arginine (L-NMMA). The purpose of these experiments was to evaluate the role of nitric oxide (NO) by inhibition of its production in control and LPS-treated kidneys. Control kidneys were perfused and the flow rate increased to a point where pO$_2$^{m} suddenly increased, and the perfusion pressure decreased (see results of 1). The system was kept at this point, and L-NMMA (1 mg/10 ml) included into the perfusion medium. In a second set of experiments, the control kidneys were perfused at 125 mmHg (as in 2 above) and L-NMMA was included in the medium. After 15 minutes, LPS was added to the system and EPR spectra recorded with time.

3.6. Our Model for the Distribution and Changes in Renal pO$_2$

Theory; According to Krogh's model describing oxygen exchange between blood and tissue[17]:

$$O_{2 \; capillary} - O_{2 \; tissue} = \frac{Flow \; (O_{2in}-O_{2out}) \; x \; (R^2 ln(R/r)^2 + (R^2-r^2)}{4 \; x \; D \; x \; Weight_{tissue}} \qquad (1)$$

where D= coefficient for diffusion of oxygen ($1.5 \times 10^{-5} cm^2/sec.$); R=distance from the capillary and r=capillary radius.

Following Kety's model[18] we assumed that

$$O_{2 \; capillary} = \frac{O_{2 \; in} + O_{2 \; out}}{2}$$

and substituting into eqn. 1 gave

$$\frac{O_{2 \; in} + O_{2 \; out}}{2} - pO_{2 \; tissue} = \frac{Flow \; (O_{2in}-O_{2out}) \; x \; constant}{4 \; x \; D \; x \; W} \qquad (2)$$

We adapted this model in order to explain oxygen supply to different regions within the kidney. We used literature values for the distribution of flow between the cortex and outer medulla region (90%:10%, respectively), where *a* represents flow into the cortex and

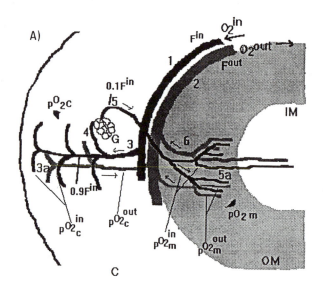

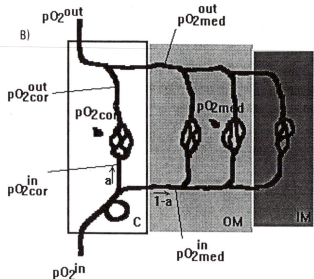

Figure 3. (a) Anatomical illustration showing blood supply to the three primary regions of the kidney; *c*=cortex, *om*=outer medulla, *im*=inner medulla. Blood enters and leaves the kidney via the arcuate artery and vein (*1* and *2*, respectively). It enters the cortical radial artery (*3*) which feeds the afferent arteriole (*4*) and supplies the Glomeruli (*G*). Blood leaves cortical glomeruli primarily via cortical radial veins (*3a*), however, the medulla is supplied by the efferent arteries of juxtamedullary glomeruli (*5*) and descending vasa recta (*5a*; taken from literature values to be 10% of the arterial supply). Blood is fed back into the arcurate vein via ascending vasa recta (*6*). pO_{2c} and pO_{2m} show the location of the LiPC crystals (measuring the pO_2 at the cortex and outer medulla, respectively). (b) A schematic cartoon illustrating the various parameters and assumptions of our model. Division of blood supply (pO_2^{in}) in the control kidney was taken from literature values to be 0.9:0.1 between the cortex and medulla, respectively (shown as *a* and *1-a* in the diagram). Values for *a'* and *1-a'* were then calculated for flow into the cortex and medulla after treatment (whether LPS, increased pressure or L-NMMA). All other labels are as for Fig.3(a).

1-a flow into the outer medulla region in the control kidney. These assumptions are illustrated in Figure 3.

From this we describe an equation system:

For the cortex region

$$\frac{O_{2in}^{c} + O_{2out}^{c} - pO_2^{c}}{2} = \frac{axF (O_{2in}^{c}-O_{2out}^{c}) \times constant^{c}}{4 \times D \times W^{c}}$$

For the medulla region

$$\frac{O_{2in}^{m} + O_{2out}^{m} - pO_2^{m}}{2} = \frac{(1-a)F (O_{2in}^{m}-O_{2out}^{m}) \times constant^{m}}{4 \times D \times W^{m}}$$

For the kidney

$$O_{2out} = (a\ O_{2out}^{c}) + (1-a)O_{2out}^{m}$$

This system had 4 unknown parameters; O_{2out}^{c}, O_{2out}^{m} and constants c and m. In order to solve this system, we assumed that O_{2out}^{m} was zero. This seemed sensible considering the low pO$_2$ that was measured in the medulla region.

We assigned the same three equations to the kidney after treatment (whether increased pressure, LPS, or L-NMMA). In this case, *a'* represented flow into the cortex and *1-a'* flow into the medulla after treatment. We also assumed that the constant (equation 2 and following equations for each region) did not change following treatment - i.e. the capillary density and capillary radius had little influence on the diversion of blood flow between large vessels at the cortico-medullary junction. The values we obtained from the control system were used to calculate the value of *a'* for each experiment.

The above equation system was applied to a program written for IBM PC, and all our calculations of *a'* were performed using this program.

Table 1. Summary of key parameters (pO$_2$ in each kidney region, total oxygen consumption, and the calculation % blood flow into the outer medulla) from control kidneys compared to those in which perfusion pressure was increased, those treated with LPS, and those treated with NO- synthase blocker, L-NMMA

	Control (n=7)	Pressure Increase (n=7)	LPS(2mg/ml) (n=4)	L-NMMA (1 mg/10 ml)(n=3)
Cortex pO$_2$(mmHg)	96.0±17.7	76.5±10.2	94.8±13.2	113.6±17.6
Outer MedullapO$_2$(mmHg)	11.2±4.1	37.6±14.2	29.6±7.0	Pre=44.0±5.6
				Post=5±7.0
Consumption O$_2$^{in}-O$_2$^{out}	245.3±24	212.0±22	173.6±28	198.4±34
1 - a(% flow into OM)	10(see[22])	32.75±11.4	17.6±3.2	45.1±8.0*

*It should be noted that this value represents the % difference in blood flow into the outer medulla pre- and post L-NMMA, and that L-NMMA caused a decrease in outer medullary blood flow.

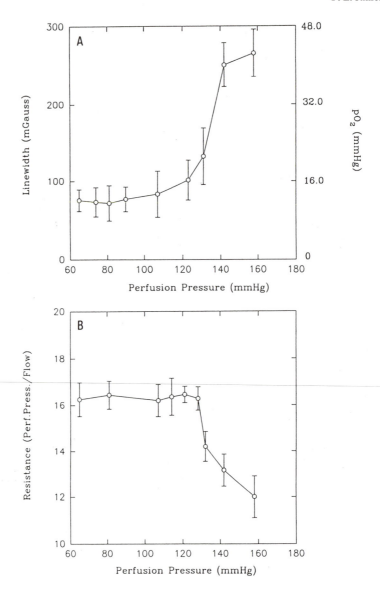

Figure 4. (a) pO_2 in the outer medulla measured at various perfusion pressures (n=7). (b) vascular resistance against perfusion pressure for the same kidneys as Fig.4(a).

4. RESULTS

The results of our renal pO_2 experiments are summarized in Table 1. We found that measurements in control kidneys showed high pO_2 in the cortex region (96.9±17 mmHg) where the crystals of LiPC were at a depth of 1 mm, and low pO_2 in the outer medulla (11.0±4 mmHg) at a depth of 2.8±0.4 mm (n=7). The separation of the two crystals was determined from the spectral splitting of the two signals in the EPR spectrum (Figure 2). This was calculated to be 2.11±0.6 mm, and was in close agreement with microscopic examination at the end of each experiment. When the perfusion pressure was 90±4 mmHg, urine flow from control kidneys was 270±44 μl/g/min.

In experiments where the arterial flow rate was gradually increased, we observed an increase in pO$_2$ measured in the cortex, whereas the pO$_2$ in the outer medulla remained unchanged (n=7). It can be seen from the data presented in Figure 4(a) however, that when the perfusion pressure reached a critical point (138±11 mmHg), the pO$_2$ in the outer medulla suddenly increased (*control*=11.0±4 mmHg, *above critical point*=37.64±14 mmHg). Above this critical point, cortex pO$_2$ decreased to 76.5±10.2 mmHg. We found that these changes in pO$_2$ were reversible, in that the flow rate could then be lowered to reduce perfusion pressure and the kidney passed through this critical point once more. Further manipulation was difficult, however, in that we could not then return to a steady equilibrium point (n=3). Figure 4(b) shows the experimental data presented in Fig.4(a) expressed in terms of the renal resistance to flow.

In a second set of experiments, perfused kidneys were passed through this critical point and the perfusion pressure (flow) maintained; in this case, medullary pO$_2$ was at a higher level than in the control (44.0±5.6 mmHg compared to 11±4 mmHg). When L-NMMA was added to the perfusion medium of these kidneys, we observed an immediate decrease in the pO$_2$ in the medulla region, followed by a slow recovery to the higher pO$_2$ level (Figure 5).

In a third group of control kidneys, where pO$_2$ in the cortex was high compared to that in the medulla and the perfusion pressure was less than the critical point (at around 125 mmHg), we added LPS into the perfusion medium (n=4). We observed a transient increase in outer medullary pO$_2$ (29.56±4 mmHg) and little to no effect on cortex pO$_2$ (94.8±13.2 mmHg). The effect on pO$_2$ in the outer medulla was reversed after 3 mins, and the pO$_2$ returned to baseline, pre-LPS values (Figure 6).

Finally, three kidneys were pre-treated with L-NMMA (1 mg/10 ml) and then LPS added to the perfusion medium as above. We were unable to detect any significant change

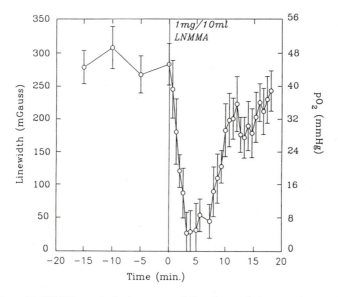

Figure 5. The effect of L-NMMA on pO$_2$ in the outer medulla when perfusion pressure was above the critical point ($\approx$140mmHg).

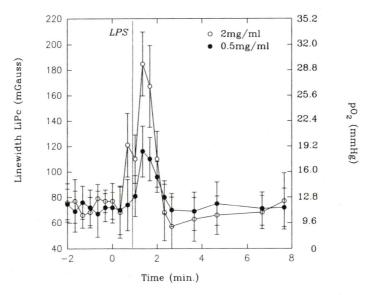

Figure 6. pO_2 in the outer medulla after inclusion of LPS into the perfusion medium. The results of two concentrations of LPS are shown (n=4 in each case).

in the pO_2 in either region of these kidneys, and all other monitored parameters remained constant. We checked that this effect was due to the antagonistic effect of the LPS and L-NMMA by further perfusing these kidneys for 30 minutes, then increasing the flow (and hence perfusion pressure) beyond the critical point. The pO_2 in the outer medulla increased as in previous control experiments.

5. DISCUSSION

Our results from EPR oximetry are consistent with those of previous studies, and depict a picture of the kidney in which the cortex region is well supplied with well-oxygenated blood compared to the medulla region[6]. This gives rise to high pO_2 in the cortex and a sharp oxygen gradient towards the medulla[5]. This was conveniently shown using EPR oximetry, since pO_2 measurements were made simultaneously at two regions within the isolated perfused kidney.

Kidneys in the control group were deemed to be functioning normally; urinary output and oxygen consumption were similar to those values quoted by other workers using similar perfusion techniques[7,10,19] and the values of the pO_2 of the renal tissue were similar to those measured using insertion of micropipettes and Clark-type electrodes[5].

In previous studies[4] we have shown that an injection of LPS in mice causes a decrease in pO_2 in the renal cortex and an increase in pO_2 in the outer medulla. EPR and MRI studies *in vivo* suggested that these changes were in part due to LPS-induced systemic hypotension, but also due to significant re-distribution of blood from the cortex to the outer medulla region. It is also possible that reduced solute delivery to the medulla reduces oxygen demand, thereby increasing medullary pO$_2$ [5,20]. It was difficult, however, to discriminate between these possible causes for the observed changes in renal pO$_2$.

The present study was unique in that it allowed pO$_2$ to be measured in the cortex and outer medulla, while other parameters (such as perfusion pressure) could be controlled and monitored. We found that in control kidneys, the pO$_2$ in the cortex region increased with perfusion pressure (increased flow) whereas that of the outer medulla remained unchanged. At a critical perfusion pressure ($\approx$140 mmHg), however, outer medullary pO$_2$ increased rapidly. The blood supply to the renal medulla is derived exclusively from the efferent arterioles of juxtamedullary glomeruli (see Fig.3(a)). The opportunity to regulate medullary blood flow thus exists at several sites. The descending vasa recta (DVR) are known to be gradually transformed such that their smooth muscle layer, which they have in the outer medulla, is gradually replaced by pericytes. Therefore contractile elements do exist in early DVR but are lost by the inner-outer medullary junction[21]. Thus the interlobular artery, the afferent and efferent arterioles, and the initial segment of the DVR could be acted on by hormonal and neural influences to alter blood flow to the renal medulla. Our results can best be explained by decreased vascular resistance at a critical perfusion pressure, causing an influx of blood into the medulla region (indicated by the decrease in a).

Addition of LPS into the perfusion medium had two observable effects; a transient increase in the pO$_2$ of the outer medulla, and a decrease in renal oxygen consumption. Although these might be explained in terms of reduced solute delivery and oxygen requirement, calculations based on our model indicated that there was increased blood flow into the outer medulla during LPS treatment. This finding is in agreement with our MRI data *in vivo* and other workers who have reported increased cortico-medullary shunting of blood after treatment with LPS[6,22], resulting in a transient period of increased blood supply (and hence oxygen) into the renal medulla. In a previous report, we have indicated that LPS does have a direct toxic effect on mitochondrial oxygen consumption of renal cells, but this delayed effect is unlikely to be the cause of the immediate changes in pO$_2$ reported here[8].

Recent studies have shown a potential role for NO in renal hemodynamics[23,24], and indicated its presence in the renal medulla[25] and its role in renal medullary oxygenation[5]. Since LPS is known to act via production of a variety of secondary molecules (interleukins, tumor necrosis factor, and NO[26,27]), it was important to establish the role of NO in our model system. By blocking the enzyme responsible for its synthesis, we demonstrated that NO is active in controlling entry of blood into the outer medulla, presumably by relaxing smooth muscle layers of the upper DVR. Moreover, we were able to block the effect of LPS on outer medulla pO$_2$ by pre-treating with L-NMMA, indicating that this was the cause of altered blood flow (and hence oxygen supply).

In summary, the data presented in this paper suggest that LPS has a direct effect on the distribution of blood between the cortex and outer medulla of the kidney. It appears that this effect may be modulated through the vasodilatory effect of LPS-induced NO in the renal medulla.

ACKNOWLEDGMENTS

The EPR Center at Dartmouth is supported by NIH grant GM 51630. The authors would like to thank Dr J. Dunn for use of the NMR Facility at Dartmouth Medical School.

REFERENCES

1. Initial management of circulatory shock as prevention of MSOF. Vincent, J.L. et al. *Critical Care Clinics* 1989;**5**:369–378.
2. Endotoxin and acute renal failure. Wardle, E.N. et al. *Nephron* 1975;**14**:321–332.
3. Relationships between endotoxemia, arterial pressure and renal function in dogs. O'Hair,D.P. et al. *Circ Shock* 1989;**27**:199–210.
4. Endotoxin induced changes in intrarenal pO_2, measured by in vivo electron paramegnetic resonance and magnetic resonance imaging. James, P.E. et al. *Submitted to Free Radical Biology and Medicine,* 1995.
5. Role of nitric oxide in renal medullary oxygenation. Breziz, M. et al. *J Clin Invest* **88**:1995; 390–395.
6. Renal Medullary Microcirculation. Pallone, T.L. et al. *Physiological Reviews* 1990;**70**(3):885–920.
7. Redox state of cytochrome a, a_3 in isolated perfused rat kidney. Epstein, E.H. et al. *Am J Physiol* 1982;**243**;F356-F363.
8. The effects of bacterial endotoxin on oxygen consumption of various cell types in vitro: An EPR oximetry study. James, P.E. et al. *Free Rad Biol Med* 1995;**18**(4):641–647.
9. Effect of endotoxemia on liver cell mitochondria in man. Schumer, W. et al. *Surg Ann* 1970;**171**;875–882.
10. Renal perfusion and metabolism in experimental endotoxic shock. Gullichsen, E. *Acta Chir Scand (Suppl.)* 1991;**560**:7–31.
11. Deterioration of renal function during hyperdynamic endotoxemia correlates with redistribution of intra-renal blood flow. Frey, L. et al., *Eur Surg Res* 1990;**22**(suppl.1):66.
12. In vivo EPR oximetry using two novel probes: fusenite and lithium phthalocyanine. Glockner, J.F. and Swartz, H.M. In: *Oxygen Transport to Tissue XIV,* edited by Erdmann, W. and Bruley, D.F. New York:1992; Plenum Publishing, 221–228.
13. Lithium phthalocyanine: A probe for electron paramagnetic resonance oximetry in viable biological systems. Liu, K.J. et al. *Proc Natl Acad Sci USA* 1993;**90**:5438–5442.
14. Selective vulnerability of the medullary thick ascending limb to anoxia in the isolated perfused kidney. Breziz, M. et al. *J Clin Invest* 1984;**73**:182–190.
15. Improved function with amino acids in the isolated perfused kidney. Epstein, F.H. et al. *Am J Physiol* 1982;**243**(12):F284-F292.
16. Effects of glucose and insulin on metabolism and function of perfused rat kidney. Gregg, C.M. et al. *Am J Physiol* 1978;**235**(4):F52-F62.
17. The supply of oxygen to the tissue and the regulation of the capillary circulation. Krogh, A. *J Physiol London* 1919;**52**:457–474.
18. Determinants of tissue oxygen tension. Kety, S.S. *Fed Proc* 1957;**16**:666–670.
19. Relation of Na^+ reabsorption to utilization of O_2 and lactate in the perfused rat kidney. Cohen, J.C. et al., *Am J Physiol* 1980;**238**(7):F415-F427.
20. Changes in cytochrome oxidation in outer and inner stripes of outer medulla. Atkins, J.L. and Lankford, S.P. . *Am J Physiol* 1991;**261**(5pt2):F849–857.
21. Urinary Concentrating Mechanism: Structure and Function. Jamison, R.L. and Kriz,W. New York: Oxford University Press,1982; p485–496.
22. Anatomic arterial-venous shunting in endotoxic and septic shock in dogs. Archie, J.P. *Ann Surg* 1977;**186**:171–176.
23. Endothelium-derived relaxing factor influences renal vascular resistance. Radermacher, J. et al. *Am J Physiol* 1990;**259**:F9-F17.
24. Control of Regional blood flow by endothelium-derived nitric oxide. Gardiner S.M. et al. *Hypertension (Dallas)* 1990;**15**:486–492.
25. Endothelium-derived relaxing factor (EDRF) in renal medulla. Biondi, M.L. et al. *Kidney Int.* 1990;**37**:364(a)(Abstr.).
26. Interleukin-1 and its biologically related cytokines. Dinarello, C.A. *Adv Immunol* 1989;**44**:153–205.
27. Nitric oxide hemoglobin in mice and rats in endotoxic shock. Wang, Q. et al. *Life Sciences* 1991;**49**:55–60.

70

MEASUREMENTS OF OXYGEN TENSION IN THE RAT KIDNEY AFTER CONTRAST MEDIA USING AN OXYGEN MICROELECTRODE WITH A GUARD CATHODE

Per Liss,[1] Anders Nygren,[1] Niels P. Revsbech,[3] and Hans R. Ulfendahl[2]

[1]Department of Diagnostic Radiology
University Hospital
Uppsala, Sweden
[2]Department of Physiology and Medical Biophysics
University of Uppsala
Uppsala, Sweden
[3]Department of Microbial Ecology
University of Aarhus
Aarhus, Denmark

ABSTRACT

The oxygen tension (PO_2) in the rat kidney was studied by modified Clark microelectrodes. Changes in PO_2 were measured in the renal cortex and outer medulla after intravenous injections of the X-ray contrast medium (CM) diatrizoate, 370 mg iodine/mg body weight. Injection of diatrizoate caused a slight fall in PO_2 in the renal cortex (from 42 ± 4 to 38 ± 4 mm Hg). In the medulla PO_2 decreased significantly (from 34 ± 6 to 20 ± 4 mm Hg). Ringer's solution did not induce any changes.

INTRODUCTION

Changes in oxygen tension in the renal medulla are considered to be of major importance for the acute renal failure (ARF) following injection of contrast media (CM) [1]. Therefore, there is a need for techniques for measuring changes in oxygen tension in the kidney. Large oxygen microelectrodes (> 10 μm) influence the measurements of tissue oxygen tension so that unstable and sometimes unreliable values may be obtained [2-6]. In this investigation we have used a modified Clark electrode [7] for measuring changes in tissue oxygen tension (PO_2) in the kidney after injection of X-ray contrast media.

Oxygen Transport to Tissue XVIII, edited by Nemoto and LaManna
Plenum Press, New York, 1997

The modified Clark microelectrode has a second cathode (a guard cathode) placed behind the O_2-sensitive cathode in order to minimize the oxygen coming to the O_2-sensing cathode from the electrolyte reservoir. Such electrodes have previously been used in environmental research by Revsbech [7].

MATERIAL AND METHODS

Animals

The studies were performed on male Lewis-DA rats with an average weight of 308 ± 7 g. Animals were anesthetized with Inactin® (Byk-Gulden, Konstanz, Germany), given intraperitoneally in a dosage of 120 mg/kg body weight (BW). Tracheostomies were performed and the rats were placed on a servo-controlled heating pad to maintain the body temperature at 37.5°C.

Surgical Procedures

A polyethylene catheter was placed in the left femoral artery for blood sampling and monitoring of BP. The left femoral vein was catheterized for infusion of Ringer's solution. The left kidney was exposed by a left subcostal flank incision and immobilized in a plastic cup. The kidney was embedded in pieces of cotton wool soaked in Ringer's solution and its surface was covered with paraffin oil. During the experiment the temperature of the kidney was monitored by a thermocouple probe.

Oxygen Microelectrode

The oxygen microelectrode was a Clark-type electrode with a guard cathode as described by Revsbech [7]. The design of the electrode is shown in Fig. 1. The electrode was made of an outer casing of soda glass pulled at one end to an outer tip diameter of about 3–10 μm and an inner tip diameter of 1–3 μm. The tip was filled with silicon rubber (Silastic, Medical Adhesive type A, Dow Corning, USA) which when cured formed a membrane. It is important to apply the silicon rubber solution within a few minutes after the tip is made, (before the glass surface starts to hydrate) otherwise there will be a risk of leakage between the glass and the cured silicone plug, which will totally invalidate the use of the electrode when measuring in tissues.

The sensing cathode was made of a platinum wire with a tip diameter of 0.5–2 μm, melted into a fine glass capillary (Schott glass 8533, Schott Glaswerke, Germany). The naked, non-glass encoated tip of the platinum wire was gold-plated [8]. The glass-encoated platinum wire was then fused into a soda glass capillary. The tip of the O_2-sensitive cathode was placed in the tip of the outer casing. The guard cathode was made of a 0.1 mm silver wire which was tapered at one end to a tip diameter of 1–2 μm. An Ag/AgCl wire was used as a reference anode. The electrolyte, consisting of 0.5 M KCl buffered with 0.05 M K_2CO_3/0.075 M $KHCO_3$ (pH 10.2), was injected into the outer casing. The electrode was then sealed with epoxy resin (Super Epoxy AB Hisingeplast, Gothenburg, Sweden).

Functionally, the PO_2 electrode consists of two separate electric circuits. The platinum cathode and the silver anode make up the true PO_2 system, while the silver cathode

a. shaft of sensing cathode (soda glass)
b. shaft of outer casing (soda glass)
c. guard cathode (Ag)
d. reference anode (Ag/AgCl)
e. electrolyte
f. platinum wire
g. Schott glass 8533 encoating the Pt wire
h. silicon membrane
i. gold-plating of the platinum wire tip
j. epoxy resin

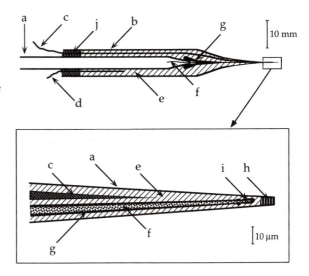

Figure 1. Oxygen microelectrode with a guard cathode (modified from Revsbech, N.P; Limnol Oceanogr. 1989; 34 (2), 474–478).

and the silver anode form the guard system. Both circuits are supplied with -0.8 V from separate voltage sources and the current in the PO_2-sensitive circuit is recorded.

The electrodes were calibrated in water at 37° C, saturated with both N_2 or air before and after the experiments.

Electrode Characteristics

Table I gives examples of some electrode characteristics. The first electrodes were built in Århus by one of the authors (PL) and the rest were made in our laboratory in Uppsala. In the wide number of electrodes used in the present study, the current at zero PO_2 amounted to 12.5 ± 0.9 pA at 37°C. The current at air saturation was 252 ± 22.9 pA. The 90% response time was 2.6 ± 0.5 sec. The stirring effect (change of electrode output in unstirred compared to stirred water) was 0.8 ± 0.2%. The average drift between the calibration of the electrodes before the 2-hour experiment and after was 1.0 ± 0.2% with N_2 gas and 1.9 ± 0.4% with air. The long-term stability of the electrodes was less than 0.5% drift per hour.

Twelve electrodes were tested (at 37°C) without and with the polarization of the guard cathode. The electrodes had been polarized without the guard for at least 4 hours before the guard cathode was polarized. The current of the sensing cathode in N_2 gas was found to be 44.0 ± 12 pA (without guard) and 14.3 ± 2.6 pA (with guard). The current in air was 297 ± 73 pA (without guard) and 207 ± 57 pA (with guard).

Experimental Protocol

When the surgical procedure was completed, the animal was allowed to recover for 30 minutes. In group A (n=6) PO_2 was measured simultaneously in the renal cortex and outer medulla after injection of CM (diatrizoate 370 mg/ml) (2070 mOsm/kg) (Urografin®. Schering, Berlin, Germany). Diatrizoate was given at a dose of 1,600 mg iodine/kg BW, a dosage not unusual in angiographic practise. Subsequently, after a 20-minute control period, a 30-minute experimental period started with an 8-minute injection of CM or control substance (Fig. 2). Ringer's solution was used as a control (group B, n=7). PO_2 was measured at a depth of 1.0 mm in the cortex and at an average depth of 3.9 mm (range 3.5–4.5) in the outer medulla. At the end of the experiments, the microelectrodes were replaced by empty outer microelectrode casings with the same shape and size, placed on the same micro-manipulator and inserted at the same depth. After injection of a small amount of India ink, the outer casings were removed and the kidney was sectioned in order to verify the sites of the measurements.

STATISTICAL EVALUATION

Values are expressed as means ± SEM. The statistical significance of the data was tested by using a multivariate analysis of variance (Manova) model. A p value of < 0.05 was accepted as significant (*) in all analyses.

RESULTS

In the renal cortex the PO_2 was 44 (range 8–88) mm Hg. In the outer medulla it was 32 (range 5–63) mm Hg and in the inner medulla it was 25 (range 3–46) mm Hg. PO_2 was significantly higher in the cortex than in the medulla.

After injection of diatrizoate there was a slight, non-significant decrease in PO_2 in the cortex, from 42.4 ± 4.1 to 38.0 ± 4.3 mm Hg (Fig. 2). In the outer medulla there was a significant decrease from 33.6 ± 5.8 to 19.9 ± 3.6 mm Hg (Fig. 3). Ringer's solution caused no significant changes in the cortex or outer medulla.

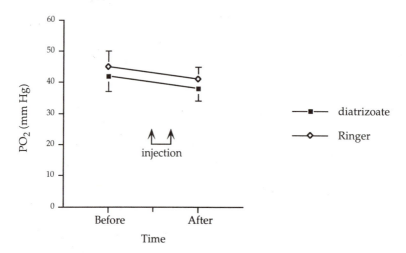

Figure 2. Effects of injection of diatrizoate and Ringer's solution (control) on PO_2 (mm Hg) in the cortex.

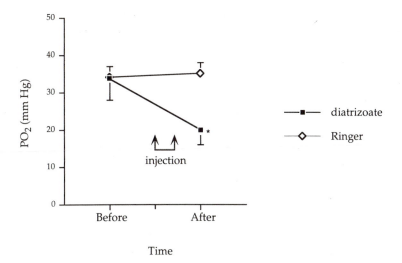

Figure 3. Effects of injection of diatrizoate and Ringer's solution (control) on PO_2 (mm Hg) in the outer medulla. * indicates a significant difference ($p<0.05$) compared with control period.

DISCUSSION

Our findings indicate that contrast media reduce the PO_2 in the outer renal medulla but leave that in the cortex unaffected. As in prior studies [9, 10], PO_2 was found to be lower in the renal medulla than in the cortex.

Heyrowsky [11] was the first to describe the polarographic method of measuring oxygen tension in electrolyte solutions. Since then, attempts have been made to develop the oxygen electrode for use in biological tissues. In 1942 Davies and Brink [12] covered the platinum tip with a collodium membrane which gave the electrodes a better stability and reproducibility. In 1956 Clark [13] presented an electrode in which he had placed both the platinum cathode and the reference anode behind an ion-impermeable membrane. The Clark electrode is now widely used. Only few reports [14, 15] have been published on miniaturised Clark electrodes (tip diameter < 5 μm). In 1989 Revsbech [7] described a modified, miniaturised Clark electrode with an in-built guard cathode. This electrode has the advantage that all oxygen diffusing towards the sensing cathode is removed from the internal electrolyte reservoir. The zero current of the electric system remains low when the guard cathode is used, even though there is a large amount of electrolyte in the outer casing. The guard cathode did not otherwise alter the characteristics of the electrode.

These electrodes have been used in environmental research since Revsbech introduced them in 1989 [7]. This oxygen microelectrode has a short stabilization period and the measurements performed in the kidney mostly show a stable value within a few seconds. Building the electrodes requires care, but most electrodes produce good stability, reproducibility and a short response time, and with gentle handling the same electrode can be used repeatedly for intratissular PO_2 measurements.

All electrodes inserted into tissues will to some extent affect the tissue [16]. In 1973 Albanese [5] showed mathematically that when measuring in tissues, an electrode with a tip of 1 μm has little error effect on PO_2 measurement, while a 10 μm outer tip diameter will have a large error effect on this measurement. It is therefore important to use an electrode with a small tip diameter [17]. A large electrode will damage the tissue and compress the

Table 1. Characteristics of some oxygen microelectrodes

	(1.)	(2.)	Average (1.)
Outer diameter (tip) (μm)	3	45	5.5 ±1.9
Inner diameter (tip) (μm)	2	40	2.1±0.1
N2 with guard (pA)	11	22	14.3 ±2.6
N2 without guard (pA)	23	62	44 ±12.0
Air, with guard (pA)	56	1486	207 ±57
Air, without guard (pA)	160	1625	297 ±73
90% response (sec)	1	4.7	2.6 ±0.5
Stirring (%)	<1	3	0.8 ±0.2
Silicon-membrane length (μm)	20	30	18 ±6
Distance membrane to cathode (μm)	90	45	43 ±4
Distance cathode to guard cathode (μm)	300	2000	471 ±50

1. Microelectrode used in this study
2. Microelectrode constructed for comparison.

capillaries, resulting in a decreased PO_2. Further, a large electrode has a high diffusion current, reflecting a high oxygen consumption [15] and in tissues where the oxygen diffusion is lower than that in a fluid [8, 18], this may affect the measurements, as the electrode is calibrated in water with different diffusion characteristics compared to that of tissues [2, 4, 6, 19]. There is a problem in obtaining absolute PO_2 values in tissues; however, these electrodes were built with a relatively large diffusion distance from the tip of the outer casing to the reducing sensing cathode. The difference between the readings in vigorously stirred and stagnant air-saturated water was thus only 0.8%, and the change in permeability of the tissue will then also have minor effect on the signal.

After injection of the ionic hyperosmolar contrast medium diatrizoate, we found a significant decrease in PO_2 in the outer medulla, while that in the cortex was not changed. There are several possible reasons for this decrease in the outer medulla.

About 80% of the O_2 extraction from the blood in the kidney, the non-basal O_2 consumption, is directly proportional to the filtration rate [20, 21] and hence to the net reabsorption of sodium. As hyperosmolar CM constitute osmotic diuretics, freely filtered by the glomeruli and poorly absorbed by the renal tubule, the high CM concentration in the tubule will reduce the reabsorption of water and sodium from the tubule and induce an osmotic diuresis. As a result of the osmotic effect, the amount of sodium arriving at mTal will increase, and hence also the active, oxygen-consuming uptake of sodium from mTal [22], leading to a further decrease in PO_2 in the outer medulla [23].

Another possible underlying cause of a decrease in PO_2 in the kidney is a decrease in blood flow. The mechanism of the vasoconstriction in the renal vessels after injection of CM and hyperosmolar compounds is unknown, although several possibilities have been proposed [24–28].

The renal blood flow may also be decreased due to the elevation of intrarenal pressure, caused by the osmotic diuresis following injection of CM [29]. Also an intratubular obstruction [30] has been suggested as a mechanism for increasing intrarenal pressure and consequently leading to a decrease in renal renal blood flow.

CONCLUSIONS

1. Injections of diatrizoate induced a PO_2 reduction in the outer medulla, while PO_2 in the cortex was unchanged.
2. The modified Clarke electrode was found to be a stable and useful instrument for intratissue PO_2 measurements.

ACKNOWLEDGMENTS

This study was supported by the Gunvor and Josef Anér Foundation and the Marcus and Amalia Wallenberg Foundation.

REFERENCES

1. Brezis M, Rosen S, Silva P, Epstein FH. Renal ischemia: a new perspective. *Kidney Int.* 26:375. (1984).
2. Grängsjö G, Ulfendahl HR. Factors influencing the properties of electrodes for continuous measurements of oxygen tension in tissues. *Acta Soc Med Upsal.* 67:107. (1962).
3. Jamieson D, van den Brenk HAS. Effect of electrode dimensions on tissue pO2 measurement in vivo. *Nature.* 201:1227. (1964).
4. Grunewald W. Diffusion error and O2 consumption of the Pt electrode during pO2 measurements in the steady state. *Pflügers Arch.* 320:24. (1970).
5. Albanese RA. On microelectrode distortion of tissue oxygen tensions. *J Theor Biol.* 38:143. (1973).
6. Baumgärtl H. Systematic investigations of needle electrode properties in polarographic measurements of local tissue pO2. In: Ehrly AM, Hauss J,Huch R, eds. Clinical oxygen pressure measurement. Springer-Verlag, 1987; 17.
7. Revsbech NP. An oxygen microsensor with a guard cathode. *Limnol Oceanogr.* 34:474. (1989).
8. Baumgärtl H, Lübbers DW. Microcoaxial needle sensor for polarographic measurement of local O2 pressure in the cellular range of living tissue-Its construction and properties. In: Gnaiger E,Forster, eds. Polarographic Oxygen Sensors. Heidelberg: Springer Verlag, 1983; 37.
9. Aukland K, Krog J. Renal oxygen tension. *Nature.* 188:671. (1960).
10. Ulfendahl HR. Intrarenal oxygen tension. *Acta Soc Med Upsal.* 67:95. (1962).
11. Heyrovsky J. The processes at the mercury dropping cathode. Part II. The hydrogen overpotential. *Trans Faraday Soc.* 19:785. (1924).
12. Davies PW, Brink F. Microelectrodes for measuring local oxygen tension in animal tissues. *Rev Scien Instr.* 13:524. (1942).
13. Clark LC. Monitor and control of blood and tissue oxygen tensions. *Trans Am Soc Art Int Org.* 2:41. (1956).
14. Fatt I. An ultramicro oxygen microelectrode. *J Appl Physiol.* 19:326. (1964).
15. Silver IA. Polarography and its biological applications. *Phys Med Biol.* 12:285. (1967).
16. Silver IA. Problems in the investigation of tissue oxygen microenvironment. *Adv Chem Sev.* 118:343. (1973).
17. Lübbers DW. The meaning of the tissue oxygen distribution curve and its measurement by means of Pt electrodes. *Progr Resp Res.* 3:122. (1968).
18. Thews G. The theory of oxygen transport and its application for gaseous exchange in the lung. In: Lübbers D-W, Luft UD, Thews G,Witzleb E, eds. Oxygen transport in blood and tissues. Stuttgart: Georg Thieme Verlag, 1968; 1.
19. Jordan J, Ackerman E, Berger RL. Polarographic diffusion coefficients of oxygen defined by activity gradients in viscous media. *J Am Chem Soc.* 78:2979. (1956).
20. Deetjen P, Kramer K. Sodium reabsorption and oxygen utilization of the kidney. *Pflügers Arch.* 273:636. (1961).
21. Lassen NA, Munck O, Thaysen JH. Oxygen consumption and sodium reabsorption in the kidney. *Acta Pysiol Scand.* 51:371. (1961).

22. Giebisch G, Klose RM, Windhager EE. Micropuncture study of hypertonic sodium chloride loading in the rat. *Am J Physiol.* 206:687. (1964).
23. Ullrich KJ, Pehling G. Active sodium transport and oxygen consumption in the outer medulla of the kidney. *Pflügers Arch.* 267:207. (1958).
24. Katzberg RW, Morris TW, Burgener FA, Kamm DE, Fischer HW. Renal renin and hemodynamic responses to selective renal artery catheterization and angiography. *Invest Radiol.* 12:381. (1977).
25. Arend LJ, Bakris GL, Burnett Jr JC, Megerian C, Spelman WS. Role for intrarenal adenosine in the renal hemodynamic response to contrast media. *J Lab Clin Med.* 110:406. (1987).
26. Ueda J, Nygren A, Hansell P, Ulfendahl HR. Effect of intravenous contrast media on proximal and distal tubular hydrostatic pressure in the rat kidney. *Acta Radiol.* 34:83. (1993).
27. Nygren A, Hellberg O, Hansell P. Red-cell trapping in the rat renal microcirculation induced by low-osmolar contrast media and mannitol. *Invest Radiol.* 28:1033. (1993).
28. Liss P, Nygren A, Erikson U, Ulfendahl HR. Effects of contrast media and mannitol on renal medullary blood flow and red cell aggregation in the rat kidney. *Kidney Int.* 49:1270. (1996).
29. Katzberg RW. Renal effects of contrast media. *Invest Radiol.* 23:S157. (1988).
30. Schwartz RH, Berdon WE, Wagner J, Becker J, Baker DB. Tamm-Horsfall urinary mucoprotein precipitation by urographic contrast agents: in vitro studies. *Am J Radiol.* 108:698. (1970).

71

OXYGEN DISTRIBUTION IN THE VASCULATURE OF MOUSE TISSUE *IN VIVO* MEASURED USING A NEAR INFRA RED PHOSPHOR

L.-W. Lo, W. T. Jenkins, S. A. Vinogradov, S. M. Evans, and D. F. Wilson

Department of Biochemistry and Biophysics and of Radiation Oncology
Medical School, and of Clinical Studies, Veterinary School
University of Pennsylvania
Pennsylvania 19104

ABSTRACT

Oxygen dependent quenching of phosphorescence has been used to measure the oxygenation of tissue in mice, including the differences between normal tissue and that of a murine tumor. Approximately 0.3 mg of the phosphorescence oxygen probe, Green 2W, was injected into the tail vein of tumor bearing mice. The mice were immobilized using an anesthetic cocktail and illuminated with flashes (< 4 μsec $t_{1/2}$) of light of 636 ± 15 nm. The emitted phosphorescence (790 nm max.) was measured using an imaging phosphorimeter with an intensified CCD camera, an instrument which provides two dimensional digital maps of oxygen pressure. Both the illumination light and the phosphorescence were in the near infra red region of the spectrum, where skin and tissue have little absorption. The light can therefore readily pass through the skin and centimeter thickness of tissue. Mice are sufficiently small that the oxygen pressure maps could be obtained by illuminating from either the same or the opposite side as the camera (and tumor). The tumors were observed as regions with oxygen pressures substantially below those of the surrounding normal tissue. Thus, it is possible to non-invasively detect these tumors and to monitor their internal oxygen pressure in real time and through cm of tissue.

INTRODUCTION

Oxygen dependent quenching of phosphorescence has been used to study oxygen metabolism and delivery in several biological systems. These include the oxygen dependence of respiration in *in* vitro suspensions of cells and mitochondria (Wilson et al, 1988;

Oxygen Transport to Tissue XVIII, edited by Nemoto and LaManna
Plenum Press, New York, 1997

Robiolio et al, 1989; Rumsey et al, 1990) as well as several tissues *in vivo*, including the brain cortex (Wilson et al, 1991), retina of the eye (Shonat et al, 1992), heart (Rumsey et al, 1994), liver (Rumsey et al, 1988), tumors (Wilson and Cerniglia, 1992), and kidney (Rumsey et al, this volume). The measurements have been limited to the surface layer of the tissue because the absorption bands of the phosphors, Pd-porphines, were all at wavelengths less than about 540 nm. At these wavelengths, absorption of the excitation light by chromophores in the tissue, notably hemoglobin, myoglobin, and cytochrome, limits measurements of phosphorescence to depths of about 1 mm or less. The emitted phosphorescence, in contrast, was maximum at 695 nm and therefore could penetrate much greater thicknesses of tissue.

Vinogradov and Wilson (1995) have recently reported synthesis of a new group of oxygen sensitive phosphors with absorption maxima near 636 nm and phosphorescence maxima near 800 nm. This communication, is a preliminary report of *in vivo* oxygen measurements using a new water soluble derivative form of these phosphors, Green 2W.

MATERIALS AND METHODS

Green 2W was prepared by sulfation of the parent Pd-meso-tetra-(phenyl)-tetrabenzoporphyrin as previously described (Vinogradov and Wilson, 1995). The absorption spectrum has a strong band at 636 nm and the phosphorescence emission is near 800 nm. Green 2W has negligable fluorescence and the emission is quantitatively due to phosphorescence. The quantum efficiency for phosphorescence was previously determined to be approximately 8% (Vinogradov and Wilson, 1995).

EMT-6 (mammary carcinoma) tumors were grown by injecting 1×10^6 cells in 0.1 ml carrier into the subcutaneous space over the muscle on the hind quarter of mice. The mice were used for phosphorescence measurements after the tumors had grown to between 3 and 8 mm diameter.

Imaging of Phosphorescence Using Green 2W Injected into the Blood of Mice

The Green 2W (0.15 mg/mouse) was injected into the tail vein and the mouse was anesthetized using an anesthetic cocktail (Ketamine at 133 mg/kg and Xylazine at 10 mg/kg). Electric hair clippers were used to remove most of the hair in the region to be measured. The mouse was then laid on its stomach on a clear plastic petri dish and illuminated with flashes of red light (636 ± 15 nm) from a flash lamp (approx. 30 μJ monochromatic light per flash) with a bandwidth at half height of less than 4 μsec. When the illumination was from the same side of the mouse as the camera, the light was directed onto the animal through a focusable ring light. For measurements through the mouse, the excitation light was carried through an 8 mm diameter light guide which directed the light upward through the bottom of the plastic petri dish.

A reference picture of the mouse was taken by reflected room light through the same system in order to allow evaluation of the position of phosphorescence to the structures of the mouse observed by eye. This picture was taken just before or after the phosphorescence was imaged without altering the position of the mouse or the camera focus.

The images of the phosphorescence were taken and analysed as previously described (Pawlowski and Wilson, 1994; Wilson et al, 1993). A series of phosphorescence images (512 x 480 pixels) were collected in which the camera was turned on at different times after the flash of excitation light (30, 50, 80, 120, 180, 240, 420 and 2,500 μsec). In each case the camera was left on for a period of 2,500 μsec effectively integrating the remaining phosphorescence signal. The images were then filtered (smoothed), the background subtracted (image taken with a delay of 2,500 μsec after the flash), and the phosphorescence lifetime calculated for each pixel position of the image set by best fit to a single exponential. The oxygen pressure at each pixel was then calculated using equation 1:

$$T^o/T = 1 + k_Q * T^o * PO_2 \tag{1}$$

where T^o and T are the phosphorescence lifetimes in the absence of oxygen and in the presence of oxygen at a pressure PO_2, respectively. The second order quenching constant k_Q is experimentally determined (see below) and is characteristic of the quenching at that temperature and pH.

RESULTS

Calibration of the Oxygen Dependent Quenching of Phosphorescence of Green 2W *in Vitro*

The Green 2W was dissolved in 0.15 M NaCl at approximately 3 mg/ml, the pH adjusted to 7.4, and then diluted as required into the final solutions (from 2 to 12 μM) for measurements of the phosphorescence lifetimes as a function of oxygen pressure. When albumin is added to the solution in a substantial molecular excess over the Green 2W, the phosphor associates with the albumin and access of oxygen to the phosphor is decreased as indicated by a decrease in k_Q. At 37°C and 2% albumin the value of T^o was 340 μsec and that of k_Q was 250 Torr^{-1} sec^{-1}. Blood contains between 2 to 4% albumin, sufficient to saturate the effect on Green 2W.

Imaging the Oxygen Distribution in the Tissue of Mice

The phosphorescence from a mouse with an EMT-6 tumor was imaged as described in Materials and Methods. A picture of the mouse was first taken using reflected room light (Figure 1A). The phosphorescence was not of equal intensity over the observed area of the mouse (Figure 1B). This asymmetric distribution resulted from a combination of several different factors. Uniform illumination cannot be achieved due to the shape of the mouse and tumor area has a lower oxygen pressure and higher blood volume than the surrounding tissue. This results in substantially greater phosphorescence intensity from the tumor than from the surrounding tissue. Calculation of the oxygen pressure map requires that there be a sufficiently high phosphorescence for accurate determination of the phosphorescence lifetime. As calculations are made for regions with progressively lower initial phosphorescence intensities, the values for the lifetime become more noisy (poorer correlation coefficients). When the phosphorescence values become very low, the lifetime values are no longer meaningful.

Imaging Oxygen Distribution through the Lower Body of a Mouse

Green 2W both absorbs and phosphoresces in the near infra-red, allowing for maximal penetration of both through tissue. Phosphorescence, and therefore oxygen distribu-

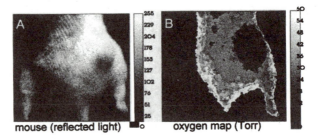

mouse (reflected light)   oxygen map (Torr)

Figure 1. A, B. Imaging the phosphorescence of mice with subcutaneous EMT-6 tumors. The mouse was imaged as described in Materials and Methods. The mouse was anesthetized and 0.3 mg Green 2 W injected into the blood. The mouse was laid on its abdomen with the tail at the top and then imaged from above using a focused ring light for illumination with the flash lamp. It was first imaged by reflected room light (1A) and then the phosphorescence was imaged with 8 different delay times after the flash (30, 50, 80, 120, 180, 240, 420 and 2,500 μsec). The phosphorescence data set was used to calculate a digital map of the pressure maps using Equation 1 and appropriate calibration constants (1B). The tumor appears as an area of relatively low oxygen pressure, with some values of less than 6 Torr (see also Wilson and Cerniglia, 1992). The oxygen pressure in regions of tissue removed from non-tumor areas show uniform values of 30 to 40 Torr.

tion, can be measured through the lower body of a mouse (about 1 cm tissue thickness) including the intact skin (Figure 2A, B). This experiment was carried out in the same manner as that in Figure 1 except that the illumination light was introduced from beneath the mouse while the phosphorescence was imaged from above. Diffusion of the light through the mouse resulted in a relatively uniform phosphorescence (Figure 2A), with sufficient

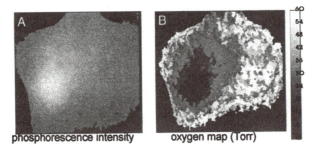

phosphorescence intensity   oxygen map (Torr)

Figure 2. A, B. Oxygen pressure maps obtained through the lower body of a mouse. The mouse was anesthetized and laid on its abdomen in a clear plastic petri dish with the tail at the center top of the map. The flash of excitation light entered the center of the lower abdomen from below and the mouse was imaged from above. The phosphorescence intensity imaged with a delay of 30 μsec after the flash is shown in A. Phosphorescence images were taken as described in the Legend of Figure 1 and used to calculate the oxygen pressure map. The combination of the excitation light and the phosphorescence passed completely through the mouse, a tissue thickness of about 1 cm. A subcutaneous EMT-6 tumor of approximately 6 mm diameter was on the flank of the mouse.

intensity to allow good quality images and calculation of oxygen pressure maps. This mouse had a subcutaneous EMT-6 tumor, approximately 6 mm in diameter, on the right side hind quarter. In this experiment the tumor was on the upper side of the mouse, closest to the camera.

DISCUSSION

Phosphorescence quenching is an accurate measure of oxygen pressure over a wide range (see for example Figure 2), with particular advantage over other methods for measurement of oxygen pressures at physiological oxygen pressures and below, i.e. less than about 40 Torr (see Vanderkooi et al, 1987; Wilson et al, 1988). The response time is only a few msec, even at low oxygen pressures, and rapid measurements are possible at all oxygen pressures. These properties have made it uniquely well suited for measuring the oxygen in biological systems. As an optical method it is also very valuable in providing non-invasive, quantitative determination of the oxygen pressure in the vasculature of tissue *in vivo*. Phosphor dissolved in the blood can provide an excellent measure of the oxygen pressure within the microvasculature of tissue.

Some of the advantages of this method for measuring oxygen pressure in biological systems can be summarized as follows:

A. Quenching of phosphorescence by oxygen occurs by well understood principles and the relationship of phosphorescence to oxygen pressure can be expressed in the form of a simple linear equation. The measured phosphorescence intensity or lifetime may be converted to oxygen pressure using equation 1, where T^o is the phosphorescence lifetime in the absence of oxygen, and T is the phosphorescence lifetime at oxygen pressure PO_2.

B. No known agents in blood, other than oxygen, affect the measured phosphorescence lifetime. Once the values of k_Q and T^o have been determined for physiological conditions, they can be used indefinitely i.e. the calibration is only dependent on the chemical structures and their microenvironment, not the measuring apparatus or other experimental conditions. Values of k_Q and T^o determined *in vitro* are equally valid for measurements *in* vivo.

C. There is no evidence for toxicity of the Pd-porphyrins probes in current use, including Green 2W. We have injected (i.v.) up to 5 mg of Green 2W into mice with no evidence of toxicity in the following 10 days. Less than 0.3 mg/mouse (10 mg/kg) is sufficient for imaging the oxygen pressure, even using trans-illumination, and measurements with light guides require < 3 mg/kg.

D. Phosphorescence lifetime is independent of probe concentration at the concentrations used for measurements in vivo.

E. Phosphorescence lifetime measurements are independent of the absorbance or fluorescence of other chromophores which may be present in the system. Chromophores and fluorophors in the tissue do not change during phosphorescence decay (< 1 msec), and therefore can not affect the measured phosphorescence lifetimes.

Phosphorescence quenching can provide high resolution digital maps of the distribution of oxygen pressure in the vasculature of tissues *in vitro* (see for example Rumsey et al, 1988) and *in vivo*, including: the cat eye (Shonat et al, 1992), the surface of the brains of newborn piglets (Wilson et al, 1991) and cats (Wilson et al, 1993), tumors in rats (Wilson and Cerniglia, 1992) and the surface of the heart of newborn piglets (Rumsey et al, 1994). In each case, the measurements were restricted to tissue after removal of the skin and to the surface (< 1 mm thickness) of the tissue by the necessity of using visible light for excitation of the phosphor. Thus, the method was limited and could not be used for the many applications which required oxygen measurements through greater depths of tissue.

Development of phosphors which absorb in the near infra red region of the spectrum (Vingradov and Wilson, 1995) has greatly extended the range of oxygen measurements possible using phosphorescence. It is no longer necessary, for example, to remove the skin in order to measure oxygen pressures in the underlying muscle, making the measurements fully non-invasive. In the near infra red region of the spectrum, tissue does not absorb light very efficiently but it does scatter the light. The light scattering process results in a rapid attenuation of the parallel component of the light beam, altering it within less than a mm to nondirectional (diffuse) light which travels through the tissue in a random walk. This causes a large increase in the distance the light must travel to pass through the tissue (see for example van der Zee et al, 1992). Oxygen measurements by phosphorescence quenching are not dependent on the light path of either the excitation or emission light *per se*. Light scattering is, however, important in determining the thicknesses of tissue through which oxygen measurements can be made since the light is attenuated as it travels through the tissue. With increasing distance from the point of light insertion the light intensity per unit volume of tissue decreases, with a proportional decrease in the efficacy of excitation of phosphorescence. The emitted phosphorescence must then diffuse through the remaining thickness of tissue to the detector. When there is equal attenuation at the wavelengths for excitation and emission, the phosphorescence decay measurement is equally sensitive to the oxygen pressure in the blood at all positions through the thickness of the tissue between the excitation source and the detector. When the tissue has different transmission coefficients for the excitation and emission light, oxygen measurements through the tissue will be weighted toward the side for which the light most rapidly attenuated. If the phosphorescence light is more strongly attenuated than the excitation, for example, the oxygen measurements will be weighted toward the side of the light detector.

Green 2W has a strong absorption at 636 nm (with an extinction coefficient of approximately 51 $mM^{-1}cm^{-1}$), providing excellent efficiency for excitation of phosphorescence. This strong absorption plus the quantum efficiency for phosphorescence of about 8% (Vingradov and Wilson, 1995), results in a high phosphorescence intensity. This greatly simplifies measurements of the phosphorescence decay and improves the quality of the resulting digital maps. In the present experiments, images of phosphorescence were obtained through the lower body of a mouse, or at least 1 cm of tissue. It is reasonable to suggest that by optimizing the instrumentation, including the use of higher intensity excitation light, it will be possible to make measurements through tissue thicknesses of 5 cm or greater. The excitation light used (< 30 µJ/flash) can be increased 10 to 100 fold with a corresponding increase in phosphorescence intensity, and intensified CCD cameras are available with 10 fold greater sensitivity than that used in our study.

An even larger increase in sensitivity can be attained by using point measurements instead of the CCD array for phosphorescence measurement. Point measurements made with a light guide can be at least 10^5 times more sensitive than imaging since the light can be measured with a single detector as compared to the 256,000 pixels (detectors) in the CCD array of the video camera. These considerations indicate that although oxygen measurements in tissue using phosphorescence quenching are already providing excellent results, technical improvements over the next few years will continue to improve the quality in the resulting data and range of applicability of the method.

ACKNOWLEDGMENTS

This research was largely supported by grant # CA-56679 from the National Institutes of Health.

REFERENCES

Pawlowski, M. and Wilson, D.F. (1994) Imaging oxygen pressure in tissue *in vivo* by phosphorescence decay. Adv. Exptl. Med. Biol. *361*, 83–93.

Robiolio, M., Rumsey, W.L., and Wilson, D.F. (1989) Oxygen diffusion and mitochondrial respiration in neuroblastoma cells. Am. J. Physiol. 256, C1207-C1213.

Rumsey, W.L., Vanderkooi, J.M. and Wilson, D.F. (1988) Imaging of phosphorescence: A novel method for measuring the distribution of oxygen in perfused tissue. Science, 241, 1649–1651.

Rumsey, W.L., Schlosser, C., Nuutinen, E.M., Robiolio, M. and Wilson, D.F. (1990) Cellular energetics and the oxygen dependence of respiration in cardiac myocytes isolated from adult rat. J. Biol. Chem. 265, 15392–15399.

Rumsey, W.L., Iturriaga, R., Spergel, D., Lahiri, S., and Wilson, D.F. (1991) Optical measurements of the dependence of chemoreception on oxygen pressure in the cat carotid body. Amer. J. Physiol. 261: C614-C622.

Rumsey, W.L., Pawlowski, M., Lejavardi, N., and Wilson, D.F. (1994) Oxygen pressure distribution in the heart in vivo and evaluation of the ischemic "border zone". Am. J. Physiol. 266: H1676–1680.

Shonat, R.D., Wilson, D.F., Riva, C.E., and Cranston, S.D. (1992) Effect of acute increases in intraocular pressure on intravascular optic nerve head oxygen tension in cats. Inv. Ophthalmology & Visual Science 33, 3174–3180.

Shonat, R.D., Wilson, D.F., Riva, C.E., and Pawlowski, M. (1992) Oxygen distribution in the retinal and choroidal vessels of the cat as measured by a new phosphorescence imaging method. Applied Optics 33: 3711–3718.

Vanderkooi, J.M., Maniara, G., Green, T.J., and Wilson, D.F. (1987) An optical method for measurement of dioxygen concentration based on quenching of phosphorescence. J. Biol. Chem. *262*: 5476–5482.

van der Zee, P., Cope, M., Arridge, S.R., Essenpreis, L.A., Potter, A.D., Edwards, J.S., Wyatt, J.S., McCormick, D.C., Roth, S.C., Reynolds, E.O.R., and Delpy, D.T. (1992) Experimentally measured optical pathlengths for the adult heart, calf, and forearm and the head of the newborn infant as a function of inter optode spacing. Adv. Exptl. Med. Biol. 316, 143–153.

Vinogradov, S.A. and Wilson, D.F. (1995) Metallotetrabenzoporphyrins. New phosphorescent probes for oxygen measurements. J. Chem. Soc. Perkin Trans. II, 2, 103–111.

Wilson, D.F. and Cerniglia, G.J. (1992) Localization of tumors and evaluation of their state of oxygenation by phosphorescence imaging. Cancer Research, 52: 3988–3993.

Wilson, D.F., Rumsey, W.L., Green, T.J., and Vanderkooi, J.M. (1988) The oxygen dependence of mitochondrial oxidative phosphorylation measured by a new optical method for measuring oxygen. J. Biol. Chem. 263, 2712–2718.

Wilson, D.F., Pastuszko, A., DiGiacomo, J.E., Pawlowski, M., Schneiderman, R., Delivoria-Papadopoulos, M. (1991) Effect of hyperventilation on oxygenation of the brain cortex of newborn piglets. J. Appl. Physiol. 70(6): 2691–2696.

Wilson, D.F., Gomi, S., Pastuszko, A., and Greenberg, J.H. (1993) Microvascular damage in the cortex of the cat from middle cerebral artery occlusion and reperfusion. J. Appl. Physiol. 74(2), 580–589.

72

IN VIVO [17]O MAGNETIC RESONANCE SPECTROSCOPY

Determination of Temperature Effects on Metabolic Rates (Q$_{10}$ Factor)

G. D. Mateescu and M. E. Cabrera

Department of Chemistry, Case Western Reserve University
Cleveland, Ohio 44106

INTRODUCTION

After the first reports on the feasibility of [17]O magnetic resonance imaging (MRI) and localized spectroscopy (MRS)[1–3] significant progress has been recorded in applications to vertebrates and invertebrates. Water diffusion in gels and time release preparations have also been reported.[4] Of particular importance are the experiments leading to the determination, *in vivo*, of the rate of oxygen consumption.[5–9] These investigations reached a new dimension with the introduction of interleave [17]O/^{31}P measurements which are yielding valuable information on the degree of uncoupling of the oxidative phosphorylation (OXPHOS) by various physical and chemical agents.[10–11] The significance of such information derives from the fact that degenerative diseases (Alzheimer, Parkinson, ischemic heart, late onset diabetes, etc) are associated to OXPHOS perturbations induced by genetic mitochondrial and nuclear DNA mutations.[12] Given the increasing interest in the elucidation of the protective mechanism of hypothermia, as compared to that of barbiturates, in traumatic or ischemic brain damage[13–16] we initiated a feasibility study for the determination of the Q_{10} factor.

There are three properties of [17]O which make it uniquely appropriate for the measurement of oxygen consumption. First, [17]O (the only stable isotope of oxygen which possesses a magnetic moment) has a very low natural abundance (0.037%). Thus, ^{17}O constitutes an excellent NMR tracer: compared to the natural abundance, an enrichment of only 4% reduces the measurement time by a factor >10,000. Second, the quadrupolar nature of the nucleus leads to very short longitudinal (T$_1$) and transverse (T$_2$) relaxation times. This means the pulse repetition rate is much shorter than that for proton, thus compensating for the low detection sensitivity of oxygen. It should be noted that the resulting line broadening is not important, since there is only one peak to be observed in the whole spectrum, namely that of water. Third, ^{17}O is neither toxic, nor radioactive. Needless to say, similar measurements are impossible with ^{1}H MRS, due to the nearly 100% natural abundance of hydrogen.

As more than 95% of the oxygen consumed by the tissue becomes metabolic *(nascent mitochondrial)*[7] water, *in vivo* quantitation of the $H_2{}^{17}O$ yields an accurate value of mitochondrial oxygen consumption. It has been shown in previous studies that this method constitutes a sensitive tool for evaluation of the effects of various factors (e.g., anaesthetics) on the rate of oxygen consumption.[7]

There are significant variations in the metabolic rate of an organism, which depend, among others, on body size and temperature.[17] For instance, smaller animals require, per unit body mass, a higher metabolic rate than larger animals. A small increase in body temperature increases the rate of all chemical processes resulting in a net increase in metabolic rate.[18] Specifically, a 10°C increase in body temperature (T) results in a 2 to 3-fold increase in the rate of oxygen consumption.[17,18] The factor Q_{10} has been used to described the effect of T on the metabolic rate expressed as the rate of oxygen consumption, MRO_2:

$$Q_{10} = \frac{MRO_2(T+10)}{MRO_2(T)}$$

The aims of this study are (a) to determine by means of ^{17}O MRS the effects of a 10°C change in temperature on the metabolic rate (Q_{10}) of small invertebrates; and (b) to evaluate the detection limits of the method.

METHODS

Tenebrio molitor larvae (6 sets of 4 larvae, 144±20 mg/larva) are placed in a minirespirator designed to introduce measured volumes of ^{17}O-labeled air and to minimize losses of $^{17}O_2$ (Fig. 1). First, the water content in a larva is measured by comparing the ^{17}O MRS signal intensity from a larva alone with that from the larva plus a known amount of water. Then, the minirespirator containing a set of four larvae is placed in the 10 mm probe of a 4.7 Tesla NMR spectrometer tuned at the ^{17}O resonance frequency (27.13 MHz). All measurements are performed using the following parameters: number of transients (pulses), 10024; pulse duration (90°), 10 µs; pulse intervals, 51 ms; spectral width, 8190 Hz; number of points, 800; zero filling, 8192 points. Three spectra are taken over a period of 25 minutes in order to obtain the natural abundance water signal at 20°C. After baseline data is collected, the atmosphere in the respirator is replaced with a mixture of 5 ml synthetic air labeled with 42% $^{17}O_2$ and 2 ml room air. The ^{17}O gas is prepared by electrolysis of water enriched in ^{17}O to 42 atom % (EG&G Mound Technologies, Miamisburg, Ohio). Five spectra are then taken in a 40 minute period at a probe temperature of 20°C, which is also the room temperature. Immediately after, the temperature of the probe is increased to 30°C and, after temperature stabilization, eight more spectra are taken.

Determination of Larval Water Content

To determine the larval water content (M_{H2O}), a larva of known weight is placed in a 10 mm NMR tube containing a 5 mm insert with a known amount of water. ^{17}O spectra are

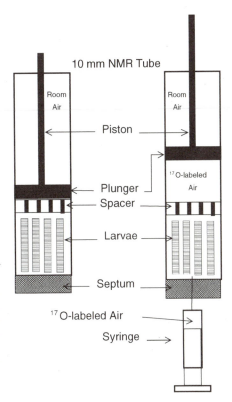

10 mm NMR Tube

Piston

Plunger

Spacer

Larvae

Septum

[17]O-labeled Air

Syringe

Room Air

Room Air

[17]O-labeled Air

Figure 1. Minirespirator designed for minimal losses of [17]O_2. In the first stage the plunger is placed against the spacer. The larvae are introduced below the spacer and the tube is capped with a rubber septum. In the second stage synthetic air containing a known amount of [17]O_2 is injected from a syringe through the septum. Under the resulting pressure the plunger retracts leaving space for the synthetic air (which is mixed with the small volume of room air remained between the larvae). The minirespirator is then inserted in the probe of the NMR spectrometer.

then taken with and without the 5 mm (spiking water) insert. The water content is determined using the folowing equation:

$$M_{H_2O} = \frac{1}{18} \cdot \frac{W_s}{(S_s / S_0) - 1}$$

where W_s is the spiking water weight (g), S_0 is the integral of the [17]O peak corresponding to the H_2[17]O present in the larva (natural abundance), S_s is the integral of known added water plus water in larva, and 18 represents the molecular weight of water.

Determination of the Rate of Formation of Metabolic Water

The fraction p of labeled nascent mitochondrial water molecules is calculated with the following equation

$$p(t) = \frac{(S_1(t) / S_0) - 1}{k - 1}$$

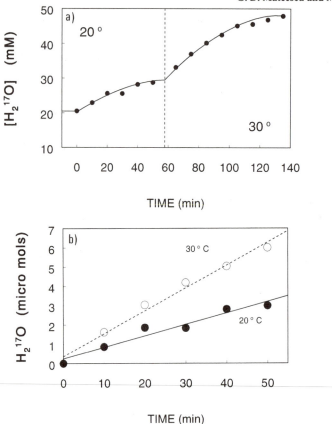

Figure 2. a) The time course of labeled mitochondrial water formation at 20° and 30° C. b) Illustration of the slope difference between the rates of metabolic water formation shown in a).

where $_{S1}$ is the intensity of the $H_2^{17}O$ signal at the time t after the animal began breathing ^{17}O-labeled air and S_o is the $H_2^{17}O$ signal intensity at natural abundance (before breathing ^{17}O-enriched air); k is the isotopic enrichment ratio (Fig. 2a).

The rate of production of metabolic water by the larvae (P_{H2O}, μ mol/min), is then determined using

$$P_{H_2O} = \frac{\Delta p}{\Delta t} \cdot M_{H_2O}$$

where $\Delta p/\Delta t$, the rate of change of the fraction of enriched water is determined from measurements of $p(t)$ at five different points in time, using linear regression (Fig. 2b). Since one molecule of O_2 produces two molecules of metabolic H_2O, the rate of oxygen consumption (MRO_2, μmol/min·g) is determined from the rate of water formation (P_{H2O}, μmol/min) and the larval weight in grams (W):

$$MR_{O_2} = \frac{P_{H_2O}}{2W}$$

The rates of oxygen consumption are calculated for each set of animals at 20°C and at 30°C. A paired *t*-test is used to determine whether the rates of oxygen consumption are significantly different at these temperatures.

RESULTS AND DISCUSSION

A 10°C increase in larval body temperature resulted in an increase of its rate of oxygen consumption (range: 1.4–3.0 fold) in all six experiments. The average larval metabolic rate increased significantly from 0.08 ± 0.02 (mean±SD) nmol/s at 20°C to 0.15 ± 0.04 nmol/s at 30°C ($p < 0.005$). Expressed per unit weight, the metabolic rate increased from 0.033 ± 0.007 µmol/g·min at 20°C to 0.064 ± 0.016 µmol/g·min at 30°C ($p < 0.005$). The average Q_{10} factor obtained from the six experiments was 1.98 ± 0.6, which represents a two-fold increase in metabolic rate with a 10°C increase in body temperature. The average body water in larvae is found to be $36 \pm 5\%$.

It is seen from Fig. 2 that variations in MRO_2 induced by large acute changes in temperature are detected noninvasively by [17]O magnetic resonance spectroscopy with adequate sensitivity. The increase in metabolic rate found in this study is comparable to that found in other insects (larval stage) of similar weight using the Warburg method[19] or a differential respirometer.[20] The absolute values for the rate of oxygen consumption however, differ from values found in the literature under similar conditions.[21,22] Loudon found values ranging from 1–3.5 nmole/s in larvae weighing 30–150 mg (1.4–2.0 µmol/g·min) at 28°C, while Johansson reported values 0.27 ± 0.03 µmol/g·min at 20°C. Since both the Warburg and differential respirometry measurements are known to yield reliable results, the lower absolute values found here by [17]O nmr are attributed to several factors: a) errors in the determination of larval body water; b) errors in the determination of the [17]O enrichment in the synthetic air; c) the presence of an unknown amount of "nmr-invisible" oxygen-17. Measurements of larval body water content ranged between 30–43% of body weight. Measurements of [17]O-enrichment ranged from 36 to 41 atom %. These errors would result in an underestimation of the rate of metabolic water formation by a factor of two. In addition, the MRS determination of the rate of oxygen consumption assumes no losses of water (e.g., excretion) during the spectroscopic measurements. If the rates of water loss were of the same magnitude as the rate of water formation, this would also result in an underestimation of the rate of water formation by another factor of two. The "invisible" oxygen-17 corresponds to the amount of water which cannot be observed due to the fact that its nmr peak is broadened to such an extent that it is incorporated into the baseline. The origin of the line broadening resides in the quadrupolar nature of the [17]O which leads to extremely short transverse relaxation times for water molecules very tightly bound to tissues.

Since both measurements of oxygen consumption (at T and T+10 C) were made in the same conditions, the errors in the absolute value mentioned above cancel out. Thus, the resulting Q_{10} values are valid; as mentioned above, they are comparable with the corresponding changes measured by the Warburg and differential respirometry methods. While the elimination of errors mentioned in a) and b) is possible, we are exploring new avenues to obtain correct estimates of the "invisible water." Thus, the magnetic resonance method provides an adequate *in vivo*, noninvasive estimation of the metabolic rate and a sensitive method to determine the effects of temperature changes on the rate of oxygen consumption. Based on MRO_2 found in the mouse, rat, cat and dog,[8,9] the MRS method for Q_{10} determination is expected to work better in larger animals and humans where the cerebral blood flow and the arterio-venous [17]O-concentration needed to calculate the $CMRO_2$ can readily be obtained.

REFERENCES

1. Mateescu, G.D., Butenhof, K.J., Benedikt, G.M., Brescic, I., High Resolution O-17 NMR and the Chemistry of Water Monomers, 1986. IX. ISMAR (Int. Soc. Magn. Reson.) Meeting, Rio de Janeiro.
2. Mateescu, G.D., Yvars, G.M. and Dular, T., Oxygen-17 MRI, 1987. Proc. Soc. Magn. Reson. Med., 6:929.
3. Mateescu, G.D., Yvars, G.M. and Dular, T., 1988. Water, Ions and ^{17}O MRI. In: Water and Ions in Biological Systems, Lauger, Packer and Vasilescu, Eds. Birkhauser: Basel-Boston, pp. 239–250.
4. Mateescu, G.D., Kinsey, R.A., Yvars, G.M., 1991. Oxygen-17 and Proton MR Microscopy in Materials Analysis, Mat. Res. Soc. Symp. Proc., 217:61–66.
5. Mateescu, G.D., Yvars, G.M.,. Pazara, D.I., Alldridge, N.A., LaManna, J.C., Lust, D.W., Mattingly, M. and Kuhn, W., ^{17}O-^{1}H MRI in Plants, Animals, and Materials. In: Synthesis and Applications of Isotopically Labelled Compounds, Baillie & Jones, Eds., 1989. Elsevier, Amsterdam, pp. 499–508.
6. Mateescu, G.D., From Materials Testing to Brain Function Testing, 1991. Spectroscopy International, 3:14–17.
7. Mateescu, G.D., LaManna, J.C., Lust, W.D., Mars, L. and Tseng, J., 1991. ^{17}O- MR: In Vivo Determination of Nascent Mitochondrial Water in Animals Breathing ^{17}O-enriched Air, Proc. Soc. Magn. Reson. Med. 10:1031.
8. Pekar, J., Ligeti, L., Lyon, R., Ruttner, Z., Gelderen, V.P., Moonen, C., Fiat, D., McLaughlin, A.C., 1991. In vivo mapping of oxygen consumption in the rat brain using ^{17}O-MRI, Proc. Soc. Magn. Reson. Med. 10:302.
9. Fiat, D., Dolinsek, J., Hankiewicz, J., Dujovny, M., Ausman, J., 1993. Determination of RCMRO2 and RCBF by noninvasive O-17 in vivo NMR and MRI, Neurol. Res., 15:237–248.
10. Mateescu, G.D. and Fercu, D., 1993. Interleave ^{17}O/^{31}P MRS: novel approach for in vivo determination of defects in oxidative phosphorylation, Proc. Soc. Magn. Reson. Med. 12:110.
11. Mateescu, G.D. and Fercu, D., 1994. Concerted ^{17}O/^{31}P magnetic resonance spectroscopy: a novel approach for in vivo correlation of oxygen consumption and phosphate metabolism, Adv. Exp. Biol. 361:234 (1994).
12. Wallace, D.C., 1992. A paradigm for aging and degenerative diseases, Science 256:628–632.
13. Nemoto, E.M., Klementavicius, R., Melick, J.A., and Yonas, H., 1996. Suppression of cerebral metabolic rate for oxygen (CMRO2) by mild hypothermia compared with Thiopental, J. Neurosurg. Anesth., in press.
14. Minamisawa, H., Nordstrom, C.H., Smith, M.L., Siesjo, B.K. 1990. The influence of mild body and brain hypothermia on ischemic brain damage. J. Cereb. Blood Flow Metab. 10:365–374.
15. Baughman, V.L., Hoffman, W.E., Thomas, C., Miletich, D.J., and Albrecht, F., Hypothermia versus ethanol: neurologic outcome after incomplete cerebral ischemia in midazolam anesthesized rats, J. Neurosurg. Anesth.: 2:290–295.
16. Clifton, G.L., Jiang, J.Y., Lyeth, B.G., Jenkins, L.W., Hamm, R.J., and Hayes, R.L., 1991. Marked protection by moderate hypothermia after experimental traumatic brain injury, J. Cereb. Blood Flow Metab. 11:114–121.
17. Weibel, E.R. 1984. The pathway for oxygen. Structure and function in the mammalian respiratory system. Harvard Univ. Press, Cambridge, MA, pp. 30–48.
18. Hochachka, P.W. and Somero, G.N., 1984. Biochemical adaptation, Princeton University Press, Princeton , NJ, pp. 355–449.
19. Knight, A.W. and Gaufin, A.R., 1966. Oxygen consumption of several species of stoneflies (Plecoptera), J. Insect Physiol. 12:347–355.
20. Petitpren, M.F. and Knight, A.W., 1970. Oxygen consumption of the Dragon Fly, Anax Junius, J. Insect Physiol. 16:449–459.
21. Loudon, C., 1986. Tracheal morphology and gas exchange in the insect Tenebrio molitor L. Ph.D Thesis, Duke University, United States.
22. Johansson, B., 1920. Der Gaswechsel bei Tenebrio Molitor und seiner Abhaengigkeit von der Nahrung. PhD Thesis, Lunds Universitets, Sweden.

73

IMAGING OF OXYGEN DISTRIBUTION IN THE SURFACE AND DEEP AREAS OF THE KIDNEY

W. L. Rumsey,[1] B. Abbott,[1] L-W. Lo,[2] S. A. Vinogradov,[2] and D. F. Wilson[2]

[1]Zeneca Pharmaceuticals
Wilmington, Deleware 19897
[2]University of Pennsylvania School of Medicine
Philadelphia, Pennsylvania 19104

1. INTRODUCTION

We have demonstrated previously that imaging of oxygen distribution based on the quenching of phosphorescence is a highly useful tool for investigating oxygen delivery in tissues at the microvascular level. The kidney offers an interesting model for the study of oxygen delivery because it receives a disproportionate amount of the cardiac output relative to its contribution to body weight. Moreover, unlike other tissues, the microvascular bed contains both afferent and efferent arterioles within its rich vascular network in order to control precisely the filtration pressure within the glomerulus. Blood flow in the kidney is markedly heterogeneous, i.e., greater in cortical regions than in medullary ones, and it can be redistributed dependent upon the volume state of the animal. Consequently, the metabolic requirements of the cortical and medullary areas may be markedly different in accordance with the capacity for sodium retention. Finally, this organ is an oxygen sensing tissue that is linked to the production of the glycoprotein hormone, erythropoietin, during hypoxia. For these reasons, we have initiated a series of experiments designed to evaluate the oxygen distribution within the kidney. In particular, we were interested in the potential effects of endothelin (ET-1), since it has been reported to produce marked reductions of renal blood flow (Badr et al., 1989) and it has been implicated in the pathogenesis of acute renal ischemic injury (Kon et al., 1989). Using both images of oxygen distribution and kinetic measurements of oxygen pressures in the microvasculature of the kidney, these preliminary data suggest that low doses of ET-1 rapidly and markedly decrease renal oxygen pressures.

Oxygen Transport to Tissue XVIII, edited by Nemoto and LaManna
Plenum Press, New York, 1997

2. METHODS

2.1. Animals

Male Sprague-Dawley rats (300–450 g) were anaesthetized (Na Pentobarbital 50 mg/kg ip) and were instrumented for administration of compounds via the left jugular vein and for measurement of systemic blood pressure by insertion of a catheter in the carotid artery. In all cases, a tracheotomy was performed either to permit the animals to respire freely or for mechanical ventilation (model 683, Harvard Apparatus, South Nadick MA). Small incisions were made at the midline of the abdomen and through its lateral aspect for viewing of the left kidney. Black cloth was draped about the periphery of the kidney to eliminate endogenous luminescence from abdominal fat.

2.2. Measurement of Oxygen Pressure in the Kidney

Two different oxygen probes, Pd-mesotetra(4-carboxyphenyl)porphine (75 mg/Kg in saline containing 6% bovine serum albumin; Porphyrin Products, Logan, Utah) and "green 2W" (4 mg/Kg), were used to obtain images of microvascular oxygen at two depths of tissue. The former compound has spectral characteristics (excitation = 530 nm, emission > 630 nm) that provide only images of oxygen pressure at the surface of tissue (500–1000 μm) whereas the latter has spectral characteristics (excitation = 636 nm, emission > 750) that enable light to penetrate to greater depths without significant absorption.

Measurement of microvascular oxygen pressures was made using a method based on the quenching of phosphorescence by molecular oxygen. This method has been described in detail previously (see for example; Lahiri et al., 1993, Rumsey et al., 1988, Rumsey et al., 1994, Wilson et al., 1989). The phosphorescence of the administered lumiphor is quenched in blood by oxygen which is free in solution (not that bound to hemoglobin) as described by the Stern-Volmer relationship:

$$I^o/I = \tau^o/\tau = 1 + k_Q\tau^o[O_2]$$

where I^o and τ^o are the phosphorescence intensity and lifetime, respectively, in the absence of oxygen; and I and τ are the phosphorescence intensity and lifetime at a given oxygen pressure. The quenching constant, k_Q, relates the rates of diffusion of oxygen to the phosphor. The oxygen measurements were primarily those obtained from blood within the capillaries and venules. The capillaries and venules contain the major portion of the total tissue blood volume. Since the phosphorescence lifetimes are independent of the probe concentration, changes in vascular volume or flow do not affect the calculated oxygen pressures.

For images of oxygen distribution, the tissue was illuminated using either a ring lamp assembly or an epifluorescence unit coupled to a 45 watt xenon flashlamp (EG & G, Salem, MA). Detection of phosphorescence emission was made using an intensified CCD camera (Xybion Electronics Systems, San Diego, CA) with appropriate optical filters in place assembled as a unit and mounted either to a stand positioned directly above the tissue or atop a Wild Macrozoom microscope, respectively. When microvascular oxygen pressures were measured on-line, the tissue was illuminated using a fiberoptic cable positioned 1 mm from the kidney. The optical cable was coupled to both a xenon flashlamp for excitation of the phosphor, in this case Pd-mesotetra(4-carboxyphenyl)porphine, and a photomultiplier tube for detection of the emitted light ("Oxyspot", Medical Systems Inc., Greenvale, NY, which was interfaced to a computer, Dell 486/66, Austin, TX)

3. RESULTS AND DISCUSSION

Figure 1 shows examples of images of renal oxygen distribution obtained from two separate animals initially ventilated on room air and then with 10% oxygen. The images in the upper portion of the panel were acquired from an animal receiving Pd-mesotetra(4-carboxyphenyl)porphine as the oxygen probe which provides data from the surface (first 0.5–1.0 mm of tissue) of the renal cortex. When ventilated with room air, it can be seen that the microvascular oxygen pressure is, in this case, about 68 Torr but there is an admixture of vascular units which deviate from this value. Reducing the level of ventilated oxygen to 10% decreases rapidly the microvascular oxygen pressures to about 36 Torr. Return to room air quickly increased these values to levels obtained prior to the hypoxic episode (data not shown). These changes were similar to those shown in the lower portion of the panel which displays images obtained from an animal administered "green 2W". Using the latter probe, the penetration of the excitation light (> 630 nm) is not markedly limited by absorption of light by endogenous pigments. It is likely, therefore, that these values represent those of microvascular units from depths of tissue greater than 1.0 mm. During ventilation with room air, the latter probe was associated with oxygen pressures of about 40–50 Torr and with 10% oxygen, oxygen pressures fell to about 24 Torr.

Although the values of renal microvascular oxygen pressure obtained using the two probes differed by several Torr using the same experimental conditions, these differences are more than likely due to variation between animal preparations. This was borne out by additional experiments using the photomultiplier system ("Oxyspot") and Pd-mesotetra(4-carboxyphenyl)porphine as the oxygen probe. Typical values were within a range of 35–45 Torr (n = 9) for animals respiring on room air. Moreover, when the levels of oxygen were compared by using the imaging system and the "Oxyspot" in the same animal,

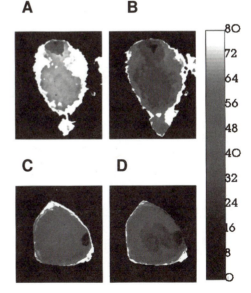

Figure 1. Response of renal oxygen pressures to hypoxia using probes for imaging surface and deeper areas of the kidney. Animals were artificially ventilated at 70 bpm (tidal volume = 2.25 ml) using either room air (left side of panel) or 10% oxygen balanced with nitrogen (right side of panel). Images in the upper portion (A & B) of the panel were obtained using Pd-mesotetra(4-carboxyphenyl)porphine whereas those in the lower aspect (C & D) were obtained with "green 2W".

the microvascular oxygen pressures were found to be similar, 30–40 Torr and 39 Torr, respectively.

Endothelin administration had marked effects on renal oxygen pressures. For example, in those animals described in Figure 1, a bolus injection of endothelin-1 (1 ηmol/kg) decreased oxygen pressures to nearly zero throughout the field of view (data not shown). By using the "Oxyspot", examination of the kinetic changes in microvascular oxygen pressures in response to endothelin (50 ρmol/kg; bolus injection) was performed. In this typical example, it can be seen that occlusion of the renal artery decreased rapidly microvascular oxygen pressures to near zero. Release of the ligature resulted in a quick increase of oxygen pressure to levels that exceeded those obtained prior to ischemia, consistent with a classic hyperemic response. In this same animal, endothelin also elicited a rapid decline of oxygen pressure to near zero but the return to pre-peptide levels was much slower, requiring several minutes. This decrease in oxygen pressure was associated initially with a depression of mean arterial pressure, a decrease of $45 \pm 3\%$ (n = 3), followed by a rise in pressure, $37 \pm 10\%$ as compared to baseline.

Endothelin has marked effects on the kidney microvasculature (for review, refer to Masaki and Yanagisawa, 1992). When radiolabeled endothelin was injected into rats, Anggard and coworkers (1989) showed that the highest uptake of the radiotracer was found in the lung, liver and kidney, suggesting a high density of endothelin binding sites. In isolated ring segments of the renal artery, endothelin displays a dose-dependent vasocontriction with ED_{50} values in the nanomolar range (Tomobe et al., 1988). When endothelin is administered in vivo, the response of the renal vasculature is dependent on the amount given. At high doses, renal blood flow and glomerular filtration rate decrease whereas at low doses of the peptide (1 ηg/kg/min), a rise in renal flow can be obtained (Masaki and Yanagisawa, 1992). At doses similar to those used presently, King and coworkers (1989) reported a fall in renal plasma flow of rats. Our results show that this peptide can reduce renal oxygen pressures to levels that are observed when the renal artery is fully occluded.

The results presented from this study indicate that it is possible to obtain images of oxygen pressure in the kidney and that these images can be obtained using two separate oxygen probes of different spectral characteristics designed for superficial and deep penetration of the exciting light. When using the former probe, oxygen pressures can be measured to be greater than 60 Torr, although this value is not typical, and when using the

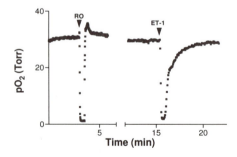

Figure 2. Comparison of kinetic changes in microvascular oxygen pressure during transient ischemia and endothelin exposure. The renal artery and vein were fully occluded (RO) for 30 sec using a suture looped around the vessels and pulled gently away from the body. Endothelin (ET-1, 50 ρmol/kg) was administered via bolus injection into the jugular vein. Data were acquired at intervals of 0.1 sec during the ischemic period and 3 sec thereafter.

latter probe, oxygen pressures were found to be markedly less, about 40 Torr. In order to evaluate regional variations in microvascular oxygen pressures from renal cortex to medulla, it may be more appropriate to inject both probes into a single animal. By using two sets of optical filters, each designed to optimize excitation and emission of the respective probes, it may be possible to obtain images of oxygen distribution from the surface of tissue and at greater depths in the same animal. Further work in this area is warranted based on the present findings.

4. REFERENCES

Anggard, E., Galton, S., Rae, G., Thomas, R., McLoughlin, L., de Nucci, G., and Vane, J.R. The fate of radioiodinated endothelin-1 and endothelin-3 in the rat. *J. Cardiovasc. Pharmacol.* 13 (Suppl 5) S46-S49, 1989.

Badr, K.F., Murray, J.J., Breyer, M.D., Takahashi, K., Inagami, T., and Harris, R.C. Mesangial cell, glomerular and renal vascular responses to endothelin in the rat kidney: Elucidation of signal transduction pathways. *J. Clin. Invest.* 83: 336–342, 1989.

King, A.J., B.M. Brenner, and Anderson, S. Endothelin: a potent renal and systemic vasoconstrictor peptide. *Am. J. Physiol.* 256 (Renal Fluid Electrolyte Physiol. 25): F1051–1058, 1989.

Kon, V., Yoshioka T., Fogo, A., and Ichikawa, I. Glomerular actions of endothelin in vivo. *J. Clin. Invest.* 83: 1762–1767, 1989

Lahiri, S. W.L.,Rumsey, D.F. Wilson, and R. Iturriaga. Contribution of in vivo microvascular PO_2 in the cat carotid body chemotransduction. *J. Appl. Physiol.* 75 (3): 1035–1043, 1993.

Masaki, T., and Yanagisawa, M. Physiology and pharmacology of endothelins. *Med. Res. Rev.* 12 (4): 391–421, 1992.

Rumsey, W.L., J.M. Vanderkooi, and D.F. Wilson. Imaging of phosphorescence: A novel method for measuring the oxygen distribution in perfused tissue *Science.* 241: 1649–1651, 1988.

Rumsey, W.L., M. Pawloski, N. Lejavardi, and D.F. Wilson. Oxygen pressure distribution in the heart in vivo and evaluation of the ischemic "border zone". *Am. J. Physiol. 266 (Heart Circ. Physiol. 35):* H1876-H1680, 1994.

Tomobe, Y., T. Miyauchi, A. Saito, M. Yanagisawa, S. Kimura, K. Goto, and T. Masaki. Effects of endothelin on the renal artery from spontaneously hypertensive and Wistar Kyoto rats. *Eur. J. Pharmacol.* 152: 373–374, 1988.

Wilson, D.F., W.L. Rumsey, and J.M. Vanderkooi. Oxygen distribution in isolated perfused liver observed by phosphorescence imaging. *Adv. Exp. Med. Biol.* 248: 109–115, 1989.

74

EXTENDED PORPHYRINS

New *IR* Phosphors for Oxygen Measurements

Sergei A. Vinogradov and David F. Wilson

Department of Biochemistry and Biophysics
School of Medicine, University of Pennsylvania
Philadelphia, Pennsylvania 19104

ABSTRACT

Tetrabenzoporphyrins (TBP) of Zn, Pd, Lu, Y, Sn and Pb show strong absorption bands in the near IR region of the spectrum. Phosphorescence in dimethylformamide (DMF) solutions at room temperature was measured for Pd and Lu complexes giving quantum yields of 7.9% and 3.5% and lifetimes of 250 μsec and 870 μsec, respectively. Pd *meso*-tetraphenyltetrabenzoporphyrin **1** (PdPh$_4$TBP) shows a red shift of the absorption Q-band to 628 nm. **1** reacted with ClSO$_3$H and obtained chlorosulfonato derivative **2** was converted to a set of water soluble chromophores: Pd meso-tetra(sulfophenyl)tetrabenzoporphyrin (Pd Ph$_4$(SO$_3$Na)$_4$TBP) **3**, corresponding sulfonamide (Pd Ph$_4$(PEG)$_4$TBP) **4** with aminopolyethyleneglycol (Av.M.W. 5,000) and sulfonamide derivatives of glucoseamine (Pd Ph$_4$(glucoseamine)$_4$TBP) **5** and aminophenylacetic acid (Pd Ph$_4$(phenac)$_4$TBP) **6**. Electronic absorption and phosphorescence spectra of **1** and some of its derivatives were recorded and phosphorescence quantum yields and lifetimes were measured for deoxygenated solutions. The oxygen quenching constants were measured for the water soluble complexes **3** and **4** and found to be suitable for oxygen measurements *in vivo*.

Tetranaphthaloporphyrin (TNP) complexes of Pd and Lu as well as Pd *meso*-tetraphenyltetranaphthaloporphyrin (PdPh$_4$TNP) were synthesized and their absorption and emission properties were examined.

INTRODUCTION

Oxygen dependent quenching of phosphorescence has become one of the most effective and accurate methods for measuring oxygen concentration. Because it is a non invasive optical technique, this method has been successfully used both *in vitro* and *in vivo* [1–3] (see ref. 4 for the latest review). It has great potential as a new clinical tool in the di-

Oxygen Transport to Tissue XVIII, edited by Nemoto and LaManna
Plenum Press, New York, 1997

agnosis and treatment of many diseased states, particularly those leading to altered oxygen pressures in tissue.

Phosphorescent probe used for biological applications in general consists of two major components: optical chromophore and surrounding environment. *Optical chromophore* (OC) is a part of the probe molecule which is responsible for the optico-physical properties necessary for adequate oxygen measurements. These properties are: i). high intensity absorption in the region of spectrum where natural chromophores of tissue, such as hemoglobin or myoglobin, do not absorb or only slightly absorb, light; ii). existence of phosphorescence with high quantum yields at room temperature (> 2%) and sufficiently long lifetimes (0.1–1 msec) for convenient measurement. *Surrounding environment* (SE) is a ligand or set of ligands linked to a chromophore skeleton to provide biological suitability of the probe: high water solubility, non-toxicity, good protection from chemically active components of tissue and appropriate size for excretion through kidney. Ideally, SE forms an inert globular structure around the chromophore, through which only small molecules, such as oxygen, can penetrate to allow phosphorescence quenching.

It is well known that porphyrins of Pd, Pt and some lanthanides have strong oxygen dependent phosphorescence [5]. Some of these porphyrins, such as Pd (*meso*-tetra-*p*-carboxyphenyl)porphyrin (PdTCPP), Pd *meso*-porphyrin (Pd*m*P), have been successfully used for oxygen measurements as complexes with bovine serum albumin (BSA). In this case BSA played the role of natural SE, providing protection for the porphyrins and increasing their water solubility [6]. However these 'first generation' probes had a major limitation: the absorption maxima of Pd porphyrins lie in the region of 520–540 nm, where other naturally occurred pigments absorb light with high molar extinctions. This limits oxygen measurements to a thin layer (< 1 mm) of tissue or to optically clear tissue, such as eye. In the present study we focused on the new OC generation, namely extended porphyrins and their metal complexes, which have absorption bands in the near IR region of the spectrum.

SYNTHESIS OF TETRABENZOPORHYRINS

Recently we have published a detailed study of the chemistry of metallotetrabenzoporphyrins [7], including a comprehensive literature review. Thus here we will describe only the major synthetic highlights.

Unlike the regular, "red" porphyrins, synthesis of TBP requires extremely drastic conditions [8]. We followed the synthetic scheme originally suggested by Linstead and Weiss [9] and later improved by Kopranenkov et al. [10, 11]. In this method, formation of the macrocycle is achieved by high temperature condensation of phthalimide with metal acetates in the presence of Zn salts. The latter most likely play the role of the ionic templates. Subsequent demetallation with AcOH/H_3PO_4 mixture followed by the metal insertion either in DMF or in imidazole melt led to the various metallo TBP complexes.

An analogous chain of transformations [12], started with 2,3-naphthalimide, resulted in the formation of Pd and Lu derivatives of TNP. In general, yields (5–10%) were poorer than in case of the corresponding TBP complexes (15–25%) and reaction mixtures required more extensive purification.

Meso-tetraphenylated TBP (Ph$_4$TBP) complexes were synthesized when phenylacetic acid was used instead of alkali metal acetates in the condensation reaction. The best results were achieved, however, when excess of Zn diphenylacetate (Zn(PhCH$_2$COO)$_2$) was used directly and no other metal salts were present in the reaction mixtures. When 2,3-naphthalimide was chosen as starting material Zn *meso*-tetraphenyl TNP ($ZnPh_4TNP$) complex formed in 4% yield.

Tetraphenylated extended porphyrins can be easily demetallated in a mixture of chloroform and trifluoroacetic acid (20:1) at room temperature and the following metal insertion also requires less rigorous conditions than in case of non-substituted TBP. Thus insertion of Pd, for example, occurs in 10 min with 100% conversion in DMF at 70°C, a process conveniently monitored by optical spectroscopy.

The reaction sequence leading to $PdPh_4TBP$ is presented as an example in Scheme 1.

The majority of the synthesized tetrabenzoporphyrin complexes were characterized by elemental analysis and ^1H NMR spectroscopy [7].

As we suggested above, certain SE has to be built around OC center and presumably covalently linked to it to provide suitable probes for biological applications. This means, in turn, that OC molecules have to bear some functional groups which would allow further chemical transformations. In case of TBP systems, introduction of such groups at the stage of macrocycle formation is limited to only very few inert substituents [11] because of extreme reaction conditions required for template condensation reaction. Therefore, such groups have to be introduced into TBP macrocycle after its initial formation. Tetraphenyltetrabenzoporphyrins (Ph_4TBP) seem to be more appropriate for this type of modification than non-substituted TBP, because the phenyl rings are more reactive toward various electrophylic agents.

We have used chlorosulfonation for modification of newly synthesized complexes. Chlorosulfonated derivative (**2**) of $PdPh_4TBP$ was prepared by treatment of $PdPh_4TBP$ with chlorosulfonic acid at 80°C (Scheme 2, A). This yielded a compound which was then converted into the water soluble sulfonato derivative **3** by alkaline hydrolysis (Scheme 2, B).

Chlorosulfonic derivative **2** formed sulfonamide **4** with NH_2-modified polyethylene glycol (Av.M.W. 5,000) (Scheme 2, C), or alternatively reacted with glucoseamine or 4-aminophenylacetic acid giving corresponding sulfonamides **5** and **6**. All obtained water soluble derivatives were tested for the presence of oxygen dependent quenching of phosphorescence.

OPTICAL PROPERTIES OF TETRABENZOPORPHYRINS

The spectra of all TBP and TNP systems show good agreement with Gouterman's four-orbital model [5], which predicts strong degenerate $S_1 \leftarrow S_0$ (Q-band) and $S_2 \leftarrow S_0$ (Soret band) absorptions. Due to the enlarged π-electron system of extended porphyrins *vs* the parent porphyrins, both bands are red shifted as expected. Spectra of some complexes are shown in Figure 1 and more detailed data on the absorption properties are summarized in Table 1.

In case of $PdPh_4TBP$ the Q-band (628 nm) lies just below the border of near-IR window of tissue, while for water soluble derivatives it is shifted even further to about 635 nm. At this wavelength light can penetrate through the *cm* depth of tissue, which suggests biological applicability of these chromophores. Another important property of TBP system is its very high extinction coefficients ($\varepsilon \approx 50$) for the Q-band absorption. This can minimize the amount of the phosphor that is actually needed to be injected for oxygen measurements *in vivo*.

As seen from Table 1, absorption bands of TNP are shifted another 70 nm to the red, which is consistent with the increase of aromatic conjugation in the molecule. Extinction coefficients for these compounds are also very high; however, relatively low synthetic yields in combination with phosphorescence maxima located too far in the IR make TNP less suitable than corresponding TBP probes.

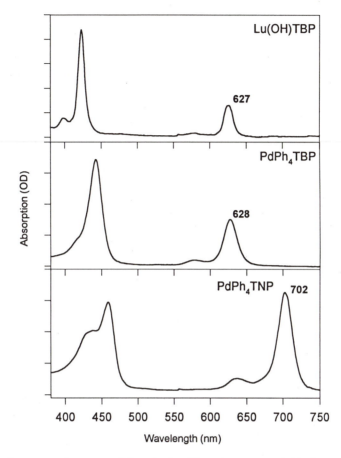

Figure 1. Absorption spectra of some extended porphyrins. All spectra were recorded in deoxygenated DMF solutions. Numbers indicate positions of the Q-band maxima.

Table 1. Absorption maxima of some metallotetrabenzoporphyrins

Compound	Soret (0,0) (nm)log ε	Q (0,0) (nm)log ε	Compound	Soret (0,0) (nm)log ε	Q (0,0) (nm)log ε
ZnTBP	433 (5.50)	628 (4.99)	Pd Ph$_4$TBP (**1**)	442 (5.07)	628 (4.70)
PbTBP	483	659	Pd (SO$_2$Cl)$_4$ Ph$_4$TBP (**2**)	443	629
Lu(OH)TBP	426 (4.98)	627 (4.49)	Pd (SO$_3$H)$_4$ Ph$_4$TBP (**3**) [b]	443	631
PdTBP	407 (5.25)	606 (5.02)	Pd (PEG)$_4$ Ph$_4$TBP (**4**) [b]	446	634
ZnTNP	444	706	Lu(OH)TNP	440 (4.64)	700 (4.86)
PdTNP	442	700	PdPh$_4$TBP	459 (4.86)	702 (4.89)

[a]Extinction coefficients could not be accurately measured. See ref. 7 for details.
[b]Spectra were recorded in aqueous media.

Table 2. Emission data for metallotetrabenzoporphyrins. (*f* and *p* indicate
fluorescence and phosphorescence, respectively)

Compound	Solvent	Emission maxim um (nm)	τ_p (μsec)	ϕ_p abs. (%) [a]	ϕ_p rel. [b]
PdTBP	DMF	767 (*p*)	260	7.9	1.1
PdPh$_4$TBP	DMF	785 (*p*)	250	8.0	1.2
Lu(OH)TBP	DMF	632 (*f*); 803 (*p*)	870	3.5	0.5
3 in H$_2$O	H$_2$O	790 (*p*)	310	2.3	0.3
3 + BSA in H$_2$O [c]	H$_2$O	790 (*p*)	320	2.8	0.4
4 in H$_2$O	H$_2$O	793 (*p*)	260	5.1	0.7
4 + BSA in H$_2$O [c]	H$_2$O	793 (*p*)	280	6.2	0.9
PdPh$_4$TNP	DMF	-	81 [d]	-	-

[a] Measured relative to H$_2$TPP or ZnTPP fluorescence quantum yields (13% and 3.3% in deaerated benzene), for which our relative values were within ±5% of published.

[b] Given relative to the phosphorescence quantum yield of PdTCPP in degassed DMF.

[c] BSA indicates 2% of bovine serum albumin present in the probe solution.

[d] The detailed data on TNP optical properties are to be published.

The emission properties of TBP and TNP complexes are summarized in Table 2. We have found that in deoxygenated solutions at room temperature the TBP complexes of Pd and Lu show susbstantial phosphorescence. The emission bands are located in IR region (790–800 nm) and do not shift much with introduction of the phenyl substituents into the core macrocycles. The same observations have been made for the water soluble derivatives.

It should be noted out that new IR chromophors are similar to the currently used "red" probes in terms of phosphorescence efficiency. Indeed, the measured quantum yield, for example, for PdPh$_4$TBP (8%) is actually higher than for the most commonly used Pd-*meso*-tetracarboxyphenylporphyrin (6.8%). The phosphorescence lifetimes for water soluble TBP derivatives all lie in the range of 220–250 μsec, which is adequate for oxygen measurements *in vivo*. The quenching constants (k_q) were determined for the water soluble derivative **3** at room temperature. The obtained values are $2.6 \cdot 10^9 \text{mol}^{-1}\text{s}^{-1}$ and $2.1 \cdot 10^8 \text{mol}^{-1}\text{s}^{-1}$ for aqueous saline solutions without and with 2% BSA, respectively. These values are consistent with the observed changes in phosphorescence quantum yields and indicate interaction of the complexes with BSA. Changes in pH, however, do not seem to have any effect on phosphorescence characteristics of the new probes.

Further modification and characterization of TBP chromophores is currently in progress.

REFERENCES

1. W. L. Rumsey, J. M. Vanderkooi and D.F. Wilson, 1988, Imaging of phosphorescence: A novel method for measuring the distribution of oxygen in perfused tissue, *Science*, **241**, 1649.

2. D. F. Wilson, W. L. Rumsey, T. J. Green and J. M. Vanderkooi, 1988, The oxygen dependence of mitochondrial oxidative phosphorylation measured by a new optical method for measuring oxygen, *Biol. Chem.*, **263**, 2712.

3. M. Pawlowski and D. F. Wilson, 1992, Monitoring of the oxygen pressure in the blood of live animals using the oxygen dependent quenching of phosphorescence, *Adv. Exptl. Med. Biol.* **316**, 179.

4. D. F. Wilson and S. A. Vinogradov, 1992, Recent advances in oxygen measurements using phosphorescent quenching, *Adv. Exptl. Med. Biol.*, **361**, 61.

5. D. Eastwood and M. Gouterman, 1970, Porphyrins. XVIII.Luminescence of (Co), (Ni), Pd, Pt Complexes, *J. Mol. Spec.*, **35**, 359.

6. J. M. Vanderkooi, G. Maniara, T. J. Green and D. F. Wilson, 1987, An optical method for measurement of dioxygen concentration based on quenching of phosphorescence. *J. Biol. Chem.*, **262**, 5476.

7. S. A. Vinogradov, and D. F. Wilson, 1995, Metallotetrabenzoporphyrins. New Phosphorescent probes for oxygen measurements. *J. Chem. Soc., Perkin Trans. 2,* 103.

8. Kobayashi, N. in *"Phthalocyanines. Properties and Applications"*, ed. C. C. Leznoff and A. B. P. Lever, VCH Publishers, New York, 1993, Vol.2, p.97.

9. R. P. Linstead, F. T. Weiss, 1950, Phthalocyanines and related compounds. Part XX. Further investigation of tetrabenzoporphin and allied substances, *J. Chem. Soc.,* 2975.

10. V. N. Kopranenkov, S. N. Dashkevich and E. A. Luk'yanets, 1981, *meso*-Tetraarylporphyrins, *J. Gen. Chem. USSR (Engl. Transl.),* **51**, 2165.

11. V. N. Kopranenkov, E. A. Tarkhanova and E. A. Luk'yanets, 1979, Phthalocyanines and related compounds. XV. Synthesis and electronoc absorption spectra of tetra(4-tert-buthylbenzo)porphin and its metal complexes, *J. Org. Chem. USSR (Engl. Trans.),* **15**, 570.

12. V. N. Kopranenkov, A. M. Vorotnikov, S. N. Dashkevich and E. A. Luk'yanets, 1985, Phthalocyanines and allied compounds. XXIV. Synthesis and electronic spectra of tetra-1,2- and tetra-2,3-naphthocyanines, *J.Gen.Chem. USSR (Engl. Transl.),* 803.

INDEX